WESTERN INFIRMARY LIBRARY
GWIG8446
WITHDRAWN

KU-508-346

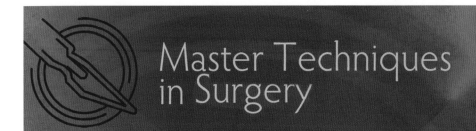


# HEPATOBILIARY AND PANCREATIC SURGERY

# Master Techniques in Surgery

Series Editor: Josef E. Fischer

Also available in this series:

**Breast Surgery**

Kirby I. Bland
V. Suzanne Klimberg

**Colon and Rectal Surgery: Abdominal Operations**

Steven D. Wexner
James W. Fleshman

**Colon and Rectal Surgery: Anorectal Operations**

Steven D. Wexner
James W. Fleshman

**Esophageal Surgery**

James D. Luketich

**Gastric Surgery**

Michael S. Nussbaum

**Hernia**

Daniel B. Jones

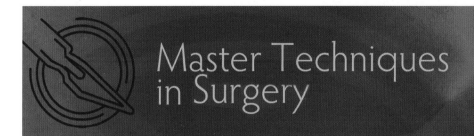

# HEPATOBILIARY AND PANCREATIC SURGERY


*Edited by:*

**Keith D. Lillemoe, MD**
W.G. Austen Professor
Harvard Medical School
Chief of Surgery
Massachusetts General Hospital
Boston, MA

**William R. Jarnagin, MD**
Chief, Hepatopancreatobiliary Service
Enid A. Haupt Chair
Department of Surgery
Memorial Sloan-Kettering Cancer Center
New York, NY

*Series Editor*

**Josef E. Fischer, MD**
Distinguished William V. McDermott
Professor of Surgery
Harvard Medical School
Chair, Department of Surgery, Emeritus
Beth Israel Deaconess Medical Center
Chair, Department of Surgery, Emeritus
University of Cincinnati College of Medicine
Boston, Massachusetts

**Illustrations by: Anne Rains,** Arains Illustration, Inc.
**BodyScientific** International, LLC.



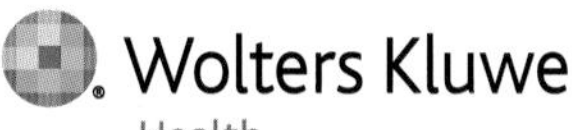
Wolters Kluwer | Lippincott Williams & Wilkins
Health

Philadelphia • Baltimore • New York • London
Buenos Aires • Hong Kong • Sydney • Tokyo

*Acquisitions Editor:* Brian Brown
*Product Manager:* Brendan Huffman
*Production Manager:* Alicia Jackson
*Senior Manufacturing Manager:* Benjamin Rivera
*Marketing Manager:* Lisa Lawrence
*Design Coordinator:* Doug Smock
*Production Service:* Aptara, Inc.


**Two Commerce Square**
**2001 Market Street**
**Philadelphia, PA 19103 USA**
**LWW.com**



Printed in China

CIP data available upon request.

ISBN: 978-1-60831-172-9

Care has been taken to confirm the accuracy of the information presented and to describe generally accepted practices. However, the authors, editors, and publisher are not responsible for errors or omissions or for any consequences from application of the information in this book and make no warranty, expressed or implied, with respect to the currency, completeness, or accuracy of the contents of the publication. Application of the information in a particular situation remains the professional responsibility of the practitioner.

The authors, editors, and publisher have exerted every effort to ensure that drug selection and dosage set forth in this text are in accordance with current recommendations and practice at the time of publication. However, in view of ongoing research, changes in government regulations, and the constant flow of information relating to drug therapy and drug reactions, the reader is urged to check the package insert for each drug for any change in indications and dosage and for added warnings and precautions. This is particularly important when the recommended agent is a new or infrequently employed drug.

Some drugs and medical devices presented in the publication have Food and Drug Administration (FDA) clearance for limited use in restricted research settings. It is the responsibility of the health care provider to ascertain the FDA status of each drug or device planned for use in their clinical practice.

To purchase additional copies of this book, call our customer service department at (800) 638-3030 or fax orders to (301) 223-2320. International customers should call (301) 223-2300.

Visit Lippincott Williams & Wilkins on the Internet: at LWW.com. Lippincott Williams & Wilkins customer service representatives are available from 8:30 am to 6 pm, EST.

10 9 8 7 6 5 4 3 2 1

RRS1207

# Dedication

*To my wife, Cheryl, and children Chris, Shannon, Becky, and Heather, for your many years of support; and to the surgical trainees who drive each of us to be at our best each and every day.*

*—K.L.*

*To my family, my colleagues, and mentors, but most of all to my trainees and patients, who motivate us to always to strive for excellence.*

*—W.J.*

# Contributors

**Peter J. Allen, MD**
Department of Surgery
Hepatopancreatobiliary Service
Memorial Sloan-Kettering Cancer Center
New York, New York

**Chad G. Ball, MD, MSC, FRCSC, FACS**
Assistant Professor of Surgery and Oncology
University of Calgary
Canada

**Joshua Barton, MD**
Department of Surgery
Methodist Dallas Medical Center
Dallas, Texas

**Kevin E. Behrns, MD**
Chairman, Edward R. Woodward Professor
Department of Surgery
University of Florida
Gainesville, Florida

**Kfir Ben-David, MD**
Assistant Professor, Chief, MIS, Gastroesophageal and Bariatric Service
Department of Surgery
University of Florida
Gainesville, Florida

**David Bentrem, MD**
Assistant Professor
Division of Surgical Oncology
Jesse Brown VA Medical Center
Feinberg School of Medicine, Northwestern University
Chicago, Illinois

**Markus W. Büchler, MD**
Professor and Chair
Department of General, Visceral and Transplantation Surgery
University of Heidelberg
Heidelberg, Germany

**Mark P. Callery, MD, FACS**
Chief, Division of General Surgery
Beth Israel Deaconess Medical Center
Associate Professor of Surgery
Harvard Medical School
Boston, Massachusetts

**William C. Chapman, MD, FACS**
Washington University School of Medicine
St. Louis, Missouri

**Daniel Cherqui, MD**
Professor of Surgery
Chief, Section of Hepatobiliary Surgery and Liver Transplantation
Weill Cornell Medical College
New York-Presbyterian Hospital
New York, New York

**Carlos U. Corvera, MD**
Associate Professor
Department of Surgery
Chief, Liver, Biliary and Pancreatic Surgery
University of California, San Francisco School of Medicine
San Francisco, California

**Steven C. Cunningham, MD**
Co-Director of Pancreatic and Hepatobiliary Surgery
Saint Agnes Hospital Center
Baltimore, MD
and
Fellow and Clinical Instructor
Hepato-Pancreato-Biliary Surgery
Johns Hopkins Hospital
Baltimore, MD

**Michael I. D'Angelica, MD, FACS**
Associate Attending Surgeon
Department of Surgery
Memorial Sloan-Kettering Cancer Center
Associate Professor
Department of Surgery
Cornell University, Weill Medical College
New York, New York

**Ronald P. DeMatteo, MD**
Attending, Hepatopancreatobiliary Service
Vice Chair, Department of Surgery
Memorial Sloan-Kettering Cancer Center
New York, New York

**Aram N. Demirjian, MD**
Assistant Professor of Clinical Surgery
Division of Hepatobiliary and Pancreas Surgery
University of California Irvine Medical Center
Orange, California

**M.B. Majella Doyle, MD, FACS**
Assistant Professor of Surgery
Section of Transplantation
Washington University in St. Louis
St. Louis, MO

**Michael B. Farnell, MD**
Professor of Surgery
Division of Gastroenterologic and General Surgery
Department of Surgery
Mayo Clinic College of Medicine
Rochester, Minnesota

**Carlos Fernández-del Castillo, MD**
Director
Pancreas and Biliary Surgery Program Massachusetts General Hospital
Professor of Surgery
Harvard Medical School
Boston, Massachusetts

**Cristina R. Ferrone, MD**
Assistant Surgeon
Department of Surgery, General Surgery
Massachusetts General Hospital
Assistant Professor in Surgery
Department of Surgery, General Surgery
Harvard Medical School
Boston, Massachusetts

**Yuman Fong, MD**
Murray F. Brennan Chair in Surgery
Department of Surgery
Memorial Sloan-Kettering Cancer Center
Professor of Surgery
Weill Cornell Medical Center
New York, New York

**Paul D. Greig, MD**
Professor of Surgery
University of Toronto
Toronto, Canada

**Alan W. Hemming, MD, MSc, FRCSC**
Professor and Chief, Transplantation and Hepatobiliary Surgery
Department of Surgery
University of California San Diego
San Diego, California

**Karen Horvath, MD, FACS**
Staff Surgeon
Department of Surgery
Division of General Surgery
University of Washington Medical Center
Professor of Surgery
Director, Residency Program
Associate Chair for Education
Department of Surgery
University of Washington
Seattle, Washington

**Michael G. House, MD**
Assistant Professor
Department of Surgery
Indiana University School of Medicine
Indianapolis, Indiana

**Thomas J. Howard, MD**
Willis D. Gatch Professor of Surgery
Indiana University School of Medicine
Indianapolis, Indiana

**William R. Jarnagin, MD**
Chief, Hepatopancreatobiliary Service
Enid A. Haupt Chair
Department of Surgery
Memorial Sloan-Kettering Cancer Center
New York, NY

**Michael L. Kendrick, MD**
Associate Professor of Surgery
Division of Gastroenterologic and General Surgery
Department of Surgery
Mayo Clinic College of Medicine
Rochester, Minnesota

**Eugene P. Kennedy, MD**
Associate Professor
Department of Surgery
Thomas Jefferson University
Philadelphia, Pennsylvania

**Adeel S. Khan, MD, MBBS**
Aurora Marinette Menominee Clinic/Bay Area Medical Center
Marinette, Wisconsin

**T. Peter Kingham, MD**
Assistant Attending, Hepatopancreatobiliary Service
Department of Surgery
Memorial Sloan-Kettering Cancer Center
New York, New York

**Michael D. Kluger, MD, MPH**
Assistant Professor of Surgery
Section of Hepatobiliary Surgery and Liver Transplantation
Weill Cornell Medical College
New York-Presbyterian Hospital
New York, New York

**Jonathan B. Koea, MD, FACS, FRACS**
Hepatobiliary Surgeon
Chief Hepatopancreatobiliary/Upper Gastrointestinal Unit
Department of Surgery
Auckland Hospital
Auckland, New Zealand

**Harish Lavu, MD**
Attending Surgeon
Assistant Professor
Department of Surgery
Thomas Jefferson University
Philadelphia, PA

**Keith D. Lillemoe, MD**
W.G. Austen Professor
Harvard Medical School
Chief of Surgery
Massachusetts General Hospital
Boston, Massachusetts

**J. Peter A. Lodge, MD, FRCS**
Professor of Surgery
HPB and Transplant Unit
St. James's University Hospital
Leeds, UK

**Ian McGilvray, MD, PhD, FRCSC**
Associate Professor of Surgery
Department of Surgery
University of Toronto
Toronto, Ontario, Canada

**W. Scott Melvin, MD**
Professor of Surgery
Chief of General and Gastro-Intestinal Surgery
Executive Vice Chair Department of Surgery
Director of the Center for Minimally Invasive Surgery
The Ohio State University
Columbus, Ohio

**James J. Mezhir, MD**
Assistant Professor of Surgery
Division of Surgical Oncology and Endocrine Surgery
University of Iowa Hospitals and Clinics
Iowa City, Iowa

**Attila Nakeeb, MD**
Professor of Surgery
Indiana University School of Medicine
Indianapolis, Indiana

**Yugi Nimura, MD**
President
Aichi Cancer Center
Nagoya, Japan

**Theodore N. Pappas, MD**
Professor
Department of Surgery
Duke University Medical Center
Durham, North Carolina

**Henry A. Pitt, MD**
Professor and Vice Chairman
Department of Surgery
Indiana University
Indianapolis, Indiana

**Florencia G. Que, MD**
Associate Professor of Surgery
Department of Surgery
Mayo Clinic
Rochester, Minnesota

**Kaye M. Reid-Lombardo, MD**
Assistant Professor of Surgery
Mayo Clinic College of Medicine
Rochester, Minnesota

**David B. Renton, MD**
Assistant Professor of Surgery
The Ohio State University
Columbus, Ohio

**Kristy L. Rialon, MD**
Research Associate
Department of Surgery
Duke University Medical Center
Durham, North Carolina

**Charbel Sandroussi, MD, MBBS(hons), MMSc, FRACS**
Uppergastrointestinal, Hepatobiliary and Transplant Surgeon
Royal Prince Alfred Hospital
Sydney, Australia

**Michael G. Sarr, MD**
James C. Mason Professor of Surgery
Mayo Clinic College of Medicine
Rochester, Minnesota

**Mark D. Sawyer, MD**
Assistant Professor of Surgery
Department of Surgery
Mayo Clinic
Rochester, Minnesota

**Richard D. Schulick, MD, MBA, FACS**
Professor and Chairman of the Department of Surgery
University of Colorado
Aurora, Colorado

**Junichi Shindoh, MD, PhD**
Postdoctoral Fellow
Department of Surgical Oncology
The University of Texas MD Anderson Cancer Center
Houston, Texas

**Lygia Stewart, MD, FACS**
Chief of General Surgery/Associate Chief of Surgery
San Francisco VA Medical Center
Professor of Clinical Surgery
University of California
San Francisco, California

**Jean-Nicolas Vauthey, MD, FACS**
Department of Surgical Oncology
The University of Texas: MD Anderson Cancer Center
Houston, Texas

**Andrew L. Warshaw, MD**
Surgeon-in-Chief and Chairman
Department of Surgery, General Surgery
Massachusetts General Hospital
Boston, Massachusetts

**Jens Werner, MD, MBA**
Professor of Surgery
Head, Division of Pancreatic Surgery
Department of General and Visceral Surgery
University of Heidelberg
Heidelberg, Germany

**Jordan Winter, MD**
Assistant Professor of Surgery
Thomas Jefferson University
Philadelphia, Pennsylvania

**Charles J. Yeo, MD**
Chief of Surgery
Department of Surgery
Samuel D. Gross Professor and Chairman
Department of Surgery
Thomas Jefferson University
Philadelphia, Pennsylvania

# Series Preface

This series of mini atlases, of which this is the fourth, is an outgrowth of Mastery of Surgery. As the series editor, I have been involved with Mastery of Surgery since the third edition, when I joined two greats of American surgery Lloyd Nyhus and Robert Baker who were the editors at that time. At that time, in addition to Mastery of Surgery, which really was, almost in its entirety, an excellent atlas of how to do operations, atlases were common and some quality atlases which existed at that time by Dr. John Madden of New York, Dr. Robert Zollinger of Ohio State, and two other atlases, with which the reader may be less familiar with is a superb atlas by Professor Pietro Valdoni, Professor of Surgery at the University of Rome, who ran 10 operating rooms simultaneously, and as the Italians like to point out to me, a physician to three popes. One famous surgeon said to me, what can you say about Professor Valdoni: "Professor Valdoni said to three popes, 'take a deep breath,' and they each took a deep breath." This superb atlas, which is not well known, was translated by my partner when I was on the staff at Mass General Hospital, Dr. George Nardi from the Italian. Another superb atlas was that by Dr. Robert Ritchie Linton, an early vascular surgeon whose atlas was of very high quality.

However, atlases fell out of style, and in the fourth and fifth editions of Mastery of Surgery, we added more chapters that were "textbooky" types of chapters to increase access to the increasing knowledge base of surgery. However, atlases seem to have gone out of favor somewhat. In discussing with Brian Brown and others of Lippincott, as well as some of the editors who have taken on the responsibility of each of these mini atlases, it seemed that we could build on our experience with Mastery of Surgery by having individual books which were atlases of 400 to 450 pages of high quality, each featuring a particular anatomical part of what was surgery and put together an atlas of operations of a sharply circumscribed area. This we have accomplished, and all of us are highly indebted to a group of high quality editors who will have created superb mini atlases in these sharply circumscribed areas.

Why the return of the atlas? Is it possible that the knowledge base is somewhat more extensive with more variations on the various types of procedures, that as we learn more about the biochemistry, physiology, genetics and pathophysiology in these different areas, there have gotten to be a variation on the types of procedures that we do on patients in these areas. This increase in knowledge base has occurred simultaneously at a time when the amount of time available for training physicians—and especially surgeons—has been diminished time-wise and continues to do so. While I understand the hypothesis that brought the 80-hour work week upon us, and that limits the time that we have for instruction, and I believe that it is well intentioned, but I still ask the question: is the patient better served by a somewhat fatigued resident who has been at the operation, and knows what the surgeon and what he or she is worried about, or a comparatively fresh resident who has never seen the patient before?

I don't know, but I tend to come down on the side that familiarity with the patient is perhaps more important. And what about the errors of hand off, which seem to be more of an intrinsic issue with the hand off which we are not able to really remedy entirely rather than poor intentions.

This series of mini-atlases is an attempt to help fill the voids of inadequate time for training. We are indebted to the individual editors who have taken on this responsibility and to the authors who have volunteered to share their knowledge and experience in putting together what we hope will be a superb series. Inspired by their experience of teaching residents and medical students, a high calling, matched only by their devotion and superb care they have given to thousands of patients.

It is an honor to serve as the series editor for this outstanding group of mini-atlases, which we hope will convey the experiences of an excellent group of editors and authors to the benefit of students, residents and their future patients in an era in which time for education seems to be increasingly limited.

Putting a book together, especially a series of books is not easy, and I wish to acknowledge the production staff at Lippincott, Wolters Kluwer's including Brian Brown, Julia Seto, Brendan Huffman and many others, and my personal staff in the office who include Edie Burbank-Schmitt, Ingrid Johnson, Abigail Smith and Jere Cooper. None of this would have been possible without them.

Josef E. Fischer, MD
Boston, MA

# Preface

Forty years ago, many of the operations described in this volume were performed rarely, if at all, and almost never outside of a few highly specialized referral centers. Over that relatively short span of time, hepatobiliary/pancreatic (HPB) surgery has progressed from a high-risk proposition, practised by a small band of pioneering surgeons, to relatively common practice, with the expectation of good outcomes for the vast majority of patients. Indeed, HPB surgical procedures are now widely performed, from academic tertiary referral centers to community hospitals, and the indications for many procedures continue to expand.

Many factors have played a role in the transformation of this field, not the least of which has been improvements in operative and perioperative care generally. Another major factor has been the evolution of HPB surgery into a recognized area of specialization. The early practitioners, many of them legendary figures in surgery, laid a solid foundation and passed on the knowledge of many hard lessons learned over the years. The next generation expanded this knowledge base and refined the surgical techniques and management approaches that propelled HPB surgery into the mainstream. With the framework established, it then became possible to shift the focus to improving outcomes in patients with HPB-related diseases, rather than merely surviving the perioperative period. It is our charge now to continue to advance the field, not only by further improving the safety of the operations, but to better align the indications with an increasing understanding of the disease processes in order to improve patient selection.

We are the beneficiaries of these several decades of hard work on the part of many surgeons, to whom we owe a large debt of gratitude. While their efforts set the stage to allow the routine performance of major HPB surgical procedures, the margin of error remains very narrow. These operations can be very challenging from a technical standpoint, and even minor miscalculations can have profound adverse consequences.

This atlas is meant to provide detailed description of the technical aspects of liver, biliary and pancreatic operations, many commonly performed but others less so. We are indebted to our co-authors, all experts in the field, who have shared their insights into these procedures based on their extensive experience. Although the focus is on the technical conduct of operative procedures, efforts are made to include discussion of indications/contraindications, preoperative assessment and perioperative management. Our aim was to provide a volume valued equally by trainees and established HPB surgeons.

We wish to express our thanks and appreciation to all who have contributed to the publication of this book, especially our esteemed publisher, Wolters Kluwer, for their patience and tremendous assistance throughout the project and for providing first class artistic support for the many illustrations.

# Contents

# 1 Pancreaticobiliary Surgery: General Considerations

Steven C. Cunningham, Aram N. Demirjian, and Richard D. Schulick

## Surgically Relevant Anatomy

The pancreas is a large, asymmetric gland lying in the central retroperitoneum, consisting of the head, neck, body, and tail. The pancreatic head lies at just right of the L2 vertebral body and extends in an oblique course to the left over the spine, cephalad, and then slightly posterior until the tail terminates near the splenic hilum, at the level of T10. The neck is often defined as that portion of the gland overlying the superior mesenteric artery and vein (SMA and SMV), and separating the head to the right from the body to the left. The dividing line between the body and tail hardly exists and is not surgically relevant. The uncinate process of the pancreas is embryologically separate from the rest of the pancreas and in adults extends from the inferior lateral head of the gland, extending slightly posterior to the SMV and terminating at the SMA (Fig. 1.1).

The arterial supply to the pancreas is abundant and comes via multiple named and unnamed vessels from both the celiac axis and the SMA, a fact largely responsible for the ability of the pancreaticoduodenectomy resection specimen to bleed abundantly until the last fibers of tissue are divided. The head is richly supplied by anastomosing branches of the pancreaticoduodenal arteries, while the body and tail are predominantly supplied by branches of the splenic artery and jejunal branches. The collateral flow often present between the SMA and the celiac axis, chiefly through the gastroduodenal artery (GDA), becomes very important at pancreaticoduodenectomy, during which the GDA is typically divided. In all cases, flow in the hepatic artery is confirmed during clamping of the GDA to detect cases in which hepatic artery flow is significantly dependent on SMA-celiac axis collaterals. In such cases, arterial bypass, preservation of the GDA, or division of a median arcuate ligament may be necessary, depending on the clinical scenario. In all cases, one must be aware of aberrant hepatic arterial anatomy (vida infra), which is common (>25% of cases) and is more commonly replaced than accessory (Fig. 1.2).

The venous drainage of the pancreas is predominantly portal, excepting small unnamed retroperitoneal veins that may drain posteriorly into the lumbar system and

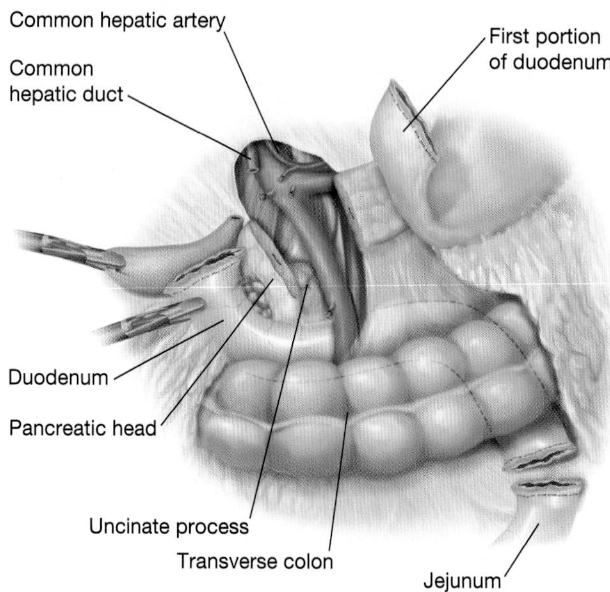


**Figure 1.1** Illustration showing the relationship of the divided duodenum, common hepatic duct, jejunum, and pancreas to its surrounding structures.

may in cases of portal hypertension become clinically relevant. The predominantly portal drainage of the pancreas accounts for the preponderance of liver metastases compared with lung metastases in cases of advanced pancreatic cancer. The pancreatic head and uncinate process drain via pancreaticoduodenal veins that run with the pancreaticoduodenal arteries and drain into the SMV and portal vein, while the body and tail drain via the splenic vein. During pancreaticoduodenectomy several prominent named veins must be ligated and divided at their confluence with the SMV in order to dissect the neck of the pancreas from the SMV. These include the gastroepiploic vein caudal and to the left, and the vein of Belcher, cephalad and to

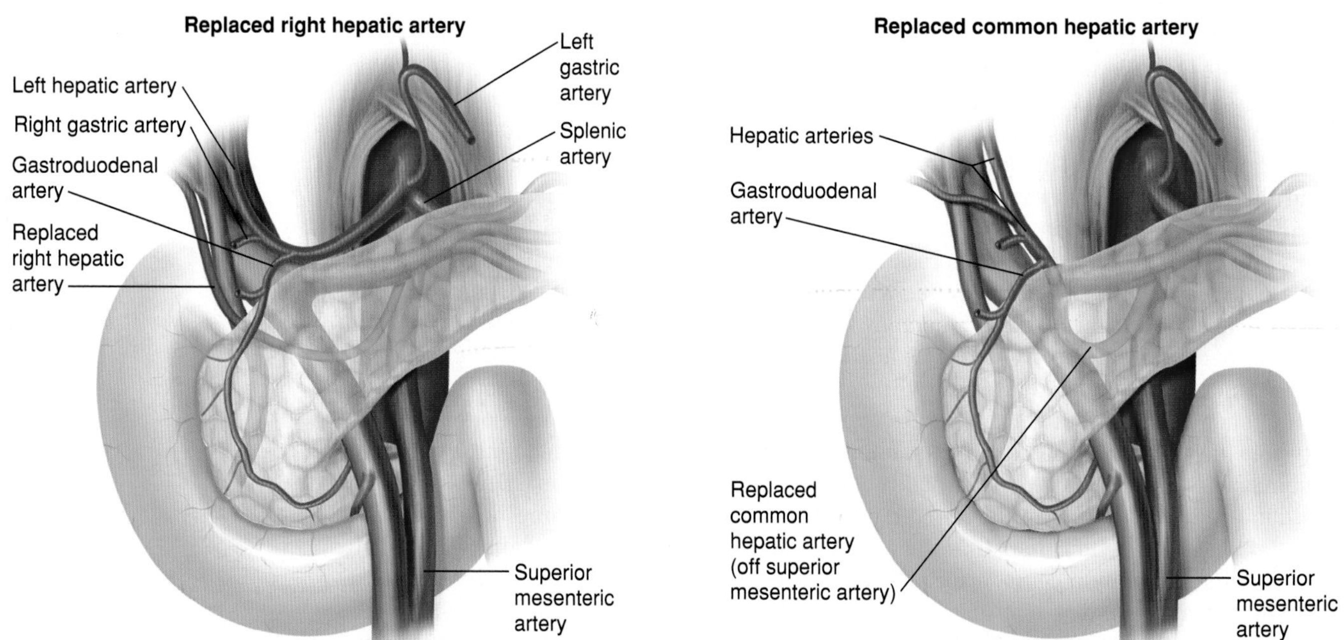


**Figure 1.2** Illustrations demonstrating the variable arterial anatomy that can be encountered during pancreaticoduodenectomy. Also noted is the relationship of the neck of the pancreas to the celiac axis, the superior mesenteric artery, the hepatic artery, and the portal vein/superior mesenteric vein confluence.

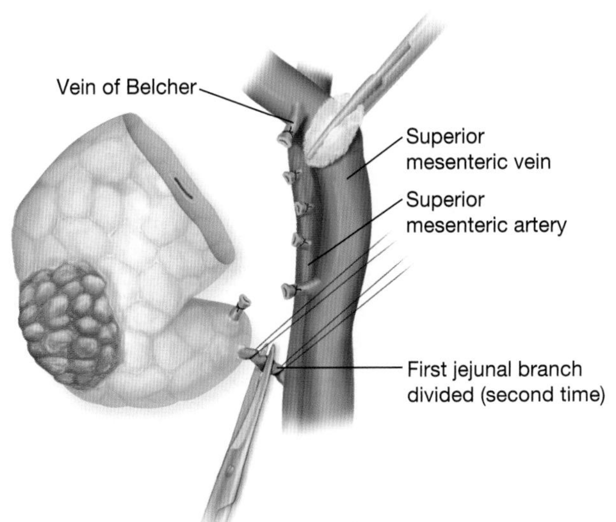


**Figure 1.3** Figure illustrating the portal vein/superior mesenteric vein confluence and the superior mesenteric artery following division of the neck of the pancreas and the uncinate process. Note the Vein of Belcher and the First Jejunal branch which can be particularly troublesome if not properly identified, ligated, and divided.

the right. After division of the neck of the pancreas, a first jejunal vein is sometimes ligated and divided at its confluence with the SMV during division of the uncinate process (Fig. 1.3).

The vascular anatomy of the pancreas and surrounding structures is crucial to the surgical care of pancreaticobiliary patients, and in fact, often determines resectability of malignant masses. Typically, patients without metastatic disease are grouped into three categories of resectability, depending on the vascular involvement by the tumors: Resectable, borderline, and unresectable. Borderline patients were first defined by the MD Anderson group and may have either encasement of a short segment of the hepatic artery (but no extension to the celiac axis) that is amenable to resection and reconstruction, or tumor abutment (viz, <180 degrees) of the SMA, or short-segment occlusion of the SMV or portal vein that is amenable to resection and reconstruction. Tumor encasement (viz, ≥180 degrees) of the SMA by the tumor typically constitutes a locally advanced, unresectable tumor.

Pancreatic lymphatic vessels travel from the acini and follow the arteries to drain into peripancreatic lymph nodes. The head and neck of the pancreas drain widely into pancreaticoduodenal nodes, superior mesenteric nodes, hepatic artery nodes, pre-aortic, and celiac axis nodes. The body and tail drain predominantly into pancreaticosplenic nodes with a minority of channels draining into pre-aortic nodes. The pancreatic islets have no lymphatics.

The exocrine pancreas is richly innervated with both sympathetic and parasympathetic fibers (the endocrine pancreas is innervated almost exclusively by the parasympathetic system). Sensory fibers from the pancreas travel through the celiac plexus, at which point they are available for ablation, typically via ethanol splanchnicectomy in cases of severe, chronic pain from pancreatitis or locally advanced malignancy.

The extrahepatic biliary tree, as well as associated arteries, is aberrant in one way or another at least as often as they are typical. Although discussion of all the variations of the hepatic, cystic, and common bile ducts, as well as the cystic and hepatic arteries, is beyond the scope of this chapter, aberrancies of the right and left hepatic arteries are worthy of further mention. The most reliable measurement of the frequency and type of hepatic artery aberrancies likely comes from autopsy studies in the 1950s by Michels, who described in a series of 200 autopsies, that 26% of bodies had aberrant right, and 27% aberrant left, hepatic arteries. On both sides, replaced was more common than accessory arteries (60% replaced on the right and 70% on the left). The practicing pancreaticobiliary surgeon must be familiar with standard as well as aberrant anatomy of the extrahepatic biliary tree and associated arteries (Fig. 1.2).

# Preoperative Considerations

## Diagnosis

Patients with pancreaticobiliary disease present in a variety of ways. In cases of extrahepatic biliary tree pathology, and processes involving the head of the pancreas, this often manifests as painless jaundice. Abdominal pain, especially in cases of pancreatitis or bile duct strictures, can also occur frequently. Regardless of the presentation, once pancreaticobiliary disease has been identified, appropriate preoperative planning is a cornerstone of a successful surgical result, and multiple tools exist.

## Imaging

### Computerized Tomography

Computerized tomography (CT) scan is one of the most reliable planning implements in the preoperative phase, providing information not only regarding the size and location of the tumor, but also more importantly about its relationship to surrounding structures. Pancreatic adenocarcinomas usually appear as hypoattenuating lesions when the pancreatic parenchyma is maximally enhanced in the early postarterial phase. CT has very high sensitivity, approaching 100%, for lesions ≥2 cm in size. There does, however, appear to be a significant decrease for smaller tumors, with sensitivities ranging from 67% to 77%. CT is a powerful tool with regard to determining resectability, as sensitivity for vascular involvement can exceed 90%. Despite continuing advances in CT technology, one drawback remains the lack of accuracy in identifying small liver metastases, small peritoneal nodules, or low-volume carcinomatosis. This can be a significant issue, and can lead to a false negative result in >30% of cases.

### Endoscopic Ultrasound

The role of endoscopic ultrasound (EUS) in the preoperative planning for pancreaticobiliary surgery is somewhat controversial. Like CT, EUS can provide information regarding the relationship of lesions to major vascular structures, but multi-detector CT scanning is of such high quality, that EUS is generally not necessary to accomplish this. Based on one study, sensitivity for EUS in detecting vascular invasion is 86%, while specificity is only 71%. EUS does, however, provide an excellent avenue for obtaining a tissue diagnosis. This may be necessary in patients with ambiguous lesions in order to determine if they should undergo pancreaticoduodenectomy, but is particularly important in marginally resectable or unresectable patients who will require chemotherapy or chemoradiotherapy. In addition, EUS may be the procedure of choice for identifying nodularity in patients with small pancreatic cysts. Lastly, EUS may be useful on occasion for identifying patients with metastatic disease, such as to the celiac lymph nodes, and this information may help guide management.

### Magnetic Resonance Imaging (MRI)

MRI also has a role in imaging the pancreatic duct and cystic lesions of the pancreas but the choice of MRI versus CT as the primary imaging modality is largely institution-dependent. The authors' institution favors CT, but recognizes that MRI can be useful in identifying pancreaticobiliary anatomy and pathology. With increasing numbers of pancreatic resections being done for intraductal papillary mucinous neoplasms, MRI has become more frequently used as a diagnostic and screening tool in some institutions. In addition, important information about the pancreatic duct can be noninvasively elucidated using MRCP. This is particularly important when assessing a distal bile duct stricture, or when planning a pancreatic drainage procedure in the setting of chronic pancreatitis.

### Positron Emission Tomography (PET)

There is currently insufficient evidence to advocate for the regular use of PET scanning in the diagnosis and staging of pancreaticobiliary disease. As with CT scan, the sensitivity of PET is closely associated with the size of the lesion, making it susceptible to missing low-volume metastatic disease.

## Patient Preparation

The sum total of risk that major abdominal surgery poses to the patient is a function of several factors, including not only medical comorbidities, but also surgeon experience and institutional capability. Multiple studies have shown a reproducible correlation between good outcomes and both institution volume and surgeon volume for complex operations such as pancreatic resections.

### Medical Considerations

The goal of the preoperative medical evaluation is not only to achieve "medical clearance" or "cardiac clearance" but also to optimize the patient's health and to minimize risk. The predominant nonsurgical contributor to postoperative morbidity and mortality is the cardiovascular system, and given that perioperative myocardial infarction has been associated with a mortality rate as high as 70%, preoperative cardiac evaluation is essential. The elective, nonemergent nature of most pancreaticobiliary procedures allows, and indeed demands, preoperative medical optimization. Major abdominal surgery is considered by the American College of Cardiology an "intermediate risk" procedure, which carries a 1% to 5% chance of myocardial infarction or death of cardiac etiology. Patient-specific factors contributing to this risk which should draw attention include recent myocardial infarction, unstable angina, symptomatic arrhythmias, severe heart block, worsening or new-onset heart failure, and advanced aortic or mitral valve stenosis. In any of these situations, it is recommended that patients have preoperative evaluation and intervention, if required, in order to define and to minimize risk.

Also important prior to major intra-abdominal surgery is consideration of pulmonary status. Perioperative complications such as pneumonia and respiratory failure requiring prolonged intubation are approximately as common as major cardiovascular complications, and can be similarly costly to the patient and to society. Those with documented chronic obstructive pulmonary disease (COPD), asthma, and an extensive smoking history, particularly in the setting of advanced age or obesity, are most at risk. Existing data do not support routine pulmonary function testing before major abdominal surgery, although it may be of benefit to properly optimize selected patients. Correct use of inhalers and steroids may be beneficial in those with COPD, and recognition of obstructive sleep apnea may be crucial in the early postextubation period. Somewhat paradoxically, cessation of smoking may be detrimental when implemented in the short term.

### Preoperative Nutrition

Nutritional status has long been recognized as a predictor of and contributor to postoperative outcome. The most pronounced degree of malnourishment is frequently seen in cancer patients, although malnutrition is likewise an important consideration in the case of chronic pancreatitis, especially if surgical intervention is considered.

There is some uncertainty and controversy involved in the assessment of nutritional status and its severity. The most rudimentary form of this assessment is clinical judgment; however, there are formulas which have been developed to assist in the process. The Nutritional Risk Index (NRI) is a mathematical formula which takes into account serum albumin levels and unintentional weight loss. The Nutritional Risk Screening (NRS) 2002 score examines nutritional status, but also takes into account the severity of the individual's illness. The NRS 2002 specifically considers body mass index (BMI), recent (unintentional) weight loss, and appetite (food intake during the week prior to surgery) to assess nourishment.

The Veterans Affairs Total Parenteral Nutrition Cooperative Study Group used the NRI in its prospective randomized study of 395 patients scheduled to undergo laparotomy or thoracotomy for noncardiac surgery. All were considered malnourished based upon the NRI, and were further subclassified as having borderline, mild, or severe malnutrition. The study group concluded that perioperative nutritional support was warranted only in those with "severe" malnutrition as this subset was the only one to demonstrate fewer complications than their control counterparts. More recently, the NRS 2002 was tested prospectively by Schiesser et al., and found to accurately portend both the occurrence and degree of postoperative complications.

### Preoperative Biliary Drainage

Unlike liver surgery, in which hyperbilirubinemia may impair or even prevent liver regeneration, pancreaticobiliary surgery is not similarly impacted by hyperbilirubinemia, provided that the operation can be performed in a timely fashion. Whether or not preoperative biliary drainage is performed often depends on referral bias, viz, depends on whether the patient was first referred to a gastroenterologist or to a surgeon. If the initial referral is to a gastroenterologist who then uses endoscopic techniques to diagnose the underlying etiology, a biliary drainage procedure will almost certainly be performed. If the first referral is to a surgeon, then much depends on the timeliness of surgery in combination with the severity of patient symptoms, primarily jaundice and pruritus. Recent studies demonstrate that preoperative biliary drainage may portend a higher rate of complications. Van der Gaag and colleagues performed a multi-institutional, randomized, controlled trial looking at preoperative biliary drainage in patients with tumors located in the head of the pancreas. This showed no difference in the rate of postoperative complications, but due to the significant rate of complications associated with the biliary drainage procedure itself, there were far more complications in the preoperative drainage group than this those who had surgery first. Clear exceptions include patients who develop acute cholangitis as a result of biliary obstruction, as well as those who will have a protracted time interval prior to surgery (as in the case of neoadjuvant therapy) and therefore require preoperative biliary drainage.

## Intraoperative Considerations

### General Considerations

With an overall trend toward less invasive procedures and attempts to shorten hospitalization, one emerging consideration in pancreaticobiliary surgery is whether or not to approach the operation laparoscopically. The minimally invasive approach has been studied most extensively with distal pancreatectomy. Various series have shown this to be a safe and effective procedure, being associated with similar rates of morbidity and mortality, as well as being oncologically sound regarding factors such as surgical margins and lymph node retrieval, as compared to the open counterpart operation. In addition, laparoscopic distal pancreatectomy has been associated with shorter hospitalization time in some series.

Laparoscopic pancreaticoduodenectomy, on the other hand, has not been widely embraced. While there are no prospective, randomized trials to compare this procedure with open pancreaticoduodenectomy, initial series report similar rates of morbidity, mortality, and similar oncologic parameters, compared to open pancreaticoduodenectomy.

### Patient Positioning

Nearly all pancreaticobiliary operations are undertaken with the patient in the supine position. It is important to have the patient properly positioned on the operating table to give sufficient room for the placement of a self-retaining retractor, while giving the surgeon and the assistant the space to move freely. Tucked arms should be well padded, especially at the elbow and wrist, and it must be certain that any intravenous line or monitoring equipment on the tucked arm(s) continue to function. If both arms are to be left untucked, they should be at a nearly 90-degree angle—but no more—from the operating table to allow for the maximum space for the retractor post and the surgeon on that side while protecting the shoulder joint from undue strain.

### Monitoring/Intravenous Access

Given the complex nature of a majority of these operations, proper monitoring is imperative to maintain patient safety and ensure a favorable outcome. All patients should have an intra-arterial catheter for continuous blood pressure monitoring, as well as arterial blood gas measurements. Central venous access can be beneficial in certain situations where peripheral access is inadequate, or if knowledge of the central venous pressure will alter the direction of the procedure. Generally speaking, two large-bore peripheral intravenous lines are adequate for patient resuscitation, and avoid the delays and complications associated with central line placement.

### Incision

A variety of incisions can be employed to approach the pancreaticobiliary system. An upper midline incision gives good access to the entire pancreas as well as the extrahepatic biliary tree. The proper exposure can also be gained using a right subcostal incision, extending across the midline to the left subcostal area if necessary.

### Staging Laparoscopy

In recent years, with steadily improving imaging technology, a trend has begun away from staging laparoscopy. This has been especially true for CT, a modality that has seen tremendous improvements since multi-detector scanners replaced helical machines at the beginning of the previous decade. The cost-benefit ratio of using diagnostic laparoscopy, which when combined with laparoscopic ultrasound can cost as much as $3,000.00 per case, has become less favorable. In cases of nonpancreatic pancreaticobiliary tumors (e.g., tumors of the distal common bile duct and ampulla), the benefit of diagnostic laparoscopy may well be so minimal as to render its use obsolete. In cases of pancreatic ductal adenocarcinoma, however, its use may affect management in 12% to 16% of cases, depending on the series. Selective use, therefore, is appropriate, especially in cases of tumors in the tail and body of the pancreas, and cases with significantly elevated CA 19–9 levels, as these may be harbingers of metastatic disease.

### Drains

The presence, number, size, and type of drains used before closing the abdomen varies widely from surgeon to surgeon. Given that one of the most common complications of pancreatic surgery is pancreatic fistula, and that this can occur with predictable regularity, most would advocate the use of intraperitoneal drainage following pancreaticoduodenectomy or distal pancreatectomy, especially after operation upon a soft gland or small-diameter pancreatic duct.

## The Normal Postoperative Pathway

Postoperative considerations begin preoperatively and are chiefly designed to prevent complications, or at least to achieve their early detection and expeditious and successful treatment, with the goal of minimizing morbidity. At Johns Hopkins Hospital a critical postoperative pathway of patients undergoing pancreatectomy has been employed since the early 1990s, and has recently been successfully transplanted from Johns Hopkins to Thomas Jefferson Hospital. Table 1.1 summarizes the current critical pathway for pancreaticoduodenectomy at Johns Hopkins Hospital.

**TABLE 1.1 Critical Pathway for Pancreaticoduodenectomy**

| | | |
|---|---|---|
| Postoperative day 0 | Before operating room | Heparin, 5,000 units SC given<br>Beta-blockade if indicated |
| | In operating room | Thromboembolic deterrent (TED) stockings and sequential compression devices<br>Arterial catheter<br>Central venous catheter if indicated<br>Perioperative antibiotics begun before incision<br>Nasogastric tube placed after anesthesia induction<br>Octreotide, 250 mcg SC given if gland soft<br>Perianastomotic drains (0–3) placed |
| | After operating room | Night of operation spent in ICU<br>Intravenous patient-controlled analgesia<br>Intravenous proton pump inhibitor (PPI) |
| Postoperative day 1 | | Remove nasogastric tube<br>Start sips of water and ice chips @ 30 ml/h<br>Out of bed ambulating<br>Discontinue sequential compression devices, continue TED stockings and heparin subcutaneously<br>Discontinue antibiotics<br>Continue intravenous beta-blockade (if indicated), octreotide (if gland soft), and PPI<br>Transfer from ICU to floor |
| Postoperative day 2 | | Clear liquid diet, ad lib or limited @ 30–60 ml/h<br>Remove Foley catheter<br>Minimize all IV fluids<br>Begin diuresis and continue until discharge or patient reaches preoperative weight<br>Erythromycin, 200 mg IV q6h<br>Ambulate TID |
| Postoperative day 3 | | Clear liquid diet, ad lib or limited @ 30–60 ml/h<br>Continue TEDs, subcutaneous heparin, blockade, and PPI until hospital discharge<br>Ambulate QID |
| Postoperative Day 4 | | Measure drain amylase level<br>Regular diet with pancreatic enzymes<br>Switch all medications to oral route including analgesics<br>Discontinue all IV fluids<br>Remove JP drain with lowest volume (if appropriate) |
| Postoperative day 5 | | Remove remaining JP drain (if appropriate)<br>Discuss pathology; Medical oncology and radiation oncology consults (if appropriate) |
| Postoperative day 6 or 7 | | Distribute preprinted discharge instructions<br>Discharge home<br>Arrange follow-up appointment for 4 weeks after discharge<br>Discharge medications: PPI, pancreatic enzymes, analgesics, stool softeners |

Modified from Kennedy EP, Rosato EL, Sauter PK, et al., *J Am Coll Surg* 2007;204:917.

# Deviations from the Pathway (Complications)

Any deviation from the ideal postoperative course as delineated by the critical pathway constitutes a complication. Defining and grading complications is an essential part of the care of pancreaticobiliary surgical patients.

## Defining and Grading of Complications

The definition and grading of postoperative complications has been greatly facilitated by several recent publications. Clavien and colleagues, for instance, have, over the course of the last several decades, developed and refined a useful complication-grading system. Since this system, unlike other systems, is based on the *intervention* required to treat the complication (Table 1.2), it is highly reproducible, and therefore more useful for comparing outcomes.

**TABLE 1.2 Classification of Surgical Complication Adopted for Pancreatic Surgery**

| Grade | Definition |
|---|---|
| I | Any deviation from the normal postoperative course without pharmacologic treatment or surgical, endoscopic, and radiologic interventions. Allowed therapeutic regimens are: Drugs as antiemetics, antipyretics, analgesics, diuretics, electrolytes, and physiotherapy. This grade also includes wound infections opened at the bedside |
| II | Requiring pharmacologic treatment with drugs other than ones allowed for grade I complications. Blood transfusion and total parenteral nutrition[a] are also included |
| III | Requiring surgical, endoscopic, or radiologic intervention |
| IIIa | Intervention not under general anesthesia |
| IIIb | Intervention under general anesthesia |
| IV | Life-threatening complication (including CNS complications)[b] requiring 1C/ICU management |
| IVa | Single-organ dysfunction (including dialysis) |
| IVb | Multiorgan dysfunction |
| V | Death of a patient |
| Suffix "d" | If the patient suffers from a complication at the time of the discharge, the suffix "d" (for disability) is added to the respective grade of complication (including resection of the pancreatic remnant). This label indicates the need for a follow-up to fully evaluate the complication |

[a]Note regarding DGE: The insertion of a central line for TPN or nasojejunal tube by endoscopy is grade IIIa. However, if a central line is still in place or a feeding tube has been inserted at the time of surgery, then a TPN or enteral nutrition is grade II complication.
[b]Brain hemorrhage, ischemic stroke, Subarachnoidal bleeding, but excluding transient ischemic attacks.
CNS, central nervous system; IC, intermediate care; ICU, intensive care unit.
Reproduced from DeOliveira M, Winter JM, Schafer M, et al. Assessment of complications after pancreatic surgery: A novel grading system applied to 633 patients undergoing pancreaticoduodenectomy, *Ann Surg*. 2006;244:6, with permission.

Specific to pancreaticobiliary patients, the International Study Group of Pancreatic Surgery (ISGPS) has recently provided consensus definitions for common complications seen in a busy pancreaticobiliary practice, including delayed gastric emptying (DGE) and pancreatic fistula (PF). Demonstration of the importance of universally accepted definitions is provided by these two common postpancreatectomy complications. DGE is defined by the ISGPS as vomiting requiring the initiation or continuation of nasogastric tube decompression beyond postoperative day 3, or the inability to tolerate solid oral intake by postoperative day 7. PF is defined by the ISGPS as the collection of any measurable volume of fluid from the pancreatic resection drain, on or after postoperative day 3 with amylase content higher than three-fold the upper normal serum value. Whereas previous series in the literature may have used nearly as many definitions for these complications as there were series, thereby precluding meaningful comparison, today's pancreaticobiliary surgeon may and should profit from the ability to compare outcomes with benchmarks in literature, and to appropriately educate patients, based on commonly accepted definitions. Although DGE and PF can and should be graded by the surgeon according to the Clavien system, these two complications—being so common in pancreaticobiliary practices—have their own ISGPS grading systems as well.

Further demonstration of the importance of defining postoperative complications is provided by the experience at Johns Hopkins Hospital. Of nearly 3000 PDs performed at Johns Hopkins Hospital from 1970 and 2006, approximately half were performed for pancreatic adenocarcinoma. A recent analysis of these cases revealed a perioperative mortality rate of 2% and morbidity rate of 38%. The mortality rate steadily decreased from 30% in the 1970s to 1% in the 2000s, reflecting improvements in surgical care. The morbidity rate, however, increased from 30% to 45% over a similar time period, likely reflecting the improved capturing of better defined complications. As such, length of stay decreased from 16 days in the 1980s to 8 days in the 2000s. The most common three complications in this series (which predated the adoption of the ISGPS definitions) were DGE, 15%; surgical site infections, 8%; and pancreatic fistula, 5%. A subsequent trial from the same institution illustrated even more explicitly the importance of defining complications, specifically illustrated the difference between the ISGPS definition and the previous Hopkins definition of PF: The PF rate during a 20-month accrual period for a RCT conducted in the mid 2000s, was 3% and 16% for hard and soft glands, respectively, according to the JHH definition, but according to the ISGPS definition those same rates were 200% to 300% higher, at 9% and 41% for hard to soft glands, respectively.

## Assessing Risk of Complications

Not all patients have an equal likelihood of suffering complications. As noted above, the clearest example of this differential risk is the risk of pancreatic fistula, which depends largely on the texture of the gland. In a recent randomized controlled trial of pancreatic duct stenting during PD, for example, patients were stratified into soft versus hard gland texture and the rate of PF was several-fold higher in the soft-gland group: 9% for patient with hard glands versus 41% for those with soft glands.

Similarly, certain biochemical markers obtained on routine blood tests have been found to predict complication rates and severity. For example, patients with peak postoperative serum amylase that is low (<100 U/L), medium (100 to 299 U/L), or high (>400 U/L) have a corresponding risk of developing a PF: 4%, 14%, and 20%, respectively (Winter 2007 biomarkers).

Elevated postoperative transaminases also predict outcome. Patients with transaminases ≥2000 U/L have a nearly logarithmic increase (56% vs. 7%) in the risk of a CT-detected cavitating hepatic infarct as opposed to mere hepatic ischemia. Risk of postoperative mortality also correlated with transaminase levels: Patients who have low (<500 U/L), medium (500 to 1999 U/L), or high (≥2000) elevations in transaminases: Bear a 0.9%, 5%, and 25% risk of mortality, respectively (Winter 2007 biomarkers).

Other factors, such as obesity and age, that have traditionally been thought to predict morbidity, have, in isolation, been shown recently to play a relatively minor role in large-volume centers.

## Detection of Complications

Most of the postoperative complications in pancreaticobiliary patients are detected as a result of routine clinical and laboratory evaluation: Vital signs and inappropriate laboratory-detected anemia indicate the possibility of hemorrhage; Visual and laboratory examinations of drain effluent detects PF or bile leaks; Inspection of surgical sites detects superficial surgical site infections; and, of course, nausea and vomiting in the appropriate clinical setting readily aids the diagnosis of DGE, which may be confirmed with an upper gastrointestinal contrast evaluation under fluoroscopy.

## Management of Complications

One of the most important aspects of complication management is patient education. Although there is a relatively wide range of acceptable management of many complications, any path of complication and management is more easily traveled by the patient and the surgeon if there exists a strong foundation of communication and trust. Specific management of selected complications is discussed below.

### Delayed Gastric Emptying

DGE virtually always resolves with time, although upper endoscopy may be performed with balloon dilation of the gastric outlet if indicated. Medical therapy, which is often concurrent with interventional therapy, consists of motility agents such as the prokinetics erythromycin and metoclopramide. Erythromycin, although found to accelerate gastric emptying, is already being taken prophylactically by patients on pathway, and metoclopramide seems to have relatively little effect on gastric emptying.

### Pancreatic Fistula

PF, like most complications, may be mild and self-limited, or severe and life threatening. Similar to DGE the medical management typically starts prophylactically, since most high-risk patients are given octreotide to prevent PF. Mild cases are treated with prolonged drainage and allowing enteral feeding if tolerated. More severe cases, however, may require the cessation of enteral feeding with the initiation of parenteral nutrition. Drains are typically left in place until effluent is low-output or low-amylase. Undrained fluid collections are detected by CT scan, usually prompted by fevers or elevated white blood cell counts, and are drained percutaneously by interventional radiology.

#### Hemorrhage

Hemorrhage following pancreaticobiliary surgery may be divided into early and late hemorrhage. Early hemorrhage (within 24 to 72 hours) is usually surgical bleeding resulting from a technical problem, whereas late hemorrhage (after 5 days) is often associated with a pancreatic leak and erosion of the GDA stump or small branches of the SMA or other vessels. Although there is little debate that clinically significant early hemorrhage is treated with emergent reoperation, there is a trend in the treatment of late hemorrhage toward management with angiographic embolization or stenting.

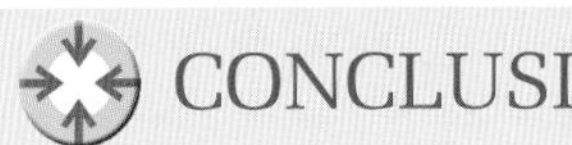

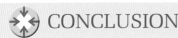

## CONCLUSION

Successful outcome of patients requiring pancreatic resections is predicated on the practitioners understanding the relevant anatomy, proper use of preoperative imaging, appropriately preparing the patient for surgery, technically precise surgical care, and recognizing and treating complications postoperatively, if and when they occur.

### Recommended References and Readings


Barabino M, Santambrogio R, Pisani Ceretti A, et al. Is there still a role for laparoscopy combined with laparoscopic ultrasonography in the staging of pancreatic cancer? *Surg Endosc.* 2011;25(1):160–165.

DeOliveira ML, Winter JM, Schafer M, et al. Assessment of complications after pancreatic surgery: A novel grading system applied to 633 patients undergoing pancreaticoduodenectomy. *Ann Surg.* 2006;244(6):931–937; discussion 937–939.

Fleisher LA, Beckman JA, Brown KA, et al. Acc/aha 2007 guidelines on perioperative cardiovascular evaluation and care for noncardiac surgery: A report of the American college of cardiology/American heart association task force on practice guidelines (writing committee to revise the 2002 guidelines on perioperative cardiovascular evaluation for noncardiac surgery) developed in collaboration with the American society of echocardiography, American society of nuclear cardiology, heart rhythm society, society of cardiovascular anesthesiologists, society for cardiovascular angiography and interventions, society for vascular medicine and biology, and society for vascular surgery. *J Am Coll Cardiol.* 2007;50(17):e159–e241.

Kennedy EP, Rosato EL, et al. Initiation of a critical pathway for pancreaticoduodenectomy at an academic institution–the first step in multidisciplinary team building. *J Am Coll Surg.* 2007;204(5):917–923; discussion 923–924.

Kinney T. Evidence-based imaging of pancreatic malignancies. *Surg Clin North Am.* 2010;90(2):235–249.

Liu RC, Traverso LW. Diagnostic laparoscopy improves staging of pancreatic cancer deemed locally unresectable by computed tomography. *Surg Endosc.* 2005;19(5):638–642.

Varadarajulu S, Eloubeidi MA. The role of endoscopic ultrasonography in the evaluation of pancreatico-biliary cancer. *Surg Clin North Am.* 2010;90(2):251–263.

Winter JM, Cameron JL, Campbell KA, et al. Does pancreatic duct stenting decrease the rate of pancreatic fistula following pancreaticoduodenectomy? Results of a prospective randomized trial. *J Gastrointest Surg.* 2006;10(9):1280–1290; discussion 1290.

Winter JM, Cameron JL, Campbell KA, et al. 1423 pancreaticoduodenectomies for pancreatic cancer: A single-institution experience. *J Gastrointest Surg.* 2006;10(9):1199–1210; discussion 1210–1211.

Winter JM, Cameron JL, Yeo CJ, et al. Biochemical markers predict morbidity and mortality after pancreaticoduodenectomy. *J Am Coll Surg.* 2007;204(5):1029–1036; discussion 1037–1038.

# 2 Pancreaticoduodenectomy With or Without Pylorus Preservation

**Harish Lavu and Charles J. Yeo**

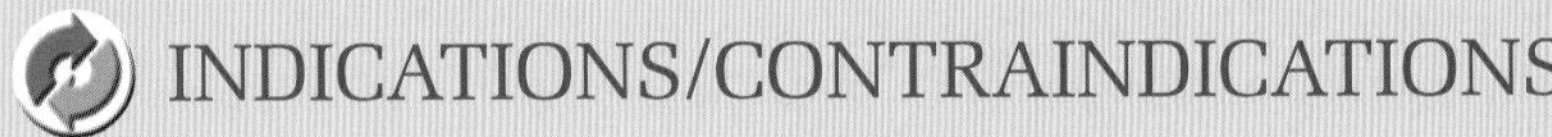

## INDICATIONS/CONTRAINDICATIONS

Pancreaticoduodenectomy (PD) is a complex surgical procedure designed to treat benign and malignant diseases of the periampullary region. (In many institutions the operation is referred to as the Whipple operation or Whipple procedure.) The most common of the malignant periampullary lesions treated by PD is pancreatic adenocarcinoma (85%), followed by distal common bile duct cholangiocarcinoma, adenocarcinoma of the ampulla of Vater, and duodenal adenocarcinoma. Taken together, these four tumors affect approximately 50,000 individuals per year in the United States. A host of other less common cancers can arise from the periampullary region including neuroendocrine tumors, pancreatic cystadenocarcinomas, acinar cell and squamous cell carcinomas, gastrointestinal stromal tumors, sarcomas, and lymphomas. In addition, a number of benign neoplasms as well as chronic pancreatitis can also be treated with PD. Finally, in rare circumstances, PD may be performed for isolated metastases to the periampullary region, or for blunt or penetrating trauma to the pancreaticoduodenal region.

Despite the differences in underlying tumor pathology, many malignant diseases of the periampullary region share similar clinical presentation, preoperative assessment, and surgical treatment strategy. Due to the difficulty and risk in obtaining a preoperative tissue diagnosis, the precise histologic tumor type is often unknown prior to surgical resection.

General contraindications to PD include known metastatic disease outside of the resection zone, locally advanced disease that is involving the mesenteric vasculature [typically the portal vein (PV) or superior mesenteric artery (SMA) or superior mesenteric vein (SMV)], and severe medical comorbidities which preclude safe anesthesia and surgery.

## PREOPERATIVE PLANNING

The goal of preoperative evaluation in patients undergoing PD is to accurately assess tumor resectability for appropriate surgical preparation and patient counseling.

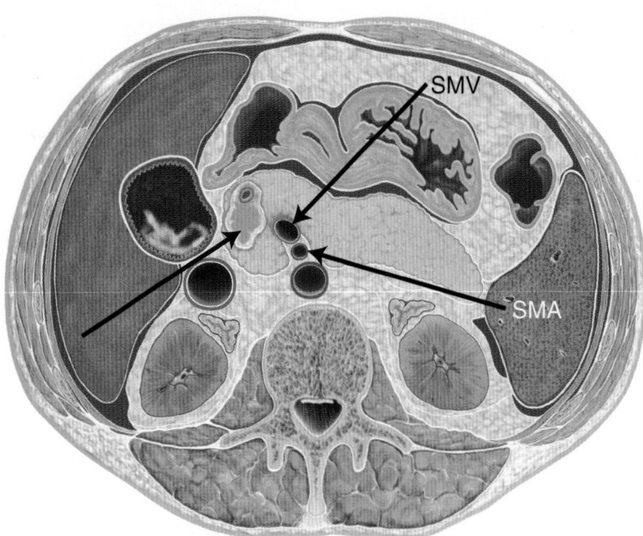


Figure 2.1 Illustration of a pancreas protocol 3D-CT scan demonstrating a 2 cm pancreatic ductal adenocarcinoma. The *arrow* highlights the characteristic hypoenhancing appearance of the lesion. Note the calcified gallstone within the adjacent gallbladder. The patient underwent a successful margin negative PD resection.

Preoperative assessment for PD should begin with a complete medical history, with special emphasis on a past history of chronic pancreatitis, or a family history of gastrointestinal cancer. A thorough physical examination may note scleral or cutaneous icterus if the patient has common bile duct obstruction. Significant weight loss is not an uncommon finding. Enlarged left supraclavicular (Virchow's) or periumbilical (Sister Mary Joseph's) lymph nodes or a perirectal tumor mass (Blumer's shelf) represent uncommon findings of disease dissemination. Laboratory evaluation should include complete blood count, electrolyte panel, liver function tests, coagulation profile, tumor markers [carbohydrate antigen 19-9 (CA 19-9) and carcinoembryonic antigen (CEA)], and serum albumin measurement to assess nutritional status.

Patients are educated at the initial office evaluation regarding the indications for surgery and undergo the informed consent process. The anatomy, operative procedure, and postoperative care plan are outlined in detail. Patients are introduced to our clinical pathway for postoperative care that is designed to improve patient safety and reduce perioperative morbidity, mortality, and length of stay.

Three-dimensional contrast enhanced thin section multidetector computed tomography (pancreas protocol 3D-CT) with oral ingestion of water has evolved to become our most valuable imaging modality for the diagnosis and preoperative staging of periampullary disease (Fig. 2.1). It allows for a finely detailed assessment of periampullary tumors, and importantly delineates their relationship to the major visceral vasculature. Patients who have tumor abutment greater than 90 degrees of the celiac axis or SMA, or who have greater than 180-degree involvement of the SMV or PV are typically considered to have locally advanced disease, because of the high likelihood of a margin positive resection if they were to undergo an attempt at PD. Patients in this locally advanced group are referred for neoadjuvant treatment (typically protocol-based chemoradiotherapy) prior to surgical resection. Pancreas protocol 3D-CT arterial reconstructions give important preoperative information by identifying vascular anatomic variants, such as replaced right hepatic artery from the SMA or atherosclerotic celiac stenosis, allowing for a safer operation (Fig. 2.2). Pancreas protocol 3D-CT may also detect distant metastatic disease to the liver or the peritoneum, though the sensitivity declines for lesions less than 1 cm in size.

Magnetic resonance imaging (MRI) is an effective tool whose use has increased in recent years in the evaluation of periampullary malignancies. MRI has an improved safety profile compared to pancreas protocol 3D-CT in patients who have an intravenous contrast allergy or chronic renal insufficiency. Magnetic resonance cholangiopancreatography (MRCP) allows for detailed imaging of the pancreatic and biliary ductal systems and is particularly useful in the assessment of pancreatic cystic disease, where it can delineate communication with the main pancreatic duct in intra-ductal papillary

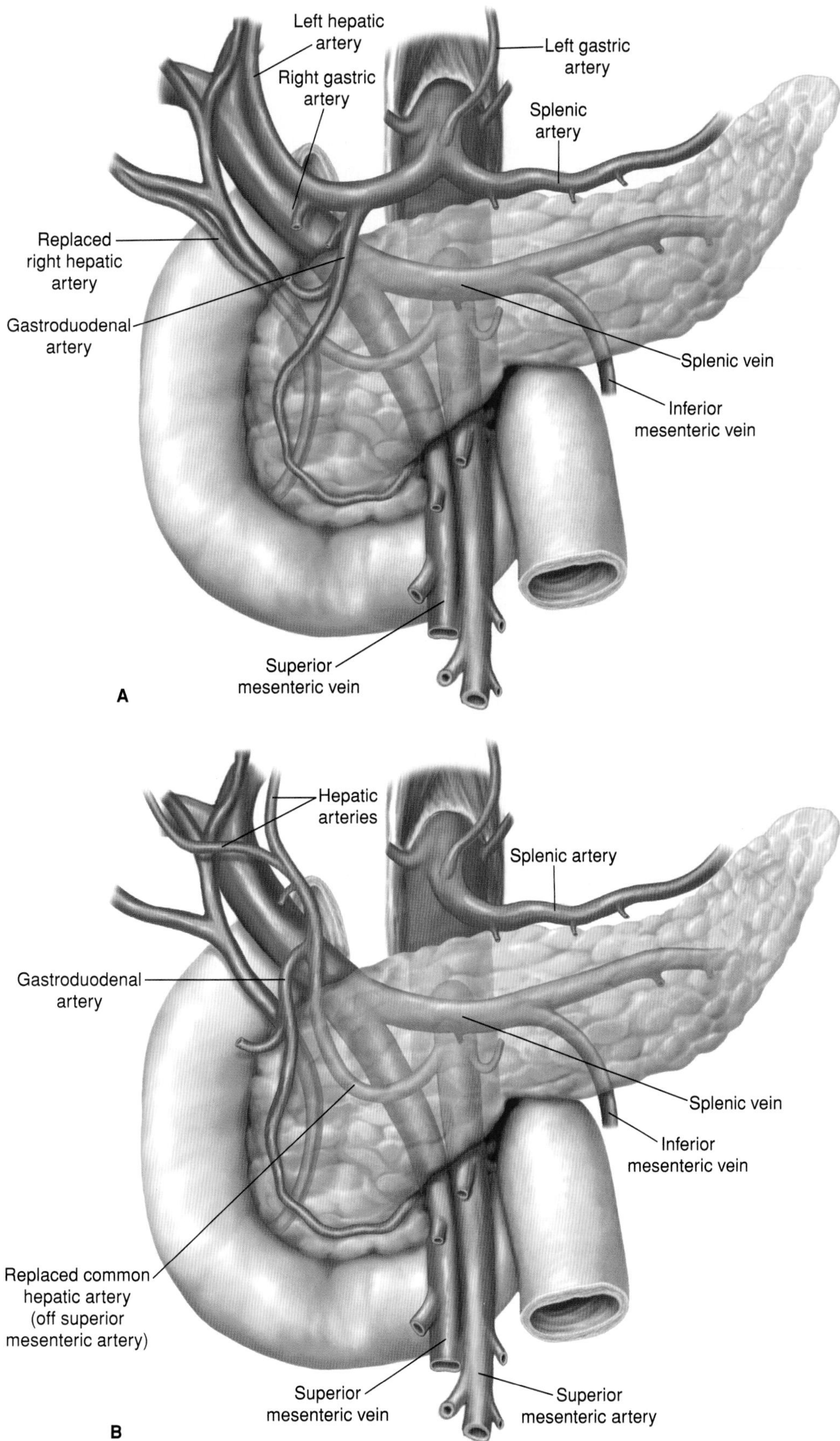


**Figure 2.2** Hepatic artery anatomic variation. On the **top** is a replaced right hepatic artery that arises directly from the SMA. On the **bottom** is a variant where the common hepatic artery trunk arises from the SMA. These hepatic arteries must be carefully preserved during PD.

mucinous neoplasms (IPMNs), or absence of ductal communication in mucinous cystic neoplasia (MCN) or serous cystic neoplasia (SCN).

Endoscopic ultrasound (EUS) is a procedure that allows for direct ultrasound imaging of the periampullary region through the walls of the gastric antrum and duodenum. It offers real-time imaging of the tumor and surrounding lymph nodes, can determine the relationship of the tumor to the visceral vasculature, and provides the ability to obtain tissue via ultrasound guided fine needle aspiration (FNA). EUS is highly operator dependent, and requires skilled application and interpretation of the ultrasound images for reliable results. EUS has a higher yield in obtaining a tissue diagnosis than cytologic biliary or pancreatic brushings from endoscopic retrograde cholangiopancreatography (ERCP). In patients with unresectable disease, EUS with FNA is an efficient and safe method for obtaining a tissue diagnosis to allow referral for protocol-based chemotherapy or chemoradiation therapy. In patients with clearly resectable periampullary abnormalities, a preoperative tissue diagnosis is not required in most cases, as the results of FNA (whether positive or negative) often do not alter the decision to proceed to surgical resection, and the low but measurable risk of procedure-related complications (pancreatitis, perforation, and bleeding) may delay surgical intervention.

Positron emission tomography (PET) scan is a diagnostic tool whose use is still being defined in the assessment of periampullary malignancy and it is not routinely recommended. PET utilizes a radio-labeled fluoro-deoxyglucose substrate which is preferentially taken up by tumor cells. This functional image can be useful in identifying occult metastatic lesions, but has a relatively high false-positive rate (typically in cases of inflammation or infection). When PET is fused with the cross-sectional images from a CT scan (PET-CT), the combined images can give functional and anatomic tumor staging details. PET scans are not currently the standard of care for preoperative staging of periampullary malignancies, but can aid in the evaluation of suspicious hepatic lesions, or in post-resectional surveillance of disease recurrence.

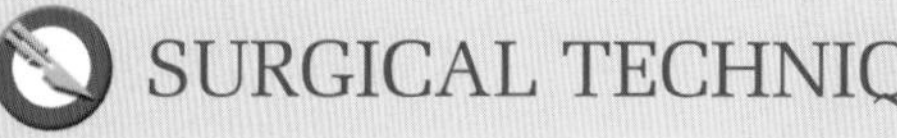

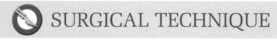

# SURGICAL TECHNIQUE

## Patient Preparation

The standard steps performed during a PD at our institution are outlined below. It is important to remember that the sequence of steps can be altered and frequently are, as needed, to facilitate the safe exposure and removal of the Whipple specimen.

The patient is prepared for PD with a clear liquid diet on the day prior to surgery. We have abandoned the use of preoperative mechanical bowel preparation in our practice. An endotracheal tube, nasogastric tube, urinary catheter, and appropriate monitoring lines are placed. Prophylactic subcutaneous heparin (5,000 units), lower extremity hose, and sequential compression devices are employed to limit the occurrence of deep venous thrombosis. Epidural catheters are not used, except in rare circumstances. Prophylactic antibiotics (typically cefoxitin 2 g intravenously) are administered within 30 minutes of the incision. The operation is performed in the supine position. The abdomen is clipped and prepped with chlorhexidine from nipples to pubis. In cases where superior mesenteric or portal venous resection or reconstruction is planned, the left neck and bilateral groins and thighs are clipped and prepped as well, to allow access to the left internal jugular vein and saphenous veins respectively, which may be needed for the visceral venous reconstruction.

## Technique—Resection (Extirpative Phase)

A midline incision is most commonly made from the tip of the xiphoid process to the umbilicus. A Bookwalter retractor™ is used for exposure. The abdominal cavity is thoroughly explored for occult metastasis, with assessment of the liver, celiac axis region, base of the transverse mesocolon, intestines, and all peritoneal surfaces. Suspicious

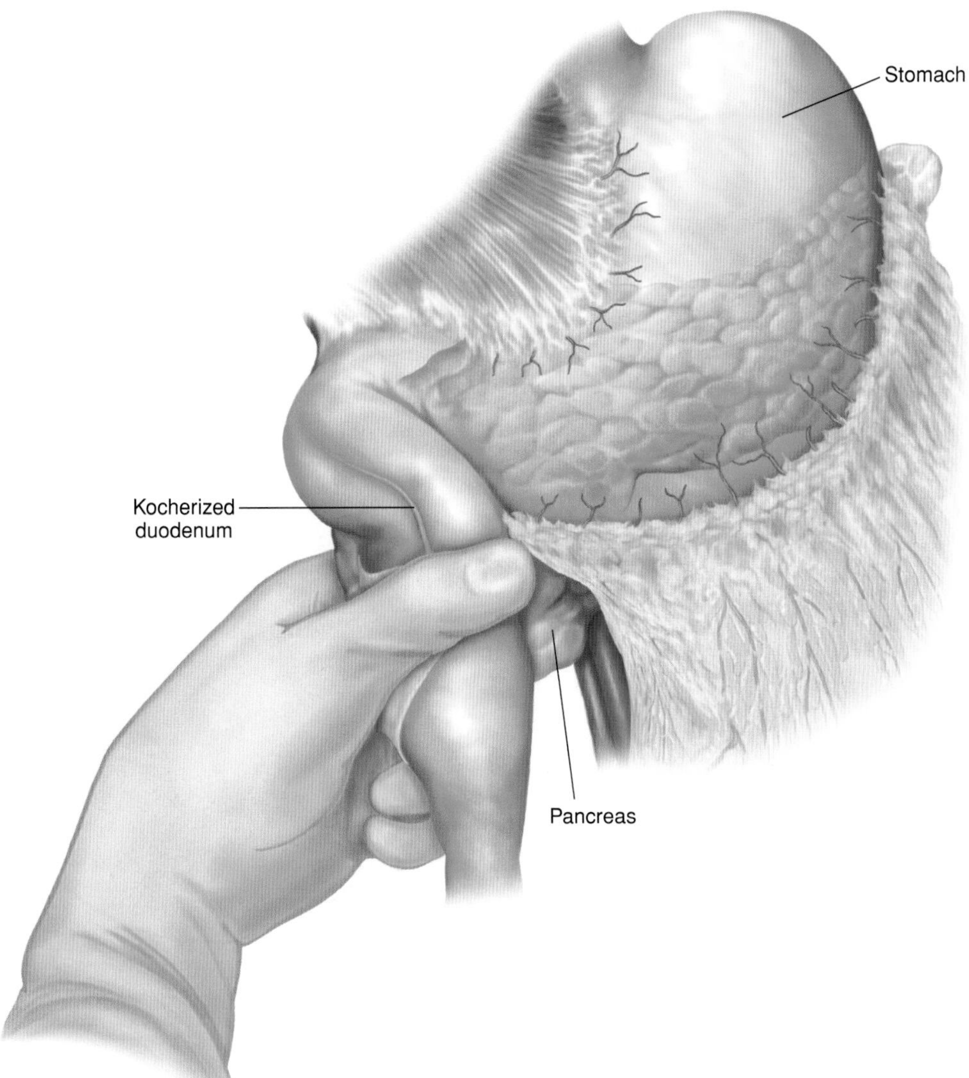


**Figure 2.3** After wide kocherization of the duodenum, the pancreatic head is elevated out of the retroperitoneum and the tumor mass is palpated, to help determine its relationship to the SMA.

lesions outside of the resection zone should be sampled by frozen section examination to rule out distant spread.

Very rarely we will perform an extended right subcostal incision which may facilitate exposure of the right upper quadrant and pancreatic head, particularly in patients who have a short trunk, are morbidly obese, or may require additional hepatic procedures.

The duodenum is widely kocherized by releasing it from the retroperitoneum and elevating the head of the pancreas ventrally off the underlying vena cava. This allows for palpation of the tumor and determination of its relationship to the SMA (Fig. 2.3). Although this is a useful step, it is important to realize that preoperative pancreas protocol 3D-CT scan imaging almost always defines the extent of vascular involvement better than such direct palpation at this point in the procedure.

The gallbladder is resected via the "dome down" technique, ligating the cystic duct and artery separately, using 2-O silk ties. The gallbladder can be removed at this point or may be left attached, to be removed later with the Whipple specimen. The gastrohepatic ligament is partially divided with electrocautery, while small vascular and lymphatic bundles are secured with 2-O silk ties and divided.

Further dissection within the hepatoduodenal ligament allows for identification of the proper hepatic artery and its branches, and encirclement of the common hepatic duct with a vessel loop. Care should be taken at this point to identify a replaced right hepatic artery if present, which often lies lateral and posterior to the common hepatic

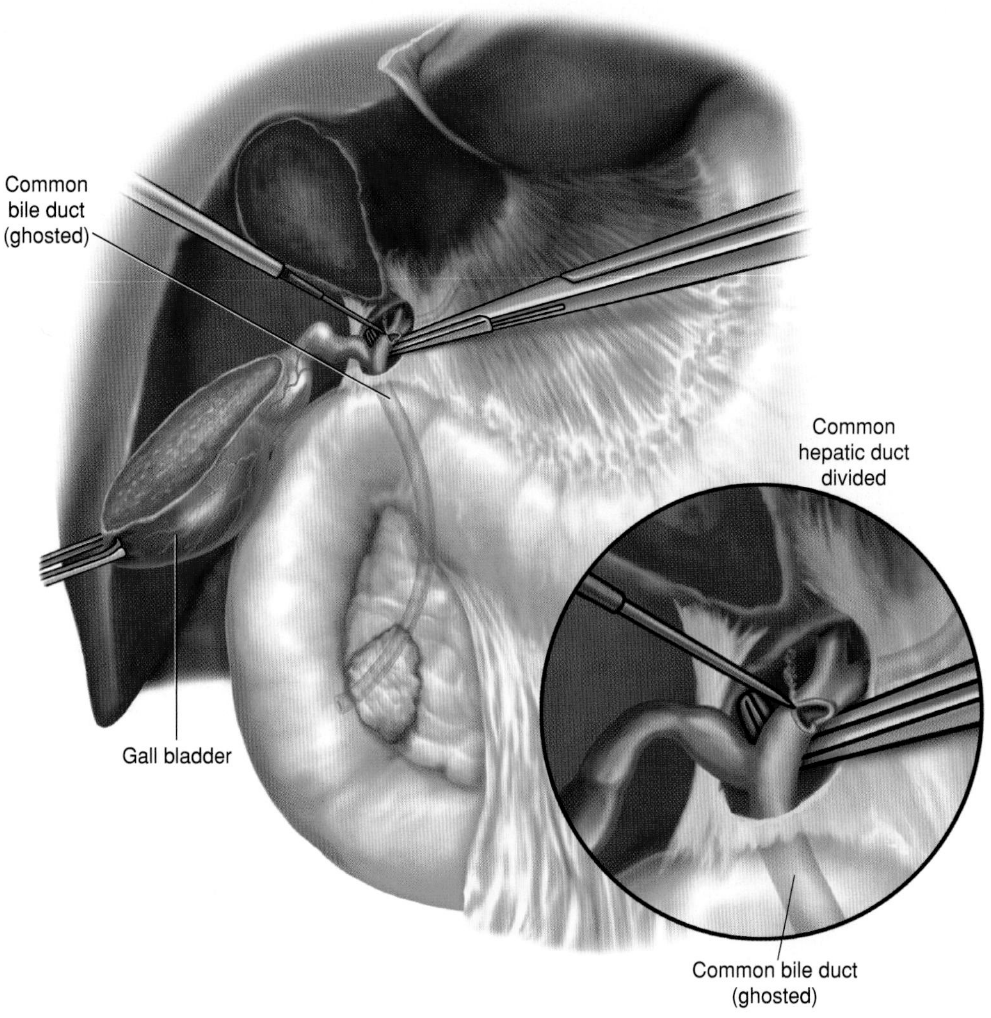


**Figure 2.4** The common hepatic duct is transected with electrocautery. For small, thin-walled ducts, we typically use a scalpel blade for the transection, to avoid thermal injury to the adjacent tissue. The gallbladder has been previously separated from its normal location in the hepatic gallbladder fossa.

and common bile ducts. The common hepatic duct is divided with a knife blade (if small) or with electrocautery (if dilated and thick walled) (Fig. 2.4). If either a plastic or metallic biliary endoprosthesis is encountered during the division of the common hepatic duct, it is removed at this point. A bulldog vascular clamp is placed on the proximal common hepatic duct to limit bile spillage until reconstruction begins. Early division of the common hepatic duct and further division of the surrounding lymphatics with their caudal retraction facilitates exposure of the anterior and lateral surfaces of the PV, which can be followed down to the superior border of the pancreatic neck.

The gastroduodenal artery (GDA) is identified within the hepatoduodenal ligament and is test clamped prior to its division, to ensure maintenance of proper hepatic artery flow to the liver. A Doppler probe may assist in this maneuver. This step ensures that there is no celiac origin occlusion with preferential proper hepatic artery filling via the GDA, originating from the SMA. The GDA is divided between 2-O silk ties and complimented by a 3-O silk suture ligature on its retained side (Fig. 2.5). A plane is then created posterior to the pancreatic neck and anterior to the PV at their interface, at the superior boundary of the pancreas.

The proximal duodenum is then separated from the pancreatic head by the creation of a tunnel approximately 2 to 3 cm distal to the pylorus. The duodenum is transected at this point with the aid of a linear stapling device (Fig. 2.6). In cases where there is tumor encroachment upon the first portion of the duodenum, or concerning lymphadenopathy in the pre-pyloric region, a classic PD should be performed, which involves up to 20% to 30% distal gastrectomy, dividing the distal stomach several centimeters proximal to the pylorus.

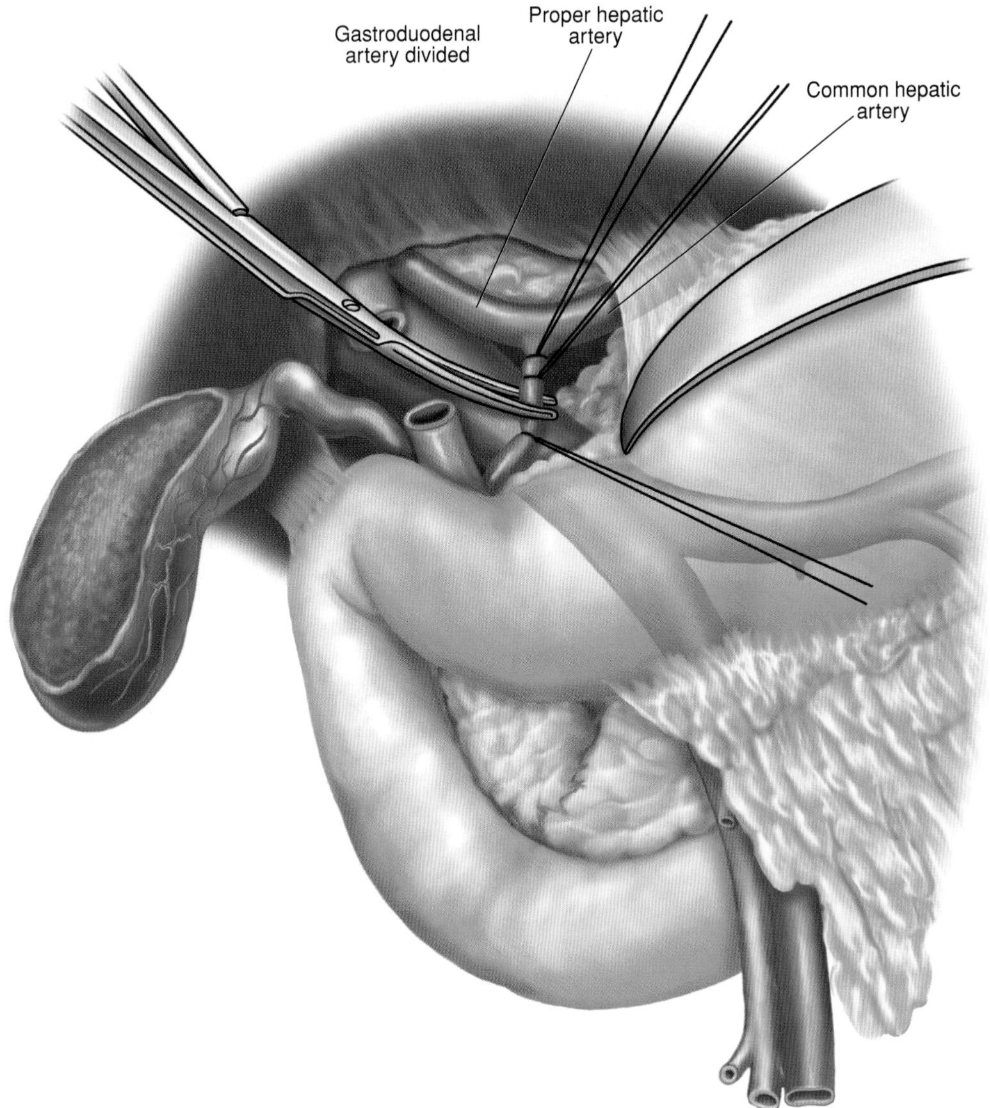


**Figure 2.5** The GDA is ligated and transected. Prior to its ligation, the GDA is test clamped, to ensure that proper hepatic artery flow is not adversely affected by concomitant celiac axis occlusion or stenosis.



The pancreatic head and uncinate process are further mobilized and the right gastroepiploic artery and vein are ligated. The SMV can be identified as it issues from under the neck of the pancreas and crosses ventrally over the third portion of the duodenum in the groove between the uncinate process and the transverse mesocolon (Fig. 2.7). Alternatively, the SMV can be identified by tracing the right gastroepiploic vein and the middle colic vein down toward the inferior border of the pancreatic neck where they may form a common "gastrocolic trunk" which enters anteriorly into the SMV. Under direct vision, the SMV exposure is continued cephalad and the tunnel posterior to the neck of the pancreas is completed, separating the neck from the SMV and PV. Care is taken at this point to avoid injury to the SMV, as control of bleeding can be difficult. A Penrose drain is passed through this tunnel, to elevate the pancreatic neck.

Four 3-O silk stay sutures are placed about the pancreatic neck (two on the superior portion of the neck and two on the inferior portion of the neck) to control intrapancreatic arterial arcades. The pancreatic neck is then divided with electrocautery over the Penrose drain, in the axis of the SMV–PV, taking care to protect the underlying SMV–PV confluence (Fig. 2.8). The location of the pancreatic duct is identified during neck transection by looking for a small gush of clear pancreatic juice (which contains substantial protein and thus bubbles when exposed to heat) when it is divided.

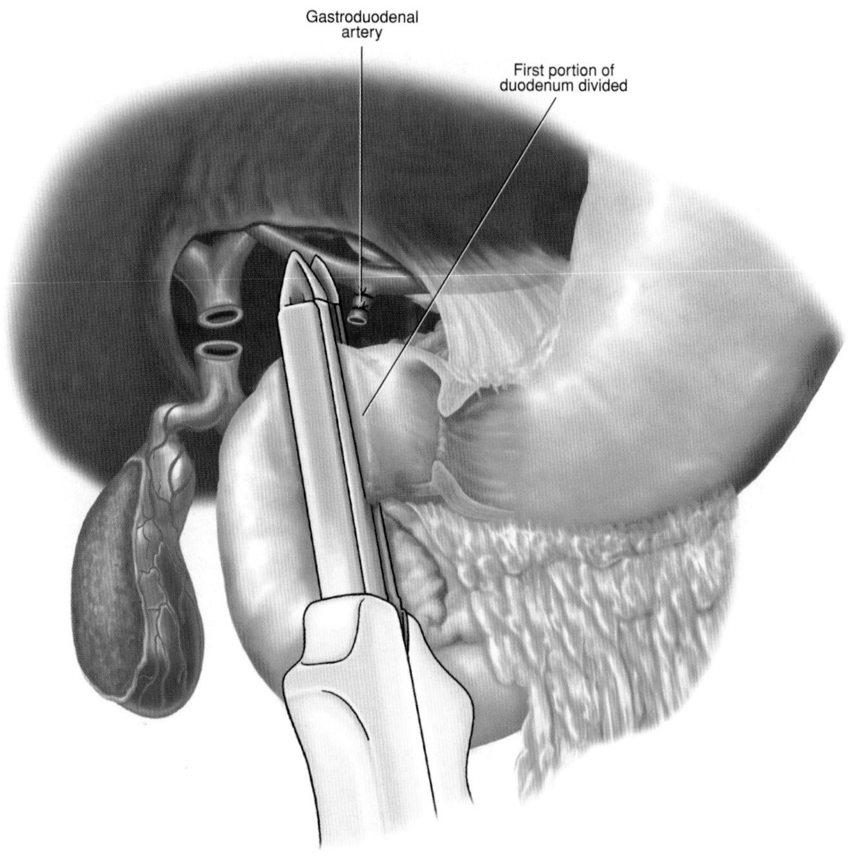


Figure 2.6 Transection of the duodenum is performed 2 to 3 cm distal to the pylorus with a linear stapling device.

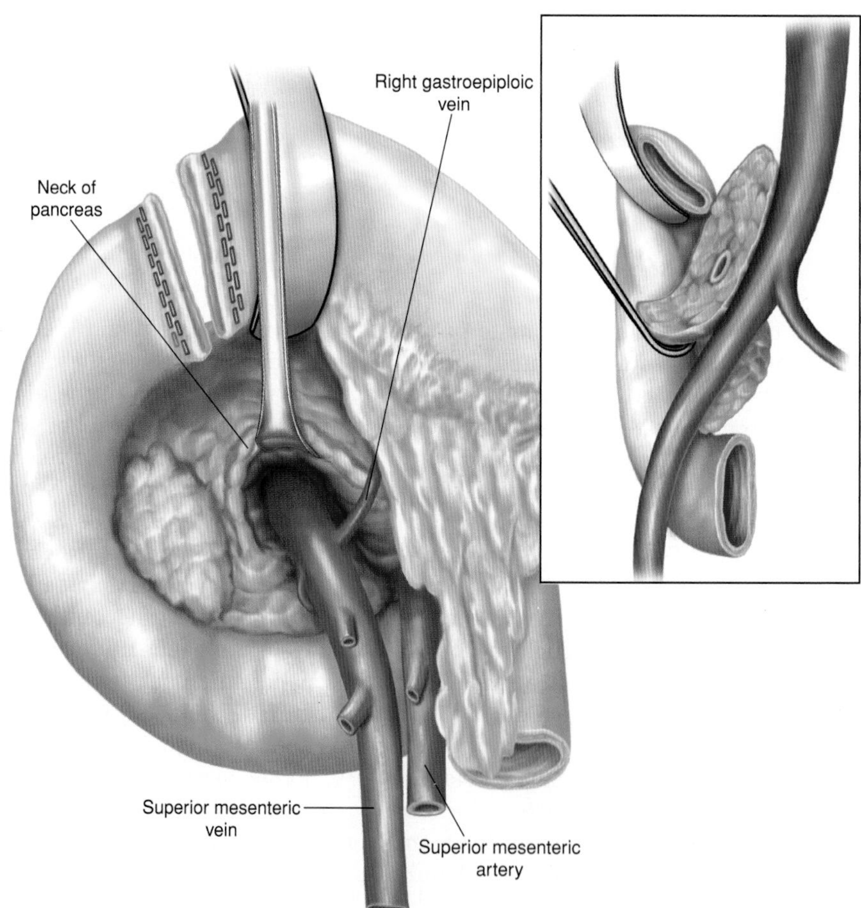


Figure 2.7 Creation of the tunnel posterior to the pancreatic neck, in the avascular vertical plane of the SMV–PV axis.

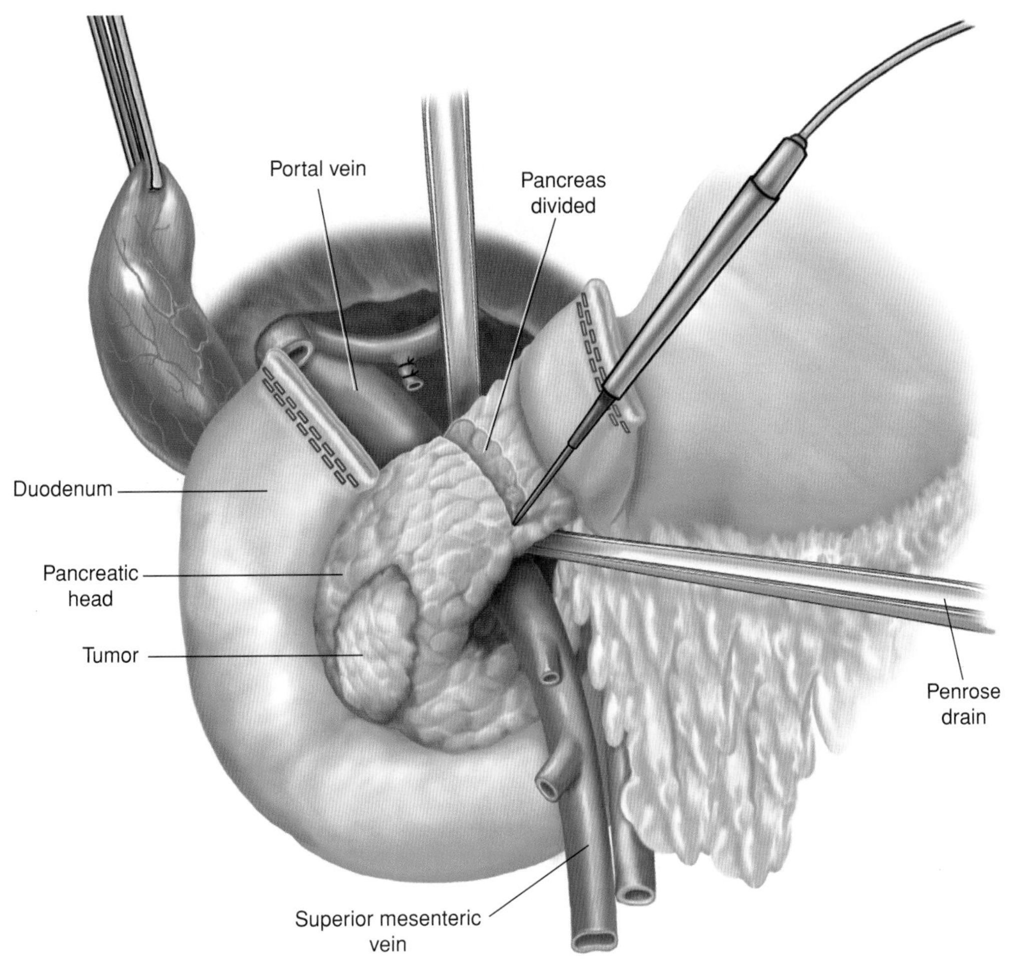


**Figure 2.8** Transection of the pancreatic neck with electrocautery. A Penrose drain is used to elevate the pancreatic neck and protect the underlying SMV–PV confluence during this step. Not shown are four 3-0 silk stay sutures which are typically placed on the superior and inferior boundaries of the pancreatic neck, to control intra-pancreatic arterial arcades.



The proximal jejunum is transected approximately 10 to 15 cm distal to the ligament of Treitz with a linear stapling device. The distal staple line is invaginated with 3-O silk Lembert sutures, as this will serve as the jejunal limb for reconstruction. The proximal jejunal mesentery is taken down between clamps and 2-O silk ties, up to the ligament of Treitz. This dissection is continued onto the mesentery of the fourth portion of the duodenum as it passes beneath the mesenteric vessels. The region is freed up enough to pass the proximal devascularized jejunum (part of the specimen) underneath the mesenteric vessels and into the right upper quadrant.

The pancreatic head and uncinate process are now gently separated from the right lateral border of the PV and SMV, and subsequently the SMA. This careful dissection is performed staying right on the plane of these visceral vessels, with serial clamping and ligation of the fine arterial and venous branches which connect the pancreatic head and uncinate process to the visceral vessels. The retroperitoneal soft-tissue margin of the uncinate is dissected free from the visceral vessels, and the right lateral margin of the SMA is skeletonized, removing all pancreatic tissue and draining lymphatics from the peri-vascular plane (Fig. 2.9).

The specimen is then removed and a hemostatic agent (we typically use Surgicel®) is applied to the area of dissection along the visceral vessels. The specimen is marked (by suture and marking pen) to identify the bile duct, pancreatic neck, and retroperitoneal soft-tissue margins and is sent for intra-operative frozen section analysis of the margins and pathologic examination of the tumor (Fig. 2.10). During every case we speak to the attending pathologist, to apprise them of the clinical scenario and our impression regarding the pathologic process at hand.

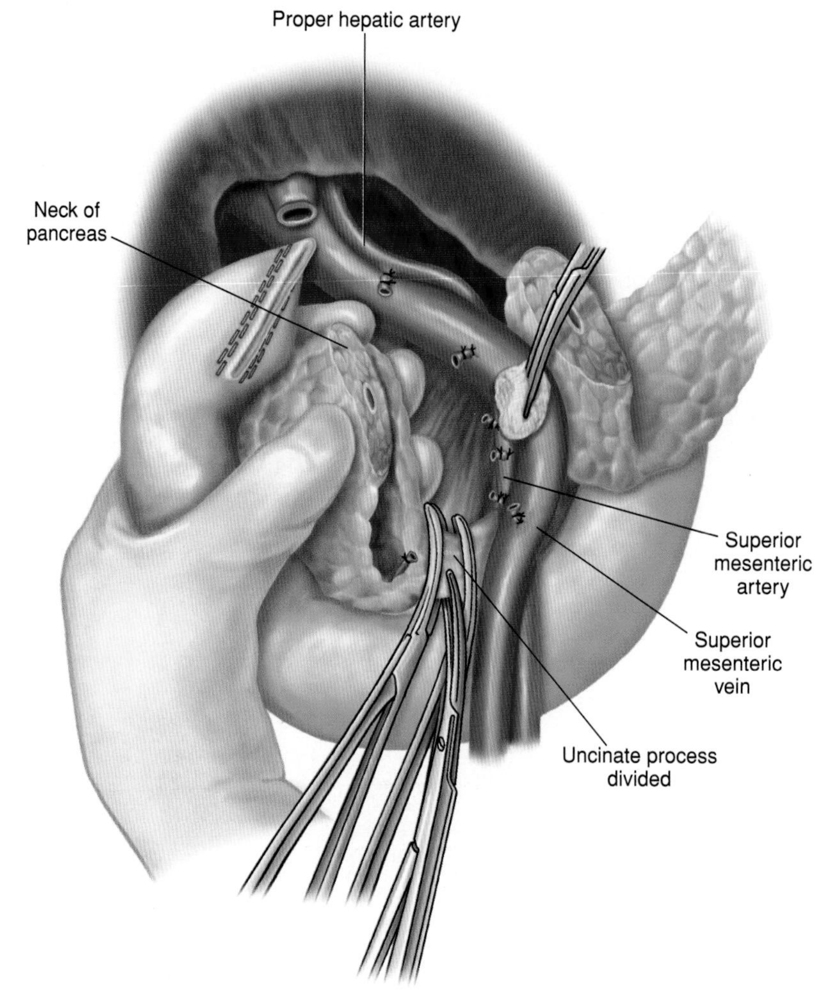


**Figure 2.9** Serial clamping and ligation along the uncinate process and retroperitoneal soft-tissue margin. Care is taken during this step to identify, palpate, and avoid injury to the underlying and adjacent SMA.

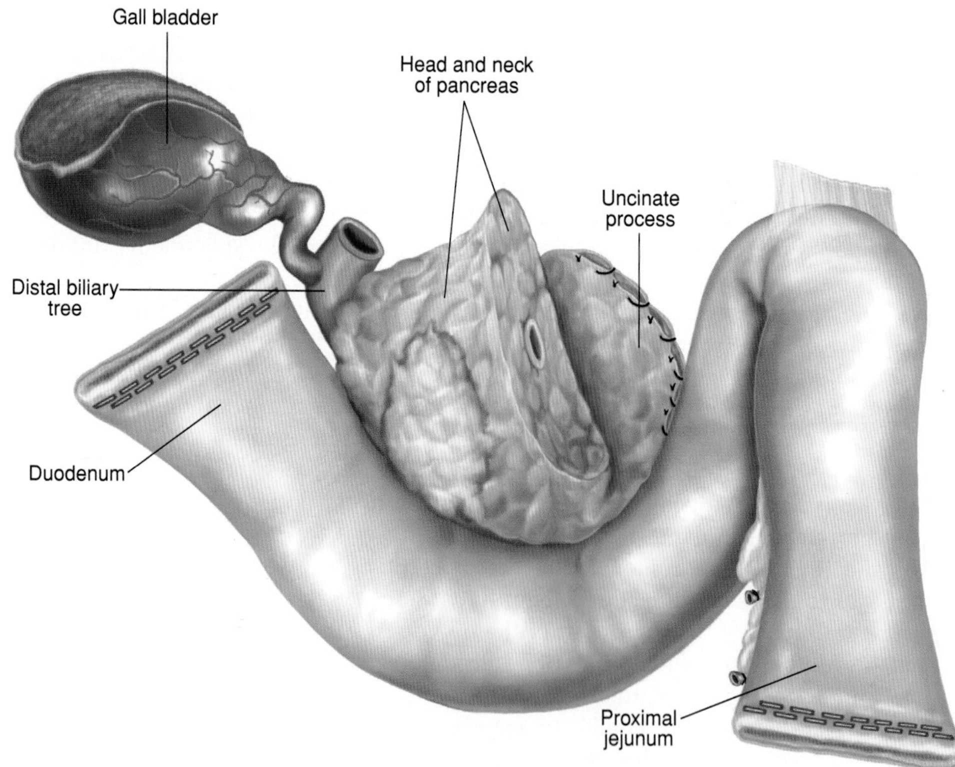


**Figure 2.10** The pylorus-preserving Whipple specimen is shown. The pancreatic neck, common hepatic duct, and retroperitoneal soft-tissue margins are marked and submitted for intra-operative frozen section analysis, as well as pathologic evaluation of the primary tumor. The patient's clinical history is communicated to the attending pathologist at the time the specimen is sent.

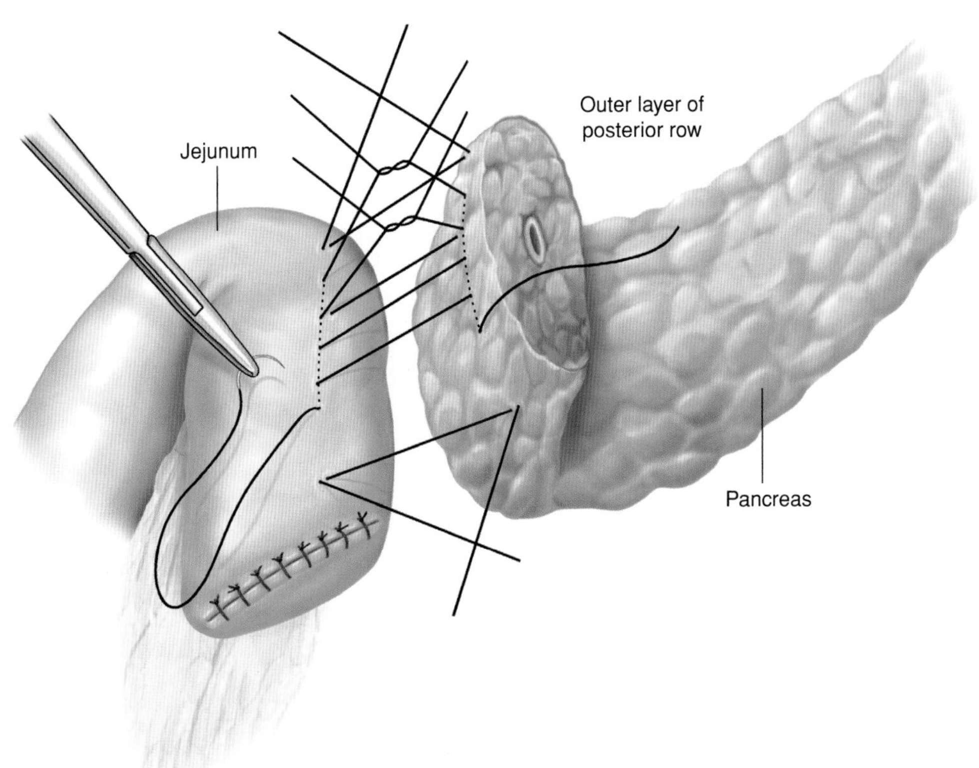


**Figure 2.11** Outer posterior row of interrupted 3-O silk sutures. These are routinely placed in a horizontal mattress fashion. A lacrimal duct probe or 5 French pediatric feeding tube can be placed within the pancreatic duct to avoid inadvertent injury to the duct while completing the pancreaticojejunostomy.



The peritoneal defect at the ligament of Treitz is closed with interrupted 3-O silk sutures to prevent internal herniation. Care is taken to avoid injury to the inferior mesenteric vein and the retained jejunal mesentery while performing this step.

## Technique—Reconstruction Phase

A defect is made in the transverse mesocolon to the right of the middle colic vessels, through which the proximal jejunal limb is delivered into the right upper quadrant. Care is taken to ensure that the jejunum lies flat without twisting or revolutions within its mesentery. All anastomoses are performed above the transverse mesocolon, in a retrocolic fashion.

The pancreatic remnant is mobilized for a distance of 2 cm ventrally off the splenic vein, to facilitate creation of the invaginated pancreaticojejunostomy.

The end-to-side invaginated pancreaticojejunostomy is performed with an outer posterior layer of interrupted 3-O silk sutures placed as a horizontal mattress between the posterior aspect of the pancreatic remnant and the seromuscular layer of the jejunum (Fig. 2.11). A jejunotomy is then made smaller than the horizontal pancreatic remnant width, as the small bowel will stretch during the creation of the anastomosis. A lacrimal duct probe or 5 French pediatric feeding tube is placed temporarily in the pancreatic duct, to avoid compromising it during suture placement. The inner posterior layer is performed in a running–locking fashion using 3-O polyglactin suture. This is brought onto the anterior portion of the anastomosis, where it is converted to a simple running suture, and tied to a second 3-O polyglactin which is brought from the other side (Fig. 2.12). The goal is to achieve full jejunal mucosal invagination, and pancreatic capsule to jejunal serosa apposition. The anastomosis is completed by placing an outer anterior row of interrupted 3-O silk sutures between the jejunum and pancreas (Fig. 2.13). These are placed in a vertical mattress fashion, and designed to roll the jejunum over the anterior inner layer (Fig. 2.14). The end result is that the invaginated pancreaticojejunostomy creates an intussusception of the end of the pancreas into the side of the jejunum, with full mucosal invagination.

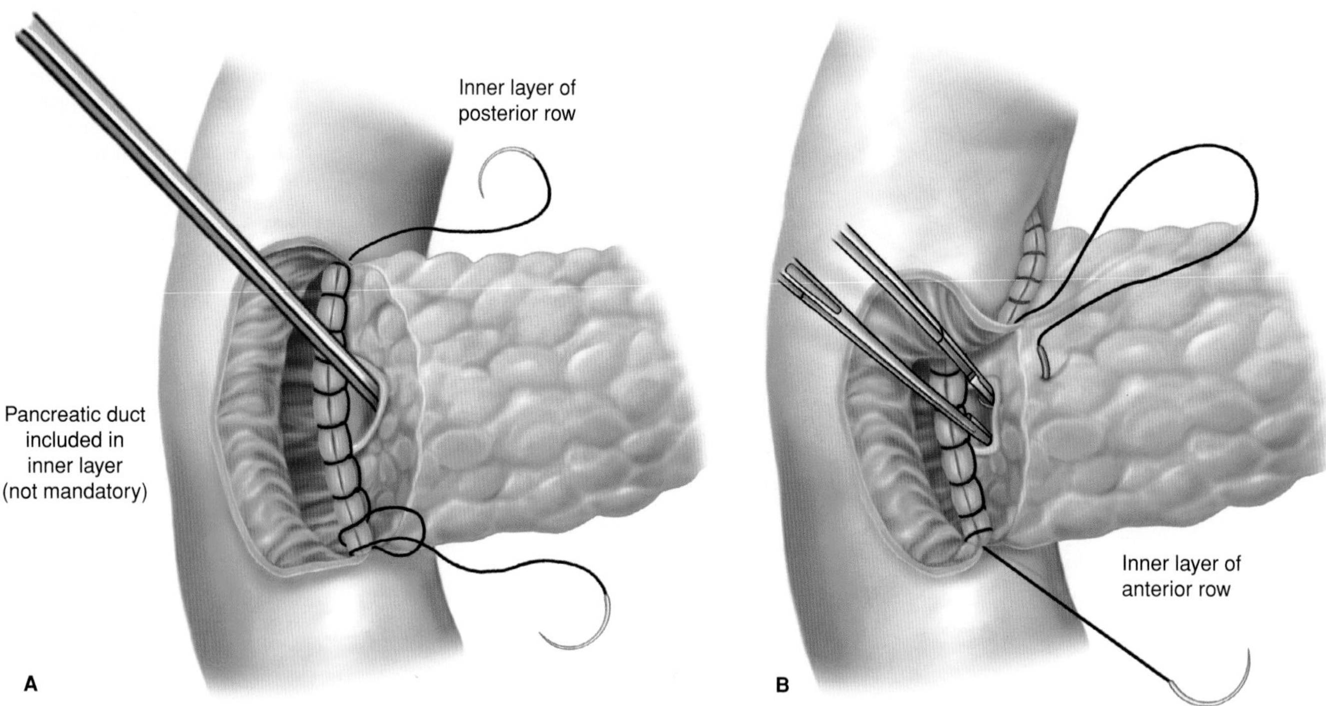


**Figure 2.12** The inner layer of continuous 3-0 polyglactin suture is placed in a locking fashion on the posterior aspect of the anastomosis **(left)** and converted to a simple running suture for the inner anterior layer **(right).**

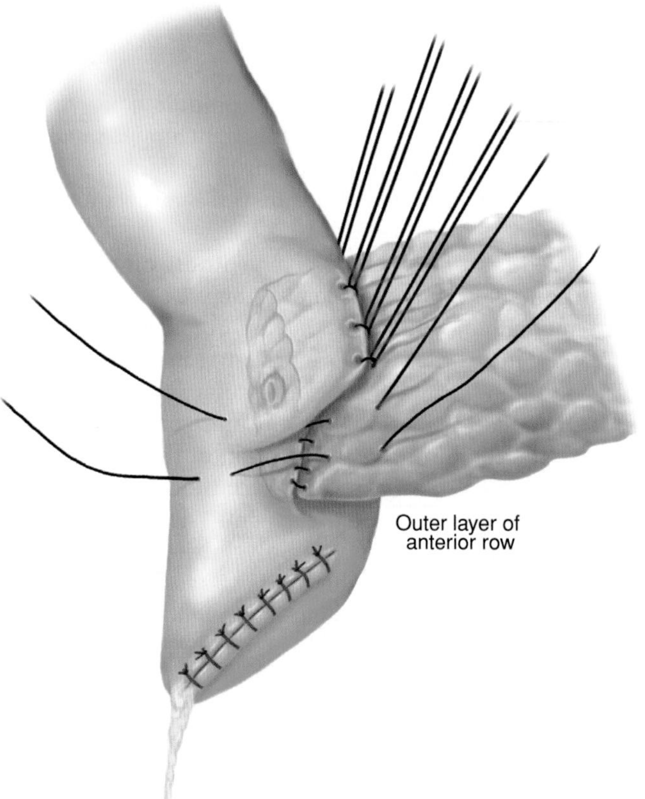


**Figure 2.13** The outer anterior layer of interrupted 3-0 silk sutures is placed as a vertical mattress. All stitches are placed before any are tied. Care should be taken when tying these to alleviate any undue tension on the suture line, which could cause the suture to tear through the pancreatic capsule. This can be accomplished while tying the suture by having the assistant cross the next successive stitch.

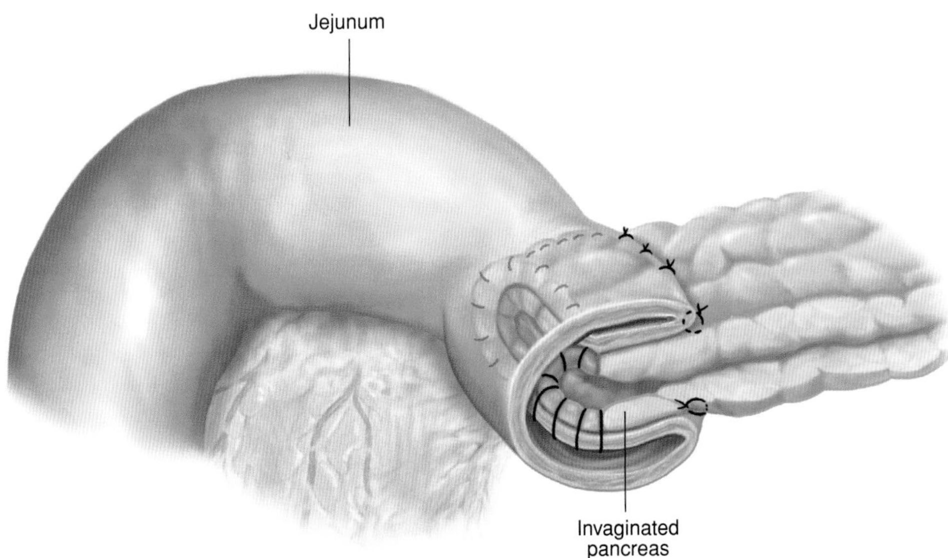


**Figure 2.14** The completed end-to-side invaginated pancreaticojejunostomy with the caudal half of the anastomosis not shown.

The hepaticojejunostomy is begun by making a small jejunotomy on the antimesenteric border of the jejunum, approximately 5 to 10 cm distal to the completed pancreaticojejunostomy. The anastomosis is created using interrupted 4-O, 5-O, or 6-O monofilament absorbable suture, depending upon the size and thickness of the bile duct (Fig. 2.15). After the posterior row of sutures is placed and tied, the long limb of a transected T-tube is temporarily placed within the anastomosis to prevent a backwall injury during placement of the anterior row of sutures. This temporary T-tube (we refer to it as I-tube) is not left in place, but rather is removed after completion of the anastomosis, when a jejunotomy is made downstream for the creation of the duodenojejunostomy. However, if a transhepatic percutaneous biliary catheter is present, it is left in place and directed through the newly created hepaticojejunostomy, into the efferent limb.

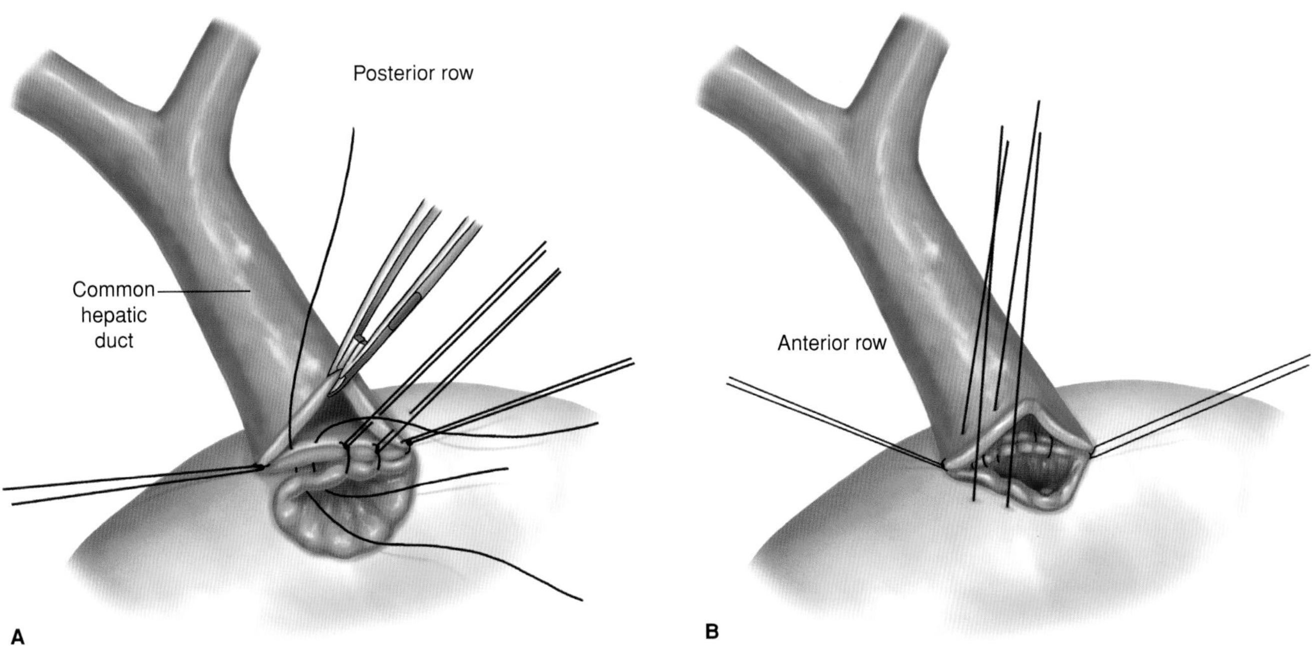


**Figure 2.15** Construction of the end-to-side hepaticojejunostomy is accomplished with fine 4-0 or 5-0 monofilament absorbable suture depending upon the size and thickness of the duct. The posterior row **(left)** is performed leaving the knots on the inside. The anterior row **(right)** leaves the knots on the outside. The long limb of a cut T-tube ("I-tube") is temporarily placed within the anastomosis before placing and tying the anterior row of sutures, to prevent inadvertent injury to the posterior row. This temporary "I-tube" is then retrieved downstream when a jejunotomy is made for the duodenojejunostomy.

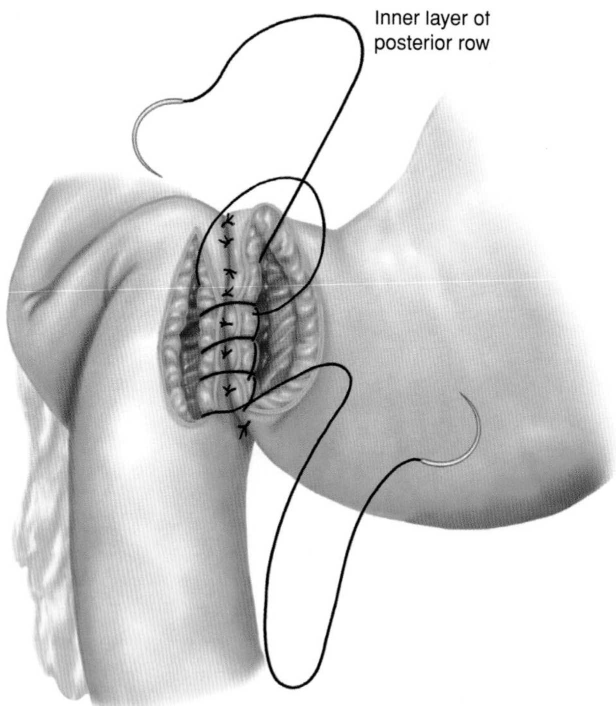


**Figure 2.16** The continuous locking inner posterior layer of the duodenojejunostomy is placed with 3-O polyglactin suture. This suture line is brought onto the inner anterior layer where it is placed as a Connell suture. The outer layer of the duodenojejunostomy is performed with 3-O silk Lembert sutures.

The duodenojejunostomy is performed 10 to 15 cm distal to the hepaticojejunostomy. It is performed in a two layer, end to side fashion, using interrupted 3-O silk Lembert sutures for the outer posterior and anterior rows. The inner rows are sewn in a continuous locking fashion posteriorly, and as a Connell stitch anteriorly with 3-O polyglactin suture (Fig. 2.16). For classic PD reconstruction, several centimeters of the gastric staple line from the lesser curvature of the stomach are imbricated with 3-O silk Lembert sutures. The remaining gastric staple line is then resected to facilitate performance of a Hofmeister type end–to-side gastrojejunostomy (Fig. 2.17). The efferent limb

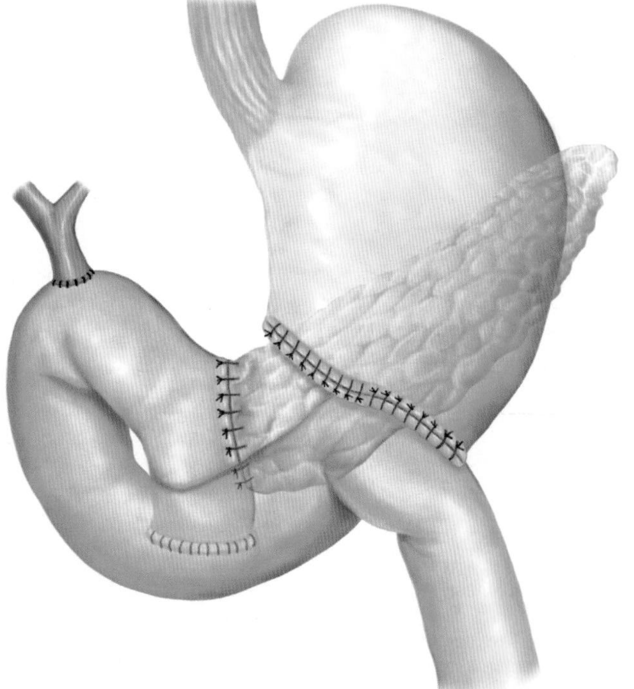

**Figure 2.17** Classic PD reconstruction showing up to 10% to 30% distal gastrectomy, and a Hofmeister type of gastrojejunostomy.

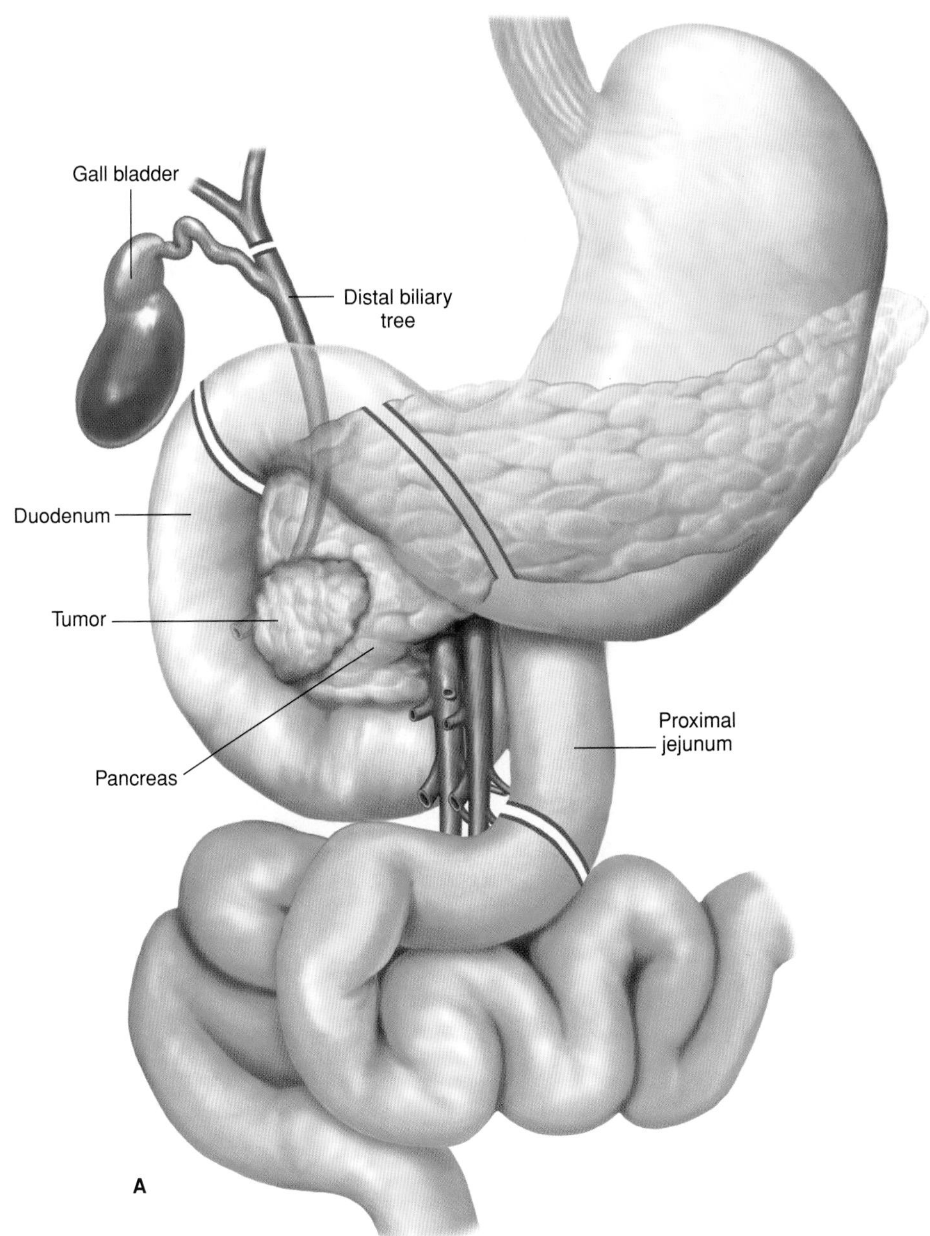


Figure 2.18 Pylorus-preserving PD. (**A**) Illustration of the lines of transection at the distal common hepatic duct, proximal duodenum, pancreas neck, and proximal jejunum.



of the duodeno- or gastrojejunostomy is tacked at its exit point through the transverse mesocolon with interrupted 3-O silk suture, approximately 5 cm below the duodenojejunostomy.

Two 3/16″ round silastic drains are placed exiting the abdomen on either side in the anterior axillary line, well below the lowest palpable rib. The right-sided drain is placed in the subhepatic space and posterior to the RUQ jejunal loops (the neoduodenum), and the left-sided drain is placed through the gastrocolic ligament and a few centimeters cephalad to the pancreaticojejunostomy. We avoid having the drains come into direct contact with any of the anastomoses. The fascia is closed with running #2 nylon or polypropylene suture and the subcutaneous tissue and skin are closed with 3-O and 4-O polyglactin or equivalent, respectively. Retention sutures are placed in those patients who are felt to be at high risk for wound dehiscence (typically recent smokers, patients on steroids, the morbidly obese, and malnourished patients), so as to avoid evisceration and the need for operative wound re-closure. The completed pylorus-preserving PD reconstruction is shown in Figure 2.18B.

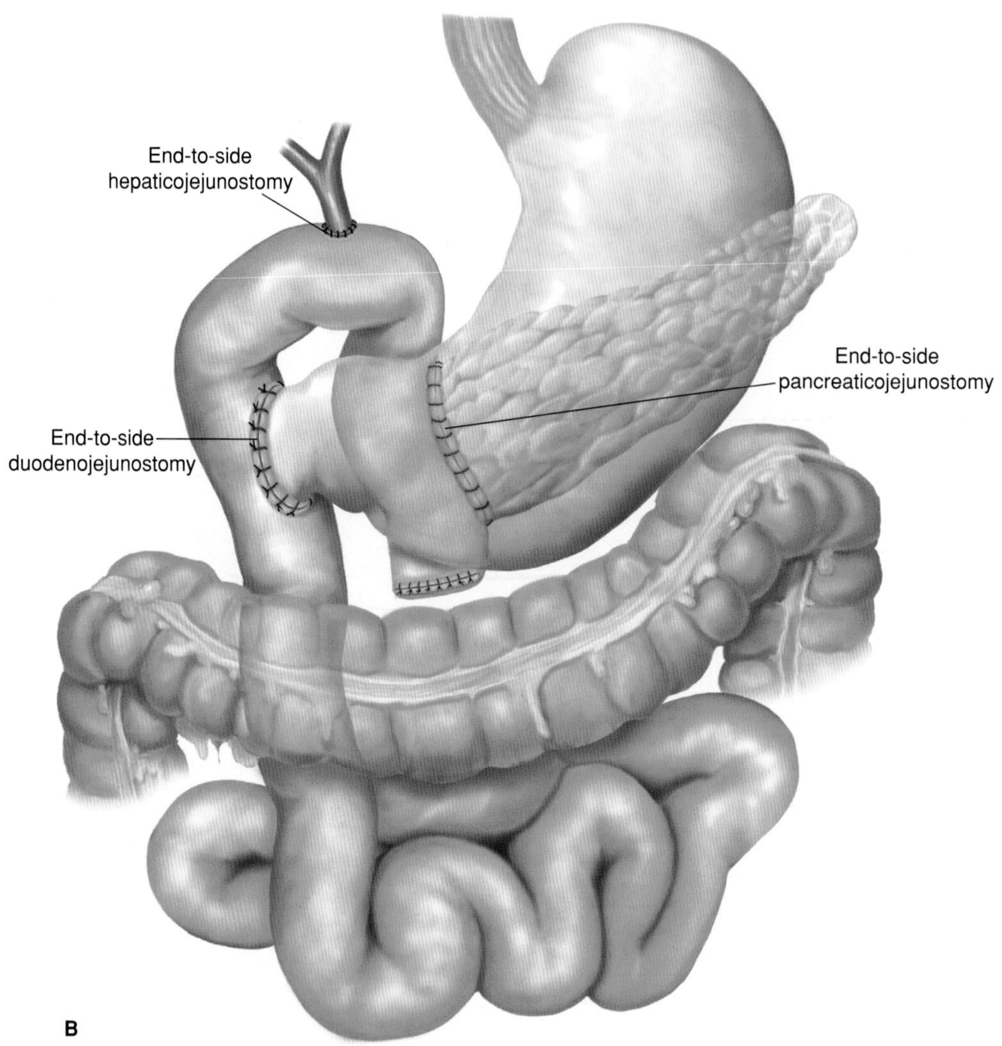


**Figure 2.18** *(Continued)* **(B)** The completed reconstruction, with all three of the anastomoses being performed cephalad to the transverse mesocolon, in a retrocolic fashion.

## POSTOPERATIVE MANAGEMENT

Patients are routinely placed in an ICU (or monitored) setting postoperatively, to allow for careful hemodynamic monitoring, an hourly assessment of urinary output, and attention to patient-controlled analgesia (PCA), incentive spirometry and early mobilization to a chair. On postoperative day #1, the nasogastric tube is removed, patients are given ice chips by mouth and encouraged to ambulate, and they are transferred (often by walking themselves!) to a stepdown unit. A clear liquid diet is started on postoperative day #2 and the urinary catheter is removed. The diet is then advanced to solids on postoperative day #3, with the commencement of oral pancreatic enzyme supplements with each meal.

The silastic drains are generally removed between postoperative days #3 to #5, depending upon the character and quantity of output. Discharge is targeted for postoperative day #6 or #7, based upon patient progress. An oncology consultation is routinely obtained for patients with malignant pathology during their index hospitalization, to allow for introduction of the topic of postoperative adjuvant therapy (chemotherapy and radiation therapy).

**TABLE 2.1 Common Post-pancreaticoduodenectomy Complications**

| | Number of Patients | Pancreatic Fistula (%) | Infection (%) | Bile Leak | Delayed Gastric Emptying (%) | Cardio-pulmonary (%) |
|---|---|---|---|---|---|---|
| Schmidt et al., 2009 | 510 | 9 | 8 | Not reported | 7 | 16 |
| Kazanjian et al., 2008 | 182 | 7 | 13 | 1 | 14 | 8 |
| Grobmyer et al., 2007 | 204 | 12 | 15 | 3 | 7 | 8.5 |
| DeOliveira et al., 2006 | 633 | 9 | 17 | 2.5 | 12.7 | 5 |

Patients are seen in follow-up between 2 and 4 weeks postoperatively for examination, counseling, and review of their final pathology and adjuvant therapy plan (if appropriate).

## COMPLICATIONS

Surgical outcomes have improved in recent years, such that the operative mortality rate for a PD has been reduced to 1% to 3%, and hospital stays are down to 6 to 10 days at most high volume institutions. These improvements in patient outcomes are due to advances in operative technique, perioperative critical care, nutritional support, and the institution of clinical pathways for postoperative management. Despite these improvements, PD still carries a formidable perioperative morbidity rate up to 40%, with the most common postoperative complications being pancreatic fistula, delayed gastric emptying, intra-abdominal abscess formation, wound infection, urinary tract infection, and cardiac arrhythmias (Table 2.1). However, when serious complications do occur, advances in interventional radiologic and endoscopic techniques have effectively reduced the necessity for operative re-intervention, and have hastened patient recovery by allowing patients to be "rescued" by non-operative interventions.

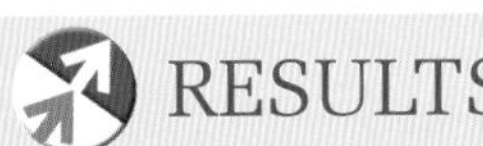

## RESULTS

Although short-term surgical outcomes are generally favorable following PD, long-term results vary widely, depending upon underlying pathology, site of tumor origin, stage at diagnosis, and the adequacy of surgical treatment. The most important factors affecting long-term survival following the resection of a periampullary adenocarcinoma include site of tumor origin (pancreas worst, duodenum best), tumor size, histologic grade, lymph node status, resection margin status, and the presence of lymphovascular and perineural invasion. For most malignant diagnoses the most powerful predictor of an adverse outcome following R0 resection is the presence of metastases to specimen lymph nodes. The most favorable outcomes in patients with pancreatic ductal adenocarcinoma are found in those with small (<2 cm), well differentiated tumors, without lymph node metastasis, who undergo R0 resection.

## CONCLUSIONS

Advances in preoperative assessment, surgical technique, and perioperative management have evolved in the last two decades to make PD a safe operation for the treatment of various periampullary diseases.

## Recommended References and Readings

Bassi C, Dervenis C, Butturini G, et al. Postoperative pancreatic fistula: an international study group (ISGPF) definition. *Surgery.* 2005;138(1):8–13.

Berger AC, Howard TJ, Kennedy EP, et al. Does type of pancreaticojejunostomy after pancreaticoduodenectomy decrease rate of pancreatic fistula? A randomized, prospective, dual-institution trial. *J Am Coll Surg.* 2009;208(5):738–747.

Cleary SP, Gryfe R, Guindi M, et al. Prognostic factors in resected pancreatic adenocarcinoma: analysis of actual 5-year survivors. *J Am Coll Surg.* 2004;198(5):722–731.

DeOliveira ML, Winter JM, Schafer M, et al. Assessment of complications after pancreatic surgery: A novel grading system applied to 633 patients undergoing pancreaticoduodenectomy. *Ann Surg.* 2006;244(6):931–937.

Fong Y, Gonen M, Rubin D, et al. Long term survival is superior after resection for cancer in high-volume centers. *Ann Surg.* 2005;242:540–544.

Greene FL, Page DL, Fleming ID, et al. *AJCC Cancer Staging Manual. American Joint Committee on Cancer.* 6th ed. New York, NY: Springer; 2002:157–164.

Grobmyer SR, Pieracci FM, Allen PJ, et al. Defining morbidity after pancreaticoduodenectomy: Use of a prospective complication grading system. *J Am Coll Surg.* 2007;204:356–364.

House MG, Yeo CJ, Cameron JL, et al. Predicting resectability of periampullary cancer with three-dimensional computed tomography. *J Gastrointest Surg.* 2002;8:280–288.

Jemal A, Siegel R, Ward E, et al. Cancer statistics, 2008. *CA Cancer J Clin.* 2008;58:71–96.

Katz MH, Wang H, Fleming JB, et al. Long-term survival after multidisciplinary management of resected pancreatic adenocarcinoma. *Ann Surg Oncol.* 2009;16(4):836–847.

Kazanjian KK, Hines OJ, Duffy JP, et al. Improved survival following pancreaticoduodenectomy to treat adenocarcinoma of the pancreas: the influence of operative blood loss. *Arch Surg.* 2008; 143(12):1166–1171.

Kennedy EP, Brumbaugh J, Yeo CJ. Reconstruction following the pylorus preserving Whipple resection: PJ, HJ, DJ. *J Gastrointest Surg.* 2010;14(2):408–415.

Kennedy EP, Rosato EL, Yeo CJ, et al. Initiation of a critical pathway for pancreaticoduodenectomy at an academic institution-the first step in multidisciplinary team building. *J Am Coll Surg.* 2007; 204:917–923.

Lavu H, Kennedy EP, Mazo R, et al. Preoperative mechanical bowel preparation does not offer a benefit for patients who undergo pancreaticoduodenectomy. *Surgery.* 2010;148(2):278–284.

Pancreaticoduodenectomy. In: Cameron JL, Sandone C, eds. *Atlas of Gastrointestinal Surgery,* 2nd edition, Vol. 1. Hamilton, ON: BC Decker; 2007:284–305.

Schmidt CM, Choi J, Powell ES, et al. Pancreatic fistula following pancreaticoduodenectomy: Clinical predictors and patient outcomes. *HPB Surg.* 2009;2009:404–520.

Winter JM, Cameron JL, Campbell KA, et al. 1423 Pancreaticoduodenectomies for pancreatic cancer: A single-institution experience. *J Gastrointest Surg.* 2006;10(9):1199–1210.

# 3 Distal Pancreatectomy—Open

**Jordan Winter and Peter J. Allen**

##  INDICATIONS/CONTRAINDICATIONS

Distal pancreatectomy, as referred to in this chapter, involves resection of the pancreas to the left of the superior mesenteric vasculature. The parenchymal margin of resection generally occurs at the level of the superior mesenteric vessels; however, when the target lesion is located in the very tail of the gland parenchymal transection may occur to the left of these vessels. When the lesion to be resected involves the pancreatic neck or body an extended resection may be performed and the parenchymal margin in this setting may be to the right of the mesenteric vessels. Regardless of the exact location of parenchymal transection, distal pancreatectomy implies that the duodenum and bile duct are not included in the resection. Splenectomy may or may not be performed.

The indications for distal pancreatectomy include both non-neoplastic and neoplastic processes. Non-neoplastic indications include focal chronic pancreatitis of the body or tail, left-sided pancreatic pseudocysts, and trauma to the distal pancreas. Neoplastic indications include benign and malignant tumors. The most common examples are ductal adenocarcinoma, intra-ductal papillary mucinous neoplasms, mucinous cystic neoplasms, and neuroendocrine tumors.

##  PREOPERATIVE PLANNING

Preoperative evaluation begins with the patient history and physical examination, with a particular focus on past medical and cancer history, familial cancer history, and the patients presenting signs and symptoms. Weight loss, abdominal pain, back pain, and new-onset diabetes are associated with a diagnosis of adenocarcinoma. Biochemical tests include liver enzymes, serum amylase, and CA 19-9. The latter test is a biochemical marker that is frequently elevated in advanced malignancy of the pancreas, and serves as a useful marker of disease recurrence after resection.

Pancreatic lesions should be evaluated preoperatively with high-quality contrast enhanced CT or MR imaging. Multidetector CT imaging using narrow collimation and precise acquisition timing during the arterial, pancreas parenchymal, and venous phases is an excellent technique for defining the nature of pancreatic lesions, their relationship to the peri-pancreatic vasculature, and whether there is concern for extra-pancreatic spread in the case of malignancy. Water is used as an oral contrast agent since visualization of the duodenum and small bowel is excellent and there is minimal interference with the peri-pancreatic vessels. Sagittal and coronal reconstructions are routinely performed at our institution. Triple-phase imaging allows for careful assessment of major visceral vessel involvement by the tumor and allows further characterization of the pancreatic mass. When there is suspicion for malignancy additional cuts through the chest and pelvis are also obtained.

Endoscopic ultrasound (EUS) with or without fine needle aspiration should be considered when the findings would influence patient management. Indications for EUS include the need for tissue diagnosis prior to neoadjuvant therapy, the desire to further characterize an asymptomatic pancreatic cyst and to obtain cyst fluid for biochemical analysis, and in any other scenario in which non-operative management of a lesion may be possible if tissue is obtained. This latter scenario often arises in the setting of focal pancreatitis in the tail of the gland. EUS may be helpful in this situation to ensure that no underlying mass is present. Core biopsy can be performed in the tail of the gland by EUS and when pancreatitis is present IgG4 staining should be considered to evaluate for lymphoplasmacytic sclerosing pancreatitis.

Although endoscopic retrograde cholangiopancreatography (ERCP) has an important role for patients with proximal pancreatic lesions, this is not usually the case for distal lesions. Diagnostic ERCP is seldom useful in evaluating distal lesions due to the risk of acute pancreatitis, and the ability to obtain high-quality imaging of the ductal system and pancreatic parenchyma with cross-sectional imaging. MRCP may be a useful alternative to ERCP when definition of ductal anatomy is desired.

After the patient has been deemed a surgical candidate from a medical standpoint and resection is indicated from an oncologic perspective, informed consent for a distal pancreatectomy with or without splenectomy is obtained and resection is scheduled. We do not routinely perform mechanical bowel preparation unless a synchronous colon resection is planned as prospective data have not found this to reduce postoperative infection.

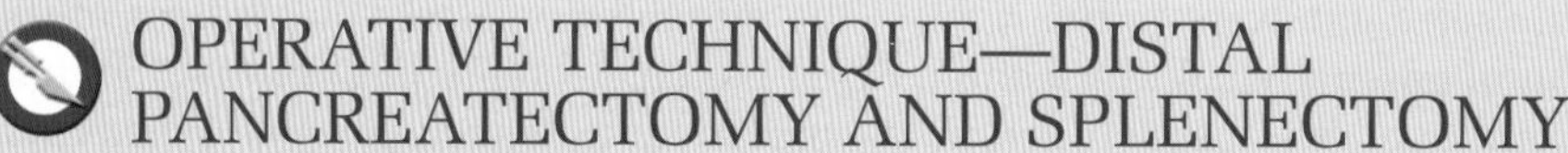

## OPERATIVE TECHNIQUE—DISTAL PANCREATECTOMY AND SPLENECTOMY

Prior to skin incision prophylactic antibiotics are administered intravenously and the abdomen is prepared with ChloroPrep® (CareFusion, Kansas, USA) from the level of the nipples down to the pubic symphysis. The operative field is squared off with towels and the remainder of the body is covered with sterile drapes. When pancreatic cancer is confirmed or suspected, an exploratory laparoscopy is generally performed to assess for metastatic disease. This can be performed in the same setting as the planned distal pancreatectomy or as a separate stage of a two-staged procedure. Laparoscopy is typically performed by utilizing a 10 mm Hasson port placed above the umbilicus or in the left upper quadrant. One or two additional 5 mm ports are added as needed to retract, perform biopsies, and do peritoneal washings.

The decision to create either a midline or subcostal incision is based on the patient's body habitus, the location of the tumor, and the surgeon preference. Midline incisions are considered for the thin patient, in the setting of a prior midline laparotomy, when access to another quadrant of the abdomen is necessary, or for the patient with an acutely angled costal margin. In obese patients, patients with a low xiphoid process, and when the tumor is located in the very tail of the pancreas, a left subcostal incision is generally utilized in order to maximize exposure to the left upper quadrant. After entering the abdomen, a self-retaining retractor system is set up such as the Bookwalter™ (Codman, Massachusetts, USA). Cephalad retraction of the costal margin is paramount. Exploration is completed to rule out metastatic disease (initiated laparoscopically), and this involves

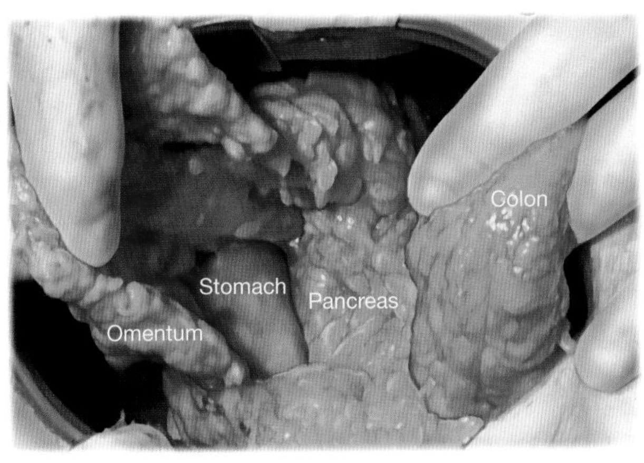


Figure 3.1 View of lesser sac after incising the greater omentum.

careful inspection of the small intestine, the liver, the pelvis, the root of the transverse mesocolon, and the peritoneal surfaces of the abdominal wall and diaphragm.

The initial step to the operation involves entering the lesser sac along the transverse colon and then dissecting the greater omentum off of the transverse colon to the splenic flexure (Fig. 3.1). The right gastroepiploic vessels and greater omentum are preserved. While many start the dissection by incising the peritoneum superior and inferior to the pancreas, we prefer to address the gland after having completely exposed the distal portion of the pancreas. Initial division of all short gastric vessels is performed so that the stomach can be retracted out of the operative field superiorly and into the right upper quadrant (Fig. 3.2). The transverse colon and splenic flexure are then mobilized inferiorly and the entire distal pancreas is then exposed.

Once the pancreas has been exposed (Fig. 3.3) and the short gastric vessels have been ligated, the pancreatic parenchyma and splenic vasculature are isolated and divided. These three structures (splenic artery, splenic vein, and pancreatic parenchyma) may be divided in any sequence depending on the location of the lesion, the patient's anatomy (particularly the relationships between the splenic vessels and the gland), and whether or not splenic preservation is being considered. Pancreatic parenchymal transection may be performed anywhere in the neck, body, or tail of the pancreas depending on the location of the lesion. When transection is to be performed at the pancreatic neck the middle colic vein serves as a useful landmark to locate the SMV, which can be found at the base of the middle colic branch. The pancreatic neck is then dissected free from its retroperitoneal attachments, the superior mesenteric vein, and the proximal splenic vein. Typically the right gastroepiploic vessels and gastroduodenal artery can be preserved. For neoplastic disease, several centimeters of gland to the right of the lesion should be mobilized in order to achieve adequate tumor clearance.

The exact method for pancreatic transection and stump closure has been the subject of much debate. Sharp transection with pancreatic duct suture ligation and oversewing

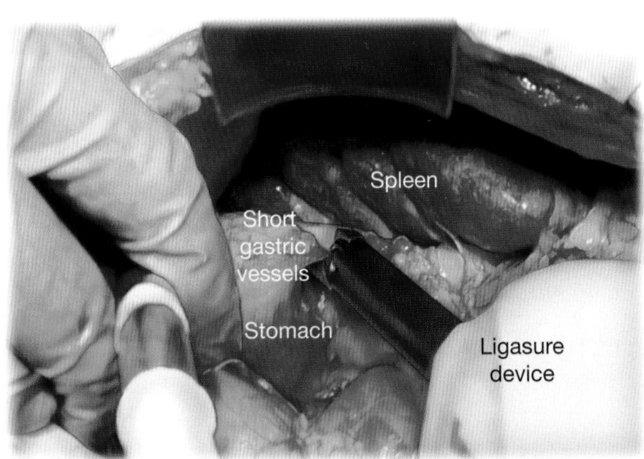


Figure 3.2 Ligation of the short gastric vessels.

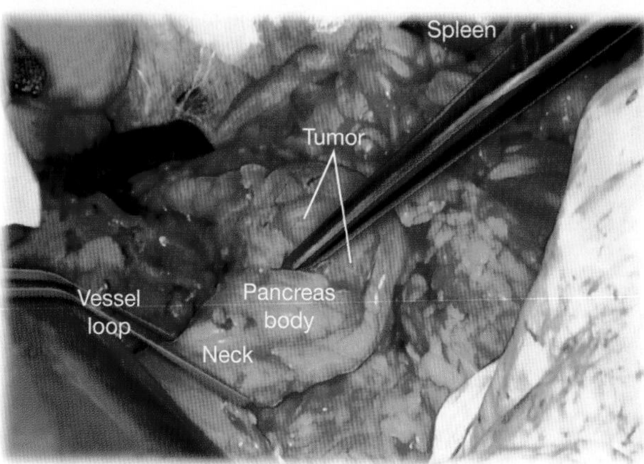


**Figure 3.3** Exposed pancreas and pancreatic tumor.

of the stump has been a frequently reported technique, however more recently division of the gland with a stapling device with or without the use of SeamGuard® (Gore, Delaware, USA) staple reinforcement has been reported. All reported studies to date evaluating these techniques have been retrospective in nature except for one prospective randomized study, and no single technique has been shown to be superior. We generally divide soft glands, particularly in the area of the neck where the gland is thinnest, using the Endo GIA™ Universal stapler (Covidien, Massachusetts, USA) with the SeamGuard®. In a firm or thick gland, particularly in the pancreatic body, we feel the stapler may be less effective. In these instances, we typically divide the gland sharply between 4-point hemostatic stay sutures positioned on the inferior and superior aspects of the gland (Fig. 3.4). During transection careful attention is paid to identify the pancreatic duct which is then ligated with a single figure-of-eight stitch (Fig. 3.5). The remaining stump is then oversewn with interrupted U-stitches.

The splenic artery, which runs along the cephalad border of the pancreas, is identified and controlled near its origin. Before dividing the splenic artery, the artery is temporarily occluded and the proper hepatic artery is palpated for a pulse to ensure that the common hepatic artery is not inadvertently ligated. If a pulse remains after occluding the vessel, the proximal splenic artery is then typically divided with an Endovascular stapler (Fig. 3.6). Alternatively, the artery can be doubly ligated with a 2-0 silk tie and then suture ligated with a 2-0 silk or Prolene stitch. Dividing the splenic artery at this juncture greatly facilitates splenic mobilization as splenic inflow has been

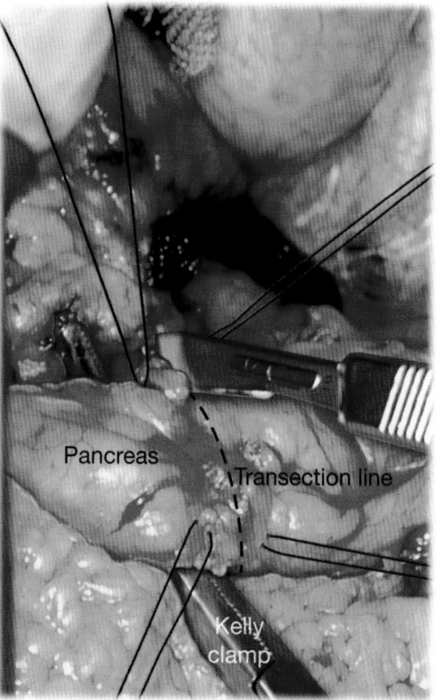


**Figure 3.4** Sharp division of the pancreas.

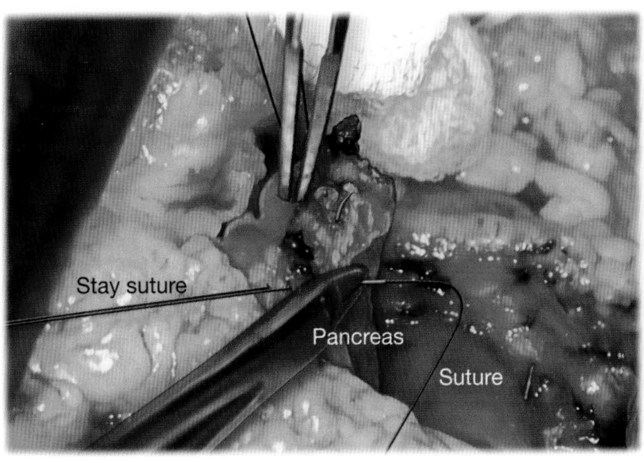


**Figure 3.5** Suture closure of the pancreatic duct.

arrested and the spleen rapidly decompresses. Small draining pancreatic branches are then ligated to fully mobilize the pancreatic neck and body off of the SMV/splenic vein confluence. If the inferior mesenteric vein drains directly into the splenic vein, it can either be preserved or ligated depending on the exact point for division of the splenic vein. The splenic vein may be divided with the endovascular stapler or by suture ligation (Fig. 3.7). Care must be taken to not narrow the SMV, nor to leave a long splenic vein stump without flow. Leaving a long splenic vein stump without flow (such as the inferior mesenteric vein) may increase the likelihood of developing thrombosis within the stump which can propagate into the SMV and compromise small bowel outflow.

Once the pancreas has been divided and the splenic vasculature ligated the spleen is then mobilized anteromedially by dividing the lateral side wall and diaphragmatic attachments. The splenocolic ligament is fully divided if it has not already. A fully mobile spleen serves as a useful handle for the remainder of the dissection. Lastly, the body and tail of the pancreas are completely mobilized out of the retroperitoneum along the superior and inferior aspects of the gland, and the specimen is removed from the operative field.

After hemostasis has been achieved, the abdomen is irrigated with saline. We do not routinely leave abdominal drains as prospective and randomized data from our institution have failed to identify benefit to routine drainage. The fascia is closed with #1 PDS suture in a running fashion, and the skin is closed with staples.

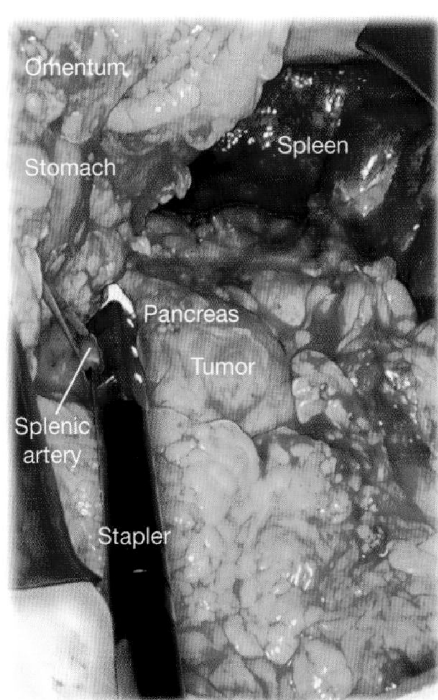


**Figure 3.6** Division of the splenic artery.

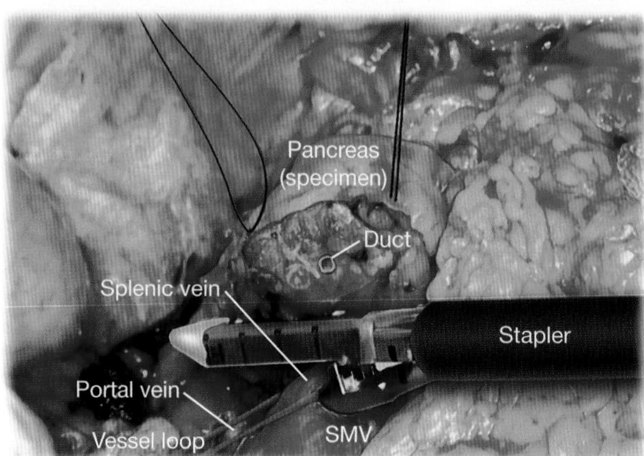


**Figure 3.7** Division of the splenic vein.

## SURGICAL TECHNIQUE—DISTAL PANCREATECTOMY WITH SPLENIC PRESERVATION

For benign disease, a spleen preserving distal pancreatectomy may be considered. The main reason to preserve the spleen in these situations is to avoid the long-term morbidity of asplenia—namely the risk of postsplenectomy sepsis. This condition is extremely infrequent in adults who undergo splenectomy for neoplastic diseases of the pancreas and in the patient with pancreatic cancer splenic preservation should in general not be considered. With splenic preservation no lymph nodes are typically removed as these lie with the vasculature, so it is undesirable if a lymphadenectomy has important diagnostic, prognostic, or therapeutic implications. While some retrospective series suggest that splenic preservation is associated with fewer postoperative complications than distal pancreatectomy with splenectomy, other studies note the contrary.

Splenic preservation can be accomplished in two ways. Classically, the splenic artery and vein are preserved through meticulous dissection and ligation of the small arterial and venous branches supplying and draining the left side of the pancreas. Alternatively, the main splenic artery and veins can be divided in the standard fashion if preservation of the short gastric and left gastroepiploic vessels is achieved.

Successful distal pancreatectomy with splenic preservation has been reported with ligation of the splenic artery and splenic vein. In this approach the inflow and outflow to the spleen is entirely through the short gastric vasculature, which in this setting must be preserved. This technique has been reported as having a similar complication rate to distal pancreatectomy with splenectomy. We have utilized this approach to splenic preservation on several occasions but have witnessed the development of splenic abscess and splenic infarction postoperatively. Because of this, our general approach is to preserve the spleen only when the splenic artery and splenic vein can be safely dissected off the pancreas and the inflow and outflow to the spleen maintained in this fashion.

When splenic preservation is performed, the initial steps of the distal pancreatectomy are the same as the steps described above, up through the division of the pancreas. Once the pancreas has been divided vessel loops are placed around the splenic artery and vein at the celiac trunk and the SMV confluence, respectively. Control of these vessels is precautionary in case hemorrhage is encountered during the dissection of the distal pancreas. The pancreatic body and tail are then mobilized in a proximal-to-distal direction (right-to-left), and the small branches of the splenic artery and vein are ligated with 4-0 silk ties or clips and divided. The peritoneum above and below the distal pancreas is incised and the specimen is removed from the operative field.

If there is desire to preserve the spleen but the splenic vasculature must be divided, the splenic artery and splenic vein are typically ligated after the pancreas has been mobilized out of the retroperitoneum along its superior and inferior borders. Next, the splenic vessels are divided proximally in the area of the transected pancreas and distally near the tail, and removed en block with the specimen. Since the spleen receives its entire blood flow from the short gastric vessels, it should be carefully examined after the specimen is removed for signs of critical ischemia such as a dark gray or black color.

## POSTOPERATIVE MANAGEMENT

While consensus in the literature exists regarding certain aspects of postoperative management in patients undergoing distal pancreatectomy, there is considerable variation amongst surgeons in other aspects. We do not perform routine postoperative nasogastric decompression in light of the evidence demonstrating a detriment with this practice. Abdominal drains are not routinely left based on data from our institution that the rate of pancreatic fistula and abdominal collections is not different with or without drains and there is emerging data that drains may actually contribute to infection and fistula formation. The role of somatostatin therapy on the development of pancreatic fistulas is less clear. There are conflicting prospective randomized data regarding somatostatin after pancreatic resection, although no such study has focused exclusively on patients undergoing distal pancreatectomy. It is not our practice to routinely give patients somatostatin after a distal pancreatectomy. Analgesia is provided via a patient-controlled pump, although there are some data to suggest that epidural analgesia provides improved pain control and is associated with fewer gastrointestinal side effects. In patients undergoing splenectomy, triple vaccination should be considered for *Haemophilus influenzae, Neisseria meningitidis,* and *Streptococcus pneumonia.* Vaccines may be administered preoperatively if the splenectomy is planned. Alternatively, they may be given prior to discharge or during follow-up.

## COMPLICATIONS

The in-hospital mortality rate for distal pancreatectomy is similar to most major abdominal operations, or about 1%. The complication rate remains high, and ranges between 20% to 40% in large series. The most common complications include new-onset insulin dependent diabetes (8% of patients), clinically significant pancreatic fistula (5% to 10%), intra-abdominal abscess (4%), small bowel obstruction (4%) and postoperative bleeding (4%).

The development of postoperative diabetes in previously non-diabetic patients is consistently under 10% across series. The low incidence of postoperative diabetes suggests that in general, oncologic principles (e.g., adequate margin, lymphadenectomy) should take precedence over pancreatic preservation (e.g., enucleation, central pancreatectomy) when planning the extent of resection. For some benign neoplasms, pancreatic preservation assumes greater importance.

Pancreatic fistula remains the most important complication in the acute postoperative period because it is a relatively frequent event and can profoundly impact recovery and the length of hospital stay. In addition to abdominal drain placement, the method of pancreatic stump closure has been cited as a contributing factor to pancreatic fistula development. A recent meta-analysis examined 15 observational studies and a single randomized prospective trial comparing sutured and stapled closure of the pancreatic remnant after distal pancreatectomy in over 2,200 patients. The authors noted that two observational studies suggested superiority of stapled closure and one favored sutured closure, while the remaining 12 observational studies did not find any statistical difference. The lone prospective randomized trial had a small sample size and did not show a benefit to either technique. When all of the studies were considered together, there was no difference observed between the two techniques, although a trend was seen favoring a stapled closure. A summary of the studies included in the meta-analysis and an additional recently published study appears in Table 3.1. The DISPACT trial is a

**TABLE 3.1 Studies of Pancreatic Remnant Closure. Suture versus Stapler**

| Study | Groups, n | Pancreatic Fistula | p |
|---|---|---|---|
| Kajiyama et al. *Br J Surg.* 1996;83:1711. | Stapler, 35<br>Suture, 175 | 40%<br>45.7% | NS |
| Bassi et al. *HPB.* 1999;1:203. | Stapler, 14<br>Suture, 15<br>Anastom., 14<br>Others, 26 | 14.3%<br>33.3%<br>7.1%<br>19.2% | NS |
| Sheehan et al. *Am Surg.* 2002;68:264. | Stapler, 16<br>Suture, 37<br>Both, 32 | 25.0%<br>13.5%<br>9.4% | NS |
| Bilimoria et al. *Br J Surg.* 2003;90:190. | Stapler, 20<br>Suture, 83<br>Both, 15<br>Others, 8 | 20.0%<br>21.7%<br>13.3%<br>8% | NS |
| Takeuchi et al. *Aust N Z J Surg.* 2003;73:922. | Stapler, 10<br>Suture, 23 | 0<br>34.8% | 0.035 |
| Sledzianowski et al. *Surgery.* 2005;137:180. | Stapler, 32<br>Suture, 26<br>Anastom., 3 | 6%<br>15.4% | NS |
| Balzano et al. *J Gastrointest Surg.* 2005;9:837. | Stapler, 32<br>Suture, 39<br>Anastom., 52 | 34.4%<br>38.4%<br>30.8% | NS |
| Pannegeon et al. *Arch Surg.* 2006;141:1071. | Stapler, 108<br>Suture, 67 | 22.2%<br>23.9% | NS |
| Lorenz et al. *HPB.* (Oxford) 2007;9:302. | Stapler, 9<br>Suture, 37 | 11.1%<br>18.9% | NS |
| Kleeff et al. *Ann Surg.* 2007;245:573. | Stapler, 145<br>Suture, 97<br>Anastom., 24<br>Others, 36 | 15.9%<br>9.3%<br>0<br>8.3% | 0.042 |
| Ridolfini et al. *World J Gastroenterol.* 2007;13:5096. | Stapler, 29<br>Suture, 35 | 24.1%<br>20.0% | NS |
| Zhao et al. *Zhonghua Wai Ke Za Zhi.* 2008;46:24. | Stapler, 56<br>Suture, 53 | 21.4%<br>41.5% | 0.024 |
| Okano et al. *J Hepatobiliary Pancreat Surg.* 2008;14:353. | Stapler, 24<br>Suture, 11<br>Others, 1 | 12.5%<br>27.3% | NS |
| Ferrone et al. *J Gastrointest Surg.* 2008;12:1691. | Stapler, 86<br>Suture, 266<br>Others, 108 | 29.1%<br>29.3%<br>27.8% | NS |
| Goh et al. *Arch Surg.* 2008;143;956. | Stapler, 21<br>Suture, 73<br>Both, 130<br>Anastom., 2 | 28.6%<br>34.2%<br>30.7%<br>0 | NS |
| Nathan et al. *Ann Surg.* 2009;250:277. | Stapler, 34<br>Suture, 578<br>Both, 66<br>Anastom., 16<br>Others, 10 | 29.4%<br>34.9%<br>19.7%<br>43.8% | NS |
| Harris et al. *J Gastrointest Surg.* 2010;14:998. | Stapler, 47<br>Suture, 69<br>Both, 91 | 27.7%<br>4.3%<br>19.8% | <0.05 |

Modified from: Zhou W, Lv R, Wang X, et al. Stapler vs suture closure of pancreatic remnant after distal pancreatectomy: a meta-analysis. *Am J Surg.* 2010;200(4):529–536.

European study expecting to accrue over 300 patients and compares the hand-sewn and stapled techniques. Pancreatic fistula is the primary endpoint of the study. The trial was opened in 2007 and results are expected in the near future.

While we have seen splenic infarction and abscesses after using the Warshaw technique of splenic preservation, an additional concern is that the majority of patients develop gastric varices. While this phenomenon is detectable either endoscopically and radiographically in most patients, the author who described the technique has not observed a single upper gastrointestinal bleed in over 100 patients with long-term follow-up.



## RESULTS

The most important metric after open distal pancreatectomy for cancer is of course survival, which varies according to the tumor pathology. For ductal adenocarcinoma, long-term survival is roughly 16 months, which is similar to the long-term survival for patients with proximal pancreatic cancers. Long-term survival is 30 months for IPMN-associated cancers and 50 months for mucinous cystadenocarcinomas after distal pancreatectomy. Pain relief is the primary outcome for patients undergoing distal pancreatectomy for chronic pancreatitis and the outcomes are generally inferior as compared to the other common resectional or drainage operations used to manage chronic pancreatitis. The main reason is that a substantial portion of the gland remains untreated after distal pancreatectomy for chronic pancreatitis and studies have shown that the disease is most commonly due to abnormalities in the pancreatic head. Good pain relief is observed in approximately 60% of patients treated with distal pancreatectomy and completion pancreatectomy is required in more than 10% of patients.

## Recommended References and Readings


Andersen DK, Frey CF. The evolution of the surgical treatment of chronic pancreatitis. *Ann Surg.* 2010;251(1):18–32.

Carrère N, Abid S, Julio CH, et al. Spleen-preserving distal pancreatectomy with excision of splenic artery and vein: a case-matched comparison with conventional distal pancreatectomy with splenectomy. *World J Surg.* 2007;31(2):375–382.

Christein JD, Kendrick ML, Iqbal CW, et al. Distal pancreatectomy for resectable adenocarcinoma of the body and tail of the pancreas. *J Gastrointest Surg.* 2005;9(7):922–927.

Conlon KC, Labow D, Leung D, et al. Prospective randomized clinical trial of the value of intraperitoneal drainage after pancreatic resection. *Ann Surg.* 2001;234(4):487–493; discussion 493–484.

Kawai M, Tani M, Terasawa H, et al. Early removal of prophylactic drains reduces the risk of intra-abdominal infections in patients with pancreatic head resection: prospective study for 104 consecutive patients. *Ann Surg.* 2006;244(1):1–7.

Klöppel G, Sipos B, Zamboni G, et al. Autoimmune pancreatitis: histo- and immunopathological features. *J Gastroenterol.* 2007;42 (Suppl 18):28–31.

Lillemoe KD, Kaushal S, Cameron JL, et al. Distal pancreatectomy: indications and outcomes in 235 patients. *Ann Surg.* 1999;229(5): 693–698; discussion 698–700.

Marret E, Remy C, Bonnet F, et al. Meta-analysis of epidural analgesia versus parenteral opioid analgesia after colorectal surgery. *Br J Surg.* 2007;94(6):665–673.

Nelson R, Edwards S, Tse B. Prophylactic nasogastric decompression after abdominal surgery. *Cochrane Database Syst Rev.* 2007; (3):CD004929.

Rodríguez JR, Madanat MG, Healy BC, et al. Distal pancreatectomy with splenic preservation revisited. *Surgery.* 2007;141(5):619–625.

Shoup M, Brennan MF, McWhite K, et al. The value of splenic preservation with distal pancreatectomy. *Arch Surg.* 2002;137(2): 164–168.

Warshaw AL. Conservation of the spleen with distal pancreatectomy. *Arch Surg.* 1988;123(5):550–553.

Warshaw AL. Distal pancreatectomy with preservation of the spleen. *J Hepatobiliary Pancreat Surg.* 2009.

Zhou W, Lv R, Wang X, et al. Stapler vs suture closure of pancreatic remnant after distal pancreatectomy: a meta-analysis. *Am J Surg.* 2010;200(4):529–536.

# 4 Laparoscopic Pancreatic Surgery

**Attila Nakeeb**

##  INDICATIONS/CONTRAINDICATIONS

Over the past decade significant advances have been made in the application of minimally invasive techniques to the management of both benign and malignant pancreatic disorders. Initially, laparoscopic pancreatic surgery was limited to diagnostic staging in patients with pancreatic cancer prior to resection. With recent advancements in laparoscopic instrumentation, an increasing number of surgeons are using laparoscopic techniques to resect benign and malignant lesions of the pancreas in carefully selected patients. Laparoscopic pancreaticoduodenectomy (PD), central pancreatectomy (CP), pancreatic enucleation (En), and distal pancreatectomy (DP) have all been described in the literature.

Potential advantages of laparoscopic surgery include decreased postoperative pain, decreased ileus, preserved immune function, decreased complication rates, shorter hospital stay and a quicker return to preoperative activity levels. While there have been no randomized prospective trials comparing laparoscopic to open pancreatic resections, several retrospective studies have shown laparoscopic resections to be associated with decreased intraoperative blood loss, lower overall complication rates, and a shorter hospital length of stay.

Laparoscopic pancreatic resections are complicated laparoscopic procedures and should be undertaken by surgeons with advanced laparoscopic skill sets. Surgeons should be comfortable with intracorporeal suturing, the use of endomechanical staplers, the use of laparoscopic ultrasound, and posses the ability to control intraoperative hemorrhage. In addition, surgeons should have experience with open pancreatic surgery in case the procedure must be converted to an open pancreatic resection.

Factors important in selecting appropriate patients for laparoscopic resections include the size of the lesion, location of the lesion within the pancreas (head/uncinate vs. body vs. tail), involvement of surrounding structures, and the suspected pathology of the lesion. Lesions that are potentially amenable to a laparoscopic pancreatic resection include benign or premalignant cystic neoplasms, small pancreatic endocrine neoplasms (neuroendocrine or islet cell tumors), pancreatic pseudocysts or isolated strictures of the pancreatic duct localized to the distal body and tail of the pancreas

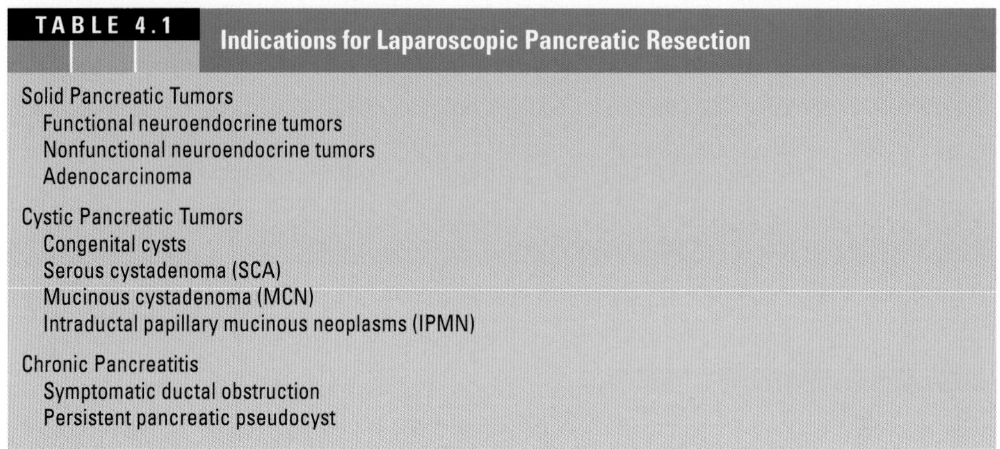

**TABLE 4.1 Indications for Laparoscopic Pancreatic Resection**

| Indications for Laparoscopic Pancreatic Resection |
|---|
| Solid Pancreatic Tumors |
| Functional neuroendocrine tumors |
| Nonfunctional neuroendocrine tumors |
| Adenocarcinoma |
| Cystic Pancreatic Tumors |
| Congenital cysts |
| Serous cystadenoma (SCA) |
| Mucinous cystadenoma (MCN) |
| Intraductal papillary mucinous neoplasms (IPMN) |
| Chronic Pancreatitis |
| Symptomatic ductal obstruction |
| Persistent pancreatic pseudocyst |

(Table 4.1). While there are a small number of reports of laparoscopic pancreatic resections for adenocarcinoma of the pancreas, it is unclear if a laparoscopic pancreatic resection should be attempted in patients with malignant neoplasms of the pancreas.

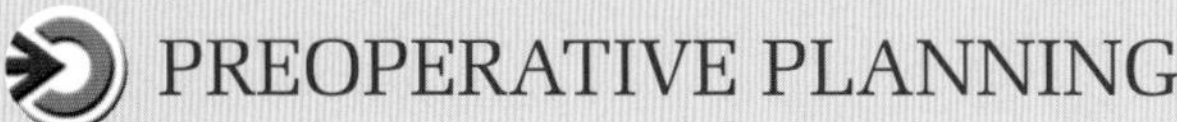

## PREOPERATIVE PLANNING

### Imaging

A number of different imaging options are available to help the surgeon determine the appropriate surgical approach to diseases of the pancreas. These options include both noninvasive (e.g., transabdominal ultrasonography, computed tomography, and magnetic resonance imaging) and invasive modalities (e.g., endoscopic retrograde cholangiopancreatography [ERCP] and endoscopic ultrasonography [EUS]).

Transabdominal ultrasonography can identify changes associated with chronic pancreatitis, biliary and pancreatic duct dilation, and the presence of pseudocysts. In the setting of malignant disease, it may demonstrate dilated intrahepatic and extrahepatic bile ducts, liver metastases, pancreatic masses, ascites, and enlarged peripancreatic lymph nodes. A malignancy of the pancreas typically appears as a hypoechoic mass; ultrasonography reveals a pancreatic mass in 60% to 70% of pancreatic cancer patients.

Helical (spiral) CT is now the preferred noninvasive imaging test for pancreatic disease, having largely supplanted ultrasonography in this context. Helical CT scan delineate the anatomy of the pancreas and the surrounding organs in considerable detail. It can also easily define pancreatic calcifications, inflammation, necrosis, and masses. Pancreatic cancer usually appears as an area of pancreatic enlargement with a localized hypodense lesion. A triple phase intravenous contrast study is ideal for the assessment. Thin cuts are obtained through the pancreas and the liver during both the arterial phase and the venous phase after the injection of IV contrast material. Besides determining the primary tumor size, CT can also identify and evaluate invasion into local structures or metastatic disease.

In general, MRI has no significant advantages over CT: Its signal-to-noise ratio is low, it is prone to motion artifacts, it does not opacify the bowel, and it has low spatial resolution. Nevertheless, magnetic resonance cholangiopancreatography (MRCP) can be quite useful for defining the anatomy and pathology of the bile ducts and the pancreatic duct noninvasively. It can be especially helpful in cases where the ampulla of Vater is not accessible (as in patients who have previously undergone Roux-en-Y or Billroth II reconstructions).

ERCP allows direct imaging of the pancreatic and bile ducts and is the gold standard for diagnosing chronic pancreatitis. It also allows therapeutic stenting of biliary and pancreatic duct strictures. The sensitivity of ERCP for the diagnosis of pancreatic cancer approaches 90%. The presence of a long, irregular stricture in an otherwise normal pancreatic duct is highly suggestive of a pancreatic malignancy. Often, the pancreatic duct is obstructed with no distal filling.

EUS now plays an important role in the evaluation of pancreatic diseases. It is a semi-invasive test that can be performed with a very low rate of complications (<0.1%). EUS can diagnose the most common causes of extrahepatic biliary obstruction (e.g., choledocholithiasis and pancreaticobiliary malignancies) with a degree of accuracy equaling or exceeding that of direct cholangiography or ERCP. It is the most sensitive modality for the diagnosis of pancreatic carcinoma. The particular strengths of EUS in the diagnosis of pancreatic cancer include its ability to (1) clarify small (<2 cm) lesions when CT findings are questionable or negative, (2) detect malignant lymphadenopathy, and (3) guide fine-needle aspiration (FNA) for definitive diagnosis and staging. The aspiration of cyst fluid and determination of cyst CEA levels and mucin can help differentiate serous from mucinous cysts.

## Patient Preparation

Every patient considered for a pancreatic resection needs a full evaluation of cardiac, pulmonary and renal function. A full array of laboratory test must be obtained including a complete blood count, renal panel, and liver panel. A nutritional assessment needs to be made to make sure that the patient can undergo surgery safely, if patient has severe weight loss or has an albumin of <3 g/dL, strong consideration for supplemental nutrition is indicated. Serum tumor markers including CEA and CA19-9 are usually measured in patients with both solid and cystic tumors. If a neuroendocrine tumor is suspected by history (symptomatic), imaging (hypervascular on CT scan), or on preoperative biopsy than serum levels of chromogranin A, insulin, proinsulin, glucagon, gastrin, vasoactive intestinal peptide (VIP), or pancreatic peptide (PP) can be measured.

For lesions involving the body and tail of the pancreas the patient should receive vaccination against encapsulated organisms to prevent post splenectomy sepsis. These include Streptococcus pneumoniae, Neisseria meningitidis, and Haemophilus influenzae vaccines. The vaccines should be administered 1 or 2 weeks prior to the operation if possible.

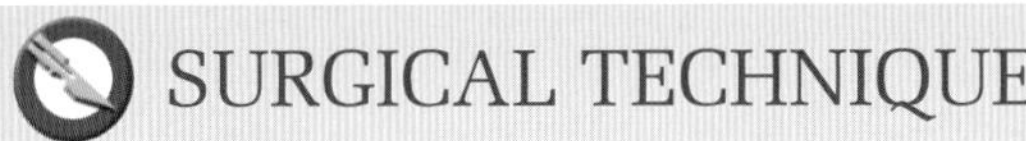

# SURGICAL TECHNIQUE

## Instrumentation

In addition to standard laparoscopic equipment available in most operating rooms, certain specialized equipment is necessary to safely carry out laparoscopic pancreatic surgery (Table 4.2). Intraoperative ultrasound is an invaluable tool during laparoscopic pancreatic resections. Ultrasound can be used to help localize lesions in the pancreas, define the relationship between the lesion and the pancreatic duct, assess for vascular invasion by the lesion, assess resection margins, and rule out metastatic disease.

**TABLE 4.2 Equipment for Laparoscopic Pancreatic Resection**

- 30° Laparoscope
- Flexible laparoscopic ultrasound probe
- Ultrasonic dissector
- Endo GIA stapler
- 5 mm and 10 mm clip applier
- Laparoscopic needle holders
- Atraumatic graspers
- Table mounted retractor

### Positioning and Room Setup

Following endotracheal intubation and general anesthesia, an orogastric tube and foley catheter are placed. Sequential compression devices and/or subcutaneous heparin are used for deep venous thrombosis prophylaxis and a first generation cephalosporin is used for infectious prophylaxis.

For lesions in the head, uncinate, or neck of the pancreas the patient is positioned supine and for lesions located in the body and tail of the pancreas I prefer to position the patient in a semilateral (30 to 45 degrees) position with the left side up. The surgeon and the camera operator stand on the patient's right side, while the first assistant and the scrub nurse stand on the patients left side. Video monitors are placed over both shoulders and the laparoscopic ultrasound monitor is placed on the patients left side near the video monitor.

## Laparoscopic Distal Pancreatectomy with or without Splenectomy

### Splenic Vessel Preserving Spleen Preserving Distal Pancreatectomy

Laparoscopic distal pancreatectomy may be performed as a splenic preserving distal pancreatectomy (SPDP) or an en bloc distal pancreatectomy plus splenectomy. Two techniques for splenic preservation have been described. The first involves preservation of the splenic artery and vein and requires a very careful dissection and ligation of the small branches from the splenic artery and vein to the pancreas (Fig. 4.1). The second technique involves the division of the splenic artery and vein proximally; followed by a second division of the vessels as they emerge from the tail of the pancreas (Fig. 4.2). The spleen is vascularized by the short gastric vessels and the left gastroepiploic vessels. Attempts at splenic preservation are appropriate for benign cystic neoplasms and neuroendocrine tumors. Splenectomy is often necessary if the tail of the pancreas extends well into the splenic hilum or there is significant peripancreatic inflammation that makes dissection of the pancreas off of the splenic vessels hazardous. Splenectomy should be performed if the procedure is being done for malignancy or there is left-sided portal hypertension secondary to splenic vein thrombosis.

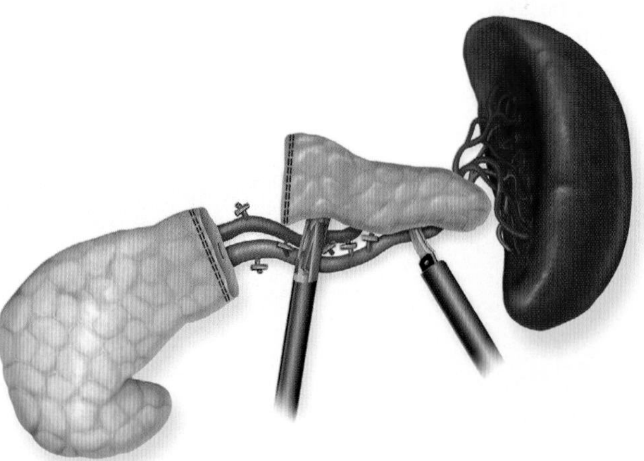

**Figure 4.1** Splenic vessel preserving spleen preserving distal pancreatectomy.

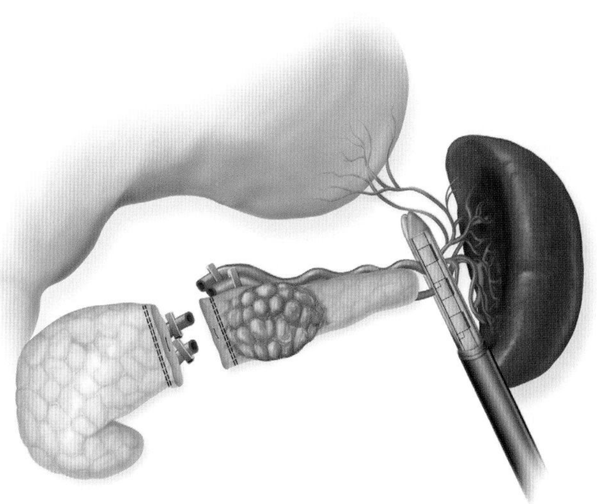

Figure 4.2 Splenic vessel ligating spleen preserving distal pancreatectomy (Warshaw Technique).

# Splenic Vessel Preserving Spleen Preserving Distal Pancreatectomy

## Port Placement

Access to the peritoneal cavity is achieved by either an open technique or via an Optiview technique. Five ports are placed (Fig. 4.3), and a 10 mm 30-degree laparoscope is used. As in all pancreatic procedures, the peritoneal surfaces, the omentum, the mesentery, and the viscera should all be carefully inspected to rule out metastatic disease. Intraoperative ultrasonography may be employed to evaluate the liver and locate the lesion in the pancreas.

## Exposure of the Pancreas

The body and tail of the pancreas are exposed by opening the lesser sac (Fig. 4.4). The gastrocolic omentum is divided and widely mobilized with an ultrasonic dissector, with

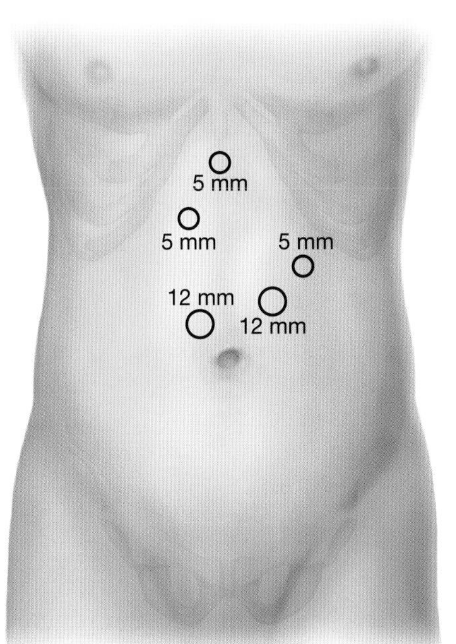


Figure 4.3 Trocar placement for laparoscopic distal pancreatectomy.

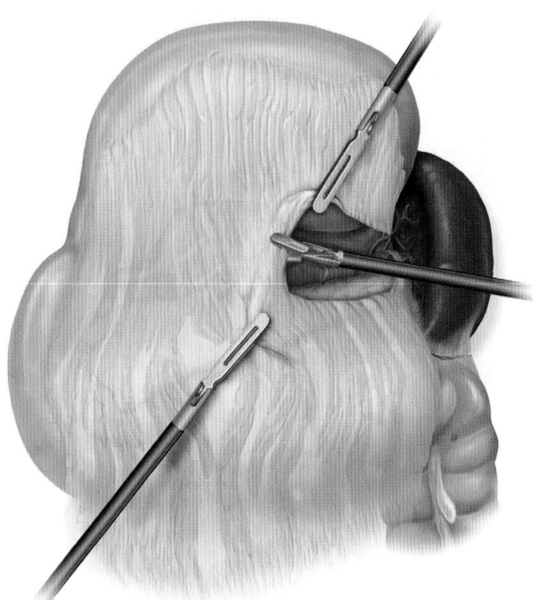

**Figure 4.4** Opening of the gastrocolic ligament for exposure of the pancreas.

care taken to stay outside the gastroepiploic vessels. The short gastric vessels should not be divided if a splenic preserving procedure is being attempted. A retractor is advanced into the lesser sac through the subxiphoid port and used to elevate the stomach anteromedially. Alternatively, the stomach can be sutured to the anterior abdominal wall with a temporary suture to obtain exposure. The splenocolic ligament is divided, and the splenic flexure of the colon is reflected inferiorly.

### Mobilization of the Pancreas

After exposure of the pancreas, the peritoneum is incised along the inferior pancreatic border, and the pancreatic body is separated from the retroperitoneum by means of sharp and blunt dissection along its inferior border. Laparoscopic ultrasonography and direct visual inspection, combined with the findings from preoperative imaging, may be employed to determine the extent of the dissection. Initially, the dissection should be directed so that it is medial to the pancreatic lesion.

### Isolation of the Splenic Vein

The pancreatic body is elevated by means of blunt and sharp dissection, after which the splenic vein should be easily identifiable (Fig. 4.5). Care must be exercised to prevent inadvertent injury to this vessel. Once the splenic vein has been identified, a careful circumferential dissection around the splenic vein is performed and a vessel loop can be placed around the vein for retraction.

### Isolation of the Splenic Artery

The splenic artery can be identified from the under surface of the pancreas by retracting on the vessel loop around the splenic vein or it can be identified along the superior border of the pancreas anteriorly (Fig. 4.5). Once it is dissected circumferentially it is also controlled with a vessel loop. These precautionary measures allow quick control of bleeding should a vascular tear occur later in the procedure.

### Parenchymal Transection

Once vascular control of the splenic artery and vein has been achieved, the pancreas is dissected off of the vessels in preparation for transaction of the gland. My preference

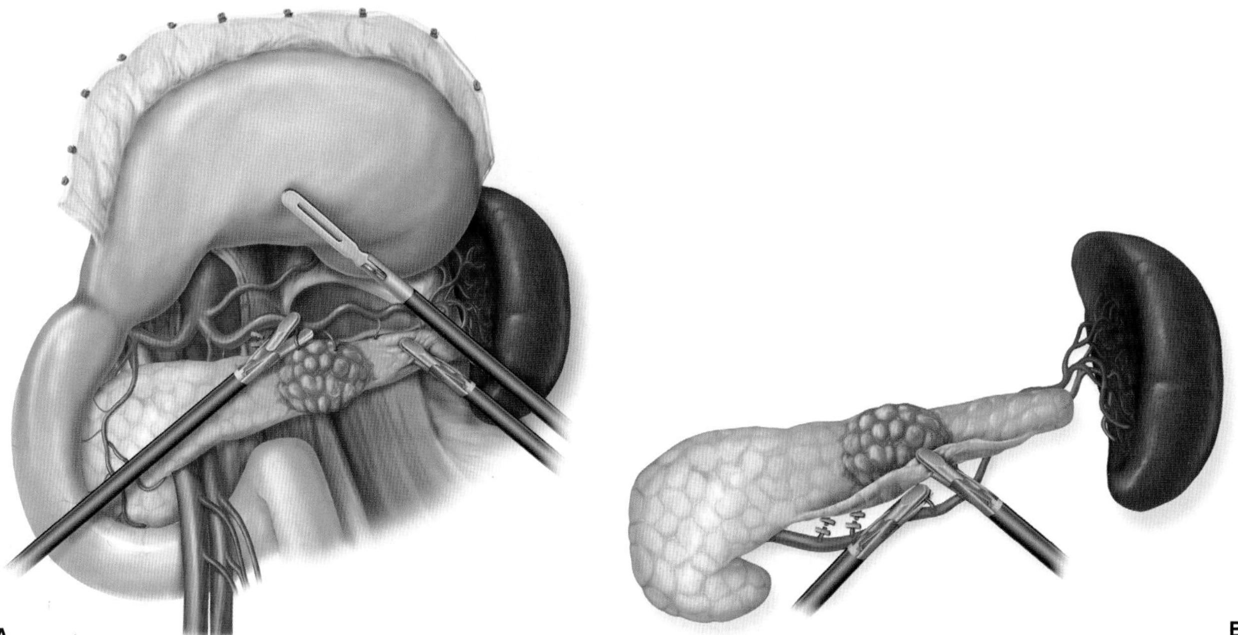


Figure 4.5 Isolation of the splenic artery and vein.

is to transect the pancreas with an ultrasonic scalpel. We have found the ultrasonic dissector to be hemostatic and to easily transect both firm and soft glands. It is important to move through the pancreas slowly and to start applying energy as the jaws are closing. If the pancreas is transected with an energy device I then treat the pancreatic remnant with a saline coupled radiofrequency sealing device (Salient Surgical Technologies) to seal the end of the remnant pancreas. Alternatively, an endoscopic stapler with or without staple line reinforcement can be placed across the body of the pancreas and used to divide the parenchyma (Fig. 4.6). If the pancreatic duct is visualized it is oversewn with a 4-0 absorbable suture.

## Medial to Lateral Dissection

Once the pancreas has been transected the specimen is grasped and gently retracted anteriorly to allow further dissection of the vessels (Fig. 4.7). The dissection proceeds toward the splenic hilum in a medial-to-lateral direction. The pancreatic branches of the splenic artery and vein are sequentially identified, dissected free and divided with

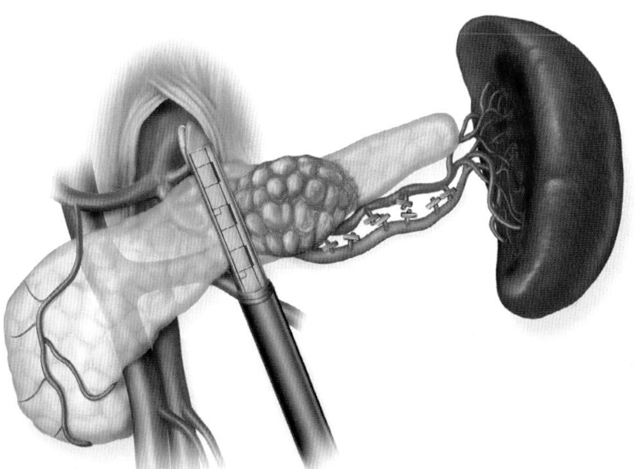

Figure 4.6 Transection of the left pancreas.

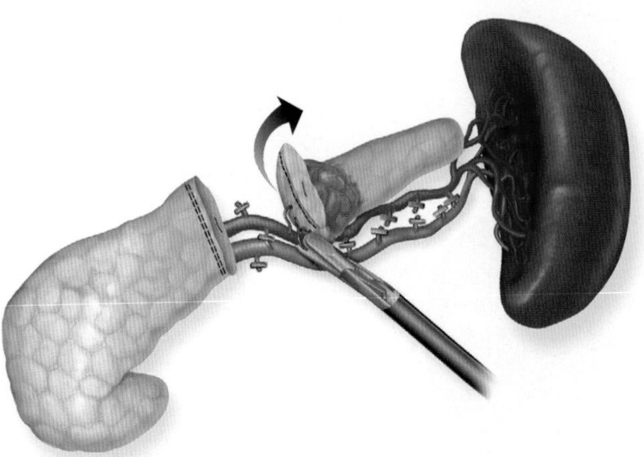

Figure 4.7 Medial-to-lateral dissection of the pancreas.

the ultrasonic scalpel or clips as appropriate. Special care must be taken as the dissection approaches the hilum of the spleen.

At the completion of an SPDP, the specimen is placed and removed in a standard endoscopic retrieval bag. A single round Jackson Pratt drain is placed near the pancreatic transaction line and brought out through one of the 5 mm lateral ports.

## Splenic Vessel Ligating Spleen Preserving Distal Pancreatectomy

An alternative approach to SPDP involves dividing the splenic vessels proximally and distally while preserving the short gastric and left gastroepiploic vessels to maintain splenic perfusion (see Fig. 4.2). The initial steps of this technique are essentially the same as those already described (see above), up to the division of the pancreas. In the vessel ligating approach to SPDP, after pancreatic transection, the splenic artery and vein are divided with an endovascular stapler, clips, or sutures. The left portion of the pancreas is lifted up and mobilized posteriorly along with the splenic artery and vein, and the vessels are again divided as they emerge from the pancreatic tail to enter the hilum of the spleen. The spleen is then supplied solely by the short gastric vessels and the left gastroepiploic vessels.

## Distal Pancreatectomy and Splenectomy

If an en bloc distal pancreatectomy with splenectomy is performed, the splenic artery and vein are divided after the pancreas is transected. The distal pancreas is dissected free in a medial-to-lateral direction. The short gastric vessels are divided with the ultrasonic scalpel, with care taken not to injure the stomach wall. The retroperitoneal attachments of the spleen and the tail of the pancreas are divided with the ultrasonic scalpel. The specimen is then placed in a specimen retrieval bag and extracted from a port site that has been enlarged to a size of 3 to 6 cm. To facilitate extraction of the specimen, the spleen may be morcellated within the bag.

## Laparoscopic Pancreatic Enucleation

Recently, laparoscopic techniques have been applied to the enucleation of small benign cysts and neuroendocrine tumors of the pancreas. This approach is indicated for tumors located in the body or tail of the pancreas or the anterior head of the pancreas that do

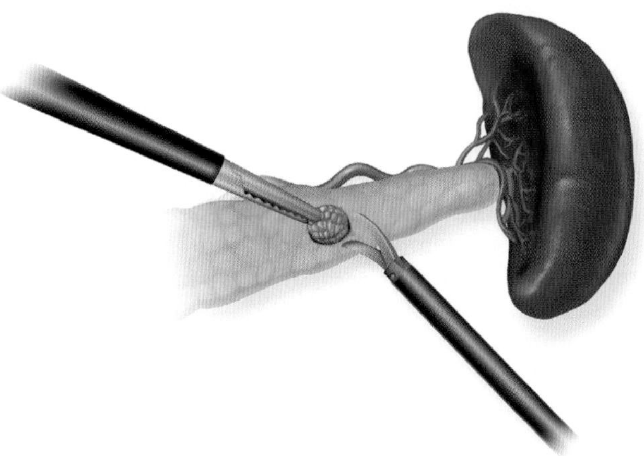

Figure 4.8 Laparoscopic pancreatic enucleation.

not appear to involve the pancreatic duct on preoperative imaging. Patient positioning and trocar placement is similar to that for laparoscopic distal pancreatectomy for lesions in the body and tail, and for laparoscopic pancreaticoduodenectomy for lesions in the head. The pancreas is widely exposed by entering the lesser sac through the gastrocolic omentum. Intraoperative ultrasound is extremely useful for the identification of the tumor and to further delineate the relationship to the splenic vessels and the pancreatic duct. The lesion can then be dissected out of the pancreatic parenchyma using the ultrasonic shears and electrocautery (Fig. 4.8). The specimen is placed in a specimen retrieval bag and removed. The enucleation bed is then inspected for hemostasis and a closed suction drain placed to control any potential pancreatic leak.

## Laparoscopic Central Pancreatectomy

Central or middle segment pancreatectomy (see Chapter 6) is another surgical option for the management of benign tumors in the neck and proximal body of the pancreas (Fig. 4.9). A central pancreatectomy may be indicated when the lesion involves or is in close proximity to the main pancreatic duct or there is fear of a duct injury with enucleation. The patient is positioned supine and the port placement is similar to distal pancreatectomy (Fig. 4.3).

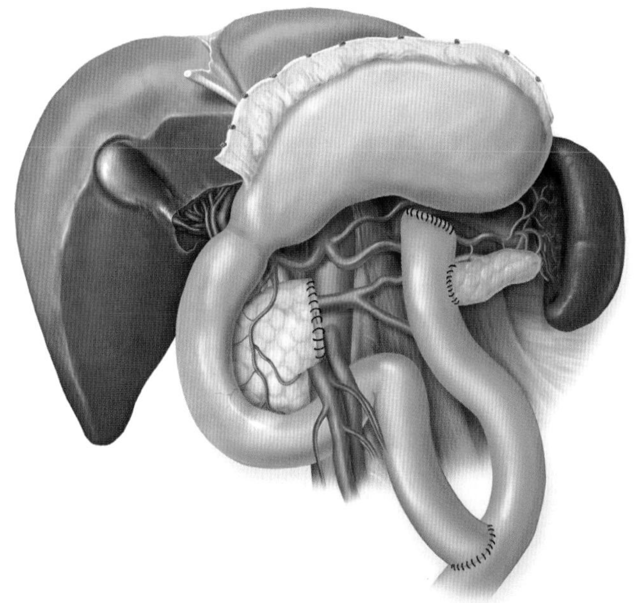

Figure 4.9 Central pancreatectomy.

### Resection of the Middle Segment

The initial steps are similar to those of spleen preserving distal pancreatectomy. The gastrocolic ligament is divided, preserving the gastroepiploic vessels, and the pancreas is fully exposed. The pancreas is then inspected with intraoperative ultrasound to define the relationship between the neoplasm and the major vascular structures. The superior mesenteric vein (SMV) and portal vein are then carefully dissected away from the posterior surface of the pancreas. The splenic artery and vein are preserved by separating them from the pancreatic segment to be resected. The pancreas is divided with an ultrasonic dissector to the left and right of the tumor. The pancreatic duct in the transected head of the gland is suture ligated if visible and the proximal pancreas is oversewn with interrupted 3-0 absorbable sutures or stapled. The distal pancreatic duct is then canulated with a 5 French pediatric feeding tube in preparation for a pancreaticojejunostomy.

### Creation of the Roux Limb

A Roux-en-Y jejunal loop approximately 45 cm long is constructed. The most proximal loop of jejunum in which there is a good vascular arcade is selected and divided with an endoscopic GIA stapler. The small bowel mesentery is divided with a vascular load of the stapler. A side-to-side stapled jejunojejunostomy is then created using a 60 mm endo GIA stapler. The enterotomy is then closed with a running 3-0 absorbable suture. The mesenteric defect should be closed with a 2-0 permanent suture. The Roux-en-Y jejunal limb is brought up into the lesser sac in a retrocolic position through a small opening in the transverse mesocolon.

### Creation of the Pancreaticojejunostomy

The anastomosis is begun by placing a series of interrupted 2-0 silk Lembert sutures between the side of the jejunum and the posterior capsule of the end of the pancreas. An enterotomy is then made approximately the same size as the pancreas and a 3-0 absorbable suture is used to complete a running anastomosis circumferentially around the entire gland. A short segment of a pediatric feeding tube is often placed across the anastomosis to be used as a temporary indwelling stent. The anastomosis is completed with an outer layer of 3-0 silk Lembert sutures placed between the anterior pancreatic capsule and the jejunum. If the pancreatic duct is greater than 3 mm a duct-to-mucosa anastamosis can also be performed (see Pancreaticojejunostomy in pancreaticoduodenectomy section below). A single round Jackson Pratt drain is placed near the pancreatic anastamosis and brought out through one of the 5 mm lateral ports.

## Laparoscopic Pancreaticoduodenectomy

In contrast to laparoscopic distal pancreatectomies and laparoscopic enucleations, the role of laparoscopic pancreaticoduodenectomy (PD) is more controversial. Laparoscopic PD is a technically demanding procedure due to the retroperitoneal location of the pancreas, its intimate association with surrounding gastrointestinal and major vascular structures, and the need for three separate anastomoses to complete the reconstruction. In addition, it is unclear whether an adequate cancer operation can be performed with respect to lymph node harvest and margin status is in patients with malignancy. Currently, laparoscopic PD is only performed in a handful of specialized centers. Many of the procedures are performed as either hand assisted or as laparoscopic assisted procedures with the resection being performed laparoscopically and the reconstruction being completed via a "mini" laparotomy or through the hand port. The technique of total laparoscopic pancreaticoduodenectomy with intracorporeal laparoscopic reconstruction will be described.

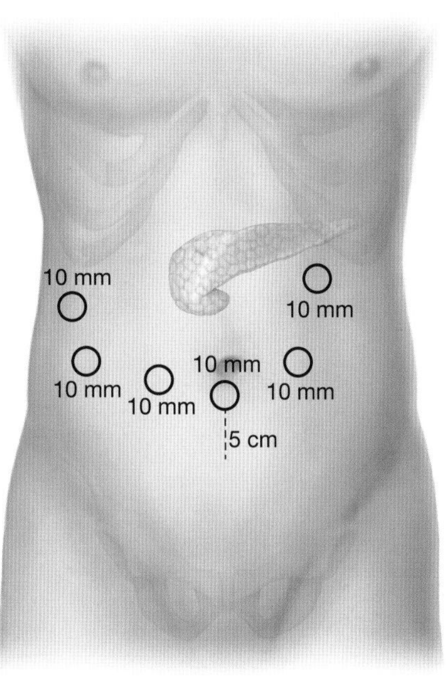


Figure 4.10 Trocar placement for laparoscopic pancreaticoduodenectomy.

## Port Placement

Laparoscopic pancreaticoduodenectomy is performed with the patient in the supine position. The surgeon and the camera operator stand on the patient's right side, while the first assistant and the scrub nurse stand on the patients left side. Trocar placement is shown in Figure 4.10.

## Exposure of the Pancreas

After establishing a pneumoperitoneum, a thorough diagnostic laparoscopy is performed inspecting all visible peritoneal and visceral surfaces. A 7.5 MHz laparoscopic ultrasound probe is used to perform ultrasonography of the liver and pancreas. The head and proximal body of the pancreas is widely exposed by dividing the gastrocolic ligament and mobilizing the hepatic flexure of the colon inferiorly with an ultrasonic shears (Fig. 4.11).

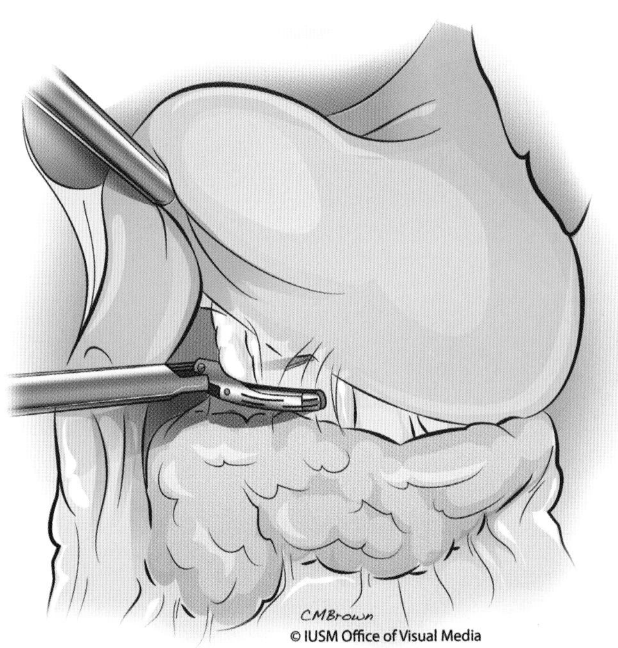


Figure 4.11 Exposure of the pancreas.

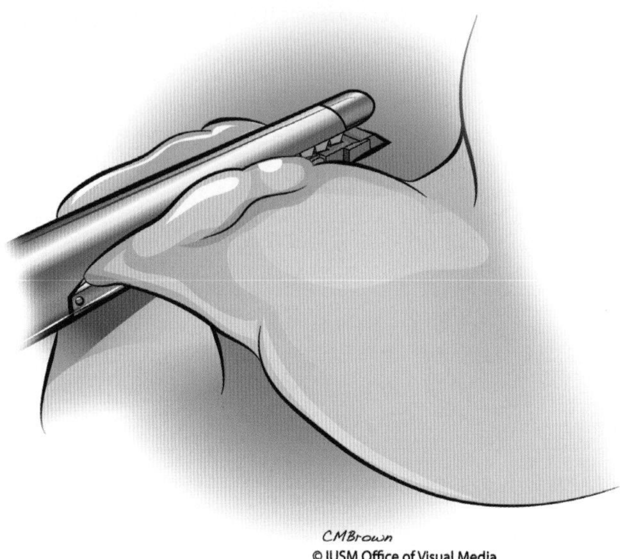


Figure 4.12 Transection of the post pylorus duodenum.

## Division of the Proximal Duodenum

The antrum of the stomach and the first portion of the duodenum are dissected away from the pancreas by dividing the small fibrovascular attachments to the head of the pancreas with the ultrasonic shears. The right gastroepiploic vessels and the right gastric artery are then divided between clips or with the ligasure. The duodenum is divided 2 cm distal to the pylorus with an endoscopic stapler (Fig. 4.12) and the proximal stomach is placed in the left upper quadrant.

## Exposure of the Superior Mesenteric Vein and Creation of the Retropancreatic Window

The SMV is identified at the inferior border of the neck of the pancreas (Fig. 4.13). The right gastroepiploic vein and the right colic vein can be followed back to the SMV to help identify it. The gastroepiploic vein is then divided between clips exposing the anterior surface of the SMV. If the anatomy permits the venous branches to the colon should be preserved. The inferior edge of the neck of the pancreas is gently retracted

Figure 4.13 Exposure of the SMV-PV confluence.

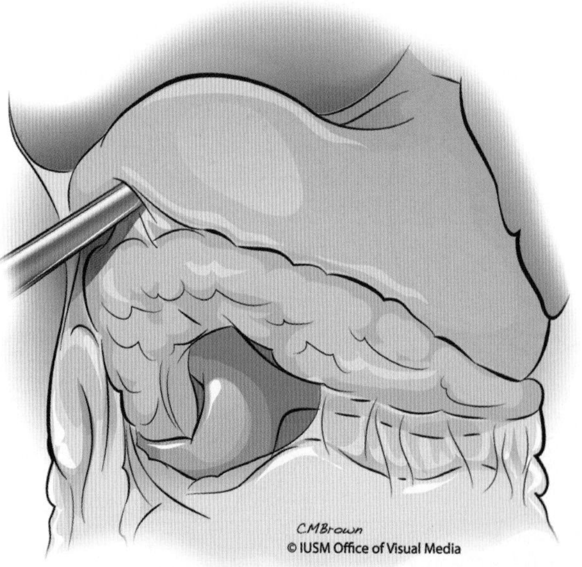

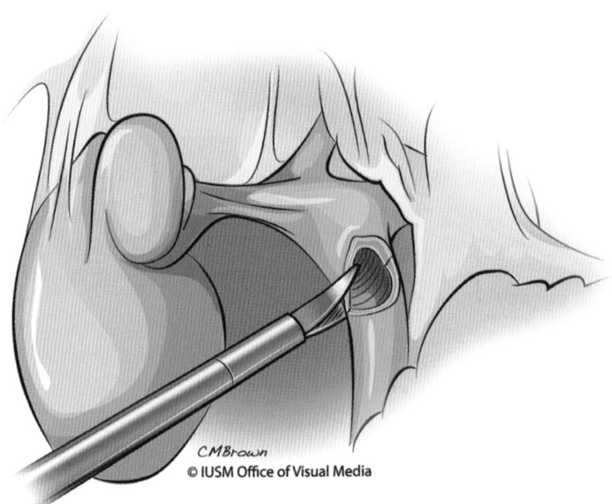


Figure 4.14 Division of the bile duct.

upward and a tunnel is carefully created between the SMV-portal vein (PV) complex and the pancreas using a combination of blunt dissection with a 5 mm suction and sharply with scissors and/or an ultrasonic shears.

## Porta Hepatis Dissection

Once the retropancreatic tunnel has been created attention is turned toward dissecting the porta hepatis. A table mounted liver retractor is inserted into the abdomen and used to elevate the liver. Calot's triangle is dissected and the cystic artery and duct are ligated. The gallbladder is kept in situ to assist with retraction and can be excised at the end of the procedure. The common bile duct is dissected circumferentially and divided sharply with a scissors (Fig. 4.14). The surgeon must be aware of variations in the hepatic arterial anatomy, including a replaced right hepatic artery during this dissection. Once divided the proximal bile duct may be temporarily clamped with a laparoscopic bulldog to prevent bile spillage. The distal bile duct is retracted caudally and the anterior surface of the portal vein cleared of all lymphovascular tissue. Finally, the gastroduodenal artery is dissected, ligated between ties, suture ligated proximally at its origin with the common hepatic artery and divided.

## Transection of the Pancreas

After completing the portal dissection and creating the retropancreatic tunnel over the SMV-PV confluence, the neck of the pancreas is divided. The inferior and superior margins of the pancreas are transected with ultrasonic shears, and the pancreatic duct is divided sharply with scissors (Fig. 4.15). The body of the pancreas is then dissected off of the splenic vein for approximately 2 cm to facilitate later reconstruction.

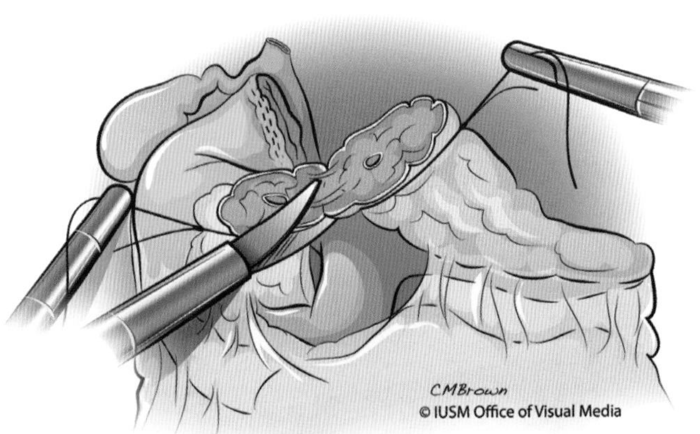


Figure 4.15 Sharp transaction of the pancreatic duct.

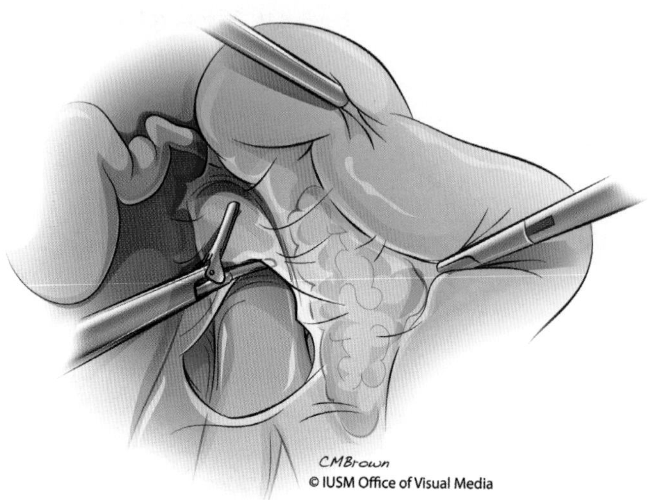


Figure 4.16 Laparoscopic Kocher maneuver.

## Kocher Maneuver and Mobilization of the Proximal Jejunum

A wide Kocher maneuver is performed by retracting the duodenum and head of the pancreas medially and the colon inferiorly. The ultrasonic shears are used to divide the retroperitoneal attachments and expose the anterior surface of the vena cava and the aorta (Fig. 4.16). The proximal jejunum is then exposed by retracting the omentum and transverse colon cephalad and identifying the ligament of Trietz. The jejunum is divided approximately 10 cm distal to the ligament of Trietz with an endoscopic stapler and the mesentery divided with the Ligasure device. The specimen is then passed posterior to the mesenteric vessels back into the right upper quadrant.

## Resection of the Head and Uncinate

The head of the pancreas is retracted laterally and the SMV and portal vein are gently retracted medially which exposes the uncinate process and the superior mesenteric artery. Dissection of the pancreatic head and uncinate process is initiated caudally and proceeds in a cephalad direction (Fig. 4.17). Small venous and arterial braches from the portal vein, SMV, and superior mesenteric artery are divided using a 10 mm Ligasure device (Tyco Healthcare Group, Dublin, Ireland). Larger tributary vessels (pancreaticoduodenal vessels) are ligated with suture or clipped as appropriate. All peripancreatic

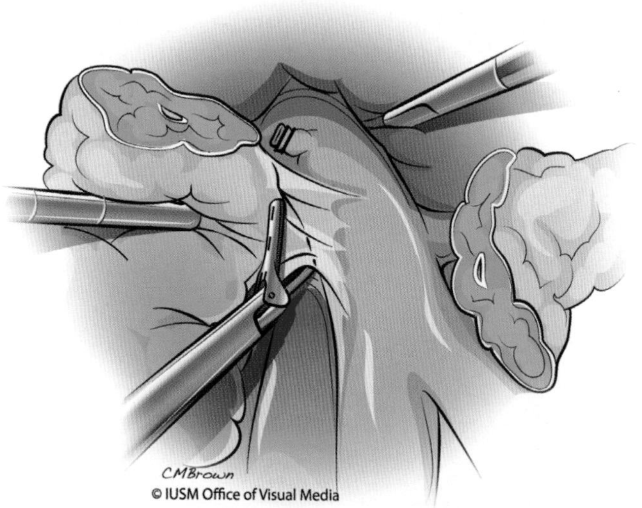


Figure 4.17 Dissection of the uncinate process off of the superior mesenteric artery and vein.

lymphatic tissue is taken en bloc with the specimen. The specimen is then removed in a specimen retrieval bag via the infraumbilical trocar site.

## Reconstruction

After fascial closure of the extraction site, the pneumoperitoneum is reestablished and intracorporeal reconstruction begun once margin status is confirmed on histology. A defect is made in the mesentery of the right colon and the jejunum is brought into the supramesocolic compartment in preparation for reconstruction.

## Pancreaticojejunostomy

An end-to-side, pancreaticojejunostomy, duct-to-mucosa anastomosis is typically performed. A row of interrupted 3-0 silk Lembert sutures is placed between the side of the jejunum and the posterior capsule of the end of the pancreas. A small enterotomy, matching the size of the pancreatic duct, is made in the jejunum, and an inner layer of interrupted 4-0 absorbable sutures is placed to create a duct-to-mucosa anastomosis (Fig. 4.18). Meticulous stitch placement is crucial and is enhanced by the magnification and visualization of the laparoscope. In small ducts, a pediatric feeding tube can be placed to insure the duct is not inadvertently sutured closed. The anastomosis is completed with an outer layer of 3-0 silk Lembert sutures placed between the anterior pancreatic capsule and the jejunum. An alternative to this duct-to-mucosa technique is to create an enterotomy approximately the same size as the pancreatic neck and to place an inner continuous layer of 3-0 absorbable synthetic suture material circumferentially around the entire gland. The neck is then invaginated 1 to 2 cm into the lumen of the bowel, and an outer interrupted layer of 3-0 silk is placed to complete the anastomosis.

## Hepaticojejunostomy

Approximately 10 cm distal to the pancreaticojejunostomy, an end-to-side hepaticojejunostomy (Fig. 4.19) is performed with a single interrupted layer of 4-0 absorbable suture (Vicryl). Alternatively larger ducts may be reconstructed with a continuous running suture. After completing the hepaticojejunostomy the loop of jejunum is tacked to the mesocolic defect with several interrupted silk sutures.

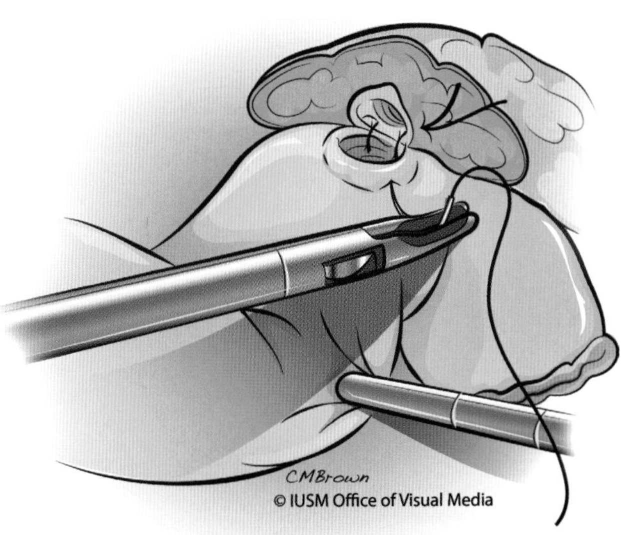


**Figure 4.18** End-to-side duct-to-mucosa pancreaticojejunostomy.

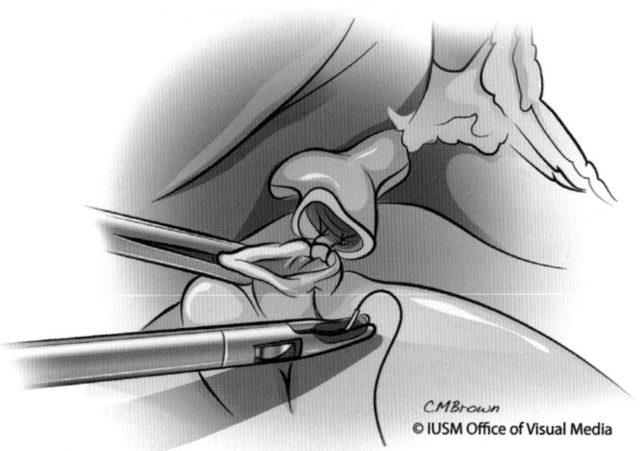


Figure 4.19 End-to side hepatico-jejunostomy.

### Duodenojejunostomy

Approximately 30 to 40 cm distal to the biliary anastomosis, an antecolic, end-to-side duodenojejunostomy is performed with two layers of running 3-0 Vicryl (Fig. 4.20). Two closed suction silastic drains are placed near the biliary and pancreatic anastamoses and brought out through the 5 mm trocar sites. The fascia is closed for all 12 mm trocar sites and all the incisions are closed with an absorbable, monofilament, subcuticular suture.

## POSTOPERATIVE MANAGEMENT

The postoperative management of patients undergoing laparoscopic pancreatic resections is similar to those undergoing traditional open resections. Laboratory test should be checked in the recovery room as well as the morning of the first postoperative day; these include a complete blood count, electrolytes, liver function tests and amylase. Mild pancreatitis can develop postoperatively and may explain the reason for an exaggerated inflammatory response. Frequent assessment of the blood glucose should be carried out and blood glucose should be kept under 150 mg/dL in the postoperative period. Prophylactic antibiotics should not be continued for longer than 24 hours. The nasogastric tube may be removed on day 1 postoperatively and the patient is allowed to have sips of liquids and the diet slowly advanced over the next few days. The peripancreatic drains

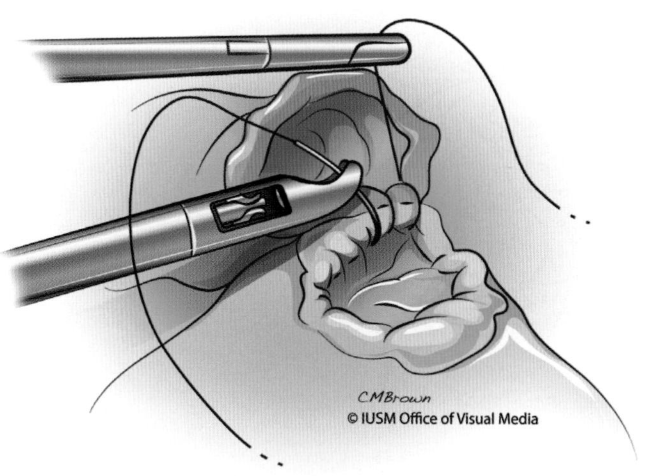


Figure 4.20 End-to side duodeno-jejunostomy.

are checked for amylase on postoperative day 1 and if the level is less than 5,000 IU are removed on postoperative day 3 if there is no evidence of a pancreatic fistula. Alternatively, the drain can be removed once the patient is tolerating a regular diet and there is no evidence of a pancreatic leak. In the event of continued leak, the patient may be discharged with the drain and instructed to record daily output, most fistulas close spontaneously without any further intervention.

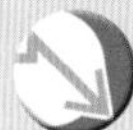

## COMPLICATIONS

Complications of laparoscopic pancreatic resections are similar to those seen in patients undergoing open pancreatic resections (see Chapters 2, 3, 6, 9). Laparoscopic resections have been associated with a slightly lower overall complication rate when compared to open surgery. However, the difference is primarily related to a lower rate of wound complications with laparoscopic surgery. There does not appear to be any significant differences in the rates of the most important complications such as operative mortality, pancreatic fistula, intra-abdominal abscess and delayed gastric emptying in the small number of reports comparing laparoscopic and open pancreatic surgery.

## RESULTS

In the past 5 years it has become clear that laparoscopic distal pancreatectomy can be performed safely by surgeons experienced in both advanced laparoscopic techniques and pancreatic surgery. Two large multi-institutional and several smaller single institution series have been published (Table 4.3). In these series the operative time ranged between 3 and 5 hours, the complication rate between 17% and 41%, the pancreatic fistula rate was between 4% and 38%, and the length of stay between 4 and 11 days. While there has not been a prospective randomized comparison of laparoscopic and open distal pancreatectomy it appears that laparoscopic distal pancreatectomy can be accomplished with a similar mortality, morbidity, and pancreatic fistula rate as open pancreatic surgery. However, laparoscopic surgery may be associated with a shorter hospital stay, blood loss, and a higher likelihood of splenic preservation.

Laparoscopic pancreaticoduodenectomy is a technically demanding procedure due to the retroperitoneal location of the pancreas, its intimate association with surrounding gastrointestinal and major vascular structures, and the need for three separate anastomoses to complete the reconstruction. In addition, it is unclear whether an adequate cancer operation can be performed with respect to lymph node harvest and margin status in patients with malignancy. Currently, laparoscopic PD is only performed in a handful of specialized centers (Table 4.4). In the two largest series reported by Kendrick and Palanivelu, where the reconstruction was completed laparoscopically, the mean operative time was slightly over 6 hours, the operative morbidity approached 40%, and

**TABLE 4.3 Laparoscopic Distal Pancreatectomy**

| Author | Year | N | Conv (%) | Spleen Pres (%) | Op time (hrs) | Fistula/absc (%) | Comp (%) | LOS (days) |
|---|---|---|---|---|---|---|---|---|
| Patterson | 2001 | 19 | 11 | 37 | 4.4 | 16 | 26 | 6.0 |
| Park | 2002 | 25 | 8 | 41 | 3.7 | 4 | 17 | 4.1 |
| Dulucq | 2005 | 21 | 5 | 76 | 4.6 | 14 | 23 | 10.8 |
| Marbut | 2005 | 96 | 15 | 71 | 3.3 | 27–38 | 41 | 7.0 |
| Fernandez-Cruz | 2007 | 82 | 7 | 64 | 3.3 | 8 | 22 | 7.0 |
| Melotti | 2007 | 58 | 0 | 55 | 2.7 | 28 | 53 | 9.3 |
| Kooby | 2008 | 159 | 13 | 31 | 4.0 | 26 | 40 | 5.9 |

**TABLE 4.4 Laparoscopic Pancreaticoduodenectomy**

| Author | Year | N | Conv (%) | Lap Recon (%) | Op Time (Min) | Comp (%) | LOS (days) | Panc Can (%) |
|---|---|---|---|---|---|---|---|---|
| Gagner | 1997 | 10 | 40 | 60 | 510 | 30 | 22.3 | 40 |
| Dulucq | 2006 | 25 | 12 | 50 | 287 | 32 | 16.2 | 44 |
| Palanivelu | 2007 | 42 | 0 | 100 | 370 | 31 | 10.1 | 21 |
| Pugliese | 2008 | 19 | 31 | 31 | 461 | 37 | 18 | 58 |
| Kendrick | 2010 | 65 | 4 | 100 | 368 | 40 | 7 | 47 |

the length of stay was 7 to 10 days. The oncologic outcomes for the patients undergoing resection for malignancy demonstrated an R0 resection rate of 89% and 100% and the mean lymph node harvest was 15 and 13 in the studies respectively. These results are comparable to those seen with open pancreaticoduodenectomy.

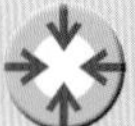

## CONCLUSIONS

The last decade has seen an increase in the application of minimally invasive surgical procedures to the management of pancreatic disease. Laparoscopic pancreatic surgery is an advanced laparoscopic procedure with a significant learning curve. It should be considered only by surgeons with extensive experience in open pancreatic surgery who possess advanced laparoscopic skills. Early reports suggest that laparoscopic pancreatic surgery can be accomplished with acceptable morbidity and mortality for the resection of small benign and low-grade malignant lesions in the body and tail of the pancreas. Its role in the management of lesions in the head, neck, and uncinate process of the pancreas is yet to be determined.

## Recommended References and Readings


Dulucq JL, Wintringer P, Mahajna A. Laparoscopic pancreaticoduodenectomy for benign and malignant diseases. *Surg Endosc.* 2006;20:1045–1050.

Dulucq JL, Wintringer P, Stabilini C, et al. Are major laparoscopic pancreatic resections worthwhile? *Surg Endosc.* 2005;19: 1028–1034.

Fernández-Cruz L, Cosa R, Blanco L, et al. Curative laparoscopic resection for pancreatic neoplasms: A critical analysis from a single institution. *J Gastrointest Surg.* 2007;11:1607–1622.

Gagner M, Pomp A. Laparoscopic pancreatic resection: Is it worthwhile? *J Gastrointest Surg.* 1997;1:20–26.

Kendrick ML, Cusati D. Total laparoscopic pancreaticoduodenectomy: Feasibility and outcomes in an early experience. *Arch Surg.* 2010;145:19–23.

Kooby D, Gillespie T, Bentrem D, et al. Left-sided pancreatectomy: a multicenter comparison of laparoscopic and open approaches. *Ann Surg.* 2008;248:438–446.

Kooby DA, Hawkins WG, Schmidt CM, et al. A multicenter analysis of distal pancreatectomy for adenocarcinoma: Is laparoscopic resection appropriate? *J Am Coll Surg.* 2010;210:779–785.

Mabrut JY, Fernandez-Cruz L, Santiago Azagra J, et al. Laparoscopic pancreatic resection: results of a multicenter European study of 127 patients. *Surgery.* 2005;137:597–605.

Melotti G, Butturini G, Piccoli M, et al. Laparoscopic distal pancreatectomy results on a consecutive series of 58 patients. *Ann Surg.* 2007;246:77–82.

Nakeeb A. Laparoscopic pancreatic resections. *Adv Surg.* 2009; 43:91–102.

Palanivelu C, Jani K, Senthilnathan P, et al. Laparoscopic pancreaticoduodenectomy: Technique and outcomes. *J Am Coll Surg.* 2007;205:222–230.

Park AE, Heniford BT. Therapeutic laparoscopy of the pancreas. *Ann Surg.* 2002;236:149–158.

Patterson EJ, Gagner M, Salky B, et al. Laparoscopic pancreatic resection: single-institution experience of 19 patients. *J Am Coll Surg.* 2001;193:281–287.

Pugliese R, Scandroglia I, Sansonna F, et al. Laparoscopic pancreaticoduodenectomy: A retrospective review of 19 cases. *Surg Laparosc Endosc Percutan Tech.* 2008;18:13–18.

# 5 Operative Palliation of Pancreatic Cancer

**Kaye M. Reid-Lombardo, Joshua Barton, and Michael G. Sarr**

## Introduction

The role of the surgeon in the palliation of patients with unresectable periampullary/pancreatic cancer has changed markedly over the last decade. In the past, most patients were treated by exploratory celiotomy and, if the lesion was unresectable (80% to 90% of patients), the surgeon would construct an intraoperative bilioenteric bypass and often a gastroenterostomy that was either therapeutic (i.e., treating established duodenal obstruction) or prophylactic [i.e., used to "prevent" gastric outlet obstruction (GOO) caused by pancreatic cancer]. More recently, marked improvements in imaging (spiral, triple-phase computed tomography and magnetic resonance imaging) and the use of staging laparoscopy have led to the majority of unresectable cancers being identified prior to celiotomy. This better selection of potentially resectable patients avoids the need for operative biliary and duodenal bypasses, because patients with non-curable disease by resection are now palliated by nonoperative means, both by endobiliary stents and, should duodenal obstruction occur, by endoduodenal stents. Moreover, the marked improvements and expertise with endoscopically placed endobiliary stents and/or percutaneous, transhepatic stents have, in most patients, all but eliminated the need for a planned, operative, palliative bilioenteric bypass. In addition, the ongoing development of intraluminal intestinal stents (partially covered duodenal endoprostheses) has, in many patients, served to relieve the duodenal obstruction from a locally advanced pancreatic cancer, thereby preventing the need for operative gastrojejunostomy. Nevertheless, the surgeon still maintains a definite role to play in the palliation of selected patients with pancreatic cancer, and the approaches/techniques described below offer different advantages for biliary and GOO.

Surgeons have and will continue to play an active role in the palliation of advanced, incurable pancreatic cancer in selected situations. Palliation should be considered from three aspects, all of which are designed to palliate specific symptoms prior to the eventual death of the patient: (1) relief of mechanical extrahepatic biliary obstruction, (2) relief or prevention of mechanical GOO, and (3) minimization/prevention of the all-too-often debilitating pain from the invasion of pancreatic cancer into the peripancreatic and celiac plexus.

*Biliary bypass*: Once the bile duct becomes obstructed by most malignant neoplasms, the progression of hyperbilirubinemia is relentless at 1 mg/dl/day up to a concentration of 20 to 25 mg/dl. At this level, the spillover into the urine and the soft tissues equals the metabolic daily production, at least for several weeks. Thereafter, the serum bilirubin concentration again increases as the hepatopathy of chronic complete biliary obstruction (biliary cirrhosis) progresses.

Relief of the biliary obstruction should be the first objective of palliation. Biliary obstruction and the absence of bile salts/lectin in the gut lumen not only lead to a maldigestion of fats (loss of solubilization of intraluminal lipids) with resultant malabsorption and exacerbation of weight loss, but also for the patient, the associated pruritus is usually the most distressing. This pruritus on occasion can be the first symptom of the disease, and in the absence of back pain, often becomes the most prominent symptom for the patient.

*Gastric outlet obstruction (GOO)*: Duodenal obstruction is a very uncommon, initial presentation of pancreatic cancer (<10%). In contrast, GOO develops later in the course of the disease in up to 15% to 30% of patients, depending on how intensely one looks for this condition; indeed, many patients ultimately die with and/or from GOO. Therefore, if GOO can be prevented without adding much morbidity, some consideration should be given to addressing its prevention in selected patients and in relieving the GOO with, if possible, a minimal access or endoscopic intervention. There is a poorly understood form of "functional" GOO that can complicate the management of unresectable pancreatic cancer that is believed to be a disorder of coordinated gastric emptying. This functional GOO is not a mechanical obstruction of the duodenal lumen but rather related presumably to local neural involvement with a subsequent gastroduodenal dysmotility. This type of GOO does not resolve with gastrojejunostomy and is difficult to treat.

*Back pain*: As the disease progresses, 60% to 80% of patients with pancreatic cancer eventually develop substantive epigastric pain and especially a "boring-through" back pain. This back pain is most prominent at night. Part of the concern of the physician/surgeon offering palliative care to the patient with unresectable pancreatic cancer must involve an aggressive approach to the patient with this horrible, often debilitating pain. As surgeons, we also have a primal role in this aspect of palliation. In addition to emotional support, provision of adequate analgesics are imperative, and many times, recruitment of the experts in this field—both the palliative care group and the hospice care team—may be the best therapy that a truly caring surgeon can administer.

In summary, palliative care provided by the surgeon should be threefold: relief of biliary obstruction, relief/prevention of GOO, and aggressive approaches to minimize or prevent pain. The remainder of this chapter will address (1) operative approaches to establish a bilioenteric bypass, (2) use of gastrojejunostomy to treat or prevent GOO, (3) intraoperative chemical splanchnicectomy or thoracoscopic splanchnicectomy to prevent the development of back pain, (4) minimal access (laparoscopic) approaches to the management of biliary and duodenal obstruction, and finally (5) several other adjunctive possibilities. A brief discussion of local ablative techniques, such as intraoperative radiation therapy, cryotherapy, and radiofrequency ablation will also be addressed.

## Operative Approaches to Establish Bilioenteric Drainage

Most pancreatic cancers arise either periampullary or within the proximal-most pancreatic duct up to the genu of the duct in the head of the gland; as they enlarge radially, they encroach on and surround the distal "intrapancreatic" portion of the common bile duct (CBD) which is only 5 to 10 mm away. Therefore, pancreatic cancer of only 2 cm diameter can lead to complete biliary obstruction before it causes any other overt symptomatology—thus, the term "painless jaundice." While most of these patients in retrospect do have some other symptoms (vague upper abdominal distress, minor weight loss, or unexplained fatigue), the symptoms bringing them to their physician are usually jaundice and pruritus.

Bilioenteric bypasses can be constructed in many ways using as the conduit either (1) the gallbladder via cholecystogastrostomy, cholecystoduodenostomy, or cholecystojejunostomy; or (2) the common hepatic duct or CBD by choledocho/hepaticoduodenostomy or choledocho/hepaticojejunostomy. The following section will discuss the technical aspects of these procedures, after which we will address considerations in selection of the optimal form of bilioenteric bypass according to the clinical situation.

## Cholecystoenteric Bypass

Technically, using the gallbladder as the biliary conduit is undoubtedly the fastest and the easiest approach to bilioenteric bypass. Distal CBD obstruction usually leads to a markedly dilated gallbladder (Courvoissier's sign), making access to the gallbladder quite easy. When choosing the gallbladder as the conduit, the surgeon must consider the proximity of the neoplasm to the entrance of the cystic duct into the extrahepatic biliary tree—this consideration will be discussed fully below in the section Selection of Bilioenteric Bypass.

Historically, *cholecystogastrostomy and/or cholecystoduodenostomy* were the early operations for bilioenteric bypass because of the proximity of the gallbladder to these organs and because of the ease (and safety) of the anastomosis. Mobilization of the fundus of the dilated gallbladder without disruption of the cystic artery will allow the gallbladder to be "folded over" for anastomosis to the stomach or duodenum. Enthusiasm for this procedure waned in the 1960's as more evidence developed showing problems with bile gastritis/esophagitis, bilious vomiting, and ongoing problems when the duodenum became obstructed from local progression of the pancreatic neoplasm. This approach to bilioenteric bypass is largely of historic interest even in benign conditions because of the reasons described above, but also because the anastomosis often strictures over time (not really a problem when used in the palliation of pancreatic cancer).

*Cholecystojejunostomy*: Due to the mobility of the jejunum, this anastomosis is the quickest, easiest, and safest form of bilioenteric drainage and does not require any mobilization of the gallbladder. A loop of proximal jejunum is brought antecolic and sewn to the anterior aspect of the gallbladder fundus; in rare cases, a retrocolic approach through the right transverse mesocolon may be easier, but usually not. The anastomosis can be created in a hand sewn, usually one layer fashion due to the thin-walled gallbladder (Fig. 5.1A), or in stapled fashion (Fig. 5.1B); if a gastrojejunostomy is also planned, an intraluminal circular stapler can be introduced in the enterotomy to be used for the gastrojejunostomy and passed distally to a site where a stapled circular anastomosis can be created (usually a 21 or 25 mm stapler is sufficient) (Fig. 5.1C). Some surgeons then create a Braun-type, side-to-side enteroenterotomy between the afferent and efferent limbs of the loop cholecystojejunostomy but most do not believe this diverting enteroenterostomy to be necessary. Overall, this is a very safe anastomosis with little morbidity.

One very important point needs to be stressed. Strong consideration needs to be directed at the possibility of future obstruction of the cystic duct where it enters the CBD as the pancreatic neoplasm enlarges; obstruction of the cystic duct will lead to recurrent biliary obstruction. If contemplating a cholecystojejunostomy, the gallbladder should be dilated or, if chronically inflamed, should contain bile. Some advocates of this easy anastomosis suggest a cholecystogram to confirm both patency of the cystic duct outflow as well as the site of entrance of the cystic duct into the CBD and its distance from tumor. If the cystic duct enters the CBD low near the duodenum, or if the neoplasm is in close proximity to the entrance of the cystic duct, using the gallbladder as the biliary conduit is contraindicated.

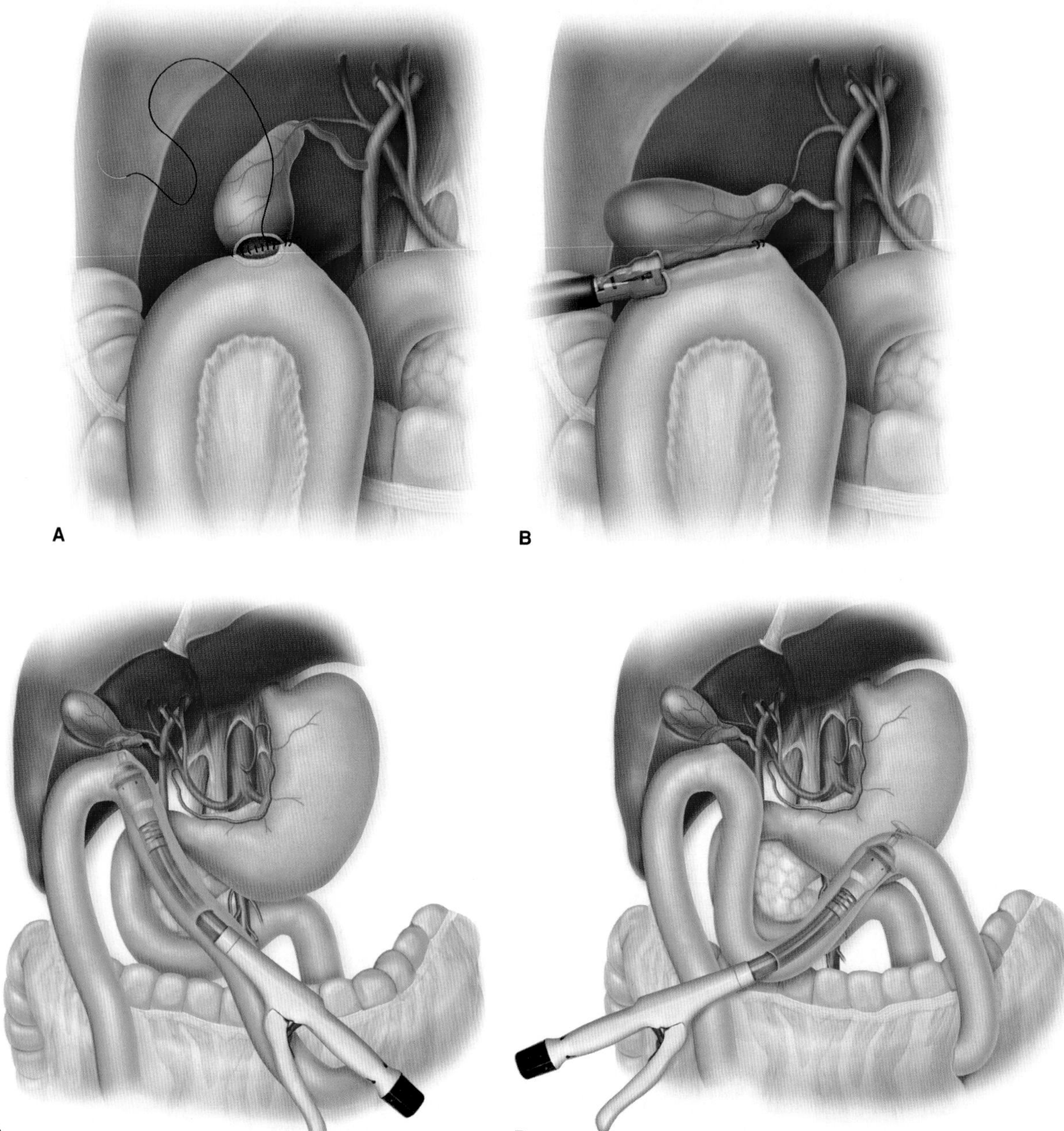


**Figure 5.1** Cholecystojejunostomy created as a loop anterior to the transverse colon. (**A**) Hand-sewn technique. (**B**) Stapled technique. (**C**) Double stapled technique in which an enterotomy is created in the jejunum and, using an intraluminal circular stapler, first a cholecystojejunostomy is created, the stapler removed and reinserted, and then (**D**) a gastrojejunostomy created, after which the enterotomy is closed.

## Hepaticoenteric Bypass

Most HPB surgeons currently use the common hepatic duct as the biliary conduit for a palliative bilioenteric bypass. The rationale behind this somewhat more involved approach than using the gallbladder or the CBD is because of worry related to local progression of the pancreatic neoplasm potentially involving the entrance of the cystic duct into the CBD and/or involving the CBD and/or any anastomosis to the CBD. Being several centimeters rostral, the common hepatic duct is involved only rarely with direct spread from a pancreatic neoplasm or only very late in the disease.

*Choledochoduodenostomy/hepaticoduodenostomy*: When possible, some groups have advocated a choledocho- or hepaticoduodenostomy. The extrahepatic biliary tree

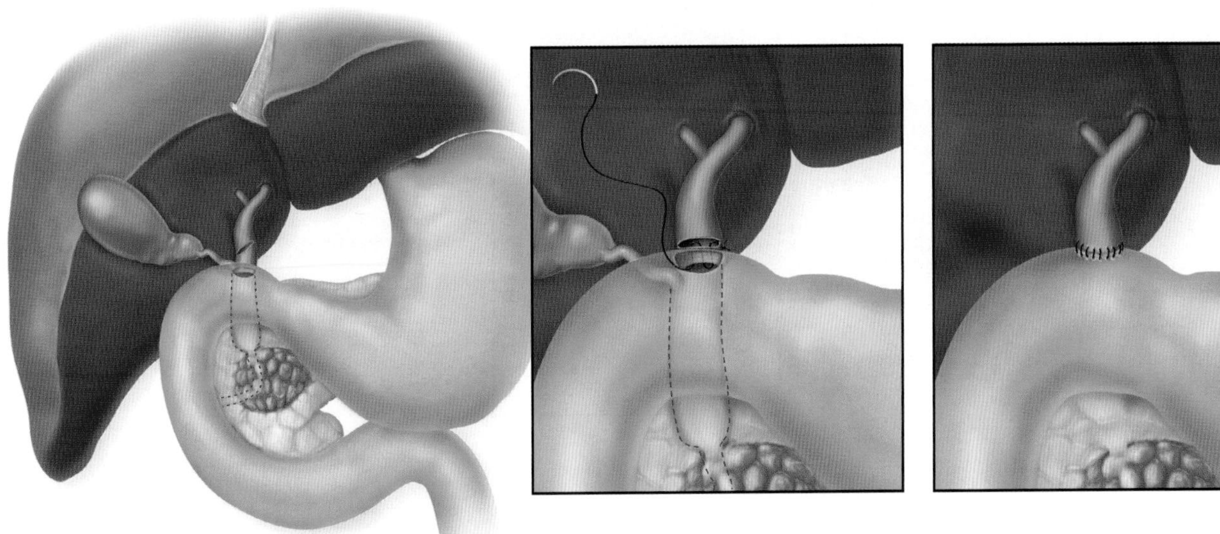

Figure 5.2 Hepaticoduodenostomy. Initially, the duodenum is approximated to the common hepatic duct and, using a diagonal incision in the hepatic duct to increase the anastomosis, a side-to-side hepaticoduodenostomy is created. The insert shows that, if the hepatic duct is of large enough diameter, the anastomosis can be done by a running suture. The second insert shows a transected common hepatic duct sewn end-to-side to the duodenum.

and the duodenum are quite close anatomically and, when the extrahepatic biliary tree is dilated, the anastomosis becomes quite easy. After a Kocher maneuver to gain duodenal mobility, this anastomosis can be done as a side-to-side anastomosis or less commonly by transecting the common hepatic duct at its junction with the CBD, oversewing the distal CBD, and carrying out an end-to-side hepaticoduodenostomy (Fig. 5.2); the latter requires circumferential dissection around the common hepatic duct and oversewing of the CBD, which seems unnecessary if a more simple, straightforward, side-to-side hepaticoduodenostomy is feasible technically. This anastomosis is straightforward, facile, and safe. Usually a cholecystectomy is also performed.

Arguments against this approach cite the potential for anastomotic obstruction in conjunction with duodenal obstruction from local extension of the pancreatic neoplasm. An increasing number of proponents with good, long-term data maintain that (1) this approach requires only one, easy, safe anastomosis, (2) late obstruction of the anastomosis is rare, and (3) when the more distal duodenum becomes obstructed, biliary drainage can still occur retrograde through the stomach and a gastrojejunostomy. The more limited reported experience appears quite good, and the arguments against hepaticoduodenostomy are largely theoretic and not actually supported by objective data.

*Hepaticojejunostomy*: Most HPB surgeons prefer enteric biliary drainage via the common hepatic duct based on the theoretic argument that the chance of future malignant obstruction by local extension of the pancreatobiliary neoplasm is much less likely—see "Selection of Bilioenteric Bypass". Hepaticojejunostomy can be carried out either to a loop of jejunum or more commonly to a Roux limb (Fig. 5.3). The latter is usually preferred for technical ease. Bringing the intestinal conduit (loop of jejunum or Roux limb) up to the hepatic duct is much easier technically and a much shorter distance via a retrocolic approach through the right transverse mesocolon rather than up and over the omentum and right transverse colon; bringing up a jejunal loop through the mesocolon is more bulky, and worry always remains about obstruction of the loop at the mesocolon; therefore, a Braun-type enteroenterostomy (a second anastomosis) is also usually created. A Roux limb is less bulky, more mobile, and easier to work with than the loop. The argument that a Roux drainage requires the potential morbidity of a second anastomosis (end-to-side jejunojejunostomy) is offset by the ease of construction of the hepaticojejunostomy and the usual construction of a Braun enteroenterostomy with the loop construction anyway. Any worry about reflux of enteric chyme into the

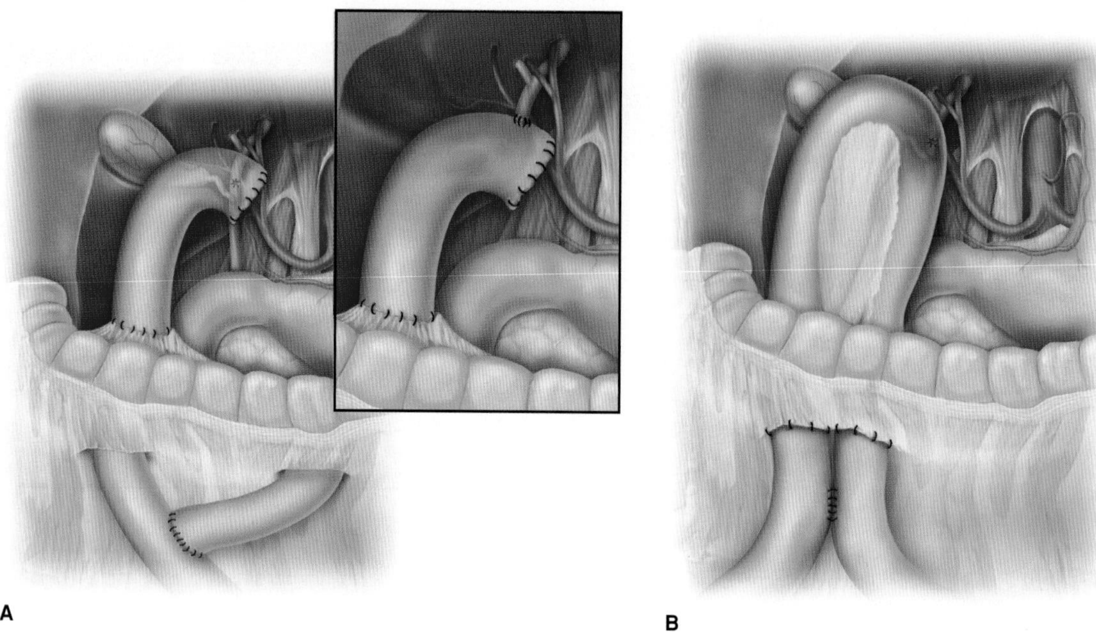


Figure 5.3 Hepaticojejunostomy. (**A**) This Roux-en-Y hepaticojejunostomy is created by immobilizing the Roux limb that passes through the right transverse mesocolon and then is sewn usually in a one-layer anastomosis to the common hepatic duct. Cholecystectomy is often done to maximize exposure. The insert shows that this can be done as an end-to-side anastomosis by transecting the common hepatic duct. (**B**) Loop hepaticojejunostomy. A loop of the jejunum is brought through the transverse mesocolon and sewn in a side-to-side fashion to the hepatic duct. The defect in the mesocolon is then sewn to the loop of jejunum and then a Braun-type enteroenterostomy is created between the ascending and descending limbs of the loop hepaticojejunostomy.

biliary tree should not be of concern, because this procedure is palliative, and prolonged survival greater than 2 years is unexpected. As with hepaticoduodenostomy, if the gallbladder is still *in situ,* most surgeons will add a cholecystectomy for several reasons: (1) the dilated gallbladder can be "in the way," and (2) by bypassing the gallbladder, there can be stasis in the gallbladder lumen, which can lead to cholecystitis requiring intervention, a condition that no one would want to develop in a patient with unresectable pancreatic cancer. Cholecystectomy is easy and adds minimal morbidity.

The hepaticojejunostomy can be constructed either in a side-to-side or end-to-side fashion (Fig. 5.3). These authors see no benefit of transecting the common hepatic duct to carry out an end-to-side hepaticojejunostomy, which requires its circumferential mobilization and oversewing of the CBD distally, although some surgeons prefer this technique. A side-to-side anastomosis is equally easy to construct. The anastomosis is usually a one-layer technique; if the biliary tree is adequately dilated, a running technique is faster. Again, because this is a palliative procedure, either absorbable or permanent 3- or 4-0 suture material is appropriate. A second serosal layer to the periductal tissues can be added if so desired. Use of any form of decompressive biliary "T-tube" or retrograde bilio-external drainage tube is unnecessary unless the surgeon is very worried about the integrity of the anastomosis for some reason. Anastomotic leak should be rare (<2%). Presence of an endobiliary stent placed preoperatively can either be removed retrograde through the hepatic ductotomy at the time of hepaticojejunostomy or, if there is any concern about the operative anastomosis, the stent can be left to provide another pathway of enteric drainage/decompression but will necessitate endoscopic removal postoperatively. Overall, this procedure has proven to be a very safe, durable anastomosis.

## Cholangiojejunostomy

The need for any type of intrahepatic enteric bypass would be extremely unusual as a technique of operative palliation. Situations that might in very rare cases justify such an approach would involve extensive nodal disease extending up the hepatoduodenal ligament. Possible operative procedures in this situation might involve a left hepatic duct-jejunostomy after taking down the hilar plate with a Hepp-Couinaud type of anastomosis, a segment 3 approach (ligamentum teres approach), or the classic Longmire, left-sided cholangiojejunostomy after excising the lateral most aspect of segment 2 of the liver. These procedures are largely of historic interest, because currently, such extensive involvement of the hepatoduodenal ligament would not have escaped notice on imaging preoperatively (i.e., intrahepatic biliary dilation with dilated extrahepatic ducts) which indicates unresectable disease; should the patient require operative palliation for some other complication (e.g., duodenal obstruction), biliary decompression would be attained by a percutaneous biliary drain without the increased morbidity of one of these intrahepatic bilioenteric bypasses.

## Selection of Bilioenteric Bypass

With the current success of either endoscopic or percutaneous techniques of bilioenteric drainage using endobiliary stents and the improved ability to select resectable patients, the need for palliative biliary bypass has become much less common. Potential situations include patients with what appears to be resectable disease explored by a full celiotomy but, on exploration, are found to have incurable (unresectable) disease, the rare patient in whom placement of an endobiliary stent is not possible for technical or other anatomic reasons (e.g., after prior gastrectomy), or the patient requiring an open duodenal bypass for GOO (also a rare situation when not amenable to a less-morbid, minimal access, laparoscopic gastrojejunostomy or endoscopically placed enteroduodenal stent. Under these situations, the surgeon must choose between a hepaticojejunostomy or, if the patient has an indwelling endobiliary stent, no biliary bypass at all. In these patients with mechanical duodenal obstruction, the local disease is more extensive and either cholecystojejunostomy or hepaticoduodenostomy are not good biliary conduits for palliation.

*Need for a biliary bypass*: Numerous studies in the recent and distant past when operative palliation was required have compared morbidity and long-term success of biliary drainage via the gallbladder versus the hepatic duct—all show similar morbidity, but all show superior long-term success with drainage via the common hepatic duct.

While cholecystojejunostomy is technically faster and much easier, the success of biliary drainage requires ongoing patency of the cystic duct. As the pancreatic neoplasm grows locally and extends into the hepatoduodenal ligament, the neoplasm invades and/or occludes any hollow viscus organs—duodenum, CBD, and cystic duct. Many patients have a low entering cystic duct that maintains a common wall with the CBD, giving the false impression on gross, external visualization of entering the CBD higher up toward the liver; this low entrance of the cystic duct predisposes to earlier obstruction as the primary neoplasm expands locally. Ideally, before using the gallbladder, the surgeon should exclude a low entering cystic duct by a cholecystogram, ERCP, or by dissecting out the real entrance of the cystic duct—currently and even in the past; such diligence in the palliative setting was done only rarely. Worry about stenosis of the cholecystojejunostomy, development of gallstones or cholecystitis, or reflux of enteric content into the gallbladder, as would be of concern when a cholecystojejunostomy is used as a long-term conduit for benign disease, is, of course, irrelevant in the palliative setting. As will be seen below, cholecystojejunostomy is a much easier procedure done laparoscopically; if contemplated, the laparoscopic surgeon really should assure a distance of 2 to 3 cm of the entrance of the cystic duct into the CBD from the neoplasm by some form of imaging before carrying out a cholecystojejunostomy.

Detailed studies in the 1980s and 1990s, including several combined reviews, unanimously are convincing and show superior patency rates of 90% to 95% after hepaticojejunostomy. In contrast, maintenance of "palliative" patency (before death) after cholecystojejunostomy is only 70% to 75% and even less in some studies, and more troublesome is that attempts to establish internal biliary drainage by an endoprosthesis can be much more difficult technically by endoscopic or percutaneous, transhepatic approaches because of more extensive local growth of the primary neoplasm; moreover, the patient is less robust physically as the disease process has progressed.

Arguments that biliary drainage via the hepatic duct is associated with greater serious morbidity have not proven to be true. Indeed, both procedures are quite safe when carried out by an experienced surgeon. Experience with hepatico- or choledochoduodenostomy as effective, long-term palliation of biliary obstruction in patients with unresectable pancreatic cancer is more limited and still remains somewhat controversial from largely a theoretic basis rather than based on data. But one of the larger series ($n = 46$ patients) from the Cleveland Clinic documented good long-term palliation with this approach, which has been echoed more recently by several other groups, which challenges by evidence-based data the assumption that hepaticoduodenostomy is subject to future obstruction by local tumor growth. Indeed, these studies show rates of recurrent jaundice of less than 8%, quite similar to that of hepaticojejunostomy. One or two groups, however, have claimed less optimistic outcomes.

Nevertheless, most HPB surgeons carry out a Roux-en-Y hepaticojejunostomy as their procedure of choice when confronted with this situation. Maintenance of effective biliary drainage is greater than 90%, the anastomosis is usually not difficult (dilated extrahepatic biliary tree), and the added time to carry out this procedure seems worthwhile; if effective, permanent palliation of the jaundice is accomplished, subsequent biliary obstruction is avoided in these unfortunate patients.

*Presence of a Functioning Endobiliary Stent*: Many (and in some institutions, most, if not all) patients with what proves at exploration to be an incurable, unresectable pancreatic cancer already have a functioning, plastic, endobiliary stent. The question then arises as to whether or not a surgically constructed bilioenteric bypass should be undertaken, because the patient already has been subjected (albeit in good faith) to the morbidity (pain, convalescence, etc) of the celiotomy (the controversy of a palliative gastrojejunostomy will be discussed later). There is no consensus amongst HPB surgeons on this question. Our ability to palliate extrahepatic biliary obstruction effectively by endoluminal stents when secondary to pancreatic cancer has improved markedly with the expandable metal stents and now readily available endoscopic experience. Construction of an operative biliary bypass in all likelihood will delay discharge a day or two and may add potential morbidity (wound infection from bacterobilia, possible anastomotic problems) which may sway some surgeons to avoid any "prophylactic" maneuvers (biliary bypass, gastrojejunostomy). Other surgeons maintain that virtually all patients with an indwelling biliary endoprosthesis have some complications eventually even if a metallic stent has been placed (occlusion, cholangitis, etc.) and, for this reason and the fact that they already are obligated to the morbidity of a celiotomy, a surgically constructed biliary bypass will virtually prevent future problems or need for readmission for biliary obstruction or cholangitis. No consensus prevails.

In contrast, if unresectability is discovered at the time of staging laparoscopy, and the patient has a functioning biliary endoprosthesis, most surgeons would not create a surgical bilioenteric bypass via a laparoscopic approach (see later) or convert to an open operative approach to construct a surgical bilioenteric bypass; the same argument holds true for a prophylactic gastrojejunostomy.

## Operative Approaches to Obtain Duodenal Bypass

### Concept of Gastrojejunostomy

The topic of performing a "prophylactic gastrojejunostomy" in patients with unresectable pancreatic adenocarcinoma in whom there is no established duodenal obstruction has been argued in the literature over the past several decades by a series of retrospective studies and reviews, prospective randomized trials, and a recent systematic review.

All these studies found that prophylactic gastrojejunostomy at the time of exploration for unresectable pancreatic head adenocarcinomas decreases the long-term incidence of GOO and does not impair short-term outcomes; the authors, therefore, support performing prophylactic gastrojejunostomy. It is important to note that these studies were conducted early in the development of endoscopic stenting of the duodenum and did not compare directly open gastrojejunostomy to endoscopic treatment by endoluminal stents. In addition, these studies were conducted at centers and/or at a time when diagnostic laparoscopy was not done routinely.

Recent studies, however, have called into question the role of prophylactic gastrojejunostomy. The use of diagnostic laparoscopy has been adopted increasingly in many centers as an adjunct in determining resectability and avoiding any non-therapeutic celiotomies. In addition, endoscopic treatment of malignant GOO appears to offer quicker resumption of an oral diet, shorter hospitalization, lesser immediate cost, and, at least, lesser short-term morbidity. It is important to note, however, that reintervention for patients who undergo endoscopic stenting appears to be needed more commonly than in patients who undergo gastrojejunostomy. The impact these reinterventions have on long-term costs and quality of life is not clear.

Although GOO traditionally has been thought to occur eventually in 10% to 25% of patients with unresectable pancreatic adenocarcinoma, other studies have shown that GOO may occur in less than 10% of patients. The wide variation in the reported occurrence of GOO is due likely to defining GOO based on clinical symptoms, radiographic findings, and the time of development of GOO (early or late in the course of the disease). The more recent appreciation of the occurrence of a functional GOO or a form of gastroparesis due to neurogenic causes likely plays a role in this wide variation as well. Several studies have shown that despite nausea and vomiting occurring as presenting symptoms in 30% to 45% of patients with pancreatic adenocarcinoma, only about 5% of patients have actual mechanical GOO. Interestingly, a more recent study found that the mean time to GOO was 15.7 months versus a mean overall survival of approximately 13 months for patients with unresectable pancreatic adenocarcinoma.

Due to the increasing role of diagnostic laparoscopy, the improvement in endoprostheses for extrahepatic biliary obstruction and for GOO, and their prior finding that GOO occurs in less than 10% of patients studied, the group at the Memorial Sloan-Kettering assessed the role of prophylactic duodenal bypass in patients with laparoscopically staged, unresectable pancreatic adenocarcinoma. They evaluated 155 patients who were found by diagnostic laparoscopy to have unresectable stage III or IV disease. Of these patients with unresectable disease, 98% did not require a subsequent, open surgical procedure to treat GOO; their conclusion was that prophylactic gastrojejunostomy has no role in treating patients with unresectable pancreatic adenocarcinoma determined at time of staging laparoscopy. What is vital in the approach to patients with unresectable pancreatic adenocarcinoma at Memorial Sloan-Kettering and other centers who share their point of view is the support of endoscopic interventionalists.

At our institution, we use diagnostic laparoscopy selectively in assessing resectability. If a patient is found to have unresectable stage III or IV disease during laparoscopy, we do not proceed to prophylactic gastrojejunostomy but do consider therapeutic gastrojejunostomy for symptomatic patients (see comments on laparoscopic gastrojejunostomy for therapeutic purposes later). In contrast, if a patient is found to have unresectable disease during an open celiotomy, we favor addition of a prophylactic gastrojejunostomy. Our opinion is that an open laparotomy by itself necessitates delay of palliative chemotherapy by at least 4 weeks and, despite disparate reports of high morbidity, addition of a gastrojejunostomy does not increase irrevocably complications or hospital stay at our institution.

## Gastrojejunostomy

The standard operation for addressing an existing or impending (in the case of prophylaxis) malignant GOO alone traditionally has been a simple loop gastrojejunostomy.

Considerable debate has occurred regarding the merits of an isoperistaltic versus an antiperistaltic gastrojejunostomy as well as placement of the anastomosis in an antecolic or retrocolic position. Experience from operations performed for peptic ulcer disease would indicate that an isoperistaltic gastrojejunostomy might be preferable but even these data are weak. In addition, some surgeons have preferred using an antecolic gastrojejunostomy with the intention of positioning the anastomosis well away from the primary malignancy and, therefore, avoiding the chance of subsequent malignant obstruction as the disease progresses locally. Several studies conducted in the 1990s, however, indicate that there is no difference in oral tolerance with reference to an isoperistaltic versus antiperistaltic anastomosis. In addition, retrocolic anastomoses appear to empty similarly or potentially better than antecolic anastomoses in these studies and are not prone to earlier malignant obstruction. Therefore, our preference to perform an isoperistaltic, retrocolic, posterior, loop gastrojejunostomy when addressing prophylaxis or management of established malignant duodenal obstructions. We also suture the stomach to the defect in the transverse mesocolon, such that the anastomosis is fixed caudad to the mesocolon. When the transverse mesocolon is involved with the tumor burden, we readily perform an antecolic anastomosis.

The process for considering a biliary bypass in conjunction with a gastrojejunostomy is a complex decision and is covered elsewhere in this chapter. The exact technique of performing a biliary bypass in conjunction with a gastrojejunostomy varies from center to center and can involve using simple double loops to a more complex Roux-en-Y reconstruction. Surgeons who advocate using two simple loops for each anastomosis cite the palliative nature of the operation and the relative ease at which this approach can be performed, because no enteroenterostomy is created. At our institution, we prefer to construct a Roux-en-Y limb for a side-to-side hepaticojejunostomy with a gastrojejunostomy to the jejunum proximal to the Roux limb in manner of a simple loop gastrojejunostomy. The gastrojejunostomy is made typically proximal to the jejunojejunostomy, thereby necessitating that the biliopancreatic limb be at least 20 to 40 cm long as measured from the ligament of Treitz.

## Operative Techniques

The actual construction of the gastrojejunostomy can be accomplished in multiple ways. The authors each have their own preferences. One technique involves a two-layer, hand-sewn anastomosis with a running inner layer of absorbable suture for hemostasis and an outer layer of interrupted, permanent suture material (Fig. 5.4).

Another technique utilizes a linear gastrointestinal stapler, often with the "green" cartridge (4.8 mm staples) because of the thickness of the wall of the stomach. A gastrotomy and jejunotomy are made, the stapler inserted, fired, and the staple line inspected for bleeding before closing the now common enterotomy. Any bleeding from the staple line can be oversewn. The common enterotomy is then closed either with interrupted sutures or with a linear stapler; in either case, the technique should not narrow the small intestinal lumen at the site of the jejunotomy.

A third technique (6) utilizes an endoluminal circular stapler on occasion in conjunction with a cholecystojejunostomy (when indicated) (Fig. 5.1-insert). An enterotomy is made about 50 cm distal to the ligament of Treitz. Through this enterotomy, a 33 mm circular stapler is introduced retrograde into the more proximal jejunum to allow a stapled gastrojejunostomy to be created about 10 cm proximal to the enterotomy. Through this same enterotomy, a 21 mm or 25 mm circular stapler can be inserted distally to create the cholecystojejunostomy. Finally, the enterotomy can either be closed or used to create a Braun-type enteroenterotomy between the afferent and efferent limbs of the loop cholecystojejunostomy. The limitation of this technique is that the anastomotic staple line of the gastrojejunostomy is much more difficult to inspect for bleeding; the possibility of bleeding from any gastric anastomosis is of concern because of the vascularity of the stomach, and this staple line needs to be inspected for bleeding at the time of its creation.

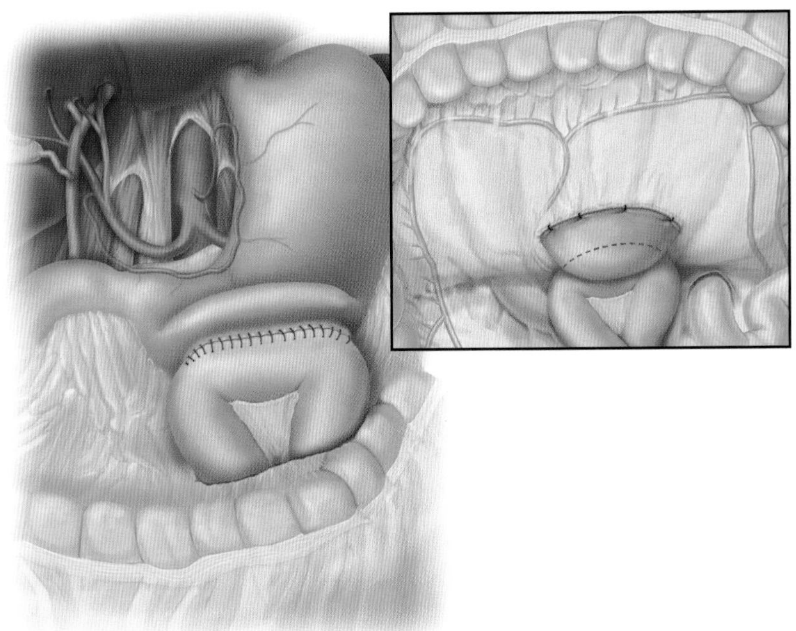


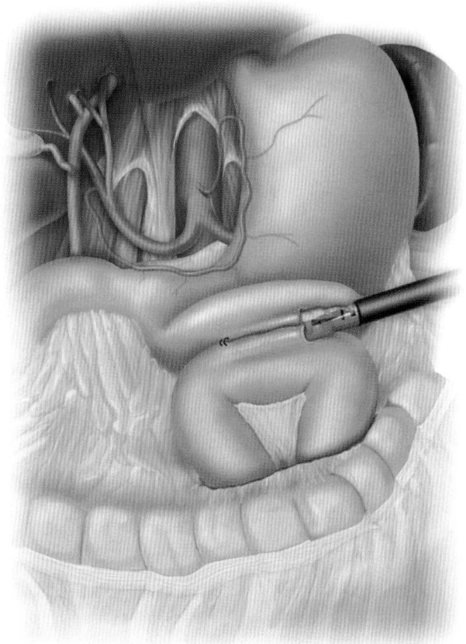


**Figure 5.4** Gastrojejunostomy. Usually a retrocolic gastrojejunostomy is created to the posterior surface of the stomach. This can be done as shown with a hand-sewn technique in (**A**) where the anastomosis is created to the posterior surface of the stomach and then the stomach is brought below the mesocolon and the stomach sewn to the defect in the mesocolon. (**B**) This anastomosis can be created with a stapler as well. Please also see Figure 1D for a double staple technique.

# Palliation of Pain

One of the most disturbing and distressing situations for the patient, the family, the home physician, and the pancreatic surgeon is the patient with unrelenting abdominal back pain related to pancreatic cancer. On rare occasions, the pain can be disabling and poorly responsive even to opiate narcotics. As the surgeon, we must be sensitive to this situation, expectant of its potential development, aggressive in its treatment, and even mindful of our potential for preventing its development. Endoscopic and percutaneous celiac plexus blocks can be incredibly effective when done by experienced personnel. Failure of effective results should, at the least, warrant consideration of referral to a center more experienced with these image-guided approaches, because these techniques are highly operator-dependent.

Although much less common today than in the past, if the patient at the time of celiotomy for potential resection is found to have incurable disease, and the focus then shifts from resection for cure to palliation, consideration should be given to performing an intraoperative celiac plexus block. A prospective, randomized trial by the Hopkins group found benefit in delaying the onset and minimizing the severity of future back pain when done "prophylactically"; morbidity was minimal.

The technique of chemical splanchnicectomy (celiac plexus block) is simple and straightforward (Fig. 5.5). The surgeon surrounds the area of the aorta containing the celiac plexus (origin of the celiac artery) between his/her index and middle finger through the lesser omentum; there is no need to transect the lesser omentum. One finger palpates the common hepatic artery and the other the splenic artery. Using a 20-gauge spinal needle (you need the added length of a spinal needle) on a 10 ml syringe, 10 ml of 50% absolute alcohol diluted with 0.9% NaCl (injectable normal saline) is injected para-aortically immediately rostral to the hepatic artery. As the needle is positioned, the surgeon will appreciate the "gritty" feeling of the neuroconnective tissue, and before injecting the solution, aspiration of the syringe will prevent intravascular injection. The needle is removed, and topical pressure is held while the syringe

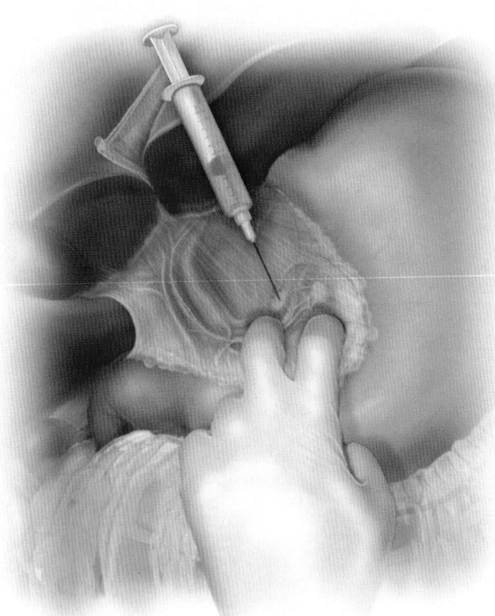

**Figure 5.5** Chemical splanchnicectomy (celiac plexus block). The surgeon positions the celiac axis between the index finger, which feels the splenic artery, and the second finger, which feels the hepatic artery. Ten milliliters of 50% alcohol is then injected rostral and caudal to the common hepatic and splenic artery.

is refilled. The same maneuver is repeated para-aortically just caudal to the hepatic artery and then, in similar fashion, rostral and caudal to the splenic artery. Using this technique, there are minimal complications, and the procedure is both easy and quick, taking no more than 2 minutes. The alternative to an intraoperative celiac axis block is either a percutaneous or endoscopic block postoperatively, which seems much less ideal when the same procedure can be done intraoperatively under direct vision, takes only 2 minutes, is cheaper, requires no repeat anesthesia or postoperative referral, and is less troublesome and less painful for the patient; remember, we are addressing patient palliation.

## Thoracoscopic Splanchnicectomy

On rare occasion, the surgeon may be approached about the possibility of carrying out a thoracoscopic splanchnic nerve transection for the unremitting pain of pancreatic cancer. Again, as surgeons we need to be sensitive and symptomatic of the severity of this pain and its impact on the future, short-lived quality-of-life of these patients. Usually, a celiac plexus block will accomplish the same outcome and is much less invasive; however, on occasion, the patient has had a good but temporary response to a celiac plexus block, but he pain has recurred, is not responsive to a repeat block, and is not well controlled pharmacologically. Under these circumstances with intractable and debilitating pain, some consideration should be given to a thoracoscopic splanchnic nerve transection. Most experience with this procedure has been for the pain of chronic pancreatitis; results in this disease have varied, and long-term effective pain relief has been disappointing. Nevertheless, in patients with the unrelenting, non-responsive disabling pain of pancreatic cancer, many HPB surgeons (and patients) would believe the risk of the thoracoscopic splanchnicectomy is worth the potential benefit despite its palliative nature.

## Radiation Therapy

Radiotherapy is used primarily as a palliative treatment to slow the local progression of the disease; radiation can also provide some relief of back pain as well. New interest in use of gamma knife technology, also called stereotactic, image-guided radiotherapy, may be applicable in this situation to focus the radiation to the celiac plexus and to deliver a therapeutic dose over only 2 to 3 days.

# Minimal Access Techniques

The use of minimally invasive surgery (MIS) was reserved originally for laparoscopic exploration to stage patients with locally advanced pancreatic cancer. Of the 15% to 20% of patients with pancreatic cancer who are deemed resectable, as many as 30% are found to be unresectable at the time of laparoscopy due to the detection of occult or metastatic disease. Therefore, laparoscopy is an important mechanism to decrease the incidence of unnecessary celiotomies in patients with advanced disease. More recently, though, experience with advanced techniques of minimal access gastrointestinal surgery as well as of laparoscopic pancreatic resections and reconstructions, have allowed expansion of laparoscopic approaches to be used for palliative procedures for malignant obstructions such as gastrojejunostomy and cholecystojejunostomy.

## Minimal Access Biliary and Gastric Bypass

At the time of laparoscopic staging, if the patient is found to have metastatic or locally advanced disease that renders the tumor unresectable, the surgeon is faced with the decision of whether to perform a palliative operation or to abort the laparoscopy and treat the patient with endoscopic stenting. The decision-making process should probably also consider the probability of concurrent or impending GOO due to the size and location of the pancreatic mass. In contemporary practices, biliary obstruction can be well and effectively palliated endoscopically with placement of a plastic stent prior to operation or a metal stent after operation, thereby rendering a laparoscopic biliary intervention unnecessary. In contrast, for GOO, although also able to be treated successfully most of the time with the use of endoscopically placed, endoluminal duodenal stents, the addition of a laparoscopic gastrojejunostomy, a technically easy procedure, should at least be entertained; laparoscopic biliary bypass is more difficult and is less attractive, and while laparoscopic cholecystojejunostomy may be easy technically, its long-term efficacy is less reliable.

## Indications for Laparoscopic Palliation

Indications for a laparoscopic biliary bypass are impending or complete biliary obstruction because of difficulty accessing the biliary tree endoscopically or transhepatically. If the surgeon chooses to proceed with a palliative procedure, then biliary palliation can be performed laparoscopically via a cholecystoenterostomy or hepaticoenterostomy. The choice depends greatly on the feasibility and technical ability of the surgeon. Some patients are not candidates for laparoscopic biliary drainage, such as patients with hilar obstruction. If biliary bypass is done using the gallbladder as the biliary conduit, there is a risk of future biliary obstruction at the cystic duct entrance.

The indications for duodenal bypass are even more restrictive, because less than 10% of patients have GOO at the time of presentation. Duodenal stents are an option but, if there are signs of impending GOO on imaging or by inspection laparoscopically, laparoscopic loop gastrojejunostomy is a safe, technically easy option.

Small, prospective, nonrandomized studies have reported the feasibility and efficacy of laparoscopic gastric and biliary bypass. An endolaparoscopic approach with endoscopically placed biliary stent and laparoscopic duodenal bypass is an option. Randomized control trials or larger prospective trials are required to determine superiority of routine laparoscopic biliary and gastric bypass when compared to double, endoluminal stenting (both biliary and duodenal).

## Technique—Laparoscopic Gastrojejunostomy

The patient is placed supine on the operating table. Three or four ports will assist with performing the procedure (Fig. 5.6). First, the decision is made to perform either an antecolic or retrocolic gastrojejunostomy. If antecolic, a loop of proximal jejunum is

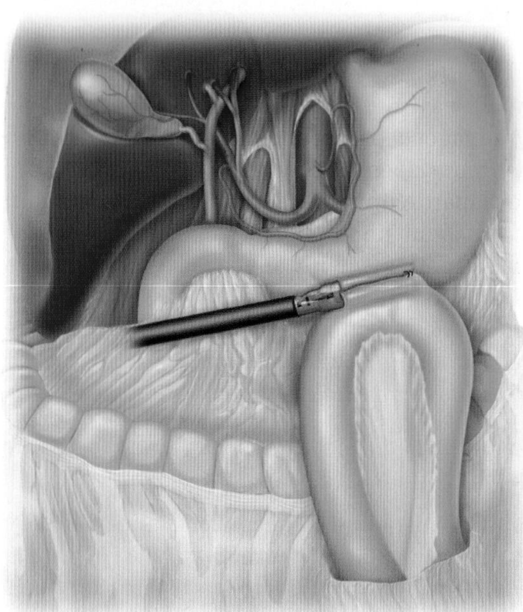

**Figure 5.6** Laparoscopic gastrojejunostomy. This anastomosis can be created most easily to the anterior surface of the stomach in an antecolic fashion by approximating the jejunum to the anterior surface of the stomach, making an enterotomy and inserting endoscopic gastrointestinal stapler. The enterostomy then can be closed with a reapplication of the stapler.

brought over the omentum and opposed to the anterior wall of the stomach; if necessary, the omentum can be split using the harmonic scalpel (Ethicon Endosurgery, Cincinnati, OH), Ligasure (Covidien, Mansfield, MA) or another form of energy. If a retrocolic anastomosis is chosen, access to the posterior wall of the stomach occurs through a rent created in the translucent part of the left transverse mesocolon with the harmonic scalpel or other form of energy. The lesser-sac can be entered through the gastrocolic ligament, or the posterior wall of the stomach pulled down through the mesocolic defect. The posterior aspect of the stomach away from the vasculature of the greater curve is sutured to a portion of jejunum 30 to 60 cm from the ligament of Treitz. This part can be done using an endostitch suturing device or via intracorporeal suturing. Using the harmonic scalpel, a gastrotomy and jejunotomy are performed, and a linear endoscopic stapler (60 mm length, 3.5 mm thickness) is introduced into the enterotomies to create a 60 mm long anastomosis. A sequential staple can be fired to lengthen the anastomosis if required. After inspecting the staple lines for bleeding, the now common enterotomy is either stapled closed or is oversewn, and a second, anterior layer of Lembert sutures can be placed. If retrocolic, the stomach near the anastomosis should be sewn to the mesocolic defect to prevent internal herniation. These procedure are easy, fast, and safe.

## Technique—Laparoscopic Cholecystojejunostomy

As mentioned previously, most surgeons do not recommend the routine use of a cholecystojejunostomy, because hepatico- or choledochojejunostomy results in superior long-term palliation of jaundice. Although a laparoscopic cholecystojejunostomy is more feasible technically, the laparoscopist should resist the urge to create a cholecystojejunostomy just because it is easier to do unless preoperative imaging confirms that the cystic duct entrance really is far away from the pancreatic neoplasm. On occasion, however, this procedure may be appropriate—multiple peritoneal or liver metastases, short-life expectancy, no indwelling biliary stent, and known appropriate biliary anatomy.

With laparoscopic cholecystojejunostomy, the goal is to create an anastomosis between the infundibulum of the gallbladder and a loop of jejunum. A minimum of three ports are needed to aid in the procedure. The first port is placed infraumbilically. The second port, if needed, is placed in the epigastric region to accommodate a liver retractor to expose the gallbladder; this port may be unnecessary if the gallbladder is

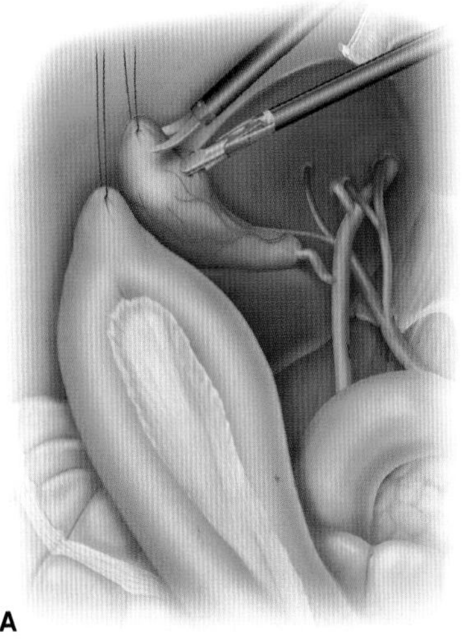
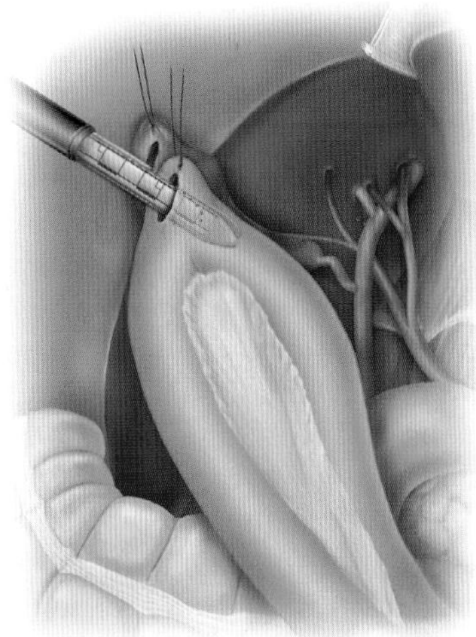
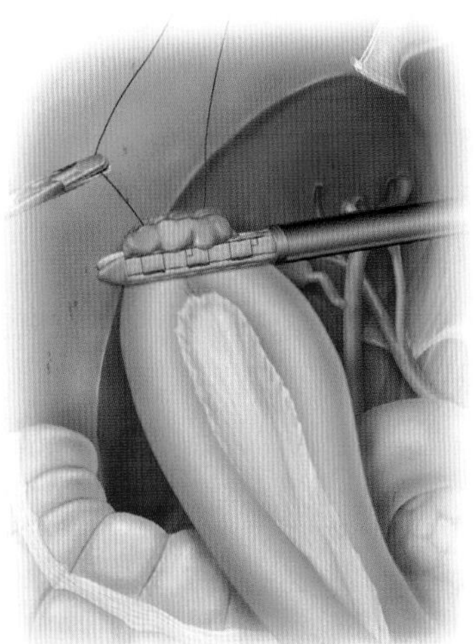

A

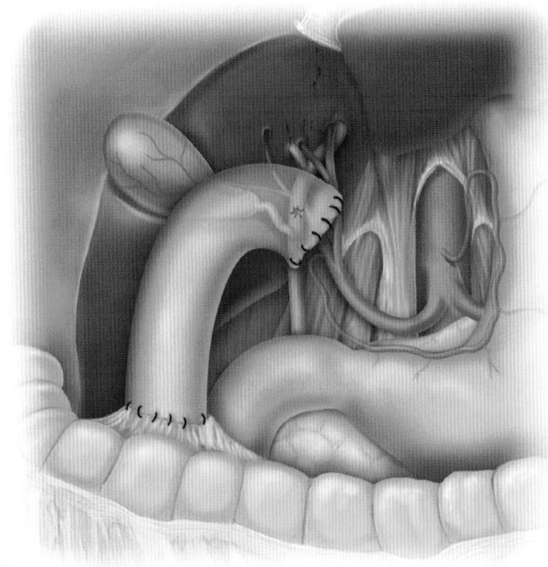

B

**Figure 5.7** Laparoscopic biliary bypass. (**A**) Laparoscopic cholecystojejunostomy. The gallbladder and the loop of jejunum brought antecolic are approximated, and then enterotomies made in each and an endoscopic stapler inserted, creating a stapled cholecystojejunostomy. The common enterotomy is then closed endoscopically. (**B**) Laparoscopic hepaticojejunostomy. This anastomosis requires advanced laparoscopic skills with hand-sewing of the Roux limb that should be mobilized and brought through the right transverse mesocolon and then by hand technique sewn to the common hepatic artery.

markedly distended. The third port is placed subcostally in the posterior clavicular line (10 to 12 mm) to accommodate a stapling device, and the fourth is placed in the left upper quadrant to assist in manipulation of the tissues (Fig. 5.7A). An aspirating needle is placed in the gallbladder to partially decompress the gallbladder if it is distended tensely. Using an atraumatic bowel grasper, a portion of jejunum, 40 to 60 cm from the ligament of Treitz is brought antecolic to the level of the infundibulum of the gallbladder. Using the harmonic scalpel, a cholecystotomy and jejunotomy are made and sutured together using intracorporeal interrupted sutures or via an endoluminal or laparoscopic stapler (45 mm length, 2.5 mm thickness). A single firing of the stapler should be adequate for patency. Closure of the common enterotomy can be made with a second tangentially placed stapler or with hand-sewn running sutures.

## Technique—Laparoscopic Hepaticoenterostomy

Laparoscopic anastomosis between the hepatic duct and either the duodenum or jejunum is a much more demanding procedure and requires advanced laparoscopic skills. Again, adequate palliation is usually available by endoscopic techniques precluding, at least currently, the need or indication for this type of a laparoscopic biliary drainage.

*Laparoscopic Hepaticoduodenostomy*: Several groups have reported this procedure. After exposing the anterior surface of the common hepatic duct and performing a limited Kocher maneuver, a single-layer anastomosis can be created using a hand-sewn technique; use of a stapler is not technically feasible with current devices. Port sites are similar to those for a cholecystojejunostomy. Cholecystectomy will increase the exposure to this area, especially if the gallbladder is distended markedly. Experience with this technique is limited; moreover, the technique requires more technical experience by the surgeon, and currently this approach is best reserved for selected situations.

*Laparoscopic hepaticojejunostomy*: As for laparoscopic hepaticoduodenostomy, the indications for this procedure should also be limited. Creation of a Roux limb laparoscopically and the subsequent enteroenterostomy are well-known, well-established technique for the bariatric surgeon, but the hepaticojejunal anastomosis, while feasible, can be a technically demanding procedure despite a dilated extrahepatic biliary tree. Again, port sites are similar as for the above procedures. A Roux limb is created 60 to 100 cm distal to the ligament of Treitz or 40 to 60 cm distal to the site planned for a gastrojejunostomy. As with open hepaticojejunostomy, a retrocolic approach through the right mesocolon the shortest, most direct routine. Similarly, a Roux limb is much less bulky and easier to work with than a jejunal loop. After opposing the Roux limb with the common hepatic duct (a cholecystectomy will facilitate the exposure), a hepatic ductotomy and jejunotomy are made, and the anastomosis is made using a one-layer hand-sewn technique (Fig. 5.7B). The defect in the mesocolon is obliterated, and a jejunojejunostomy is created about 40 to 60 cm distal to the hepaticojejunostomy. Again, while feasible for the accomplished laparoscopic surgeon, this procedure should be used in highly selected patients and is not recommended currently as the routine form of operative palliation of extrahepatic biliary obstruction, even if a robotic system is available.

# Other Potential Palliative Procedures

## "Palliative" Pancreatectomy

While potentially arguable by the zealots, there appears to be no justifiable role for a truly "prophylactic" proximal pancreatectomy (pancreatoduodenectomy) and especially for a distal pancreatectomy in the typical patient with unresectable-for-cure, ductal adenocarcinoma or intraductal papillary mucinous neoplasm (IPMN). The authors caution the reader to be careful when reading the literature claiming the benefits of "prophylactic pancreatectomy." Most times, these articles have reviewed the outcomes of patients who were explored for resection, deemed "resectable" on local clinical findings at operation, and after undergoing what was thought to be a curative resection are only then found to have either R-1 or R-2 disease. In these patients, the surgeon did not really carry out a premeditated, "palliative" pancreatectomy. This situation happens from 15% to 70% of the time after a pancreatoduodenectomy, depending on your definition of "R-1 disease;" for R-2 disease, the occurrence is less common, but still approaches 10%, usually related to residual disease at the uncinate margin not amenable to removal with a portal or superior mesenteric vein resection or the pathologic presence of a peritoneal metastasis having gone unnoticed.

The authors believe that there is no evidence to support the practice of a truly "palliative" pancreatoduodenectomy or "palliative" distal pancreatectomy for ductal adenocarcinoma or for IPMN; i.e., patients know to have incurable disease (liver or peritoneal metastases, distant nodal metastases, or local unresectable invasion). While several anecdotal reports have surfaced entertaining pancreatic resection with metastasectomy for localized distant disease (liver metastases) for ductal adenocarcinoma of the pancreas, the reader is cautioned to remember that no evidence-based work (or even suggestion of benefit) is available as yet. Evidence-based arguments can potentially be made for islet cell neoplasms or other neoplasms that are more responsive to chemotherapy, especially if they release vasoactive or hormonal products that cause systemic problems or extensive local involvement of the celiac axis/paraaortic nodes, but not for typical ductal adenocarcinoma or IPMN in these authors' opinions. There is no justification in the literature, and this practice, at least currently with our nonoperative treatment modalities, cannot be condoned.

### Local Ablative Palliation

With improvements in tumor response to palliative chemotherapy, an interest has emerged recently in the possibility of local ablative techniques (alcohol ablation, cryoablation, radiofrequency ablation, and even again, intraoperative radiation therapy) in an attempt to provide debulking for a longer-term survival in patients with locally advanced but unresectable disease. Currently, these techniques should be considered experimental and not state-of-the-art; however, with further improvements in palliative chemotherapy and radiation therapy or in patients who experience a marked response to chemoradiation therapy, these techniques may offer some advantages, especially if these newer approaches of aggressive palliation can be carried out with a minimal access approach. Need for a full celiotomy just to trial these techniques cannot be condoned outside of formal clinical trial until good evidenced-based data are available.

There is an increasing role of MIS in treating hepatobiliopancreatic malignancies. The role for these MIS approaches is limited by the surgeon's technical abilities, and we do not advice routine use of these procedures unless a surgeon has adequate experience. Data is limited in the application of MIS in palliative surgery warranting more studies in the area.

## Acknowledgments

Dr. Reid Lombardo was funded by Grant Number 1 UL1 RR024150 from the National Center for Research Resources (NCRR), a component of the National Institutes of Health (NIH), and the NIH Roadmap for Medical Research. Its contents are solely the responsibility of the authors and do not necessarily represent the official view of NCRR or NIH. Information on NCRR is available at http://www.ncrr.nih.gov/. Information on Reengineering the Clinical Research Enterprise can be obtained from http://nihroadmap.nih.gov.

### Recommended References and Readings

Ghanem AM, Hamade AM, Sheen AJ, et al. Laparoscopic gastric and biliary bypass: a single-center cohort prospective study. *J Laparendosc Adv Surg Tech A.* 2006;16:21–26.

Kuhlmann KFD, van Poll D, de Castro SMM, et al. Initial and long-term outcome after palliative surgical drainage of 269 patients with malignant biliary obstruction. *Eur J Surg Oncol.* 2007;33:757–762.

Lillemoe KD, Barnes SA. Surgical palliation of unresectable pancreatic carcinoma. *Surg Clin N Am.* 1995;75:953–968.

Lillemoe KD, Cameron JL, Hardacre JM, et al. Is prophylactic gastrojejunostomy indicated for unresectable periampullary cancer? A prospective randomized trial. *Ann Surg.* 1999;230:322–328.

Lillemoe KD, Cameron JL, Kaufman HS, et al. Chemical splanchnicectomy in patients with unresectable pancreatic cancer: a prospective randomized trial. *Ann Surg.* 1993;217:447–455.

Nagorney DM, Edis AJ. A use of the stapler in pancreatic surgery. *Am J Surg.* 1981;142:384–385.

Neuberger TJ, Wade TP, Swope TJ, et al. Palliative operations for pancreatic cancer in the hospitals of the U.S. Department of Veterans Affairs from 1987 to 1991. *Am J Surg.* 1993;166:632–636.

Sarfeh IJ, Rypins EB, Jakowatz JG, et al. A prospective, randomized clinical investigation of cholecystoenterostomy and choledochoenterostomy. *Am J Surg.* 1998;155:411–414.

Sarr MG, Cameron JL. Surgical palliation of unresectable carcinoma of the pancreas. *World J Surg.* 1984;8:906–918.

Sarr MG, Lillemoe KD, Singh B, et al. Denervation: pain management. In: Clavien P-A, Sarr MG, Fong Y, eds. Atlas of Upper Gastrointestinal and Hepato-Pancreato-Biliary Surgery. Heidelberg: Springer Verlag GmbH & Co., KG, 2007;745–751.

Shibamoto Y, Manabe T, Ohshio G, et al. High-dose intraoperaive radiotherapy for unresectable pancreatic cancer. *Int J Radiatioin Oncology Biol Phys.* 1996;34:57–63.

Spiliotis JD, Datsis AC, Michalopoulos NV, et al. Radiofrequency ablation combined with palliative surgery may prolong survival of patients with advanced cancer of the pancreas. *Langenbecks Arch Surg.* 2007;392:55–60.

Stuart M, Keo T, Hermann RE, et al. Palliation of malignant obstruction of the common bile duct by side to side choledochoduodenostomy. *Am J Surg.* 1971;121:505–509.

Tinoco R, El-Kadre L, Tinoco A. Laparoscopic choledochoduodenostomy. *J Laparoendosc Adv Surg Tech A.* 199:9:123–126.

van Hooft JE, Uitdehaag MJ, Bruno MJ, et al. Efficacy and safety of the new WallFlex enteral stent in palliative treatment of malignant gastric outlet obstruction (DUOFLEX study): a prospective multicenter study. *Gastrointest Endosc.* 2009;69:1059–1066.

# 6 Central Pancreatectomy

**Cristina R. Ferrone, Carlos Fernández-del Castillo, and Andrew L. Warshaw**

##  INDICATIONS/CONTRAINDICATIONS

Central pancreatectomy provides patients and surgeons an alternative to an extended pancreatic resection or enucleation of lesions located in the neck or body of the pancreas (Fig. 6.1). Central pancreatectomy was first described by Guillemin and Bessot in 1957 and was first performed for a neoplasm by Dagradi and Serio in 1984. The procedure was popularized in North America by Warshaw et al. after publishing their experience of 12 middle pancreatectomies for 7 cystic lesions, 4 neuroendocrine tumors and 1 intraductal papillary mucinous tumor. Segmental resection has been adopted by many for benign or borderline lesions, focal chronic pancreatitis, and trauma. If a central pancreatectomy is not performed, lesions located in the mid portion of the pancreas would require an aggressive surgical resection, such as an extended pancreaticoduodenectomy or extended distal pancreatectomy. The main advantage of central pancreatectomy compared to an extended resection is the ability to conserve more pancreatic parenchyma, thereby preserving exocrine and endocrine function. The long-term incidence of new onset diabetes mellitus ranges from 50% to 57% of patients undergoing distal pancreatectomy in comparison with 11% for patients undergoing central pancreatectomy. Exocrine insufficiency requiring enzymes occurs in 27% of patients undergoing distal pancreatectomy as opposed to 10% of patients undergoing central pancreatectomy. An additional advantage is the preservation of normal upper gastrointestinal and biliary anatomy. Central pancreatectomy also assures preservation of the spleen. Splenic preservation not only decreases operative duration, morbidity and length of stay, but also reduces the risk of post splenectomy sepsis, malignancy, and reactive thrombocytosis which can result in a myocardial infarction. While enucleation of a pancreatic lesion also preserves pancreatic parenchyma and upper gastrointestinal anatomy, it can result in disruption or compromise of the pancreatic duct. We do not recommend a central pancreatectomy for patients with ductal adenocarcinoma due to potentially inadequate elimination of the relevant lymphatic drainage. Adequate lymph node dissection is essential for accurate staging of patients with malignant lesions and may influence their long-term survival.

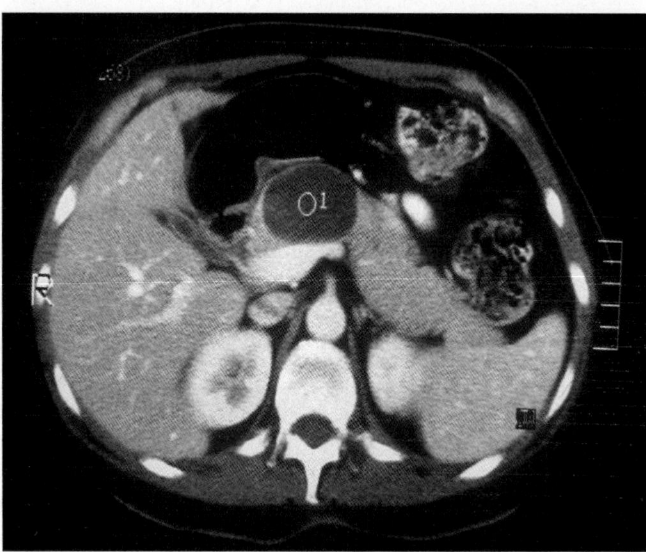


**Figure 6.1** Cystic lesion in the neck of the pancreas.

Important points to evaluate when considering a central pancreatectomy are as follows.

1. The lesion should be benign or borderline (pathologic frozen section at the time of surgery is essential to assure that the margins are free of tumor).
2. The lesion should be located in the neck or proximal body of the pancreas.
3. Enucleation is an undesirable option if the main pancreatic duct is close and likely to be disrupted.
4. The distal pancreatic stump should be at least 6 cm in length to make its conservation worthwhile.

## PREOPERATIVE PLANNING

Abdominopelvic contrast-enhanced computed tomography (CECT) or magnetic resonance cholangiopancreatography (MRCP) should be performed for preoperative evaluation. These imaging studies are essential to determine the anatomic relationship of the neoplasm to the pancreatic duct, portal vein, superior mesenteric vein, superior mesenteric artery, common hepatic artery, and splenic vessels. Understanding the relationship of the lesion to these landmarks is essential to determine if a central pancreatectomy is the appropriate operation and to performing a safe operation.

For patients in whom the precise diagnosis of the pancreatic neoplasm is unclear, an endoscopic ultrasound with fine-needle aspiration may be desirable. The fine-needle aspirate will provide tissue to make a histologic diagnosis, while the endoscopic ultrasound assists in outlining anatomic landmarks.

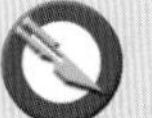

## SURGICAL TECHNIQUE

The pancreatic lesion needs to be deemed resectable. Therefore, the lesion needs to be evaluated relative to pertinent anatomical landmarks as noted above. Central pancreatectomy is only recommended for benign or borderline lesions; therefore vascular involvement or adjacent organ invasion should be absent. For a central pancreatectomy to be worth this added effort and risk of complications, the distal pancreas should

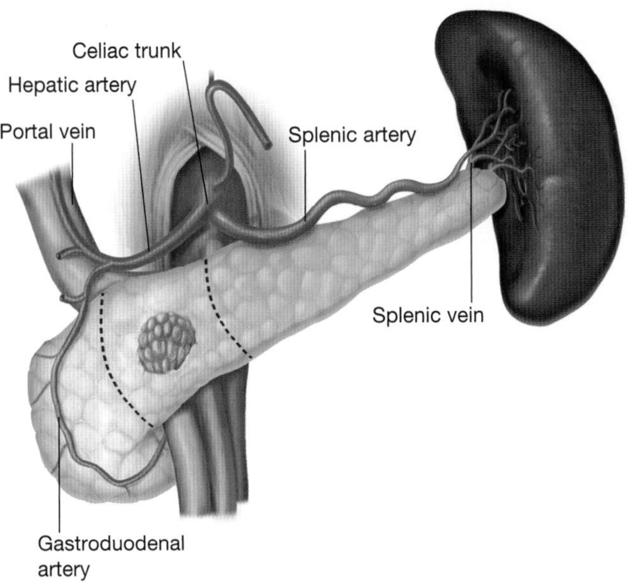


**Figure 6.2** Pancreatic lesion in the neck of the pancreas.

measure at least 6 cm in length to ensure adequate length for an anastomosis and to add significant endocrine and exocrine capacity over what would be lost with a distal resection.

## Positioning

The patient is placed in the supine position with both arms out. All patients should have adequate intravenous access, a Foley catheter, deep venous thrombosis prophylaxis and receive appropriate antibiotic prophylaxis, depending on the individual's allergies.

## Technique

An upper midline incision is made from the xiphoid to the umbilicus. The abdomen is inspected to rule out metastatic disease or any other pathologies. The gastrocolic omentum is divided outside the gastroepiploic vessels, and the lesser sac is entered. The stomach is retracted cephalad and the transverse colon and omentum caudad. Adhesions in the lesser sac are lysed. The neck, body, and tail of the pancreas will then be visible (Fig. 6.2). The peritoneum along the superior and inferior borders of the pancreas is incised, and the pancreatic neck is mobilized. The relationship of the lesion to the portal vein, superior mesenteric artery and vein, and the common hepatic artery must be clarified (Fig. 6.3). Attention must be given not to avulse branches between the

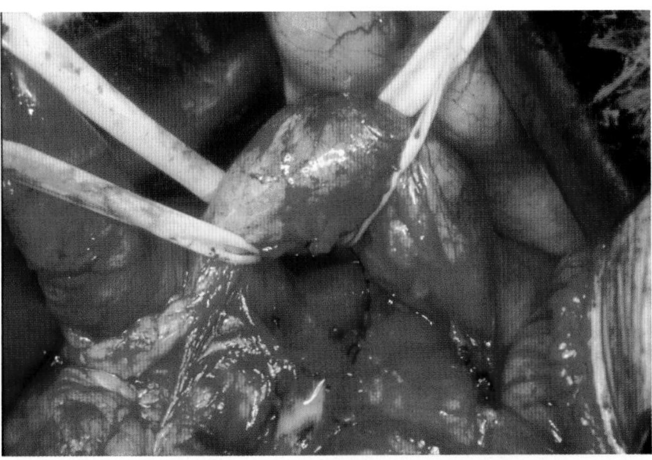

**Figure 6.3** Cystic lesion in the neck of the pancreas being retracted between the two penrose drains. The pancreas has been separated from the uninterrupted splenic artery and vein.

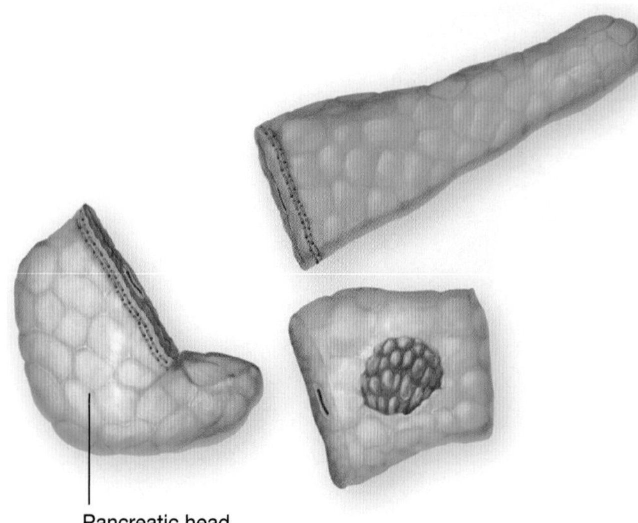


Figure 6.4 Proximal pancreatic neck is stapled and the distal pancreas is transected, leaving the splenic vessels intact.

splenic artery or vein and the pancreas; careful ligation of some of these branches may be required for adequate mobilization of this pancreatic segment. Usually the splenic vessels can be preserved. If this is not possible, we either suture ligate or staple the splenic vessels and rely on the short gastric vessels for splenic perfusion.

1. Once the area of the pancreas containing the lesion is mobilized, the proximal pancreas is transected with a stapler (Fig. 6.4). Depending on the thickness of the pancreas, we utilize either a 3.5 mm staple or 4.8 mm staple cartridge which is 60 mm in length. Bioabsorbable staple line reinforcement can be utilized, but we have not found that it decreases the risk of a pancreatic fistula. Before transecting the pancreas distal to the lesion, we place two simple stay sutures to control the vascular supply along the superior and inferior pancreatic margins. The pancreas is then transected with either a scalpel or electrocautery. The specimen is sent for frozen section to confirm the diagnosis and to confirm negative margins. We drain the distal pancreas either into the stomach (pancreaticogastrostomy) or into the jejunum (Roux-en-y pancreaticojejunostomy)—see later. Some surgeons describe ligation of the pancreatic duct in the remnant body/tail and over-sewing the transected pancreas by imbricating the pancreatic capsule but the risk of persistent pancreatic fistula is substantial. We utilize this technique only if the pancreatic stump measures less than 4 cm in length.

## Management of the Pancreatic Remnant

A. Our preferred technique is a pancreaticogastrostomy (Figs. 6.5 and 6.6). Pancreaticogastrostomy requires the pancreatic body to be mobilized off the splenic vessels

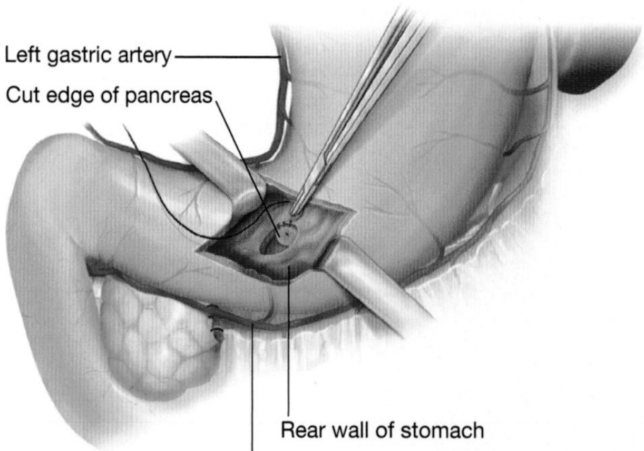


Figure 6.5 Pancreaticogastrostomy through the anterior wall of the stomach.

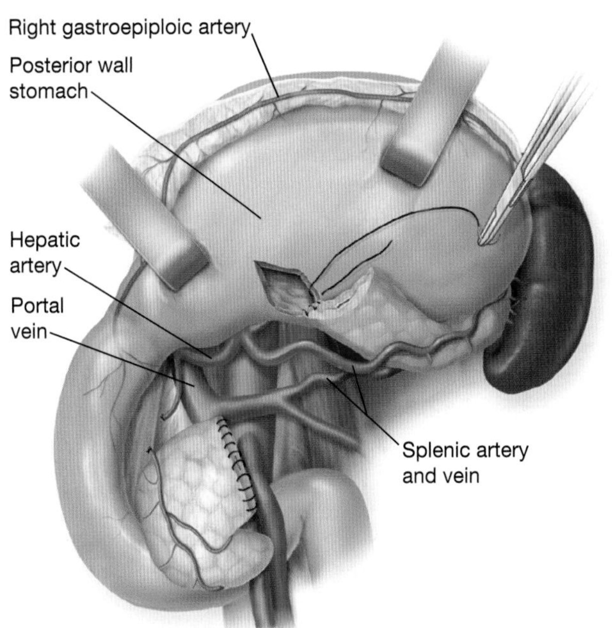


Figure 6.6 Pancreaticogastrostomy to posterior wall of the stomach.

for a distance of approximately 2 to 3 cm by dividing and ligating the communicating vascular branches. This additional mobilization facilitates the rotation of the stump anteriorly into the stomach. Anterior and posterior gastrostomies are made so that the pancreatic stump can be delivered into the stomach without tension. Either running or interrupted full thickness bites are taken through the posterior gastric wall and the capsule of the pancreas with 3-0 polydioxanone (PDS; Ethicon; Johnson & Johnson) or silk suture. The anterior gastrotomy is then closed in two layers with running 3-0 PDS followed by interrupted 3-0 silk suture. A round 19 Blake or Jackson-Pratt drain is then placed next to the anastomosis and the pancreatic stump. The abdomen is closed according to the surgeon's preference.

B. An alternative approach for the remnant pancreas is a pancreaticojejunal anastomosis (Fig. 6.7). A Roux-en-Y jejunal limb is created by transecting the jejunum 15 to 20 cm distal to the ligament of Treitz. A limb of jejunum approximately 40 cm long is passed through the mesocolon to the remnant pancreas. Jejunal continuity is

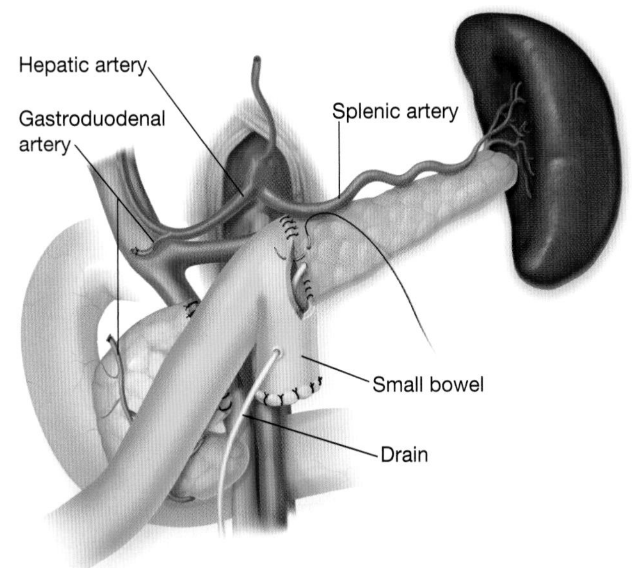


Figure 6.7 Pancreaticojejeunostomy to a roux-en-y loop of jejeunum.

restored with a jejunojejunostomy below the mesocolon. An end-to-side duct-to-mucosa pancreaticojejunostomy is constructed in two layers. The posterior row of interrupted seromuscular bites on the jejunum and the pancreatic capsule are made with 3-0 silk or PDS suture. A small enterotomy opposite the pancreatic duct is made in the jejunum. The pancreatic duct and the mucosa, including the seromuscular wall of the jejunum, are approximated with interrupted sutures of 5-0 vicryl (polyglactin 910; Ethicon; Johnson & Johnson) or PDS. A 5-french pediatric feeding tube is left through the anastomosis into the pancreatic duct and brought out through a tunnel in the jejunal loop. This tube functions as a stent, but probably more important, it assures that the duct cannot be inadvertently obstructed by the sutures of the duct-to-mucosa anastomosis (especially when the pancreatic duct is small/normal). The tube is anchored to the jejunum with a 2-0 chromic purse-string suture. The anastomosis is completed with an anterior row of 3-0 PDS or silk to appose the pancreatic capsule to the seromuscular layers of the jejunum. A round Blake or Jackson-Pratt drain is then placed next to the anastomosis and the pancreatic stump. The abdomen is closed according to the surgeon's preference.

C. A second anastomosis between the proximal pancreas and the jejunal limb may be desirable if the proximal pancreas is too thick to allow a secure staple line closure or turn-in, or if there is concern for a proximal pancreatic duct stricture. Performing a second jejunal anastomosis utilizing the same Roux loop will provide the pancreatic head with an alternative outflow and perhaps obviate a pancreatic fistula. This anastomosis is performed as has been described above, or a larger enterotomy can be created in the jejunal limb, and the remnant can be invaginated into the jejunum. This requires either running or interrupted full- thickness jejunal bites with 3-0 PDS or silk suture to the pancreatic capsule, the same drain can serve both anastomoses.

## POSTOPERATIVE MANAGEMENT

A nasogastric tube is placed at the time of the operation and is removed on postoperative day (POD) #1. Patients are started clear liquids after removal of the nasogastric tube, and the diet is advanced as tolerated, usually by POD#4. The drain output and amylase are evaluated on POD#4. The drain is removed if the amylase is less than 300 units/liter, no matter what the volume of output is, or if the amylase is high and the drain output is less than 30 cc/24 hours. If these two criteria are not met, the patient is discharged with the drain in place. If a pediatric feeding tube has been placed in the pancreatic duct, the patient is discharged with the tube in place. Patients return on POD #21 to have the tube removed.

## COMPLICATIONS

Postoperative pancreatic fistula is the most common complication after this operation, with rates ranging from 25% to 35%. Most of these fistulas are grade A fistulas requiring only continued drainage until spontaneous healing and closure. Occasionally patients will require an additional percutaneous drain (grade B) or another operation (grade C) to address the fistula. Postoperative hemorrhage from a splenic vessel pseudoaneurysm is almost unheard of if the main splenic artery has not been transected, leaving a vulnerable vascular stump.

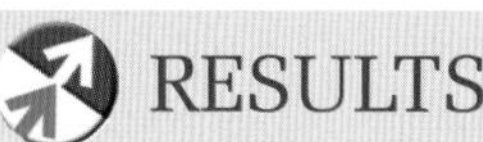

## RESULTS

Central pancreatectomy will result in removal of a benign or borderline lesion with negative margins in most patients. The most common indications include cystic lesions of the pancreas and neuroendocrine lesions. Several series of central pancreatectomies

**TABLE 6.1 Published Series of Central Pancreatectomy**

| Authors | Patients (N) | Complications N (%) | Fistula N (%) | Mortality N (%) | Follow-up (months) |
|---|---|---|---|---|---|
| Rotman et al. 1993 | 14 | 4 (29%) | 2 (14%) | 0 | 36 |
| Ikeda et al. 1995 | 24 | 3 (13%) | 0 | 0 | 40 |
| Sauvanet et al. 2002 | 53 | 22 (41%) | 16 (30%) | 1 (2%) | 26 |
| Warshaw et al. 1998 | 12 | 3 (25%) | 2 (16.7%) | 0 | 18 |
| Goldstein et al. 2004 | 12 | 3 (25%) | 0 | 0 | 20 |
| Efron et al. 2004 | 14 | 7 (50%) | 5 (36%) | 0 | 12 |
| Iacono et al. 2005 | 20 | 7 (35%) | 5 (25%) | 0 | 0 |
| Crippa et al. 2007 | 100 | 58 (58%) | 44 (44%) | 0 | 54 |
| Adham et al. 2008 | 50 | 18 (36%) | 4 (8%) | 0 | 68 |
| LaFemina et al. 2010 | 23 | 16 (70%) | 6 (26%) | 0 | 13 |

have been published (Table 6.1). Postoperative complications occur in 13% to 70% of patients, with pancreatic fistula rates ranging from 8% to 44%. Although the median length of stay for patients undergoing central pancreatectomy is longer than for those undergoing extended left pancreatectomies, the rate of endocrine and exocrine insufficiency is significantly lower. Endocrine insufficiency after a central pancreatectomy ranges from 4% to 11%. The incidence of clinically apparent exocrine insufficiency is reported to be 3% to 10% of patients.

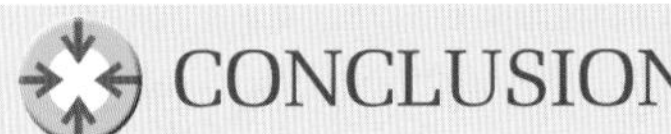

## CONCLUSIONS

Central pancreatectomy is a safe operation which should be considered for patients with benign or borderline lesions located in the neck or proximal body of the pancreas. This technique allows for maximal sparing of normal pancreatic parenchyma, thereby preserving endocrine and exocrine function of the pancreas.

## Recommended References and Readings


Crippa S, Bassi C, Warshaw AL, et al. Middle pancreatectomy: indications, short- and long-term operative outcomes. *Ann Surg.* 2007;246:69–76.

Iacono C, Bortolasi L, Serio G. Indications and technique of central pancreatectomy-early and late results. *Langenbecks Arch Surg.* 2005;390:266–271.

LaFemina J, Vagefi PA, Warshaw AL, et al. Transgastric pancreaticogastric anastomosis: an alternative operative approach for middle pancreatectomy. *Arch Surg.* 2010;145(5):476–481.

Roggin KK, Rudloff U, Blumgart LH, et al. Central pancreatectomy revisited. *J Gastrointest Surg.* 2006;10:804–812.

Warshaw AL, Rattner DW, Fernandez-del Castillo C, et al. Middle segment pancreatectomy: a novel technique for conserving pancreatic tissue. *Arch Surg.* 1998;133:327–331.

# 7 Total Pancreatectomy

**Michael L. Kendrick and Michael B. Farnell**

## Introduction

Total pancreatectomy (TP) in both benign and malignant pancreatic disease remains an acceptable alternative in selected patients. Whereas the significant operative sequela and morbidity of this procedure has limited general enthusiasm, increasingly aggressive diabetic management, pancreatic enzyme replacement, surgical techniques, and auto islet cell transplantation continue to spark interest for TP.

In theory, a more radical operation would be expected to provide a more favorable outcome with regard to disease such as intractable pain from chronic pancreatitis or disease free survival after resection of malignancy. In practice, however, superior outcomes have not been consistently demonstrated in cohort studies and Level I evidence does not exist. The treatment of intractable pain in patients with chronic pancreatitis, recurrent acute pancreatitis, and pancreatic malignancy, remains challenging with either medical or surgical approaches and the search for methods to improve outcomes continues. In selected patients, TP appears to be a valid and occasionally necessary alternative and indications may be expanding. Several series have demonstrated increasingly favorable outcomes of TP with appropriate patient selection, surgical technique, and postoperative care.

The potential advantages of TP include:

- Elimination of pancreatic leak from the pancreatic remnant observed after partial pancreatectomy.
- Amelioration or elimination of intractable pain in recurrent or chronic pancreatitis.
- Elimination of recurrent disease such as pancreatitis or intraductal papillary mucinous neoplasm (IPMN).
- Avoidance of parenchymal transection with potential tumor spillage in malignancy.
- Negates the need for surveillance imaging for potentially recurrent disease of the remnant pancreas.

Disadvantages of TP include complete pancreatic exocrine and endocrine insufficiency as well as the morbidity of the procedure itself. Diabetes after TP may result in considerable morbidity as "brittle diabetes" sets the stage for difficult diabetic management where readmission for hypoglycemic episodes and suboptimal nutrition are not uncommon. With the lack of a pancreatic anastomosis, one would also expect reduced perioperative morbidity compared to partial pancreatectomy. In most series, however,

**TABLE 7.1 Possible Indications for Total Pancreatectomy**

- Chronic pancreatitis with intractable pain or recurrent acute pancreatitis
- Hereditary pancreatitis
- Diffuse main-duct intraductal papillary mucinous neoplasm
- Diffuse branch-duct intraductal papillary mucinous neoplasm
- Recurrent pancreatic neoplasm after partial pancreatectomy
- Intrapancreatic extension of localized pancreatic malignancy preventing R0 resection with partial pancreatectomy
- Technical factors or intraoperative complications after partial pancreatectomy

morbidity after TP ranges from 40% to 60% and is comparable to that observed in partial pancreatectomy and historically, mortality has been higher than for pancreaticoduodenectomy.

## INDICATIONS/CONTRAINDICATIONS

Indications for TP are listed in Table 7.1. For benign disease such as chronic or recurrent acute pancreatitis, the indication for TP may include relief of intractable pain or prevention of recurrent pancreatitis. In hereditary pancreatitis, TP prevents recurrent pancreatitis and addresses the potential increased risk of pancreatic adenocarcinoma in these patients. In a premalignant condition such as IPMN, TP may be warranted when the disease is diffuse and is considered high risk for malignancy such as in main-duct and multicentric large (>3 cm) branch-duct disease. In addition, completion TP may be indicated for recurrent neoplasm after previous partial pancreatectomy. Whereas the need for TP in the setting of pancreatic adenocarcinoma is uncommon, a completion pancreatectomy to achieve an R0 resection has gained general acceptance. Local factors may occasionally warrant TP for resection of pancreatic neoplasms such as tumor size, location, and presence of marked atrophy of the body and tail with preoperative pancreatic insufficiency. Completion pancreatectomy may also be indicated for management of complications after partial pancreatectomy or to address recurrent neoplasia in the remnant pancreas.

## PREOPERATIVE PLANNING

Patients with indications for TP should be screened for prohibitive comorbidities and have an appropriate cardiopulmonary evaluation based on a thorough history and physical examination. Existing comorbidities such as hypertension, diabetes, and cardiopulmonary conditions should be adequately assessed and optimized prior to TP. Appropriate selection of patients for TP also includes assessment of the patient's ability to comprehend the implications of complete pancreatic endocrine and exocrine insufficiency, and ability to follow the nutritional recommendations and comply with necessary treatment. Ideally, the patient should receive diabetes education preoperatively which facilitates the assessment of patient understanding, may identify compliance issues and enhances the education process in the postoperative period. The patient should also be vaccinated against common encapsulated bacteria (*Streptococcus pneumoniae, Haemophilus influenzae,* and *Neisseria Meningitidis*) 2 weeks preoperatively when splenectomy is anticipated and should be educated regarding the entity of postsplenectomy sepsis. The anesthesiologist should be alerted to the need for intraoperative glucose monitoring and continuous infusion of insulin. Prophylactic (<24 hours) antibiotics and deep venous thrombosis prophylaxis are used routinely.

# SURGICAL TECHNIQUE

## Positioning and Exposure

The patient is positioned supine with arms padded and tucked at their side (preferred) or at 90 degrees. A fixed retractor is positioned to allow bilateral cephalad retraction of the costal margins.

An initial right subcostal or limited upper midline incision is made. A thorough exploration is performed focusing on all peritoneal and visceral surfaces. In the absence of metastatic disease, the subcostal incision is extended to the left. The subcostal retractors are placed and secured to the frame of the fixed retraction system chosen. To maximize the exposure, the inferior abdominal wall flap is secured with a heavy suture to the inferior abdominal wall. Initial dissection is performed to identify evidence of any local findings that would preclude resection. Mobilization of the hepatic flexure of the colon optimizes exposure for kocherization and the eventual distal duodenal dissection. A full kocherization of the duodenum is then performed, extending medially to the aorta (Fig. 7.1). This maneuver allows assessment of the pancreatic head and exclusion of retroperitoneal extension of inflammation or tumor. The left hand is placed around the pancreatic head and the tips of the fingers assess for involvement of the superior mesenteric artery (SMA). In the current era of improved CT imaging, these maneuvers will rarely identify evidence of local unresectability, however, they optimize initial exposure and allow improved control needed during dissection of the superior mesenteric and portal vein. Careful inspection of the lesser sac is performed to exclude peritoneal metastases and assess for adjacent organ involvement by inflammation or malignancy. The omentum is dissected off the transverse colon in the avascular plane and the lesser sac is widely exposed (Fig. 7.2). With the anterior surface of the pancreas exposed, the avascular attachments between the stomach and pancreas are divided. The middle colic vein is followed to the superior mesenteric vein (SMV) and the gastrocolic venous trunk is identified, ligated, and divided (Fig. 7.3A). This allows safe exposure of the SMV and the inferior border of the pancreas. The middle colic vein is occasionally divided on the basis of necessary exposure or suspected proximity to tumor. Retraction of the colon inferiorly without division of the gastrocolic trunk can lead to inadvertent avulsion and

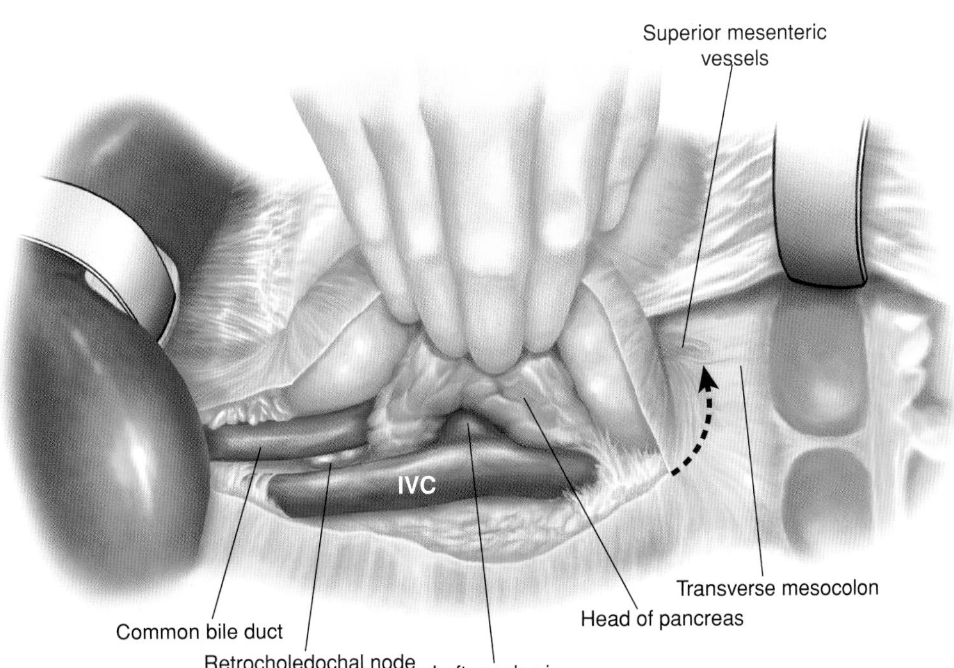


**Figure 7.1** The hepatic flexure of the right colon is released inferiorly to aid in performing a Kocher maneuver, which elevates the duodenum and the head of the pancreas (view from right lateral side of the patient). IVC, inferior vena cava. Adapted from illustrations by David Factor from "The Role of Total Pancreatectomy in the Treatment of Pancreatic Cancer" **Pancreatic Cancer,** edited by Von Hoff, Evans and Hruban, 2005. By permission of Mayo Foundation for Medical Education and Research. 

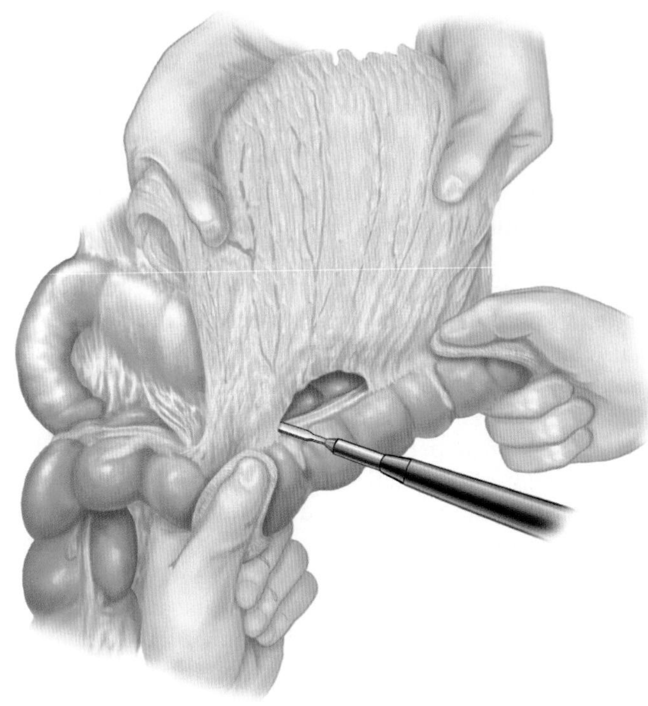

Figure 7.2 The lesser sac is entered by freeing the greater omentum off the transverse colon. Adapted from illustrations by David Factor from "The Role of Total Pancreatectomy in the Treatment of Pancreatic Cancer" **Pancreatic Cancer,** edited by Von Hoff, Evans and Hruban, 2005. By permission of Mayo Foundation for Medical Education and Research. 

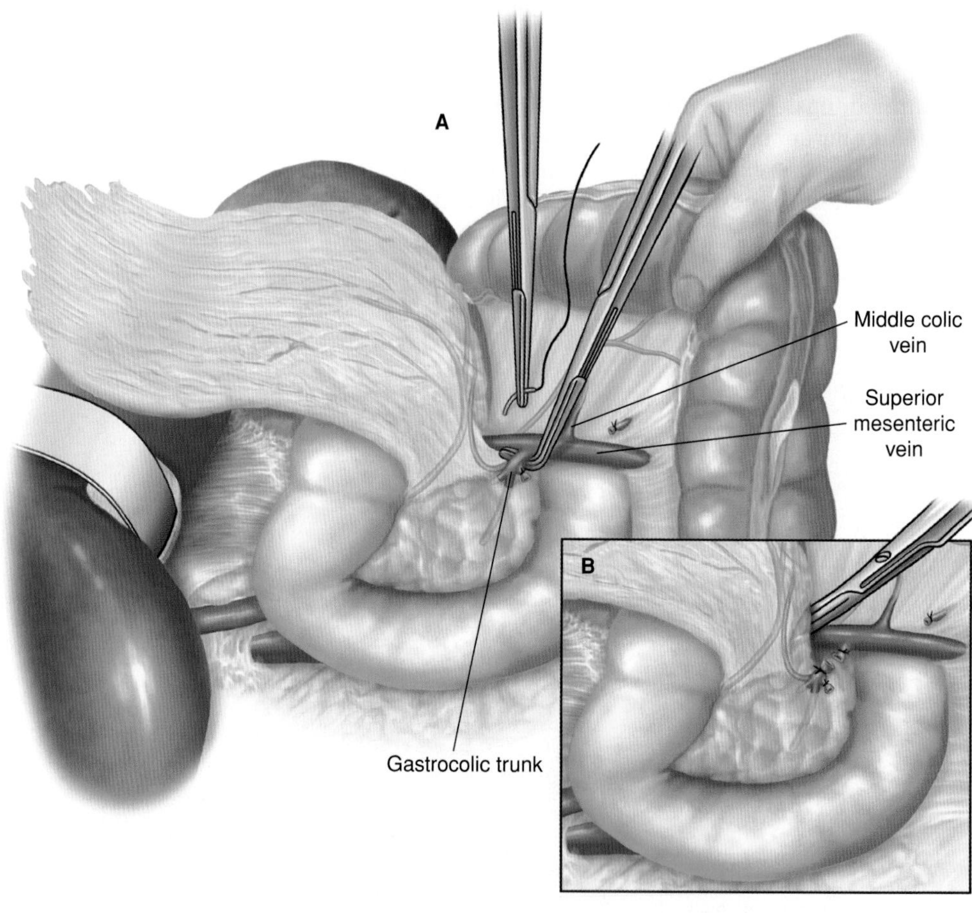


Figure 7.3 (**A**) The anterior and lateral exposure to the superior mesenteric vein is facilitated by ligation of the gastrocolic venous trunk. (**B**) Careful dissection with a blunt clamp anterior to the superior mesenteric vein/portal vein confluence aids in assessing the relationship of the neck of the pancreas to the vein (view from right lateral side of the patient). Adapted from illustrations by David Factor from "The Role of Total Pancreatectomy in the Treatment of Pancreatic Cancer" **Pancreatic Cancer,** edited by Von Hoff, Evans and Hruban, 2005. By permission of Mayo Foundation for Medical Education and Research. 

bleeding. If bleeding is encountered during dissection or ligation of the gastrocolic trunk, the left hand placed posterior to the pancreatic head with the thumb anteriorly will allow direct compression of the SMV to control hemorrhage and facilitate venorrhaphy.

With the gastrocolic trunk divided, the SMV can easily be followed to the inferior border of the pancreas. A curved, blunt clamp is used to develop the plane between the SMV and the posterior aspect of the pancreatic neck (Fig. 7.3B). The clamp should advance easily. Difficulty in passing the clamp posterior to the neck of the pancreas should prompt consideration of malignant invasion or significant inflammatory involvement of the superior mesenteric or portal vein. After an initial assessment of the pancreatic neck from the inferior approach, assessment at the superior aspect is performed. The gastrohepatic ligament is incised and the right gastric artery ligated and divided (Fig. 7.4A). The common hepatic artery is dissected at the

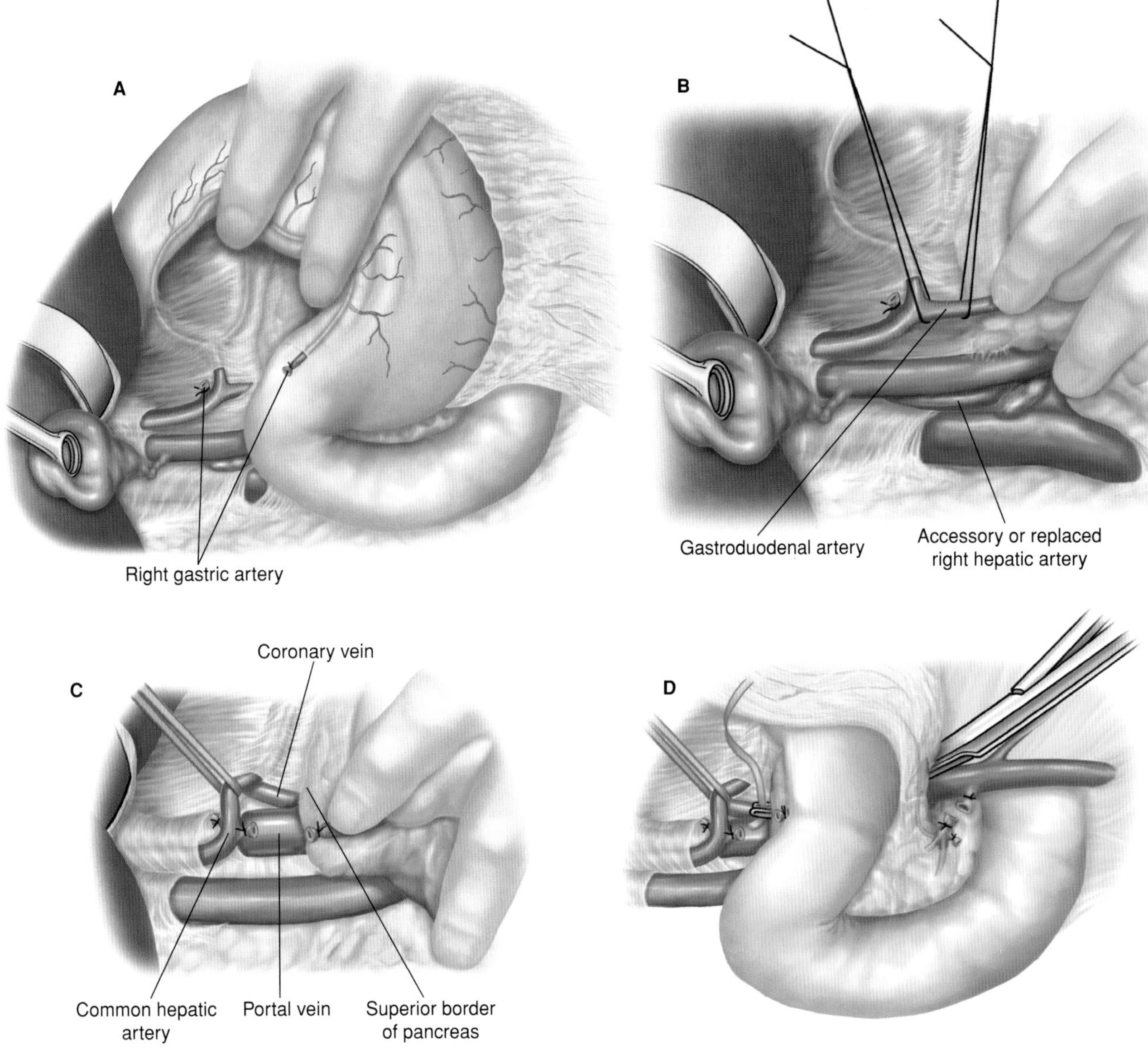


Figure 7.4 (**A**) Placement of inferior traction on the lesser curvature of the stomach allows incision of the gastrohepatic ligament and exposure and ligation of the right gastric artery. (**B**) Inferior traction on the neck of the pancreas allows for optimal dissection and ligation of the gastroduodenal artery. An accessory or replaced right hepatic artery can be seen or palpated posterior to the common bile duct. (**C**) Superior retraction of the common hepatic artery allows exposure of the anterior surface of the portal vein as well as identification of the coronary vein. (**D**) A tape is passed around the neck of the pancreas (view from right lateral side of patient). Adapted from illustrations by David Factor from "The Role of Total Pancreatectomy in the Treatment of Pancreatic Cancer" **Pancreatic Cancer,** edited by Von Hoff, Evans and Hruban, 2005. By permission of Mayo Foundation for Medical Education and Research. 

superior border of the pancreatic neck and the consistent lymph node in this region is excised. This allows excellent exposure of the origin of the gastroduodenal artery and the insertion of the coronary vein. Ligation and division of the gastroduodenal artery is performed (Fig. 7.4B). Careful dissection at the inferior border of the common hepatic artery near the origin of the gastroduodenal artery will identify the portal vein (Fig. 7.4C). From an inferior approach, a clamp is now advanced anterior to the SMV with the tip oriented in the same direction as the exposed portal vein. Care should be taken to avoid veering to the medial aspect of the vein, as inadvertent injury to the insertion of the coronary vein or splenic vein can occur. A cloth "tape" is passed around the neck of the pancreas which facilitates exposure and retraction of the pancreas (Fig. 7.4D).

## Resection

With adequate assessment and exposure of the pancreatic head and neck, the mesocolon is dissected off the caudal aspect of the pancreatic body and tail and the splenic flexure of the colon is mobilized inferiorly (Fig. 7.5). The short gastric vessels are ligated and divided. With medial traction on the spleen, the splenic peritoneal attachments are divided and the spleen and distal pancreas are mobilized medially off the retroperitoneum (Fig. 7.6). An avascular dissection plane is developed between the pancreas anteriorly and the left kidney and the adrenal gland posteriorly. All peripancreatic adipose and lymphatic tissue is resected with the specimen. Mobilization continues to medially to the origin of the splenic artery and insertion of the splenic vein. The splenic artery is then ligated and divided at its origin. The confluence of the inferior mesenteric vein

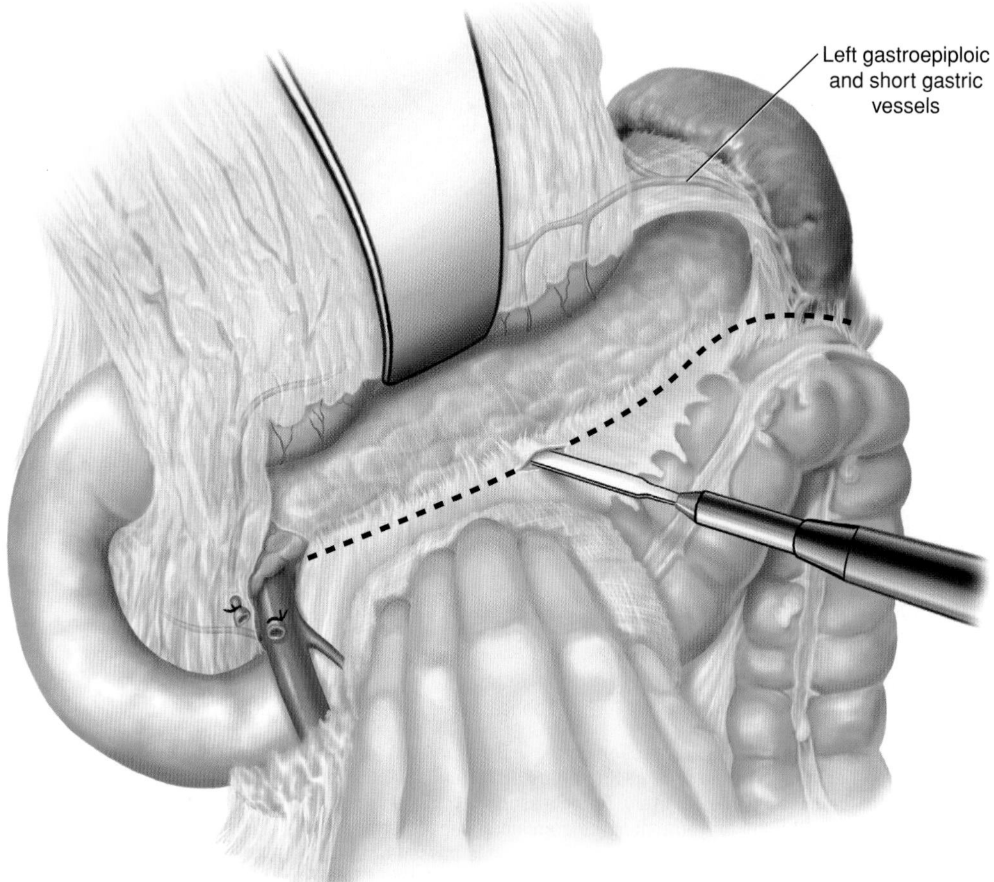


Figure 7.5 The transverse mesocolon is retracted in an inferior direction as the peritoneum at the inferior border of the pancreas is incised. The inferior mesenteric vein is identified and at this stage preserved. Adapted from illustrations by David Factor from "The Role of Total Pancreatectomy in the Treatment of Pancreatic Cancer" **Pancreatic Cancer,** edited by Von Hoff, Evans and Hruban, 2005. By permission of Mayo Foundation for Medical Education and Research. All rights reserved.

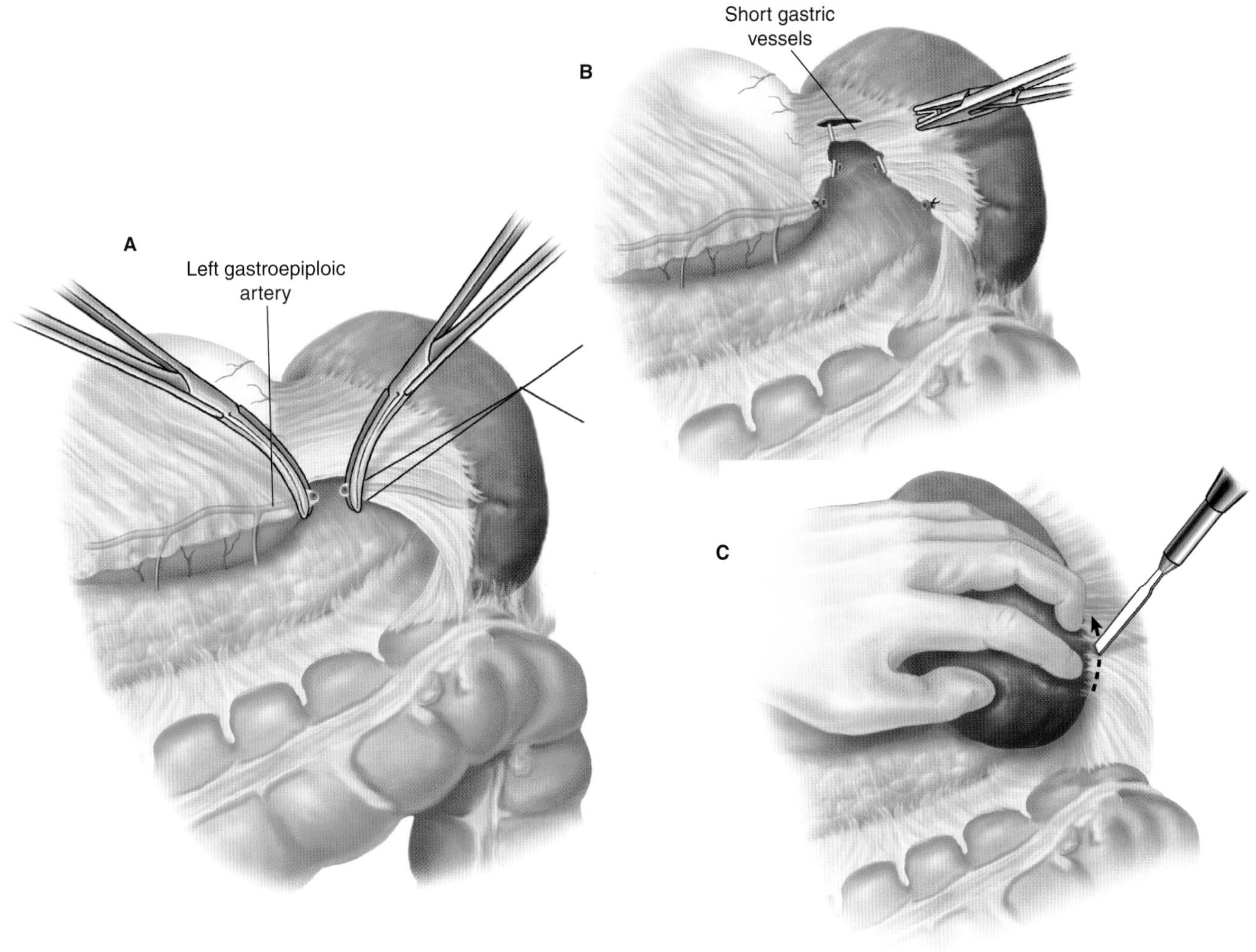


Figure 7.6 (**A**) Ligation of left gastroepiploic vessels allows access to the gastrosplenic ligament in anticipation of dissecting the short gastric vessels. (**B**) Ligation of short gastric vessels. (**C**) Retraction of the spleen to the right allows incision of the lateral and superior peritoneal attachments. Adapted from illustrations by David Factor from "The Role of Total Pancreatectomy in the Treatment of Pancreatic Cancer" **Pancreatic Cancer,** edited by Von Hoff, Evans and Hruban, 2005. By permission of Mayo Foundation for Medical Education and Research. All rights reserved.

and splenic vein should be identified. If technically feasible, the splenic vein should be ligated just proximal to the confluence of the inferior mesenteric vein, otherwise it should be ligated and divided flush with the portal vein (Fig. 7.7). Moreover, care should be taken to preserve the coronary vein if pylorus preservation is planned as venous congestion of the distal stomach may occur. Alternative venous drainage routes (short gastric, right gastric, right and left gastroepiploic veins) are routinely sacrificed underscoring the need to preserve the coronary vein.

A cholecystectomy is performed, mobilizing the gallbladder from its hepatic fossa. The cystic artery and cystic duct are ligated and divided. The hepatic hilum is then carefully inspected to assess for a replaced or aberrant right hepatic artery, which usually lies posterior and lateral to the common bile duct within the hepatoduodenal ligament (Fig. 7.4B). The common hepatic duct is ligated distally and divided (Fig. 7.8). A bulldog clamp is placed on the proximal duct to prevent continuous biliary drainage throughout the remainder of the dissection. All hilar adipose and lymphatic tissue at the level of the duct transection is mobilized inferiorly with the pancreatectomy specimen. The first portion of the duodenum is then skeletonized and transected 3 cm distal to the pylorus with a stapler.

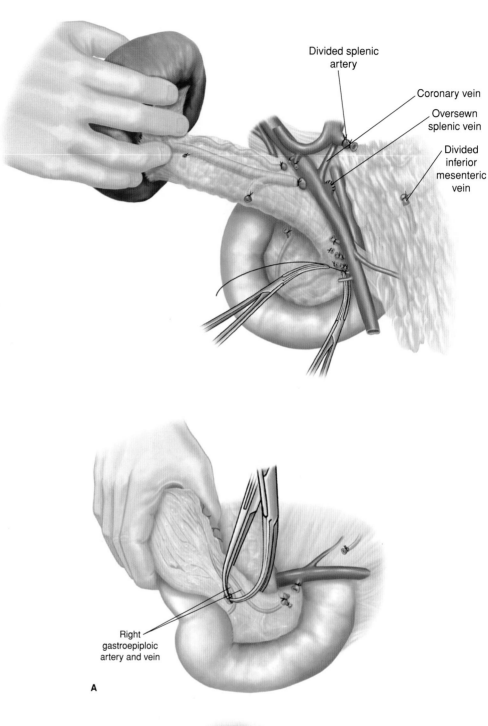

**Figure 7.7** After the spleen is mobilized from its bed, the plane posterior to the pancreas is dissected to allow for proximal ligation of the splenic artery and vein. The splenic artery and vein are individually ligated with transfixing sutures. Careful dissection of the splenic vein/portal vein confluence prevents injury to the coronary vein. If the inferior mesenteric vein enters the splenic vein remote from the portal vein, the inferior mesenteric vein is clamped, divided, and ligated. Venous branches draining the uncinate are ligated in continuity and divided. This enables leftward traction of the portal vein/superior mesenteric vein to expose the superior mesenteric artery. Adapted from illustrations by David Factor from "The Role of Total Pancreatectomy in the Treatment of Pancreatic Cancer" **Pancreatic Cancer,** edited by Von Hoff, Evans and Hruban, 2005. By permission of Mayo Foundation for Medical Education and Research. All rights reserved.



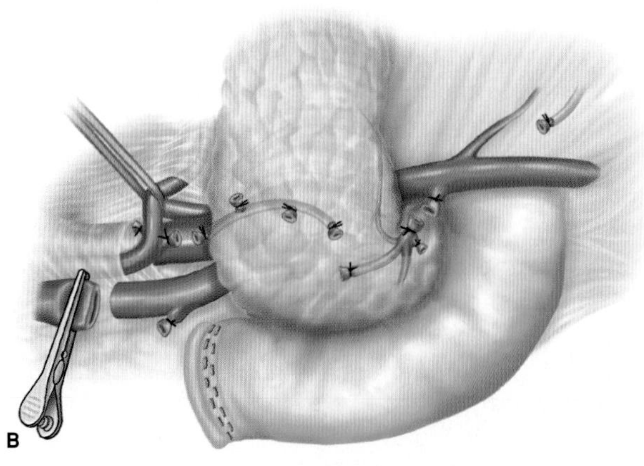


**Figure 7.8** (**A**) Before division, the proximal duodenum is skeletonized on its inferior border by clamping, dividing, and ligating the right gastroepiploic vessels. (**B**) After the gallbladder is mobilized from its bed, the common hepatic duct is transected proximal to the cystic duct. Control is achieved with a bulldog clamp (view from right lateral side of patient). Adapted from illustrations by David Factor from "The Role of Total Pancreatectomy in the Treatment of Pancreatic Cancer" **Pancreatic Cancer,** edited by Von Hoff, Evans and Hruban, 2005. By permission of Mayo Foundation for Medical Education and Research. All rights reserved.

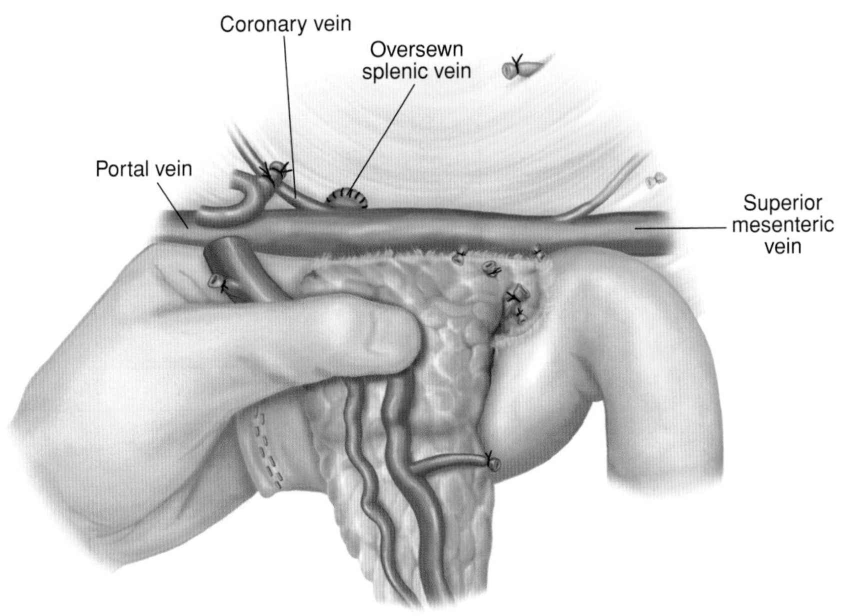


Figure 7.9 The spleen and tail of the pancreas are retracted to the patient's right exposing the portal vein/superior mesenteric vein confluence. Venous branches from the head and uncinate process are dissected and ligated. Adapted from illustrations by David Factor from "The Role of Total Pancreatectomy in the Treatment of Pancreatic Cancer" **Pancreatic Cancer,** edited by Von Hoff, Evans and Hruban, 2005. By permission of Mayo Foundation for Medical Education and Research. All rights reserved.

The ligament of Treitz is mobilized and the jejunum is divided approximately 10 cm distally with a stapler. The jejunal and duodenal mesentery is then clamped, divided, and ligated until the uncinate process is encountered. The jejunal stump is then passed posterior to the superior mesenteric vessels into the supramesocolic compartment. The defect created by this mobilization is closed with suture to prevent possible internal herniation and subsequent small bowel obstruction.

The previously mobilized distal pancreas and spleen are then reflected rightward exposing the interface of the pancreatic head and uncinate process with the mesenteric vessels. Identification and careful dissection of the venous branches of the pancreatic head and uncinate are necessary to avoid avulsion of these tenuous vessels during traction (Fig. 7.9). Ligation and division of these venous branches allow sufficient mobility of the portal vein and SMV for exposure of the SMA. With gentle left lateral retraction of the PV/SMV with vein retractors and rightward retraction of the specimen, a periadventitial dissection of the SMA is performed. Care is taken to identify the pancreaticoduodenal arteries which are ligated and divided (Fig. 7.10A, B, C, D). The retroperitoneal soft tissue is divided, skeletonizing the right lateral aspect of the SMA. This critical dissection ensures that a maximal uncinate/SMA margin is obtained.

The specimen is then inspected on the back table and the portal vein groove and uncinate/SMA margins are inked to assure accurate margin assessment. Margins are reviewed by frozen section and include the bile duct, duodenal and uncinate/SMA margin. While the uncinate/SMA margin is of staging benefit, if the original dissection skeletonized the SMA, no further resection is possible. Although en-bloc venous resection is performed when necessary to ensure negative margins in the setting of malignancy, we do not generally advocate en-bloc arterial resection and reconstruction.

## Reconstruction

Once margin status has been confirmed and the resection bed is carefully inspected for hemostasis, reconstruction is performed. A small window is made in the avascular portion of the right mesocolon and the jejunum passed into the supramesocolic compartment. An end-to-side hepaticojejunostomy is performed with a single layer of continuous Vicryl or PDS suture. When the duct is small (≤6 mm) or is thin walled, the anastomosis is constructed with interrupted sutures; otherwise, a running suture is utilized. The jejunum is then fixated to the mesocolon with interrupted suture. Approximately 40 cm

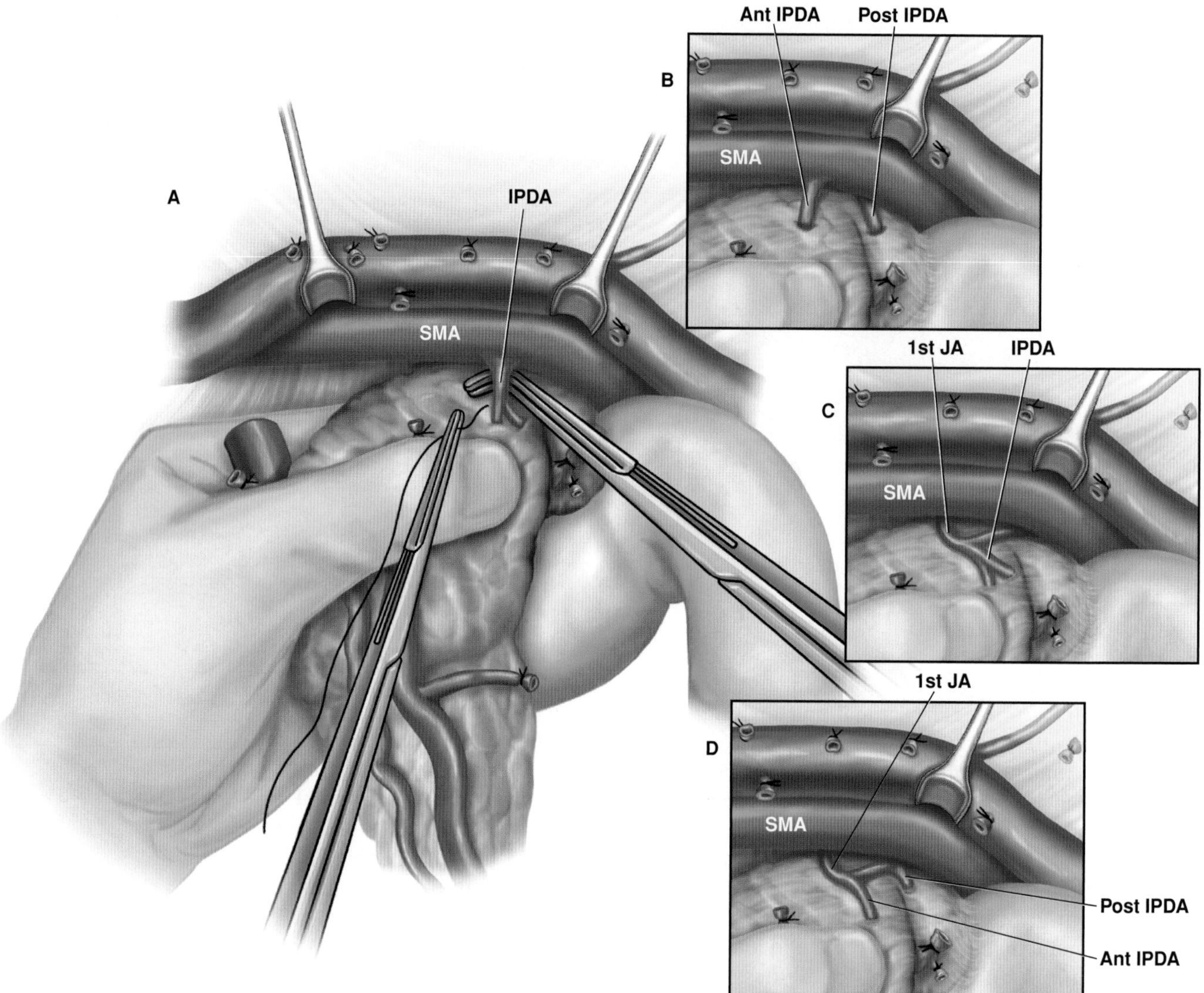


Figure 7.10 (**A**) Once the portal vein is mobilized, further traction anterior and to the patient's left allows for a periadventitial dissection of the superior mesenteric artery (SMA). The inferior pancreaticoduodenal artery (IPDA), which often arises as a single vessel before it bifurcates into the anterior and posterior inferior pancreaticoduodenal arteries, should be sought and carefully ligated and divided. (**B**) It should be noted that there may be more than one arterial vessel coursing into the uncinate process of the pancreas as the anterior (ANT) and posterior (POST) inferior pancreaticoduodenal arteries may arise from the superior mesenteric artery separately as in **B,** from the first jejunal artery (1st JA) either as a single trunk as in **C,** or as separate branches as in **D.** Care should be taken to preserve the first jejunal artery lest ischemia of the proximal jejunum result. Adapted from illustrations by David Factor from "The Role of Total Pancreatectomy in the Treatment of Pancreatic Cancer" **Pancreatic Cancer,** edited by Von Hoff, Evans and Hruban, 2005. By permission of Mayo Foundation for Medical Education and Research. All rights reserved.

distal to the hepaticojejunostomy, an antecolic end-to-side duodenojejunostomy is constructed with an inner layer of running Vicryl suture and an outer layer of interrupted silk suture in a Lembert fashion. A single closed suction drain is placed in Morison's pouch and is brought out through the right lateral abdominal wall (Fig. 7.11).

## Laparoscopic Approach

TP can be performed with a total laparoscopic approach in selected patients. Few case reports exist in the current literature and although this approach appears feasible, limited data with regard to outcome is available. The authors have experience with this approach in fifteen patients to date. Indications have included multicentric branch-duct IPMN, main-duct IPMN, and isolated multicentric renal cell metastases. The technique

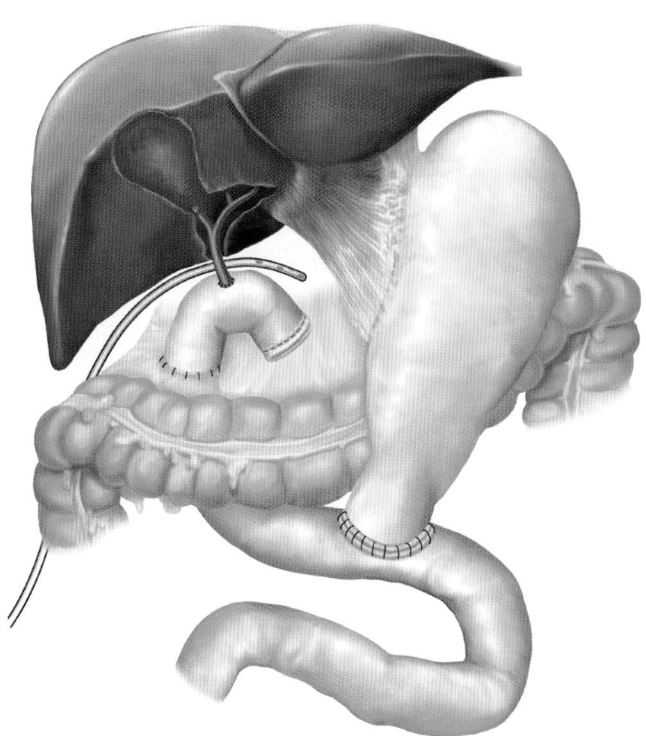

**Figure 7.11** The proximal jejunum is passed through the transverse mesocolon to the right of the middle colic vessels, and an end-to-side hepaticojejunostomy is performed with a single layer of interrupted or continuous absorbable suture. An antecolic end-to-side duodenojejunostomy is performed in two layers. A surgical drain is routinely placed in the subhepatic space behind the hepaticojejunostomy. Adapted from illustrations by David Factor from "The Role of Total Pancreatectomy in the Treatment of Pancreatic Cancer" **Pancreatic Cancer,** edited by Von Hoff, Evans and Hruban, 2005. By permission of Mayo Foundation for Medical Education and Research. All rights reserved.

of the procedure is patterned after the open approach described above with few modifications. The major difference is the use of coagulation devices such as Harmonic Scalpel and Ligasure for transection of the omentum, jejunal mesentery, and uncinate/SMA margin. When these devices are used for the uncinate dissection, we still advocate identification and ligation of the pancreaticoduodenal arteries. Reconstruction is identical with end-to-side hepaticojejunostomy and antecolic end-to-side duodenojejunostomy.

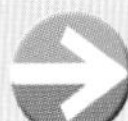

## POSTOPERATIVE MANAGEMENT

Hourly monitoring of glucose levels and continuous infusion of insulin is continued in the initial postoperative period. The nasogastric tube is typically removed the first postoperative day and the patient is started on clear liquids with advancement to a diabetic soft diet over several days. Once the glucose levels have stabilized, the frequency of glucose monitoring is decreased and the transition is made from continuous infusion to intermittent percutaneous injection. When the patient is tolerating an oral diet, pancreatic enzyme supplementation is initiated and diabetes education is intensified. The prophylactic operative drain is removed when output is low and non-bilious in character. Patients are discharged when there is no evidence of complication and they demonstrate understanding and competence with diabetic management. Close postoperative follow-up is recommended to assure an uncomplicated convalescence and monitor the management of diabetes and nutritional status. Post splenectomy vaccinations are given 2 weeks postoperatively if they were not given preoperatively.

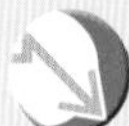

## COMPLICATIONS

Although TP avoids the significant complications resulting from pancreatic leak that are observed with partial pancreatectomy, the postoperative morbidity and mortality remain substantial (Table 7.2). Postoperative morbidity occurs in 30% to 40% of patients after TP and includes delayed gastric emptying, intra-abdominal abscess, biliary anastomotic leak, intra-abdominal hemorrhage, sepsis, hypoglycemic episodes and wound complications. These complications are treated as with partial pancreatectomy and

TABLE 7.2 Selected Large (>30 Patients) Series of Total Pancreatectomy

| Author | Year | Study Period | Total Patients (n) | Malignancy (%) | IAT (n) | Hospital Stay (days) | Morbidity (%) | Mortality (%) |
|---|---|---|---|---|---|---|---|---|
| Karpoff | 2001 | 1983–1998 | 35 | 80 | 0 | 32 | 54 | 3 |
| Billings | 2005 | 1985–2002 | 99 | 68 | 0 | n/a | 32 | 5 |
| Jethwa | 2006 | 1989–2003 | 47 | 64 | 0 | n/a | n/a | 21.7 |
| Schmidt | 2007 | 1992–2006 | 33 | 100 | 0 | 10 | 36 | 6 |
| Muller | 2007 | 2001–2006 | 147 | 78 | 0 | 11 | 35 | 4.8 |
| Sutherland | 2008 | 1977–2007 | 173 | 0 | 173 | n/a | n/a | 5[a] |
| Fujino | 2009 | 1994–2006 | 36 | 94 | 0 | n/a | 39 | 6 |
| Garcea | 2009 | 1996–2006 | 85 | 0 | 50 | 20 | n/a | 3.5 |
| Reddy | 2009 | 1970–2007 | 100 | 100 | 0 | 10 | 69 | 8 |

[a]one-year survival.
IAT; islet cell autotransplantation.

early identification and prompt treatment are necessary. In a recent update from our institution evaluating 99 patients undergoing TP, overall morbidity was 32% with reoperation for hematoma or small bowel obstruction in two patients. The overall hospital or 30-day mortality was 5%.

The diabetic state induced after TP is characterized by complete insulin deficiency, pancreatic polypeptide deficiency, and absence of functional glucagon. In the apancreatic state, the therapeutic window is narrow and episodes of mild-to-severe hypoglycemia following insulin administration are not uncommon. Despite these difficulties, recent reports demonstrate improved glycemic control with current management strategies. In our institutional experience, a mean $Hb_{A1c}$ level of 7.4% was observed, reflecting glycemic control close to that advocated for decreasing complications of hyperglycemia and is lower than reported in earlier series of TP.

In addition to pancreatic exocrine deficiency, other factors such as delayed gastric emptying, anorexia, intra-abdominal complications and poorly controlled diabetes contribute to the potential for poor nutritional status after TP. Patients with inadequate nutritional intake in the postoperative period should prompt investigation for correctable causes. Appropriate education with regard to use of pancreatic enzyme supplements and proper nutritional intake may reduce nutritional complications. In patients with preoperative malnutrition or those with anticipated postoperative difficulties, consideration may be given to jejunostomy tube placement at the time of TP and early postoperative supplemental enteral nutrition.

Operative mortality rates of less than 5% are consistently reported in more recent series from tertiary centers specializing in pancreatic disease. In a review of 100 patients undergoing TP at a single institution, observed mortality rates decreased over time from 40% between 1970 and 1989, to only 2% from 2000 to 2007. Several factors including refined surgical techniques, improved noninvasive diagnostic and therapeutic options for management of complications and improved diabetic management and medical care account for the reduction in operative mortality.

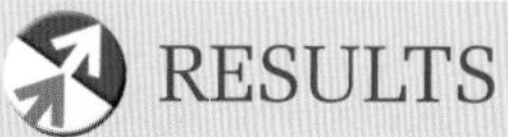

## RESULTS

### Malignancy

The first successful TP for neoplasm was performed at the Mayo Clinic in 1944. Initial enthusiasm for TP was fostered by the theory that it would control local recurrence and avoid the high mortality observed with pancreaticoduodenectomy from pancreatic anastomotic leak. This theory was soon disproved with the understanding that most recurrence is from distant metastases and that local recurrence is predominantly due to a positive retroperitoneal margin which is not improved with TP. In addition, overall morbidity after TP is comparable to pancreaticoduodenectomy despite absence of a pancreatic remnant and operative mortality for both procedures has decreased over time. In a retrospective cohort study using data from the Surveillance, Epidemiology, and End Results (SEER) Program database, perioperative mortality and long-term survival were similar after TP or partial pancreatectomy for pancreatic adenocarcinoma. Finally the supposition that TP would improve oncologic outcomes has not been substantiated compared to partial pancreatectomy.

While the general use of TP for adenocarcinoma is not advocated, it is warranted from an oncologic basis when the only barrier to a R0 resection is the pancreatic parenchymal margin. Reddy and colleagues reported a comparative series of patients undergoing TP or pancreaticoduodenectomy for adenocarcinoma. Patients undergoing TP had larger tumor size relative to patients undergoing partial pancreatectomy but similar rates of N1 disease, vascular invasion and perineural invasion. The rates of R0 resection and 30-day mortality were higher in the TP group, yet the five-year survival was similar (18.9% vs. 18.5%).

In evaluation of intraoperative conversion TP to achieve negative margins, Schmidt and colleagues evaluated 28 patients who underwent PD with an isolated positive neck margin were compared to 33 patients who underwent conversion to TP after isolated positive neck margin to achieve R0 resection. Patients undergoing TP had greater median survival (18 vs. 10 months; $p = 0.04$). Morbidity (36% vs. 54%, $p = 0.2$) and mortality (6% vs. 7%) were similar.

### Chronic or Recurrent Acute Pancreatitis

Surgical intervention for chronic pancreatitis is reserved for patients with intractable abdominal pain or pancreatitis-related complications when other methods have failed. Total pancreatectomy for intractable pain or prevention of recurrent pancreatitis has been advocated for patients with hereditary pancreatitis and other causes of chronic or recurrent acute pancreatitis. Several series have described favorable outcomes after TP for patients with chronic pancreatitis. Reductions in opioid requirement, hospital admissions and pain (based on visual analogue scales) have all been demonstrated. These outcomes are comparable to those reported for partial pancreatectomy with or without drainage and randomized trials are needed to substantiate any potential advantages of TP over other accepted procedures for patients with chronic pancreatitis and intractable pain.

TP with islet autotransplantation (IAT) for patients with chronic or recurrent acute pancreatitis has attracted attention with the hope of ameliorating or alleviating both the disease and the diabetic sequela of the apancreatic state. Sutherland and colleagues have performed TP with IAT in over 170 patients and outcomes appear promising. After IAT, 65% of patients have functioning islets in the first year and 32% were insulin independent. Of those with initial islet function (full or partial) 85% continued to have functioning islets at 2 years. While insulin independence is the most desirable outcome, this measure overlooks the potential benefit of IAT in prevention of "brittle diabetes" that may be observed in patients with partial function. Although sufficient experience is limited and is focused to relatively few centers, TP with IAT appears feasible and beneficial for selected patients. Since higher islet recovery rates correlate with improved outcomes of IAT, proponents argue for early pancreatectomy in patients with chronic pancreatitis prior to significant loss of β-cell mass. Ongoing evaluation and investigation of the role of IAT after TP is warranted.

### IPMN

Intraductal papillary mucinous neoplasm is a premalignant condition with variable presentation with regard to its malignant potential, distribution and symptomatic sequela. TP may be indicated for IPMN in selected patients with main-duct disease or diffuse branch-duct disease based on risk of malignancy or symptoms. For main-duct disease we prefer a focused operative approach (pancreaticoduodenectomy or distal pancreatectomy) when possible with immediate frozen-section margin assessment. In the setting of high-grade dysplasia and the inability to obtain a negative margin, TP is warranted. For branch-duct disease that is either diffuse or is multicentric with increased risk of malignancy (size >3 cm or mural nodules) TP may also be indicated. Because of the malignant potential of IPMN and the need to complete a thorough histologic evaluation of the entire specimen, IAT is contraindicated.

We recently published experience in 40 patients undergoing TP for IPMN. In nine patients TP was performed as a conversion procedure due to persistent microscopically positive margins. While it appears that TP is increasingly utilized, we favor a targeted, subtotal resection when feasible as the morbidity and reduction of quality of life (QoL) seen with TP outweigh the risk of recurrent IPMN in our opinion. Ongoing surveillance is indicated after partial pancreatectomy as the radiographic recurrence of IPMN after resection of noninvasive IPMN is approximately 8%. If recurrent IPMN does occur, similar indications for resection are based on type (main- or branch-duct), size, and symptoms. We have performed completion pancreatectomy for recurrent IPMN in several patients and find this a valid approach to patients as opposed to initial TP.

### Quality of Life

While it has been perceived that the QoL after TP would be significantly worse having both endocrine and exocrine deficiency, there is a paucity of data in the current era. Using the European Organization for Research and Treatment of Cancer Quality of Life Questionnaire (EORTC QLQ), the University of Verona reported QoL scores and health scores after TP were similar to age-matched patients with type II diabetes. In 88% of patients, HbA1c was normal although 72% of patients claimed to have hypoglycemic episodes at least weekly. More recently, our institution reported QoL assessment after TP using the Short Form-36 (SF-36), Audit of Diabetes Dependent QoL (ADD QoL) and European Organization for Research and Treatment in Cancer Pancreas 26 (EORTC PAN 26) and demonstrated that the role physical and general health domains were decreased after TP compared to an age and gender-matched national population ($P < 0.05$). When compared with insulin-dependent diabetics from other causes, however there was no significant difference in QoL.

In a matched-pairs analysis of patients undergoing TP and pancreaticoduodenectomy, global health status was not different, however, on a functional scale, role functioning and social functioning were reduced for patients after TP compared to pancreaticoduodenectomy. As further refinements in care exocrine and endocrine deficiency in the apancreatic patient continue, corresponding improvements in the QoL of these patients is expected.

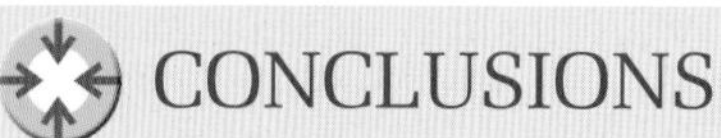

## CONCLUSIONS

Total pancreatectomy is an appropriate option in selected patients where subtotal procedures are insufficient to treat the disease or symptoms. Careful attention to the technical details of the procedure and postoperative care of these patients is necessary to reduce the morbidity and mortality. Islet autotransplantation is a reasonable consideration when total pancreatectomy is performed for chronic pancreatitis albeit long-term outcomes of IAT remain unclear and ongoing evaluation is necessary. For premalignant or malignant disease, the sequela of TP should be weighed against the risk of recurrence or residual disease. Current outcomes justify the use of TP in selected patients with benign and malignant disease.

## Recommended References and Readings

Argo JL, Contreras JL, Wesley MM, et al. Pancreatic resection with islet cell autotransplant for the treatment of severe pancreatitis. *Am Surgeon.* 2008;74:530–537.

Billings BJ, Christein JD, Harmsen WS, et al. Quality-of-life after total pancreatectomy: Is it really that bad on long-term follow-up? *J Gastrointest Surg.* 2005;9:1059–1067.

Dixon J, Delegge M, Morgan KA, et al. Impact of total pancreatectomy with islet cell transplant on chronic pancreatitis management at a disease-based center. *Am Surgeon.* 2008;74: 735–738.

Garcea G, Weaver J, Phillips J, et al. Total pancreatectomy with and without islet cell transplantation for chronic pancreatitis: a series of 85 consecutive patients. *Pancreas.* 2009;38:1–7.

Kulu Y, Schmied BM, Werner J, et al. Total pancreatectomy for pancreatic cancer: indications and operative technique. *HBP.* 2009;11:469–475.

Landoni L. Salvia R, Festa L, et al. Quality of life after total pancreatectomy: Ten year experience. *J Pancreas* 2004;5(5 suppl):441.

Muller MW, Friess H, Kleef J, et al. Is there still a role for total pancreatectomy? *Ann Surg.* 2007;246:966–975.

Muller MW, Fries H, Kleef J, et al. Is there still a role for total pancreatectomy? *Ann Surg.* 2007;246:966–976.

Nathan H, Wolfgang CL, Edil BH, et al. Peri-operative mortality and long-term survival after total pancreatectomy for pancreatic adenocarcinoma: A population-based perspective. *J Surg Oncol.* 2009;99:87–92.

Ong SL, Gravante G, Pollard CA, et al. Total pancreatectomy with islet autotransplantation: an overview. *HPB.* 2009;11:613–621.

Priestley J, Comfort M, Rancliff J. Total pancreatectomy for hyperinsulinism due to an islet cell adenoma. *Ann Surg.* 1944;199:211–221.

Reddy S, Wolfgang CL, Cameron JL, et al. Total pancreatectomy for pancreatic adenocarcinoma: evaluation of morbidity and long-term survival. *Ann Surg.* 2009;250:282–287.

Schmidt CM, Glant J, Winter JM, et al. Total pancreatectomy (R0 resection) improves survival over subtotal pancreatectomy in isolated neck margin positive pancreatic adenocarcinoma. *Surgery.* 2007;142:572–580.

Schnelldorfer T, Sarr MG, Nagorney DM, et al. Experience with 208 resections for intraductal papillary mucinous neoplasm of the pancreas. *Arch Surg.* 2008;143:639–646.

Sutherland DER, Gruessner AC, Carlson AM, et al. Islet autotransplant outcomes after total pancreatectomy: A contrast to islet allograft outcomes. *Transplantation.* 2008;86:1799–1802.

Webb MA, Illouz SC, Pollard CA, et al. Islet auto transplantation following total pancreatectomy: A long-term assessment of graft function. *Pancreas.* 2008;37:282–287.

# 8 Debridement for Pancreatic Necrosis

**Karen Horvath**

##  INDICATIONS/CONTRAINDICATIONS

### Introduction

There are approximately 210,000 cases of acute pancreatitis per year in the United States. Ninety percent of patients will have a mild form of interstitial edematous pancreatitis, but about 10% will develop severe acute pancreatitis. Some patients will develop acute peripancreatic fluid collections (APFC) that will resolve with medical support alone or will go on to develop a pancreatic pseudocyst (Chapter 12). The subject of this chapter concerns those patients who develop necrotizing pancreatitis. These patients develop acute post-necrotic collections (APNC) involving necrosis of the pancreatic parenchyma and the peripancreatic tissues, the pancreatic parenchyma alone, or the peripancreatic tissue alone. When APNC persists beyond 4 weeks from the onset of pancreatitis, the term walled-off necrosis (WON) can be applied. These terms represent morphologic abnormalities noted on contrast-enhanced CT scan that are used for classification purposes and to guide treatment (Fig. 8.1).

When treating patients with necrotizing pancreatitis it is important to be cognizant of the time from onset of symptoms since recent data demonstrates that delayed intervention leads to lower morbidity and mortality rates. Over a four-week period, APNC's evolve: the peripancreatic tissue inflammation subsides, the tissue within the collection demarcates into viable and non-viable components and the perimeter of the collection matures into the defined wall of WON. A distinction should also be made between sterile and infected necrosis, since the presence of infection means a different prognosis, natural history and approach to treatment. Patients with sterile WON will usually resolve over time without any intervention. In fact, a percutaneous drain should generally *not* be placed into sterile collections unless there is a very good indication since it will iatrogenically infect the collection after a short time and complicate the patient's management. A small subset of patients with sterile WON will require pancreatic necrosectomy either because of persistent symptoms such as anorexia, early satiety, vomiting, pain, fever, or failure to thrive. All patients with WON who become infected require treatment with parenteral antibiotics in combination with effective drainage/necrosectomy.

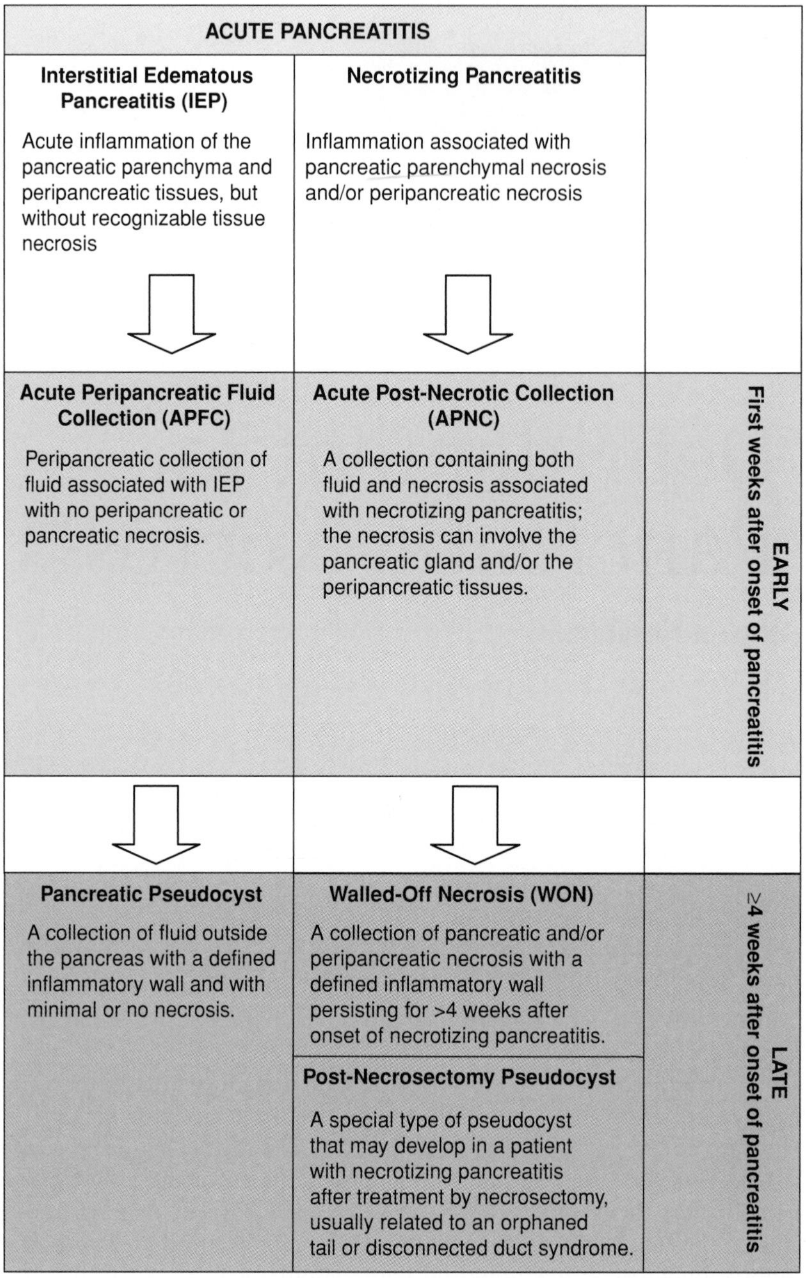

Figure 8.1 Spectrum of Acute Pancreatitis.

| ACUTE PANCREATITIS | | |
|---|---|---|
| **Interstitial Edematous Pancreatitis (IEP)**<br>Acute inflammation of the pancreatic parenchyma and peripancreatic tissues, but without recognizable tissue necrosis | **Necrotizing Pancreatitis**<br>Inflammation associated with pancreatic parenchymal necrosis and/or peripancreatic necrosis | |
| **Acute Peripancreatic Fluid Collection (APFC)**<br>Peripancreatic collection of fluid associated with IEP with no peripancreatic or pancreatic necrosis. | **Acute Post-Necrotic Collection (APNC)**<br>A collection containing both fluid and necrosis associated with necrotizing pancreatitis; the necrosis can involve the pancreatic gland and/or the peripancreatic tissues. | **EARLY**<br>First weeks after onset of pancreatitis |
| **Pancreatic Pseudocyst**<br>A collection of fluid outside the pancreas with a defined inflammatory wall and with minimal or no necrosis. | **Walled-Off Necrosis (WON)**<br>A collection of pancreatic and/or peripancreatic necrosis with a defined inflammatory wall persisting for >4 weeks after onset of necrotizing pancreatitis.<br>**Post-Necrosectomy Pseudocyst**<br>A special type of pseudocyst that may develop in a patient with necrotizing pancreatitis after treatment by necrosectomy, usually related to an orphaned tail or disconnected duct syndrome. | **LATE**<br>≥4 weeks after onset of pancreatitis |

Infection develops in 30% to 70% of patients with necrotizing pancreatitis and accounts for more than 80% of deaths from acute pancreatitis. The risk of infection increases with the amount of pancreatic glandular necrosis and the time from the onset of acute pancreatitis, peaking at 3 weeks. Infection is presumed when there is gas present in the WON on CT scan. It is also diagnosed definitively with an image-guided fine needle aspiration (FNA) showing a positive Gram stain and culture. Since patients carry a significant risk of converting from sterile to infected tissue over time, patients should be followed closely and an FNA performed if clinically indicated with a change in abdominal pain, fever, or leukocytosis. Since FNA has a false-negative rate of about 10%, a negative FNA may be repeated after appropriate intervals, such as 5 to 7 days, if a clinical suspicion of infection persists. FNA has a low iatrogenic infection rate along with a high sensitivity and specificity.

Once the patient is determined to be infected, they require complete external drainage or face a near 100% mortality. While deciding amongst percutaneous, laparoscopic, endoscopic, or open surgical options, a percutaneous drain should be placed within

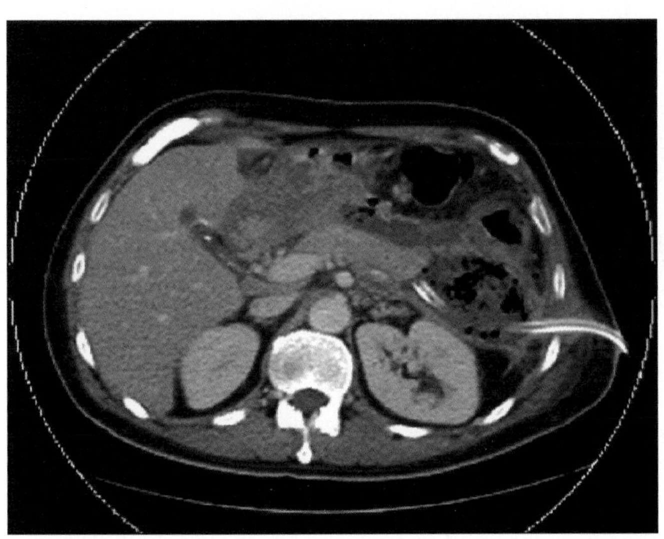

Figure 8.2 Contrast-enhanced CT scan of a patient with infected WON. A percutaneous drain is present in the collection.



24 hours of a positive FNA to initiate external drainage (Fig. 8.2). Once a percutaneous drain has been placed, we aggressively upsize the catheters every 3 to 4 days to an 18-20Fr goal. A CT is repeated about 2 weeks after the first drain was placed. If the patient has a remaining large collection and at least 4 weeks have elapsed since onset of disease, plans are made for surgery. In general, surgery for APNC should be delayed until the WON phase due to lower morbidity and mortality. While waiting for this safer time, sepsis control can be temporized with percutaneous drains and when necessary, the addition of parental antibiotics. Careful attention must be paid to the protein and calorie requirements in these patients which are very high. Most patients are unable to consume their total caloric needs and almost all will require supplemental enteral or parenteral nutrition and close monitoring of their nutritional status with serum markers. Enteral nutrition (nasogastric or nasojejunal) is the preferred route when tolerated, since it has been shown to be associated with significant decreases in the risk of pancreatitis associated morbidity and mortality.

A small subset of necrotizing pancreatitis patients will require emergent surgery for organ failure and acute decompensation due to an intra-abdominal catastrophe such as visceral ischemia. Acute decompensation is most often due to a reactivation of the SIRS response or a non-surgical source of infection. Because of this, intensive support should be given for 24 to 48 hours along with a search for the cause, but if an intra-abdominal catastrophe is suspected the patient will need an emergency laparotomy.

## Indications for Surgery

- Severe acute pancreatitis with APFC or APNC, less than 30 days from the onset of pancreatitis, with organ failure and suspected intra-abdominal catastrophe unresponsive to 24 to 48 hours of intensive support.
- WON, by definition greater than 30 days from the onset of necrotizing pancreatitis, that is:
  - Infected, with infection documented by gas seen in the collection on contrast-enhanced CT scan or with a positive FNA.
  - Sterile but symptomatic.

# PREOPERATIVE PLANNING

There are many excellent surgical options for pancreatic debridement. Transgastric endoscopic methods and percutaneous drains can also be used as primary or adjunctive methods. Minimally invasive methods are increasingly being used as a first step for operative necrosectomy in patients with infected WON with open necrosectomy reserved for patients who fail minimal access techniques or require an emergent exploration. The three most popular minimally invasive retroperitoneal debridement methods are:

- *Step-Up Approach consisting of percutaneous drainage followed by Videoscopic-assisted retroperitoneal debridement (VARD)*
- Percutaneous Necrosectomy
- Minimal Access Retroperitoneal Pancreatic Necrosectomy (MARPN)

There are four methods for open surgical necrosectomy:

- *Necrosectomy followed by continuous postoperative lavage.*
- Conventional drainage with placement of standard surgical drains and reoperation as needed.
- Open management technique with necrosectomy followed by scheduled relaparotomies through a marsupialized open abdomen.
- Open retroperitoneal approach through the base of the 12th rib.

The two techniques described here will be the Step-Up Approach which now has phase I feasibility, phase II safety and efficacy, and phase III randomized controlled data supporting its use and open necrosectomy followed by continuous postoperative lavage which is the open method upon which VARD is based.

Once the patient with a WON is determined to be infected a percutaneous drain is placed. If this drain is not effective a VARD will be needed. The patient will need a minimum of one percutaneous drain placed into the collection from the flank, to be used as an intraoperative guide. When doing the VARD procedure, the surgeon follows the path of this drain through the retroperitoneum and into the collection. Even if another drain is already in place, it is important for the interventional radiologist to place a drain *as close as possible to the left mid-axillary line just under the costal margin* for operative guidance (Fig. 8.3). A CT scan should be repeated showing this drain in place and a hard copy made for use in the OR. The position of this drain inside the collection and its location to nearby anatomical structures will be used in the OR by the surgeon to guide operative debridement. Necessary OR equipment is shown in Table 8.1.

All patients with necrotizing pancreatitis should have an ultrasound of the gall bladder performed. If gallstones or sludge are present, a cholecystectomy should be planned. Patients undergoing a VARD should have a laparoscopic cholecystectomy within 6 months following complete resolution of the peripancreatic collections and inflammatory process. Patients undergoing an open necrosectomy may have a cholecystectomy attempted at the time of their surgery; however, it may not be possible to perform a safe cholecystectomy when there is a large amount of necrosis because of significant inflammation in the porta hepatis.

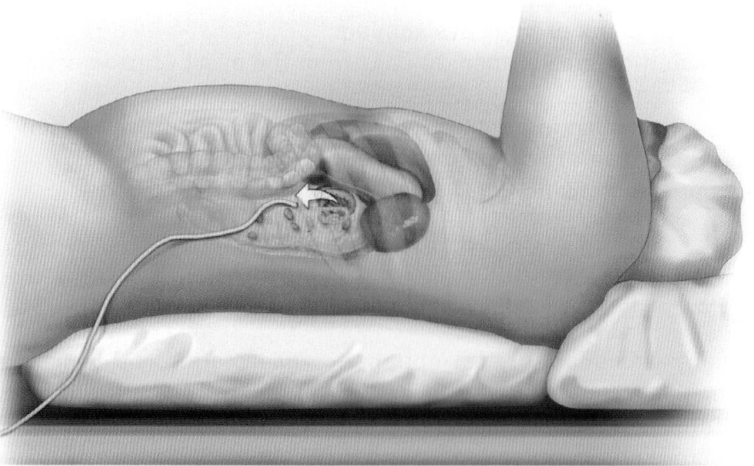

**Figure 8.3** Percutaneous drain entering flank near mid-axillary line under left costal margin to be used as an operative guide into the collection.

**TABLE 8.1 Necessary OR Equipment**

| | VARD | Open necrosectomy |
|---|---|---|
| Bean Bag for obese patients | ✓ | |
| Extra-long 10 mm blunt laparoscopic port | ✓ | |
| Christmas-tree connector to facilite gas insufflation via a lure-lock percutaneous drain | ✓ | |
| 10 mm, 0-degree laparoscope | ✓ | |
| Laparoscopic "spoon" or "stone" 10 mm forceps for debridement | ✓ | |
| Ring forceps | ✓ | ✓ |
| Yankauer suction device | ✓ | ✓ |
| Pulse jet irrigator/lavage system | ✓ | ✓ |
| Two one-inch penrose drains | ✓ | ✓ |
| Urostomy appliance and Foley urimeter for post-op lavage system | ✓ | ✓ |
| Open laparotomy set | ✓ | ✓ |
| 4 units of typed and cross-matched blood | ✓ | ✓ |

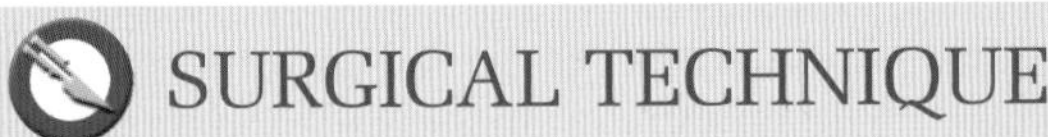

## SURGICAL TECHNIQUE

### Pertinent Anatomy and General Operative Principles

The pancreas is a retroperitoneal organ and the areas of WON almost always respect this anatomic compartmental boundaries. Whether the collections extend down the paracolic gutters and into the pelvis or into the leaves of the small or large bowel mesenteries, the collections usually remain bounded by peritoneum. Some patients may also develop ascites but this is most often a separate, sterile process. Thus, the overarching goal of any pancreatic debridement procedure should be to limit intrusion into the peritoneal cavity and protect the visceral contents from infection and injury as much as possible. Another important operative principle for pancreatic necrosectomy follows the dictum, "Perfect is the enemy of good." The goal of a necrosectomy is to break up loculations and debride large pieces of necrotic tissue but *not* to completely clean out the cavity. The postoperative lavage system and the percutaneous drains will generally be able to take care of remaining bits of necrosectum once the bulk of the disease is removed.

The use of a pulse lavage irrigator to promote hydrodissection periodically throughout the procedure is a very useful tool, even during a VARD. With many advanced laparoscopic operations irrigation is minimized until the end of the operation, so the recommendation for earlier use of pulse lavage here represents a deviation from laparoscopic convention. A final word of advice concerns band-like structures coursing through a cavity which should be treated as blood vessels and avoided. The pancreatic enzymes released in the acute pancreatitis event do a remarkable job of digesting pancreatic gland, adipose and connective tissue while skeletonizing blood vessels and other vital structures (e.g., ureters). Whether the cavity being debrided is in the lesser sac or the paracolic gutters, the idea of relevant anatomy should be constantly kept in the forefront of the surgeon's mind.

### Positioning

*Before positioning and draping* it is important to mark the following anatomic landmarks with the patient in the supine position: xiphoid, bilateral costal margins to the table,

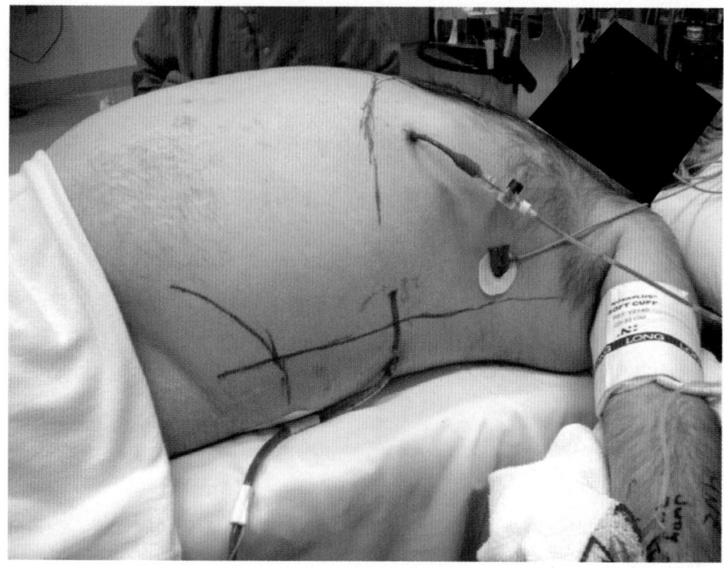

**Figure 8.4** Photo of patient showing important anatomic landmarks and incision (marked before positioning and draping).

anterior superior iliac spine, mid-axillary line, and planned incision site (Fig. 8.4). The 4 to 5 cm incision is placed one finger breadth below the left costal margin over the mid-axillary line. The mid-axillary line generally approximates the junction of the posterior peritoneal sac with the retroperitoneum where access is gained into the collection. Once the patient is positioned and draped, it can be difficult to accurately determine these important landmarks.

The patient is positioned as shown in Figure 8.5. A roll is placed under the left flank and the patient is placed in a modified right lateral decubitus position at about 30 degrees. The patient's flank should be centered over the kidney flex in the bed to facilitate opening of the costal margin. For obese patients, a bean bag may be needed to help stabilize the patient on the bed. The left arm is strapped into an airplane device. Sequential compression devices are used. The thighs are slightly flexed with a pillow between the legs. A strap is used over the hips and the patient is taped into position at the chest and lower extremities since extreme table angles may be used. An active body-warming device is placed.

The entire abdomen and left flank, including the percutaneous drains are prepped into the field from table-to-table and nipple-to-pubis. The table is placed into reverse

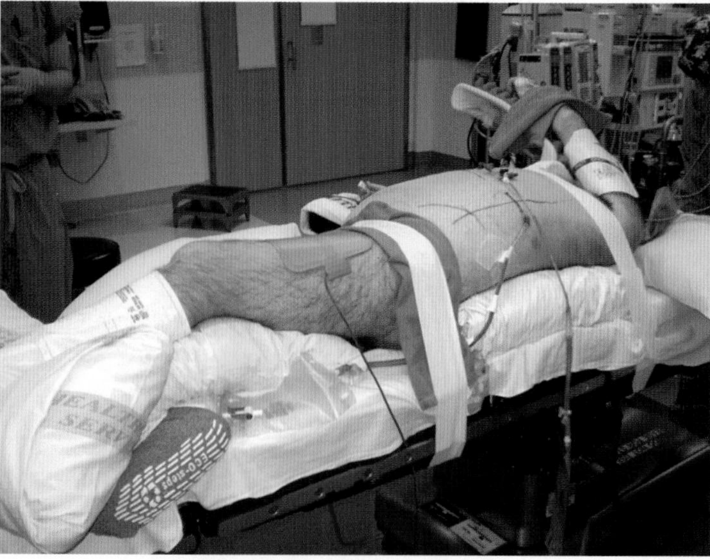

**Figure 8.5** Patient Position. The patient is in a modified lateral decubitus position with a roll under the left flank. The left arm is secured in an airplane device.

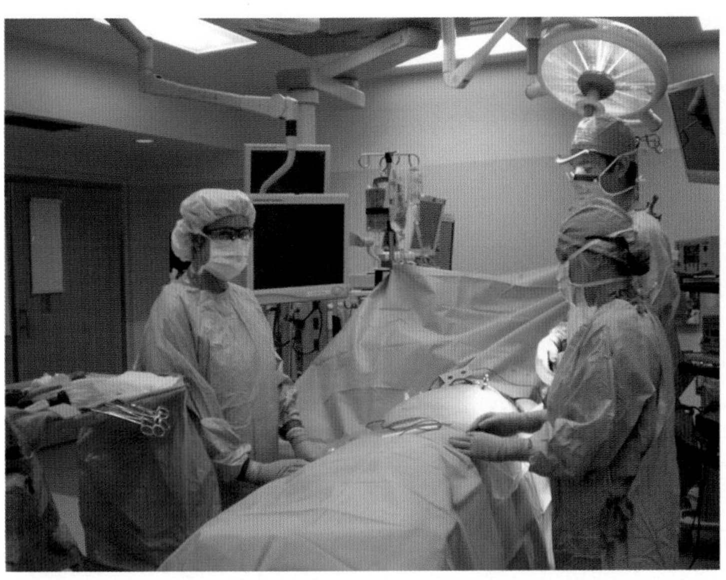

Figure 8.6 Room set-up for a VARD.



Trendelenburg and rolled right side down about 15 to 30 degrees. If conversion to an open laparotomy is required, the bed can be rotated to neutral and the previously marked anatomic landmarks will be helpful. The monitor is placed near the right shoulder (Fig. 8.6).

An open necrosectomy is done with the patient in the supine position.

## VARD Technique

The CT scan is reviewed before making the incision and frequently throughout the procedure. It is important for the surgeon to have a mental image of the precise location of the percutaneous drain(s) within the cavity, and their relationship to the inferior pole of the spleen, the splenic vessels, the colon and other vital structures. A 4 to 5 cm incision is made transversely over the mid-axillary line, immediately below the left costal margin. It is essential to place this incision high under the costal margin and near the site of an existing percutaneous drain since this will guide digital access into the cavity. Cautery is used to divide the lateral abdominal wall muscles, but each layer should be identified and divided separately. The thickness of the external oblique, internal oblique, and transversus abdominis varies greatly between patients. The transversus abdominis muscle should be divided under clamp-control so that the peritoneal cavity, which lies right below this muscle, is not inadvertently entered and the bowel injured (Fig. 8.7). If the peritoneum is entered, it should be closed with an absorbable suture. The bed should now be rolled left side down about 20 degrees and remain in reverse Trendelenburg.

The junction between the peritoneal sac anteriorly and the retroperitoneum can be appreciated as a thin white line approximating the position of the previously marked mid-axillary line. A finger is placed into the retroperitoneum and the track of the drain is located in a triangulated manner (Fig. 8.8). The peritoneal contents and the colon are located immediately anterior. The drain is followed to the wall of the necrotic sac which will be palpated as a firm, fibrous structure. Gentle application of pressure with the digit staying right next to the drain will lead into the cavity itself. Following the drain into the sac usually takes several minutes of diligent work. Entry is usually followed by the exodus of a large amount of purulent effluent through the wound. *Gentle* debridement of nearby necrosectum can be done with finger fracture of any soft, mushy tissue, Yankauer suction, and use of the ring forceps through the wound. It is essential that this blind maneuver be done *gently and in a minimal fashion.* We have seen large skeletonized blood vessels course through the center of a cavity and inadvertent debridement of a blood vessel could lead to significant hemorrhage.

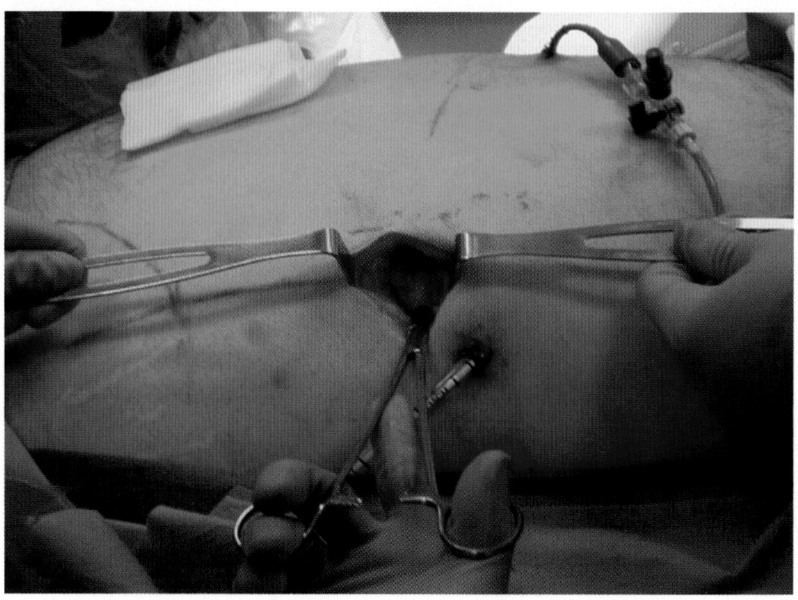

Figure 8.7 Clamp-controlled division of the transversus abdominis muscle.

Debridement under direct visualization of the laparoscope is then performed. A gas insufflation line is connected to one of the percutaneous drainage catheters and a pneumoretroperitoneum achieved to a pressure of 20 mm Hg. Next, an *extra-long* blunt 10/12 mm port *without the trocar,* is placed through the wound into the retroperitoneum with digital guidance. A second port is not required and makes the operation more difficult. A 10 mm, 0-degree laparoscope is used. Because of the parallel arrangement of the scope and forceps, an angled laparoscope (30 or 45 degrees) is *not* recommended. To minimize smudging of the scope two technical maneuvers are helpful. The first is to have the assistant stabilize the port against the external body wall with their hand throughout the procedure. The second is to make sure the laparoscope remain within the gray walls of the port at all times—a very different goal than in other laparoscopic operations. The cavity is debrided utilizing a laparoscopic stone forceps alternating with a Yankauer suction device inserted directly into the wound and parallel to the scope (Fig. 8.9). The pulse-lavage suction irrigator is used periodically throughout the operation to promote hydrodissection of the necrotic tissue. Frequent correlation with the CT scan throughout the

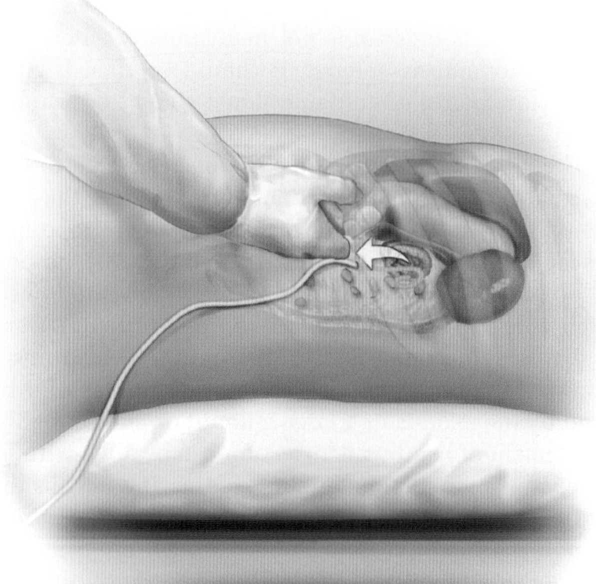

Figure 8.8 A finger is placed into the incision and the drain is located and followed into the thick wall of the WON.

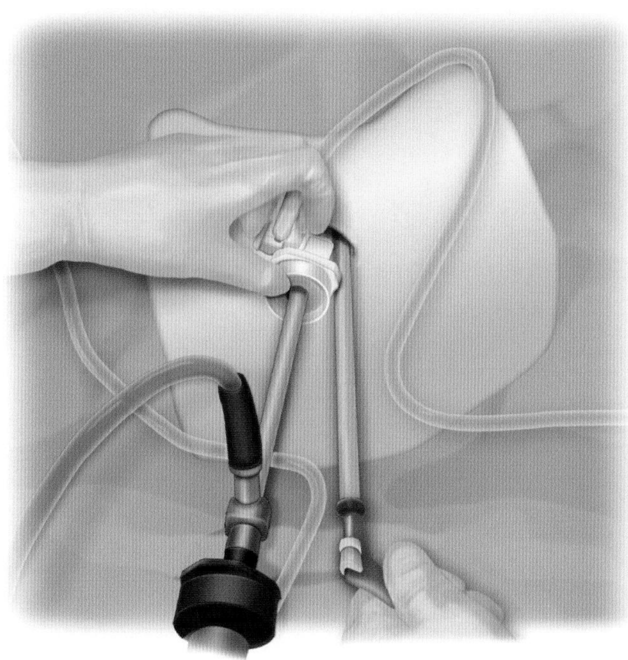

**Figure 8.9** Illustrations of parallel set-up of port and debridement stone forceps inserted directly through the wound.

operation is important to determine the adequacy of debridement. This is assessed by locating the tip of a drain on the CT scan and correlating this with the progress of debridement of the cavity as seen with the laparoscope. The goal of debridement is to remove larger pieces of necrotic tissue and break up loculations, not to strive for a completely clean cavity. It is important to not remove tissue that does not fracture or debride easily. Aggressive debridement can lead to bleeding complications.

Following necrosectomy the cavity is irrigated one last time with the pulse-lavage suction irrigator utilizing 3 L of saline. The port and scope are then reintroduced and the cavity inspected one last time. One or two soft penrose drains are then placed under the direct vision as far medially as is possible and brought out through the dependent part of the wound (Fig. 8.10). All percutaneous drains are left in place for use in delivering the post-operative lavage.

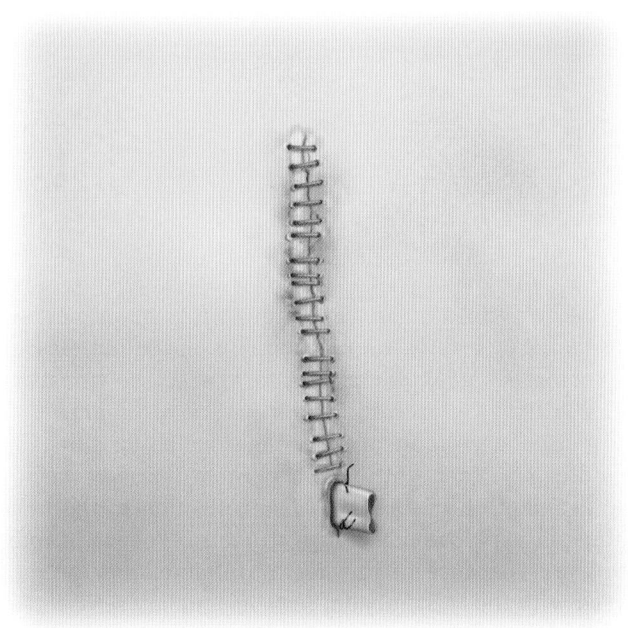

**Figure 8.10** Position of penrose drain(s).

Figure 8.11 Postoperative lavage set-up.

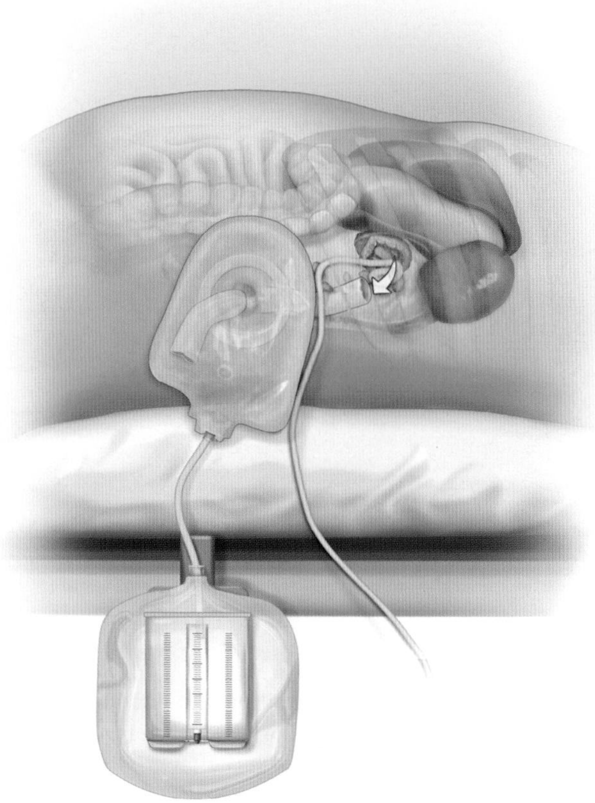

The wound is closed in three separate layers (transversus abdominis, internal oblique, and external oblique) with interrupted 0 absorbable sutures. En masse muscle closure leads to a high rate of flank hernias. The penrose drains are secured posteriorly at the skin and the skin is closed with skin staples. A urostomy appliance is placed over the wound with the penrose drains going into the urostomy appliance and the bag hooked up to a foley urimeter (Fig. 8.11).

The principles of the VARD technique can be applied to collections extending down right flank or into the paracolic gutters or the pelvis. For right-sided collections the operation described above is reversed. For pelvic extensions the monitor should be placed near the patient's knees. The port is simply rotated inferiorly. The penrose drain should be brought out through the same incision.

## Open Necrosectomy Technique

Open necrosectomy is performed through a bi-subcostal incision (Fig. 8.12). Even though this is an open procedure the concept of a "minimally invasive" debridement should be used. Once inside the abdominal cavity, most of the operation can be performed through small incisions with minimal disturbance of nearby vital structures. A Bookwalter retractor is placed and the transverse colon with attached omentum lifted anteriorly and superiorly. It is preferable to debride through the avascular window of the left mesocolon (Fig. 8.13). Retractors and laparotomy pads are placed to expose the transverse mesocolon. The necrotic sac with the light yellow-white color typical of saponified fat will typically "point" through the avascular window of the left mesocolon for a distance of about 2 cm. The "pointing" and can be seen with a thin peritoneal cover over the discolored area just lateral to the ligament of Treitz. The WON collection in the lesser sac on the other side of the peritoneum is palpated as a firm structure. The small intestine is sometimes adhered to this area because of the nearby inflammatory process. Adhesions should be carefully lysed with the Metzenbaum scissors and any serosal tears repaired at the time they are made. Once the avascular window in the mesocolon is

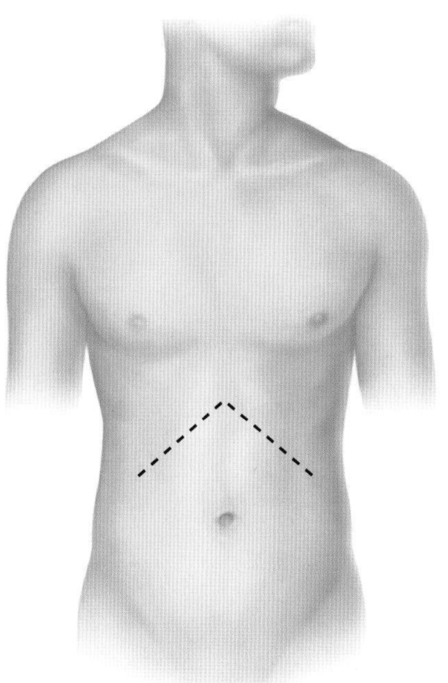

Figure 8.12 Bi-subcostal incision for open necrosectomy.

exposed a small incision in the anterior–posterior direction of about 3 cm is all that is required to enter the necrotic sac (Fig. 8.14). A finger can be inserted into the sac to gently mobilize the necrosectum. Debridement is done through this incision using a combination of the finger, Yankauer suction, empty ring forceps and the pulse lavage irrigator similar to the VARD procedure. Given the small incision, it is helpful to have an open common bile duct exploration set on hand because the curved gall stone forceps are useful for debridement around corners. For necrotic sacs extending into the head and uncinate process area, a similar incision is made into the avascular window of the right transverse mesocolon. Duodenal injuries can occur here so only medium to large collections should be accessed. We have found that if the majority of the necrosectum is removed from other areas that small head/uncinate process collections can be effectively resolved with a combination of post-operative lavage, catheter drainage and time.

Sometimes, the small bowel is very densely adherent to the transverse mesocolon access sites or the collections do not seem to be pointing toward the transverse mesocolon. In this case it is best to avoid adhesiolysis since this can lead to small bowel enterotomies and fistulas. An alternate approach to the pancreas can be made through

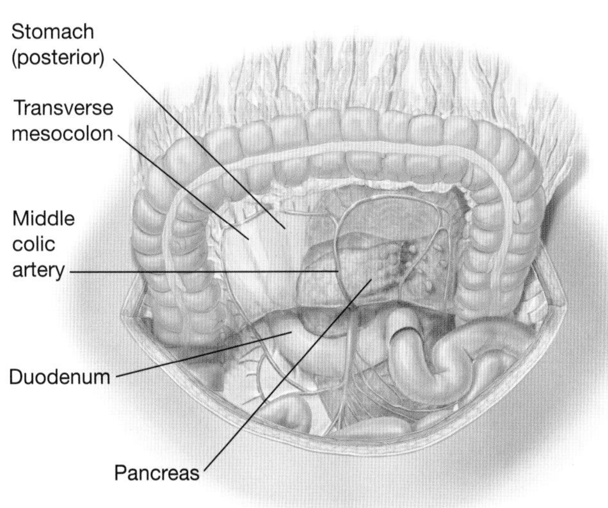


Figure 8.13 The omentum and transverse colon are retrated superiorly and the retractors placed to expose the avascular window in the transverse mesocolon lying just to the left (or right) of the middle colic vessels.

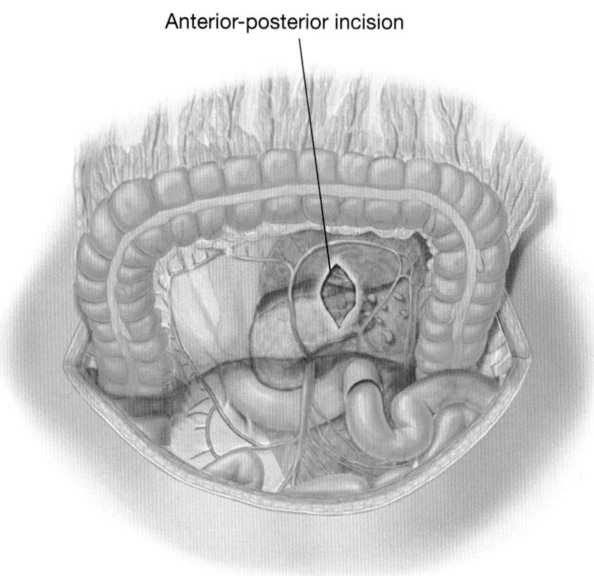


Figure 8.14 Only a small incision is needed for debridement.

the gastrocolic ligament into the lesser sac. In this case the omentum and the transverse colon are rotated back down into their normal anatomic position. The greater curvature and gastroepiploic vessels should be identified and preserved. There is often a large amount of inflammation present and normal anatomy is obscured. If entry into the lesser sac is difficult, it is safest to stay closer to the stomach and avoid potential injury to the transverse colon and middle colic blood vessels. A small 5 cm incision is made in the gastrocolic ligament and the firm walls of the necrotic sac palpated inferiorly (Fig. 8.15). The sac is then entered through a small hole of 2–4 cm in size and debrided using the same principles as above. It is essential that the CT scan is used as an intraoperative map to guide access to and debridement of the collections. In this disease, every patient is slightly different.

Following necrosectomy the cavity is irrigated one last time with the pulse-lavage suction irrigator utilizing 3 to 6 L of saline. Penrose drains are then placed into the

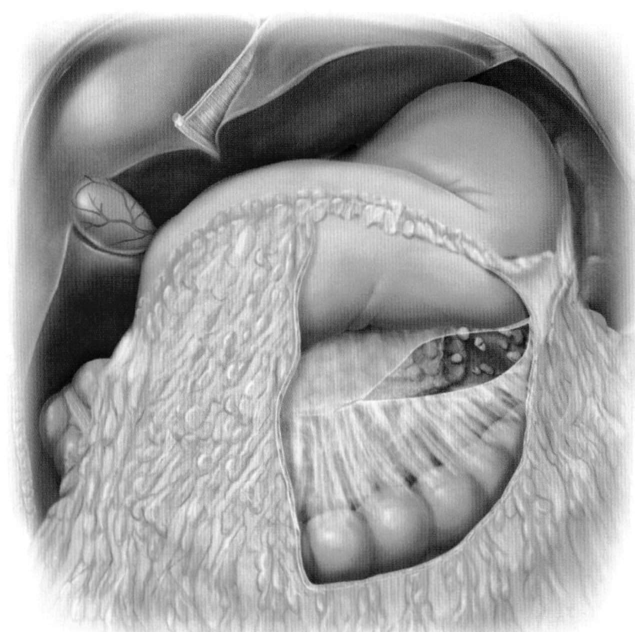

Figure 8.15 Alternate approach: entering the cavity through the gastrocolic ligament. Only a small incision into the necrotic cavity is needed for debridement.

cavity as far medially as is possible and brought out through the flank in a dependent area. All percutaneous drains are left in place for use in delivering the lavage. The penrose drains are secured at the skin and a urostomy appliance is placed. The penrose drains are directed into the urostomy appliance and the bag hooked up to a foley urimeter (Fig. 8.11).

Patients that have collections extending down the paracolic gutters can also be debrided through the bi-subcostal incision. Most patients with paracolic gutter collections also have peripancreatic collections which are in continuity with the more inferior extensions so it is best to first debride the peripancreatic collections. Usually the more superior aspects of the paracolic gutter extensions can be accessed through these incisions. Any remaining collections in the paracolic gutters or pelvis not debrided from above can be debrided by mobilizing the colon in a medial direction for a few centimeters. A separate penrose drain is placed into this more inferior space and brought out through a flank incision.

Open necrosectomy performed for suspected visceral ischemia should be performed through a midline laparotomy.

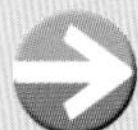

## POSTOPERATIVE MANAGEMENT

With both the VARD and open necrosectomy procedures described, postoperative lavage is performed. Saline or Ringers Lactate is continuously infused in through a percutaneous drain at 200 cc/hr and passively drains out through the penrose and other drains. Postoperative lavage is continued for up to 5 days or until the effluent is clear. Following the lavage period, all drains are opened to gravity drainage. A CT scan is first obtained 2 weeks postoperatively to evaluate the collections. Criteria for drain removal include all of the following:

- Complete resolution of retroperitoneal collections on contrast-enhanced CT scan
- Drain outputs of 10 cc/day or less
- Absence of elevated amylase levels in the drain effluent

## COMPLICATIONS

The main complications of pancreatic necrosectomy include:

- Perioperative hemorrhage
- Enteric fistulas (including gastric, small bowel, and large bowel)
- Pancreatic fistulas, most often from a disconnected duct (aka "orphaned tail")
- Incisional hernias
- Pancreatic endocrine and exocrine insufficiency

Bleeding occurs if vessels traversing the cavity are debrided or disrupted or by using the Yankauer suction too aggressively. Structures traversing the cavity that do not easily fracture with gentle blunt pressure are blood vessels unless proven otherwise and should be left undisturbed. If significant hemorrhage is detected, the first step is to tightly pack the retroperitoneal wound and wait. This is often sufficient to stop most bleeding and to gain hemodynamic stability. Adjunctive use of angiographic embolization should also be strongly considered. Dissection of the indurated and inflamed tissues of the retroperitoneum is discouraged as this will frequently result in further hemorrhage. The distorted anatomy also makes routine exposure techniques extremely difficult. If packing does not quickly control bleeding in a VARD, there should be a low threshold for performing an open laparotomy with retroperitoneal packing followed by angiographic embolization.

Visceral injury to the left colon during a VARD is best avoided by accessing the retroperitoneum under direct vision and utilizing preoperatively placed drainage catheters as a digital manual road-map into the cavity. Blunt finger dissection also facilitates safe entry into the cavity, minimizing the risk of visceral injury. Despite careful technique, patients will still develop enteric fistulas. Fistulas may require prolonged percutaneous drainage but almost all fistulas will close without surgery. Patience is required since most enteric fistulas will not close until all collections are drained, and the patient is anabolic and has a normal serum albumin which may take months. Most pancreatic fistulae can also be treated with patience and percutaneous drainage. Persistent pancreatic fistulas are treated with a distal pancreatectomy of the orphaned tail.

## RESULTS

The pre and postoperative CT scan from a VARD patient is seen in Fig. 8.16. Though most often the debrided necrosectum comes out in small pieces, large pieces of necrotic pancreatic gland can also be easily debrided through the small VARD incision (Fig. 8.17). The feasibility of the Step-Up procedure has been established. Safety and efficacy have been demonstrated in a multi-center, Phase II trial. This study demonstrated that for patients needing surgery, VARD was possible in almost two-thirds of patients with most patients requiring just one operation. The most common reason for crossover from VARD to open was a centromedial collection with extension into the small bowel mesentery that could not be accessed via the flank. The safety profile reported in this prospective study was excellent with a 7.5% hemorrhage rate, a 17.5% enteric fistula rate, and a 2.5% mortality rate, using intention to treat. These low mortality and complication rates compare favorably to pooled open necrosectomy literature reporting incisional hernia formation (25% to 50%), hemorrhage (10%), enteric fistula (17% to 20%) and mortality (6% to 34%). The Phase III results from the Dutch PANTER trial have provided additional data in support of the Step-Up approach. In this randomized controlled trial, 88 patients with infected pancreatic or peripancreatic tissue were randomized to either open necrosectomy or a minimally invasive Step-Up approach. Patients randomized to the Step-Up arm had a lower rate of incidence of post-operative organ failure, a lower rate of major complications, and a lower risk of death or complications (primarily attributable to the decreased complication rate). Postoperatively, the Step-Up arm had fewer incisional hernias (7 vs 24%), less diabetes (16 vs 38%), less exocrine insufficiency with need for pancreatic enzyme supplementation (7 vs 33%), and lower healthcare utilization and medical costs. In addition, surgical intervention (other than drain placement) was avoided in one third of patients in the Step-Up arm.

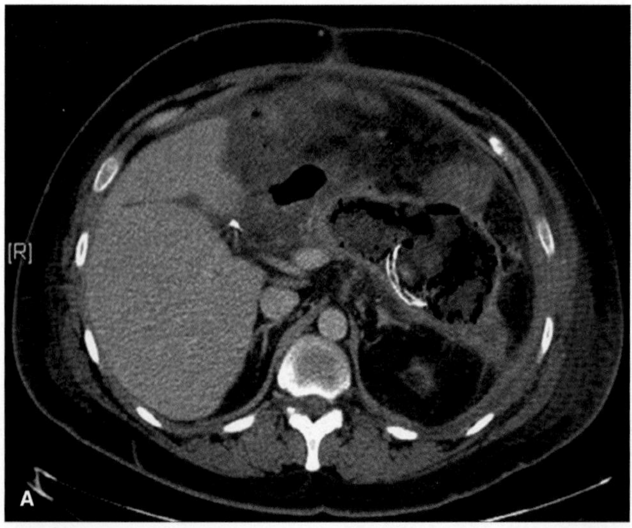


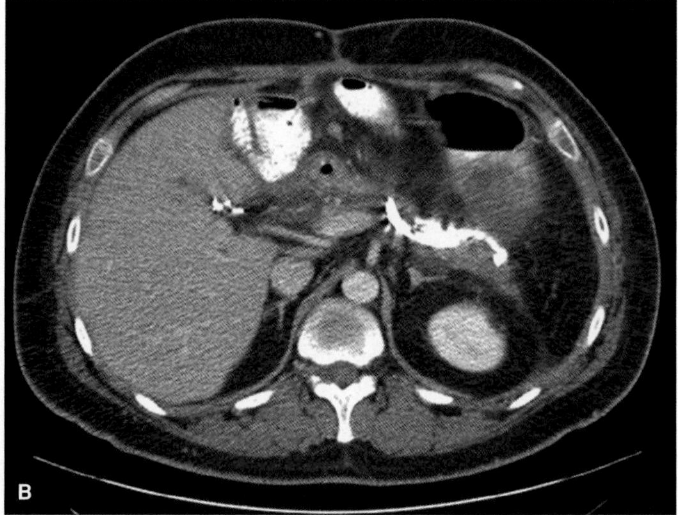


**Figure 8.16** Pre **(A)** and postoperative **(B)** CT scan from the same VARD patient with drains in place.

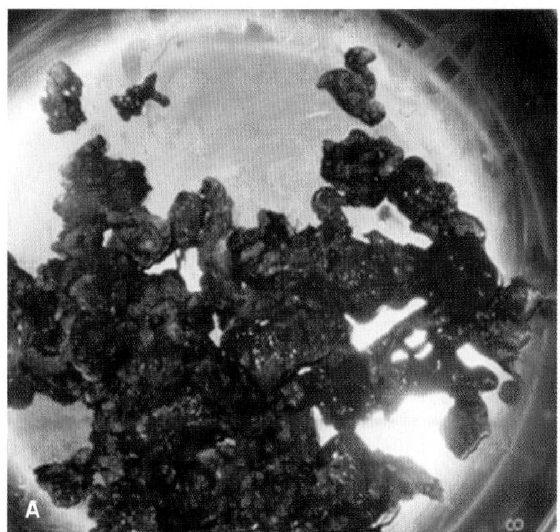
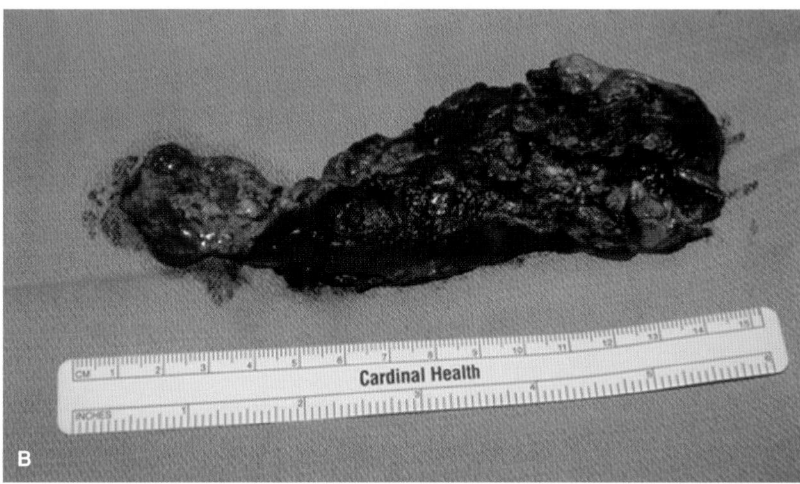


**Figure 8.17** Debrided fragments of necrosectum **(A)** or the necrotic pancreas in one large piece **(B)** can both be removed through the small VARD flank incision.

## CONCLUSIONS

The treatment of necrotizing pancreatitis has undergone significant advances. Many lessons have been learned from the stalwart work done by surgeons in the 1970s, 1980s, and 1990s. Changes over the past century include improved ICU care, a move toward delayed surgery to after 30 days from the onset of symptoms, and the use of percutaneous drains and other minimal access techniques. With these advances, patients are experiencing a much lower morbidity and mortality than in the past.

# Acknowledgments

VARD technique development and evaluation was done with the support of the National Institutes of Health: 5R03DK061362.

## Recommended References and Readings

Beger HG, Buchler M, Bittner R, et al. Necrosectomy and postoperative local lavage in patients with necrotizing pancreatitis: results of a prospective clinical trial. *World J Surg.* 1988;12:255–262.

Besselink MG, Verwer TJ, Schoenmaeckers EJ, et al. Timing of surgical intervention in necrotizing pancreatitis. *Arch Surg.* 2007; 142(12):1194–1201.

Carter CR, McKay CJ, Imrie CW. Percutaneous necrosectomy and sinus tract endoscopy in the management of infected pancreatic necrosis: an initial experience. *Ann Surg.* 2000;232(2):175–180.

Fernandez-Del Castillo C, Rattner DW, Makary MA, et al. Debridement and closed packing for the treatment of necrotizing pancreatitis. *Ann Surg.* 1998;676–684.

Horvath KD, Freeny P, Escallon J, et al. Safety and efficacy of Videoscopic Assisted Retroperitoneal Debridement (VARD) for infected pancreatic collections: a multicenter, prospective, Single-Arm Phase II Study. *Arch Surg.* 2010;145(9):817–825.

Mier J, León EL, Castillo A, et al. Early versus late necrosectomy in severe necrotizing pancreatitis. *Am J Surg.* 1997;173(2):71–75.

Papachristou GI, Takahashi N, Chahal P, et al. Peroral endoscopic drainage/debridement of walled-off pancreatic necrosis. *Ann Surg.* 2007;245(6):943–951.

Raraty MG, Halloran CM, Dodd S, et al. Minimal access retroperitoneal pancreatic necrosectomy: improvement in morbidity and mortality with a less invasive approach. *Ann Surg.* 2010;251(5): 787–793.

Rattner DW, Warshaw AL. Acute pancreatitis. In: Bell RH, Rikkers LF, Mulholland MW, eds. *Digestive Tract Surgery: A Text and Atlas.* Philadelphia, PA: Lippincott-Raven Publishers, 1996: 817–834.

Tsiotos GG, Luque-de León E, Söreide JA, et al. Management of necrotizing pancreatitis by repeated operative necrosectomy using a zipper technique. *Am J Surg.* 1998;175(2):91–98.

Uhl W, Warshaw A, Imrie C, et al. IAP guidelines for the surgical management of acute pancreatitis. *Pancreatology.* 2002;2(6):565–573.

van Santvoort HC, Besselink MG, Bakker OJ, et al. A step-up approach or open necrosectomy for necrotizing pancreatitis. *N Engl J Med.* 2010;362(16):1491–1502.

# 9 Enucleation of a Pancreatic Tumor

**Henry A. Pitt**

## Introduction

Over the past four decades, the mortality of pancreatic resection has improved significantly at high-volume centers. As a result, the most common procedures performed for small neuroendocrine and cystic tumors of the pancreas are pancreatoduodenectomy and distal pancreatectomy. However, the short- and long-term morbidity of a major pancreatic resection remains high. Thus, debate continues as to whether small benign and premalignant lesions of the pancreas should be observed or resected. In comparison, enucleation is a low-risk procedure that preserves pancreatic parenchyma and function. Thus, pancreatic enucleation may be an underutilized procedure that should be considered for small, frequently asymptomatic, pancreatic lesions that, if observed, have the potential to grow and metastasize.

##  INDICATIONS/CONTRAINDICATIONS

The relative indications for and contraindications against pancreatic enucleation are presented in Table 9.1. The most frequent indication for pancreatic enucleation is a neuroendocrine tumor. Pancreatic neuroendocrine tumors (PNETs) that are small with a low Ki67 and/or mitotic index have a low potential for spread and, therefore, are an appropriate indication for enucleation (Fig. 9.1A). However, considerable debate exists regarding what represents a "small" PNET. In a recent analysis of well to moderately differentiated PNETs LaRosa and colleagues determined that 3 cm provided the best discriminative power for a size cutoff. Both Lee et al. and Pitt and associates also used 3 cm as the size limit in their analyses.

In addition to size, other considerations in PNETs include whether the tumor is (a) functioning or nonfunctioning, (b) sporadic or part of a multiple endocrine neoplasia syndrome, (c) solitary or multiple and/or (d) isolated or associated with liver metastases. In general, functioning tumors present when they are smaller and, therefore, may be more amenable to enucleation. Similarly, sporadic, solitary, nonmetastatic tumors may be more appropriate for enucleation. However, enucleation also may be reasonable if the primary tumor is small, and the patient has multiple liver metastases that are not

**TABLE 9.1 Indications and Contraindications for Pancreatic Enucleation**

| Indications | Contraindications |
|---|---|
| Neuroendocrine tumors[a] | Neuroendocrine tumors[b] |
| Side-branch IPMN | Mixed IPMN |
| Mucinous cystic neoplasms | Mucinous cystadenocarcinoma |
| Serous cystadenomas | Pancreatic cancer |
| Solid pseudopapillary neoplasms | Proximity to main duct |
| Lymphangiomas | Pancreatic tail |

[a]Small, Low Ki67 and/or Mitotic Index.
[b]Large, High Ki67 and/or Mitotic Index.
IPMN, Intraductal Papillary Mucinous Neoplasm.

amenable to resection and/or ablation. Since the Ki67 and/or mitotic index usually are not known at the time of surgery, one strategy that may be employed intraoperatively is sentinel lymph node removal. If a lymph node metastasis is found, enucleation may be abandoned in favor of resection with local lymph node dissection.

In a recent analysis from Indiana University side-branch intraductal papillary mucinous neoplasms (IPMNs) were the second most common indication for enucleation (Fig. 9.1B). However, because of the increased risk of carcinoma *in situ* or invasive cancer in main duct IPMNs, enucleation should not be undertaken in patients with mixed IPMNs which involve both the main duct and side branches. Enucleation also should be considered in patients with small mucinous cystic neoplasms (MCNs) (Fig. 9.2A). On the other hand, enucleation is not an adequate operation for mucinous cystadenocarcinomas.

Debate also continues regarding whether serous cystadenomas (SCAs) should be observed or removed. SCAs (Fig. 9.2B) have negligible malignant potential and generally grow slowly. However, enucleation is usually straight forward when SCAs are small. On the other hand, if a SCA is allowed to grow, resection in an otherwise normal pancreas

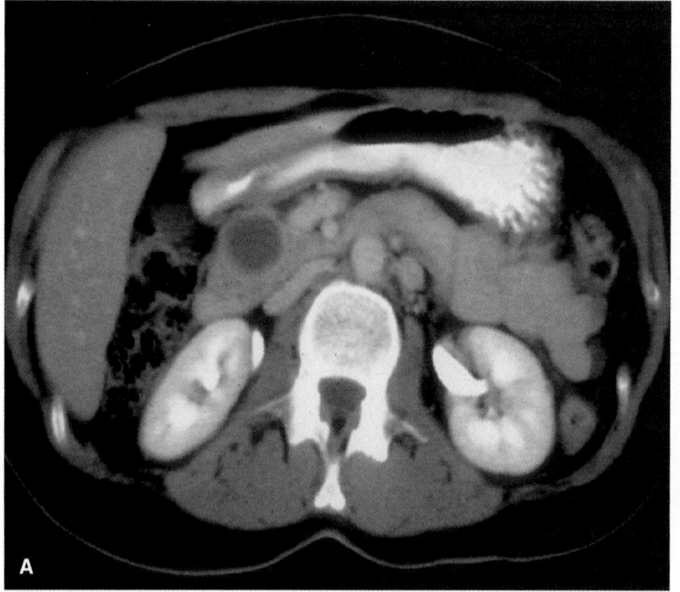


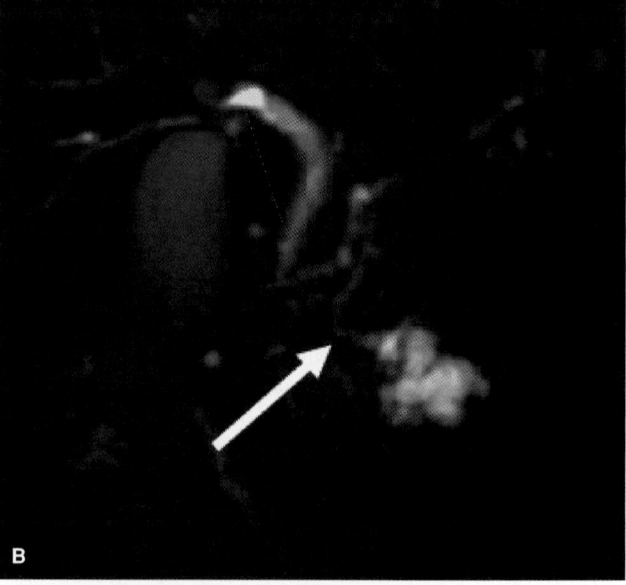


**Figure 9.1** **(A)** Computerized tomography (CT) scan demonstrating a cystic neuroendocrine tumor (NET) in the pancreatic head that was enucleated. Note the hypervascular rim on the arterial phase. Reprinted with permission from: Kiely JM, Nakeeb A, Komorowski RA, et al. Cystic pancreatic neoplasms: enucleate or resect. *J Gastrointest Surg.* 2003;7:890–897. **(B)** Magnetic resonance cholangiopancreatography (MRCP) demonstrating a side-branch intraductal papillary mucinous neoplasm (IMPN) of the uncinate process that was enucleated. White arrow shows the communicating duct. Reprinted with permission from: Turrini O, Schmidt CM, Pitt HA, et al. Side-branch intraductal papillary mucinous neoplasms of the pancreatic head/uncinate: resection or enucleation? *HPB (Oxford).* 2011;13:126–131.

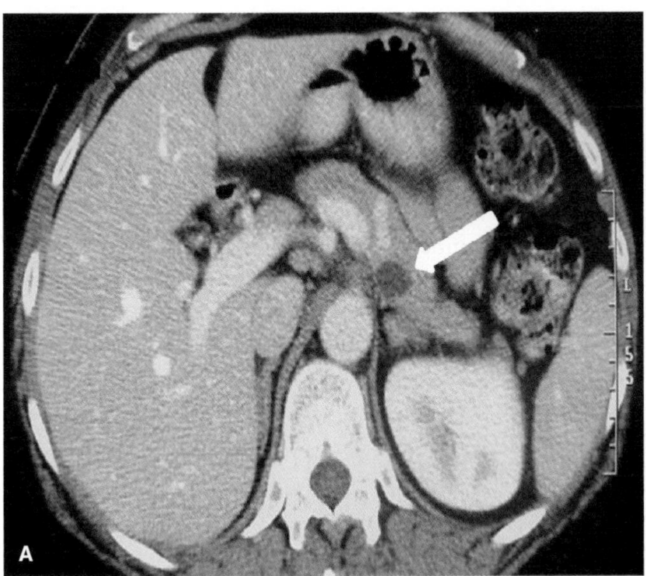


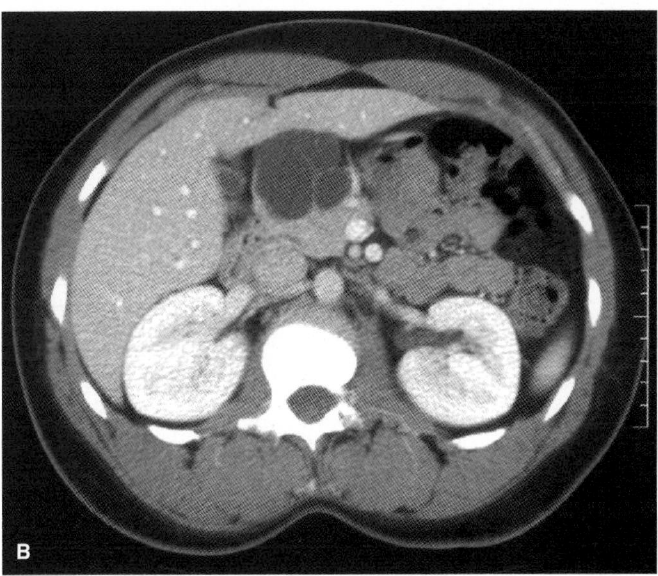


**Figure 9.2** **(A)** Computerized tomography (CT) scan demonstrating a mucinous cystic neoplasm (MCN) of the body of the pancreas (*white arrow*) that was enucleated. **(B)** Computerized tomography (CT) scan demonstrating a serous cystadenoma (SCA) of the head of the pancreas that was enucleated.

may be the only option but is associated with increased short- and long-term morbidity. At the other end of the spectrum, enucleation is not an appropriate operation for adenocarcinoma of the pancreas. Solid pseudopapillary neoplasms (SPNs) lymphoepithelial cysts and lymphangiomas also may be adequately removed by enucleation. However, for all of the pancreatic lesions that may be enucleated, proximity to the main pancreatic duct as well as placement in the pancreatic tail are relative contraindications.

## PREOPERATIVE PLANNING

The most common pancreatic lesions that may be enucleated are small, functioning neuroendocrine tumors. The diagnosis of insulinoma, gastrinoma, vasoactive intestinal peptide producing tumor (VI Poma) and glucagonoma may be established with a careful history, physical examination (for the rash with glucagonoma) and appropriate laboratory studies. For nonfunctioning PNETs, a serum chromogranin A also may be elevated. For the remaining lesions where enucleation may be indicated, no serum markers are available (Table 9.1).

A pancreatic lesion that may result in enucleation is most often discovered on a computerized tomography (CT) of the abdomen (Fig. 9.2). This study may be performed for vague symptoms, usually pain, or for other reasons such as an evaluation for kidney stones. As concern increases for the over exposure to radiation with repeated CT scans, magnetic resonance imaging (MRI) also is detecting more small pancreatic lesions. Magnetic resonance cholangiopancreatography (MRCP) also may be more sensitive than CT at detecting small cystic pancreatic tumors. In addition to CT and MRI, percutaneous ultrasound (US) may detect small pancreatic lesions, but percutaneous US is not as sensitive as CT and MR.

Endoscopic ultrasound (EUS) with fine needle aspiration (FNA) for cytology, the presence of mucin, amylase, carcinoembryonic antigen (CEA) and chromogranin A (CGA) is being performed more frequently to decide whether to observe or to operate. However, the accuracy of CT, MRI or EUS, even with FNA, is at best 75% to 85% in establishing a correct diagnosis. All of these imaging modalities are able to accurately locate the lesion within the pancreas. However, MRCP may be the best at demonstrating the relationship between the lesion and the main pancreatic duct as well as the communicating duct in side-branch IPMNs (Fig. 9.1B).

The remainder of the preoperative preparation for pancreatic enucleation does not differ significantly from other pancreatic surgery. Evaluation of the patient's general health, including cardiopulmonary, renal and hepatic function is indicated. However, the relative risk to life is significantly less for enucleation than for pancreatic resection. Data from the American College of Surgeons—National Surgical Quality Improvement Program suggest that the relative risk of mortality following enucleation is one-sixth that of distal pancreatectomy and one-tenth of pancreatoduodenectomy. Thus, the decision to operate in elderly patients with comorbidities may favor surgery if enucleation is the planned operation. Blood loss is less with enucleation than with resection, and the need for a blood transfusion is unlikely. Nevertheless, typing and cross matching blood is reasonable. Pancreatic enucleation is a "clean" operation so preoperative administration of a first generation cephalosporin is adequate antibiotic prophylaxis. As the operative time for enucleation is less than for resection antibiotic redosing intraoperatively usually is not necessary.

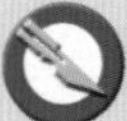

## SURGICAL TECHNIQUE

The first decision is whether to perform the operation minimally invasively or open. This choice will be based on surgeon expertise, patient preference and location of the lesion. For potentially malignant lesions, the first step is to examine the peritoneum and surface of the liver for metastases. If none are found, ultrasound of the liver also should be performed. Again, in the absence of metastatic disease, the next step is to widely expose the pancreas. In general, tumors and/or cysts that are anterior to the pancreas will be more amenable to enucleation. However, lesions that lie posteriorly in the head and/or uncinate can be enucleated but an extensive Kocher maneuver will be required. Once the lesion has been exposed, intraoperative ultrasound imaging is performed to further assess (a) involvement/relationship to the main pancreatic duct, (b) whether the lesion is cystic or solid, (c) if cystic, whether mural nodules are present, and (d) whether other pancreatic lesions are present. If concern exists that enucleation will result in injury to the main pancreatic duct or if a mural nodule is encountered, resection should be undertaken.

To proceed with enucleation of a deep lesion, the pancreatic parenchyma overlying the tumor or cyst should be carefully opened with small vessels being ligated with fine sutures or cauterized. However, most lesions that are amenable to enucleation are on or close to the surface of the pancreas. As a result, dissection is begun at the edges of the lesion and continues with care being taken to stay close to but not entering the tumor or cyst. For neuroendocrine tumors, staying in the correct plain between the pancreas and the tumor is usually straight forward (Fig. 9.3A). This goal may be somewhat more difficult for mucinous cystic neoplasms (Fig. 9.3B) and for side-branch IPMNs because the wall of the cyst may be quite thin.

When enucleating neuroendocrine tumors, mucinous cystic neoplasms, serous cystadenomas, solid pseudopapillary neoplasms and lymphangiomas, no direct connection exists between the lesion and the pancreatic ductal system. However, when enucleating side-branch intraductal papillary mucinous neoplasms, a goal is to identify and, when possible, ligate the communicating duct (Fig. 9.4). In general, frozen section is performed to (a) make a final diagnosis and (b) for cystic lesions, to be sure that no carcinoma *in situ* or invasive cancer is present. However, the likelihood of discovering cancer at this stage is extremely low as the presence of invasion will generally preclude enucleation. For neuroendocrine tumors, injection of 1 or 2 ml of methylene blue dye into the cavity to determine the location of sentinel node(s) may be appropriate.

After the lesion has been removed, checking the integrity of the main pancreatic duct with ultrasound is advisable. If suspicion exists about a pancreatic duct injury, intravenous secretin may be given to determine whether a major ductal injury has occurred. If no concern exists, closure of the parenchymal cavity with one or two figure-of-eight absorbable sutures on a relatively large, fine needle also may reduce the likelihood of developing a pancreatic fistula. A soft closed suction drain is then placed close to the operative field. To begin prophylactic octreotide intraoperatively in the hope of

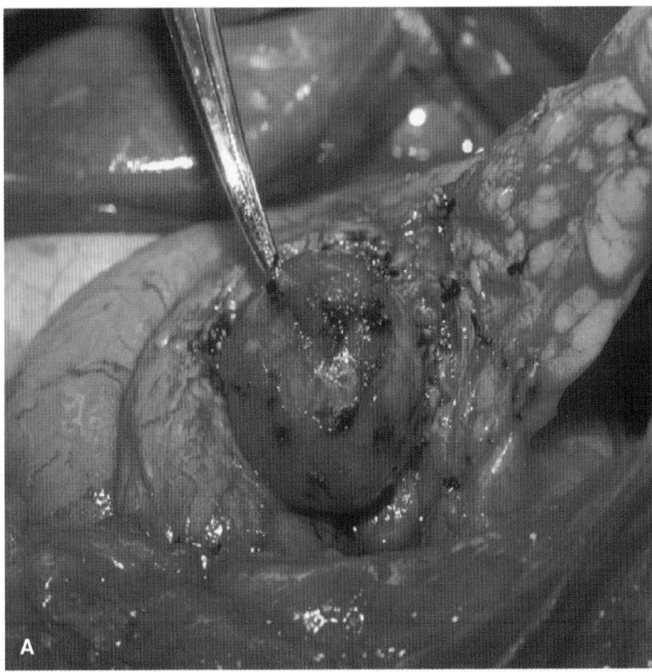


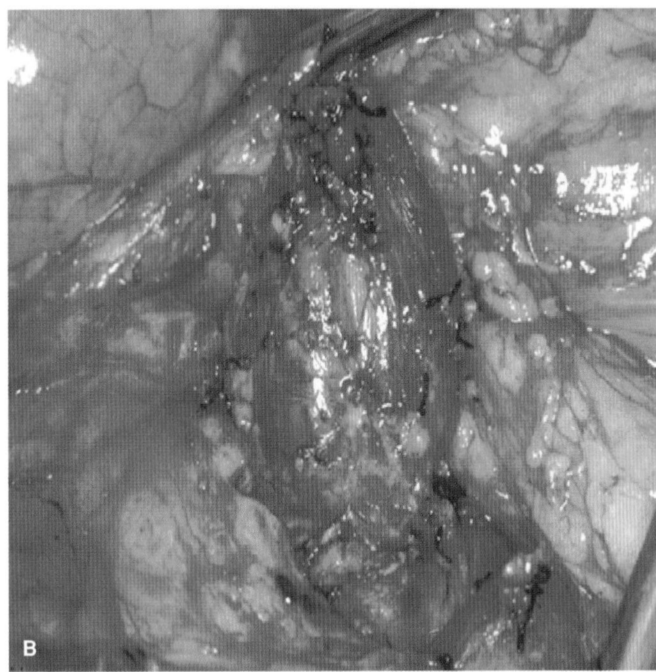


Figure 9.3 **(A)** Operative picture of the cystic NET in the pancreatic head (see Fig. 9.1A) being enucleated. Reprinted with permission from: Pitt SC, Pitt HA, Baker MD, et al. Small, low-risk neuroendocrine tumors of the pancreas, ampulla, and duodenum: resect or enucleate? *J Gastrointest Surg.* 2009;13:1692–1698. **(B)** Operative picture of a MCN in the uncinate being enucleated.

reducing the chance of developing a pancreatic fistula, is an individual surgeon decision as no good data exist in patients undergoing enucleation.

Major advantages of pancreatic enucleation over resection are reduced operative time and blood loss (Table 9.2). Four comparative analyses of enucleation versus resection in neuroendocrine tumors, cystic tumors, side-branch IPMN, and all lesions have documented significantly shorter operative times (90 to 110 minutes, $p < 0.05$) with enucleation. Similarly, these same four comparative analyses have demonstrated that enucleation is associated with significantly less blood loss (320 to 580 ml, $p < 0.05$). These operative advantages clearly save money and reduce the likelihood of transfusion.

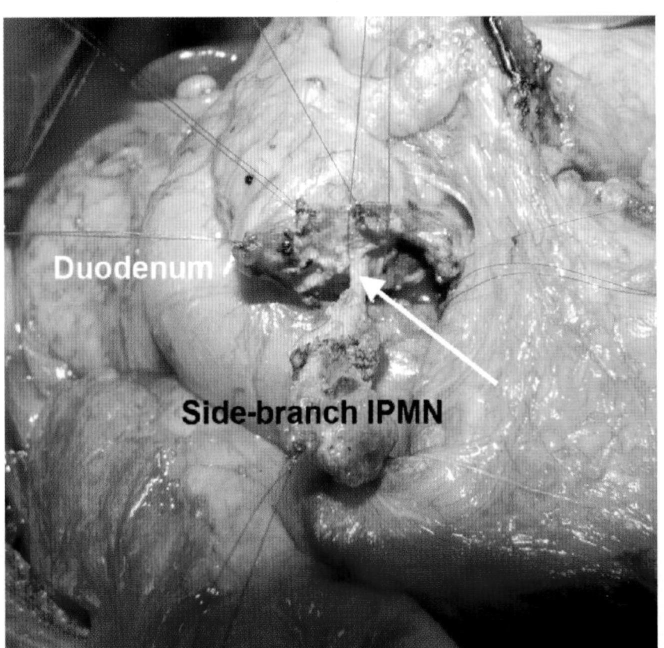


Figure 9.4 Operative picture of a side-branch IPMN of the uncinate (see Fig. 9.1B) after enucleation. The white arrow demonstrates the communicating duct being ligated. Reprinted with permission from: Turrini O, Schmidt CM, Pitt HA, et al. Side-branch intraductal papillary mucinous neoplasms of the pancreatic head/uncinate: resection or enucleation? *HPB (Oxford).* 2011;13:126–131.

TABLE 9.2 Operative Time and Blood Loss for Pancreatic Enucleation and Resection

| | | Operative Time (Minutes) | |
|---|---|---|---|
| **Authors** | **Lesions** | **Enucleation** | **Resection** |
| Pitt et al. | Neuroendocrine[a] | 230[b] | 330 |
| Kiely et al. | Cystic tumors | 190[b] | 280 |
| Turrini et al. | S-B IPMN[a] | 200[b] | 300 |
| Cauley et al. | All | 220[b] | 330 |
| | | **Blood Loss (Milliliters)** | |
| **Authors** | **Lesions** | **Enucleation** | **Resection** |
| Pitt et al. | Neuroendocrine[a] | 290[b] | 870 |
| Kiely et al. | Cystic tumors | 100[b] | 420 |
| Turrini et al. | S-B IPMN[a] | 290[b] | 840 |
| Cauley et al. | All | 150[b] | 690 |

[a]Head and uncinate.
[b]$p < 0.05$ vs. Resection.
S-B IPMN, Side-Branch Intraductal Papillary Mucinous Neoplasm.

## POSTOPERATIVE MANAGEMENT

The decision to place the patient in an intensive care or progressive care unit should be based on the patient's comorbidities. Checking laboratory data shortly after surgery and the next morning is advisable, primarily for amylase to determine whether the operation has caused pancreatitis. Sending the fluid from the drain for amylase on postoperative day (POD) one also is appropriate to predict whether a pancreatic fistula will or has occurred. If the drain amylase is low in the first few days postoperatively, removal of the drain on POD 3 will usually preclude the development of a pancreatic fistula. As mentioned above, no postoperative antibiotics are indicated, but prophylaxis for deep vein thrombosis and stress ulceration is appropriate.

If the surgeon has chosen to leave a nasogastric tube postoperatively, the decision to remove this tube on POD 1 can be based on the results of the serum and drain amylase. In general, foley catheters and central lines, if present, should be removed by POD 2 to prevent infection. Pain management and diet advancement should be undertaken as with other upper abdominal operations and differ if the operation was performed minimally invasively or open.

If a pancreatic fistula occurs after enucleation, the most likely possibility is that Type A, rather than Type B or C, fistula will develop. The facts that no anastomosis to the intestine has been undertaken and usually no severe pancreatitis has developed, make Type A fistula most likely. In this setting nutrition options include (a) making the patient npo and starting total parenteral nutrition, (b) providing liquid enteral nutrition either orally or via a nasojejunal tube or (c) advancing to a low fat diet. Similarly, octreotide therapy may be (a) given intravenously, (b) injected subcutaneously three times a day, (c) provided as a depot injection or (d) withheld. In addition, the drain may be managed with (a) continuous suction, (b) gravity drainage, (c) gradual advancement, (d) replacement after a track has formed or (e) removal when the output diminishes or stops. Various combinations of these options are appropriate, and no good level of evidence favors one technique over another.

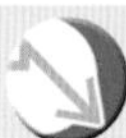

## COMPLICATIONS

Following pancreatic enucleation, the most frequent complication is pancreatic fistula. However, most of the fistulas that occur after enucleation are Type A, which have relatively little clinical consequence. The fact that the pancreatic parenchyma is normal in

**TABLE 9.3 Morbidity of Pancreatic Enucleation and Resection**

| | | Overall Morbidity (Percent) | |
|---|---|---|---|
| **Authors** | **Lesions** | **Enucleation** | **Resection** |
| Pitt et al. | Neuroendocrine | 49 | 44 |
| Kiely et al. | Cystic tumors | 37 | 48 |
| Turrini et al. | S-B IPMN | 43 | 36 |
| Cauley et al. | All | 56 | 61 |
| | | **Pancreatic Fistula (Grade A, B, and C)** | |
| **Authors** | **Lesions** | **Enucleation** | **Resection** |
| Pitt et al. | Neuroendocrine | 38%[a] | 15%[b] |
| Kiely et al. | Cystic tumors | 28% | 28% |
| Turrini et al. | S-B IPMN | 43% | 25% |
| Cauley et al. | All | 33% | 28% |

[a] $p < 0.05$ vs. Resection, 43% B and C.
[b] 77% B and C.
SB-IPMN, Side-Branch Intraductal Papillary Mucinous Neoplasm.

the vast majority of patients undergoing enucleation explains why 30% to 40% of these patients develop a pancreatic fistula (Table 9.3). In comparison, when these patients undergo resection, a pancreatic fistula occurs in 25% to 30% (Table 9.3) and is more likely to be Type B or C fistula.

This point regarding the severity of the pancreatic fistula is clearly illustrated by the analysis performed by Cauley et al. In their comparative analysis of 45 patients undergoing enucleation with 90 resected patients matched for multiple parameters, the pancreatic fistula rate was slightly higher with enucleation (33 vs. 28%, NS), but serious complications, as defined by the American College of Surgeons—National Surgical Quality Improvement Program (ACS-NSQIP) was significantly lower (12 vs. 29%, $p < 0.05$) in the enucleated patients (Fig. 9.5A). However, in four comparative analyses the overall morbidity of enucleation was the same as resection because of the relatively high incidence of Type A fistulas with enucleation (Table 9.3).

The other major advantage of enucleation over resection is significantly reduced mortality. Parikh et al. have analyzed the ACS-NSQIP database to define the risk factors for patients undergoing pancreatectomy. Many of the factors that predict mortality, serious morbidity and overall morbidity are patient related. Factors such as age, male gender, obesity, underlying cardiac or pulmonary disease and a bleeding disorder clearly are related to patient outcomes. However, in this analysis the procedure performed also was statistically significantly related to postoperative morbidity and mortality. Compared to pancreatoduodenectomy, the Odds Ratio of mortality for enucleation was only 0.10 ($p < 0.01$). Similarly, compared to distal pancreatectomy the Odds Ratio of mortality for enucleation was 0.17 ($p < 0.01$) (Fig. 9.5B).

## RESULTS

As documented above, enucleation is associated with reduced operative time (Table 9.2), blood loss (Table 9.2), serious morbidity (Fig. 9.5A) and mortality. While the pancreatic fistula rate in high (30% to 40%) with enucleation, the majority are Grade A fistulas with little clinical consequence. In comparison, resection in patients with an otherwise normal pancreas also is associated with a high pancreatic fistula rate as well as a high incidence of serious complications (Fig. 9.5A). Cauley et al. also have documented that patients undergoing enucleation are less likely to require a stay in an intensive care unit. They also have reported that patients undergoing enucleation have a median hospital stay that is 2 days shorter. Pitt et al. also have reported that the length of

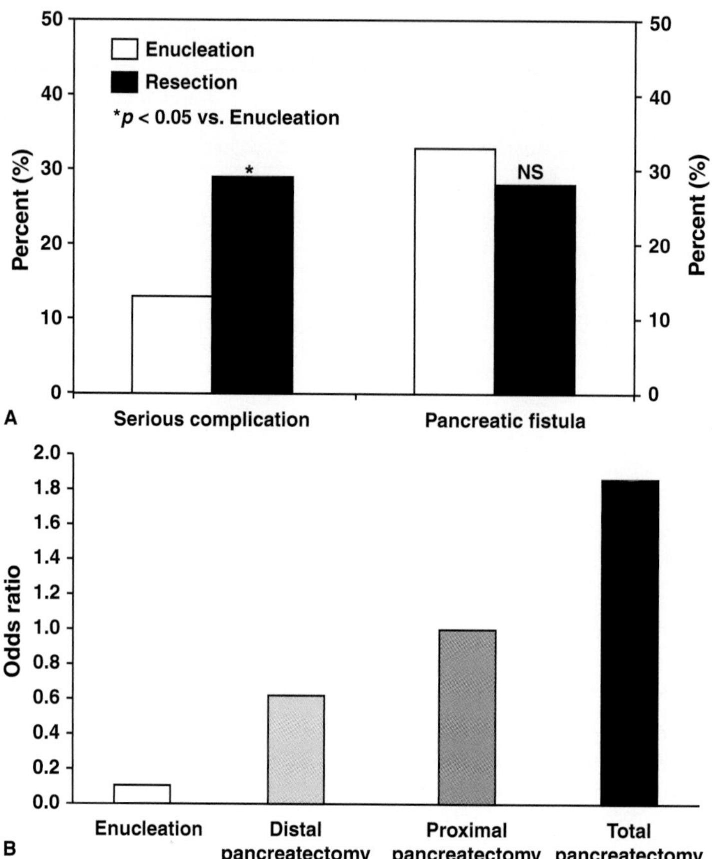


**Figure 9.5** **(A)** Serious complications (*left*) and pancreatic fistula rates (*right*) in patients undergoing enucleation (*open bars*) versus resection (*dark bars*). Serious complications occurred less frequently ($p < 0.05$) after enucleation. Reprinted with permission from: Cauley CE, Pitt HA, Ziegler KM, et al. Pancreatic enucleation: improved outcomes compared to resection. *J Gastrointest Surg.* 2012;16:1347–1353. **(B)** Odds ratios for mortality composing enucleation to distal pancreatectomy, proximal pancreatectomy and total pancreatectomy. Reprinted with permission from: Parikh PY, Shiloach M, Cohen ME, et al. Pancreatectomy risk calculator: an ACS-NSQIP resource. *HPB (Oxford).* 2010;12:488–497.

hospital stay was significantly shorter (6.9 vs. 9.3 days, $p < 0.03$) for patients with neuroendocrine tumors of the pancreatic head or uncinate managed with enucleation.

Another key outcome for the patient is whether they develop endocrine or exocrine insufficiency. While preserving pancreatic parenchyma would intuitively lessen these long-term consequences of resection, little data are available to document this concern. However, Cauley and associates have recently documented that both new endocrine and exocrine insufficiency are significantly less ($p < 0.05$) when enucleation is compared to resection. With a mean follow-up of approximately 4 years, they discovered new exocrine and endocrine insufficiency in only 4% and 2% of patients, respectively, after enucleation. In comparison, both new endocrine and exocrine insufficiency were documented in 17% of patients undergoing resection. Almost all of these resected patients had undergone a proximal as opposed to a distal pancreatic resection.

Another key issue is whether premalignant lesions such as neuroendocrine tumors, mucinous cystic neoplasms, and side-branch IPMNs will recur after enucleation. In this author's 20-year experience with enucleation, recurrence either locally or systemically has not been observed. For patients with serous cystadenomas and lymphangiomas with negligible malignant potential, one CT scan is performed at 3 or 6 months postoperatively to document the pancreas' appearance after surgery. However, for premalignant lesions, annual CT scans have been performed for 5 years after enucleation to document that no recurrence has occurred (Fig. 9.6).

Another important issue with respect to enucleation is whether survival is compromised in patients with premalignant lesions. For patients with neuroendocrine tumors, Pitt et al. compared 36 patients undergoing enucleation with 86 undergoing resection (Fig. 9.7A). The overall 5-year survival in this analysis was 92% with no significant difference between enucleation and resection. While all patients in this analysis had small (<3 cm) tumors without evidence of metastatic disease at the time of resection, five resected patients developed a systemic recurrence. Cauley et al. also have calculated 10-year survival in their patients with premalignant lesions (Fig. 9.7B). Again, they demonstrated that long-term survival was similar with enucleation and resection.

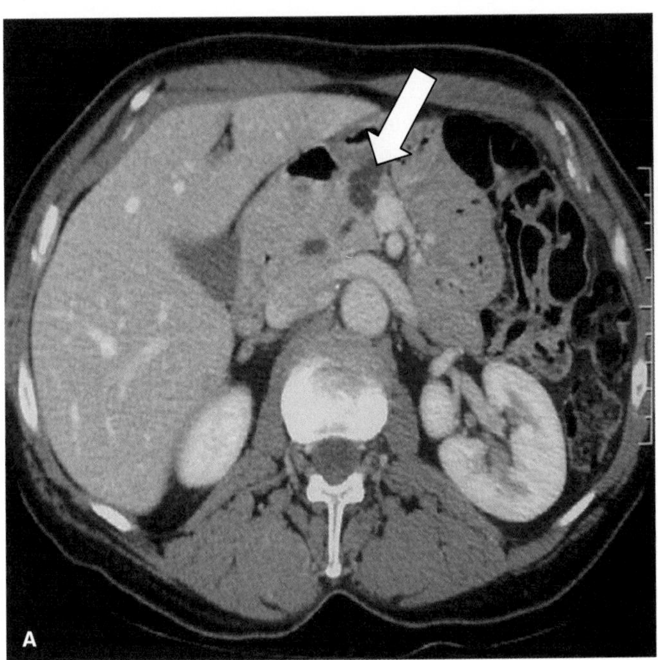


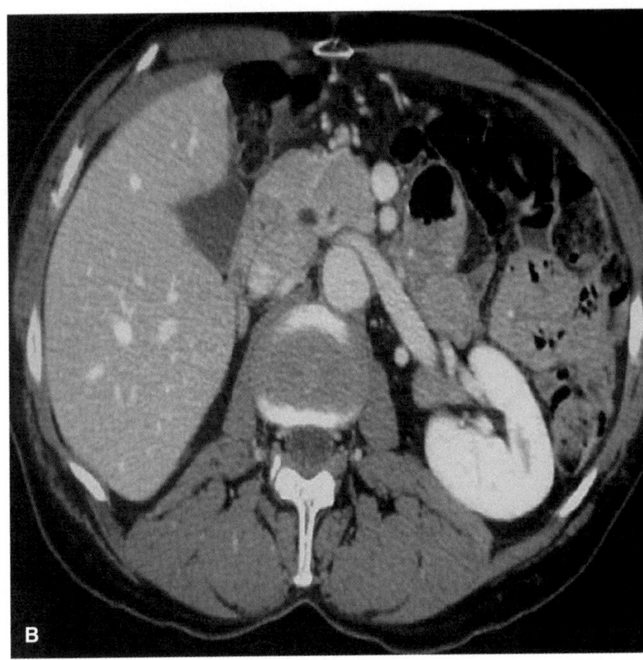


**Figure 9.6** **(A)** Computerized tomography (CT) scan demonstrating a MCN in the pancreatic neck (*white arrow*) before enucleation. **(B)** Computerized tomography (CT) scan demonstrating the same area of the pancreas 2 years after enucleation.

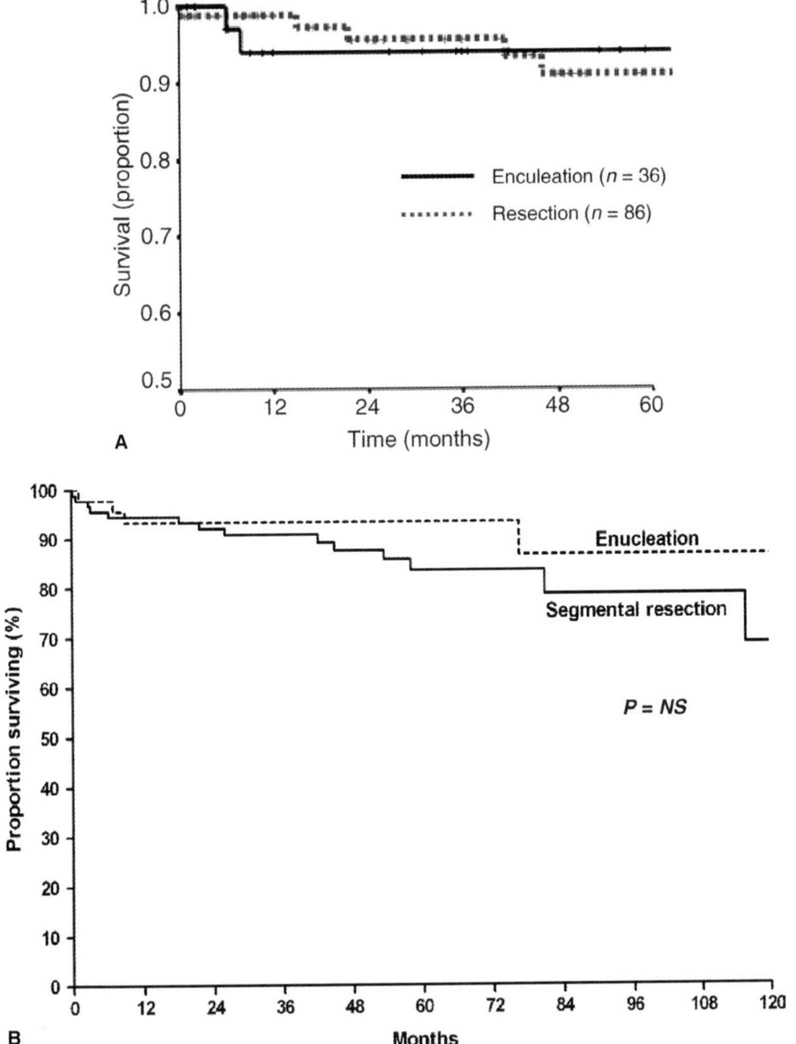


**Figure 9.7** **(A)** Five-year survival of 122 patients with small (<3 cm) neuroendocrine tumors of the pancreas undergoing enucleation ($n = 36$, *solid line*) or resection ($n = 86$, *dotted line*). Reprinted with permission from: Pitt SC, Pitt HA, Baker MD, et al. Small, low-risk neuroendocrine tumors of the pancreas, ampulla, and duodenum: resect or enucleate? *J Gastrointest Surg.* 2009;13:1692–1698. **(B)** Ten-year survival of patients with premalignant pancreatic tumors or cysts who underwent enucleation (*dotted line*) or resection (*solid line*). Reprinted with permission from: Cauley CE, Pitt HA, Ziegler KM, et al. Pancreatic enucleation: improved outcomes compared to resection. *J Gastrointest Surg.* 2012;16:1347–1353.

## CONCLUSIONS

Pancreatic enucleation should be considered for relatively small, benign or premalignant lesions of the pancreas. Both short- and long-term advantages of enucleation over resection have clearly been demonstrated for lesions in the pancreatic head, uncinate and neck. For lesions in the pancreatic body, the primary advantage of enucleation is preservation of pancreatic function. The advantages of enucleation are less clear for small lesions of the pancreatic tail where limited distal pancreatectomy with splenic preservation can routinely be performed by minimally invasive techniques.

In summary, compared to pancreatic resection, enucleation of small, benign or premalignant lesions has multiple advantages. Enucleation has clearly been demonstrated to take less time in the operative room and is associated with less blood loss. Fewer patients undergoing enucleation require an ICU stay or experience serious complications. In addition, for patients with proximal lesions, enucleation is associated with relatively fewer Grade B and C pancreatic fistulas, shorter length of hospital stay and less endocrine and exocrine insufficiency. Moreover, enucleation is not associated with local recurrence, and long-term survival is not compromised. For all of these reasons, pancreatic enucleation should be considered the procedure of choice for small, benign, or premalignant pancreatic pathology.

## Recommended References and Readings


Ahrendt SA, Komorowski RA, Demeure MJ, et al. Cystic pancreatic neuroendocrine tumors: is preoperative diagnosis possible. *J Gastrointest Surg*. 2002;6:66–74.

Assalia A, Gagner M. Laparoscopic pancreatic surgery for islet cell tumors of the pancreas. *World J Surg*. 2004;28:1239–1247.

Baker MS, Knuth JL, DeWitt J, et al. Pancreatic cystic neuroendocrine tumors: preoperative diagnosis with endoscopic ultrasound and fine-needle immunocytology. *J Gastrointest Surg*. 2008;12:1548–1553.

Bilimoria KY, Tomlinson JS, Merkow RP, et al. Clinicopathologic features and treatment trends in pancreatic neuroendocrine tumors: analysis of 9,821 patients. *J Gastrointest Surg*. 2007; 11:1460–1467.

Cauley CE, Pitt HA, Ziegler KM, et al. Pancreatic enucleation: improved outcomes compared to resection. *J Gastrointest Surg*. 2012;16:1347–1353.

Crippa S, Bassi C, Salvia R, et al. Enucleation of pancreatic neoplasms. *Br J Surg*. 2007;94:1254–1259.

Fernández-Cruz L, Glanco L, Cosa R, et al. Is laparoscopic resection adequate in patients with neuroendocrine pancreatic tumors? *World J Surg*. 2008;32:904–917.

Kiely JM, Nakeeb A, Komorowski RA, et al. Cystic pancreatic neoplasms: enucleate or resect. *J Gastrointest Surg*. 2003;7:890–897.

LaRosa S, Klersy C, Uccella S, et al. Improved histologic and clinicopathologic criteria for evaluation of pancreatic endocrine tumors. *Human Pathol*. 2009;40:30–40.

Lee CJ, Scheiman J, Anderson MA, et al. Risk of malignancy in resected cystic tumors of the pancreas less than or equal to 3 cm in size: is it safe to observe asymptomatic patients? *J Gastrointest Surg*. 2008;12:234–242.

Parikh PY, Shiloach M, Cohen ME, et al. Pancreatectomy risk calculator: an ACS-NSQIP resource. *HPB (Oxford)*. 2010;12:488–497.

Pitt SC, Pitt HA, Baker MD, et al. Small, low-risk neuroendocrine tumors of the pancreas, ampulla, and duodenum: resect or enucleate? *J Gastrointest Surg*. 2009;13:1692–1698.

Talamini MA, Moesinger R, Yeo CJ, et al. Cystadenomas of the pancreas: is enucleation an adequate operation. *Ann Surg*. 1998; 227:896–903.

Turrini O, Schmidt CM, Pitt HA, et al. Side-branch intraductal papillary mucinous neoplasms of the pancreatic head/uncinate: resection or enucleation? *HPB (Oxford)*. 2011;13:126–131.

Ziegler KM, Nakeeb A, Pitt HA, et al. Pancreatic surgery: evolution at a high-volume center. *Surgery*. 2010;148:702–710.

# 10 The Beger, Frey, and Bern Procedures for Chronic Pancreatitis

**Jens Werner and Markus W. Büchler**

## Introduction

In chronic pancreatitis (CP) a benign inflammatory process in the pancreas results in progressive structural changes with replacement of functional exocrine and endocrine parenchyma by a fibrotic and inflammatory tissue. The consequences are diabetes mellitus, exocrine insufficiency, and severe recurrent upper abdominal pain, often resulting in a significant reduction of the quality of life. In addition, the inflammatory process or the formation of pseudocysts can cause local complications such as obstruction of the pancreatic duct, bile duct, duodenum, as well as the portal vein. In most patients with CP the trigger of the disease is an inflammatory mass of the pancreatic head, and surgical resection provides good short and long-term results including pain relieve and improvement in the quality of life in patients with CP. Despite adequate surgical resection, exocrine and endocrine insufficiency may progress. In contrast, ductal drainage operations have limited effects and poor long-term outcomes.

While the partial pancreatoduodenectomy (Kausch–Whipple procedure), in its classical or pylorus-preserving variant, has been the procedure of choice for pancreatic head resection in CP for many years, the duodenum-preserving pancreatic head resections (DPPHR) and its variants (Beger procedure, Frey procedure, Bern procedure) represent less invasive, organ-sparing techniques with better perioperative, better short-term, and at least equally good long-term results. The present chapter describes the different types of DPPHR in detail and elucidates the individual advantages and disadvantages.

##  INDICATIONS

A summary of the common surgical indications for chronic pancreatitis are listed in Table 10.1.

**TABLE 10.1 Indications and Techniques for Surgery in Chronic Pancreatitis**

| | |
|---|---|
| **Indications for surgery in chronic pancreatitis:** | Intractable pain<br>Symptomatic local complications<br>Unsuccessful endoscopic management<br>Suspicion of malignancy |
| **Surgical techniques** | **Indications and recommendations** |
| **Pure drainage operations:** | |
| Zystojejunostomy | Surgical procedure of choice for isolated pseudocysts<br>Caution: intraoperative frozen section to exclude cystic neoplasm! |
| Laterolateral pancreaticojejunostomy: | Ductal dilation >7 mm, without inflammatory mass |
| Partington–Rochelle procedure | |
| Puestow Procedure | |
| **Resection procedures:** | |
| Pancreatic head resections | Always include a ductal drainage<br>Procedures of choice if inflammatory mass in the head of the pancreas<br>All techniques have comparable results (see Table 10.2) |
| PD and ppPD | Procedure of choice in suspected malignancy and in irreversible duodenal stenosis |
| DPPHR techniques: | Caution: intraoperative frozen section to exclude malignancy |
| DPPHR, Beger (Fig. 10.2A, B) | Procedures of choice if inflammatory mass in the head of the pancreas |
| DPPHR, Bern (Fig. 10.4A, B) | Bern technically less difficult than Beger but equal long-term outcome. |
| DPPHR, Frey (Fig. 10.3A, B) | Patients with ductal obstruction in the head and tail and a smaller inflammatory mass in the head. |
| V-shaped excision: | Small duct disease (diameter of pancreatic duct <3 mm) |
| Pancreatic left resection | Rare cases, e.g., isolated CP in the tail (e.g., posttraumatic)<br>Rare cases of large pseudocysts in the tail |
| Segmental resection | Rare cases, e.g., isolated ductal stenosis in the body (e.g., posttraumatic) in patients without diabetes. |
| Total pancreatectomy | Rare cases with severe changes in the entire pancreas and preexisting IDDM |

PD: pancreatoduodenectomy, ppPD: pylorus-preserving pancreatoduodenectomy, DPPHR: duodenum-preserving pancreatic head resection, IDDM: insulin-dependent diabetes mellitus.

Pain remains the most important and most frequent indication for surgery in CP, followed by the local complications of CP as shown in Figure 10.1. Most of the patients with chronic pancreatitis present with a ductal obstruction located in the pancreatic head, frequently associated with an inflammatory mass. In cases of portal vein obstruction and secondary portal hypertension with the formation of collaterals, the transection of the pancreas is technically challenging and sometimes not possible. In those cases, the Bern procedure which omits the transection of the pancreatic neck, is the only option to resect the pancreatic head.

Suspicion of malignancy is another important indication for surgery. In those cases, a DPPHR should be avoided and a primary partial pancreatoduodenectomy in its classical or pylorus-preserving form should be performed to adequately address the malignancy.

In very rare cases, diffuse small duct disease of the whole gland, segmental or distal pancreatitis is present. These changes need different surgical approaches including V-shape resection, segmental resections, or left resections.

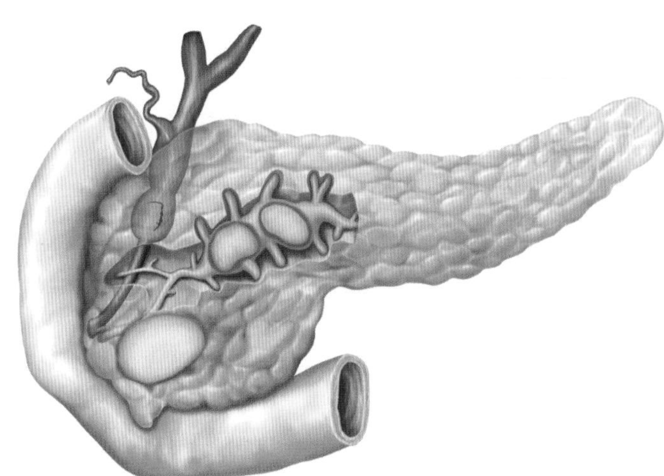

**Figure 10.1** Local complications of chronic pancreatitis. Fibrosis and the inflammatory mass can result in stenosis and prestenotic dilatation of the pancreatic duct, the common bile duct and the duodenum. Intraductal concrements result in ductal obstruction. Formation of pseudocysts results in local compression of neighboring structures. Not shown: Parenchymal calcifications and portal vein thrombosis.

## PREOPERATIVE PLANNING

A thorough medical history and physical examination is pivotal for the diagnosis and adequate therapy of patients with CP. In the medical history, evaluation of etiologic factors (especially alcohol) and of pancreatic pain is crucial to select patients for the different therapeutic options as discussed below.

Besides routine parameters, laboratory data should include cholestasis parameters, and tumor markers for pancreatic adenocarcinoma. In order to adequately inform patients about the course of their disease and possible consequences of surgery (e.g., need of insulin), the endocrine and exocrine function have to be evaluated. Exocrine function test is often provided by gastroenterologists but not required for surgical decision-making, except for patients with uncertain diagnosis due to atypical clinical presentation.

For tailored therapy and especially for planning of surgical therapy, imaging studies play a central role in the diagnostic workup of patients with CP. Most of the patients with CP first consult general practitioners and gastroenterologists. For the general practitioner abdominal ultrasound is an effective screening method, which may help to establish the diagnosis in patients with a thickened pancreas or head mass, a dilated duct, or pseudocysts. Gastroenterologists frequently use endoscopic ultrasound, which is more sensitive and specific than transabdominal ultrasound. Many patients undergo multiple endoscopic retrograde cholangiopancreatographies (ERCP) for diagnosis and therapeutic intervention. The gold standard of imaging for diagnosing CP and for the design of surgical therapy is cross section imaging by contrast-enhanced computed tomography (CT) and magnetic resonance imaging (MRI). The superiority of CT or MRI is still a matter of debate but either imaging study is adequate if performed with sufficient quality. If a patient presents without ERCP, the MRI offers the additional possibility to evaluate the ductal system by MR cholangiopancreatography. Only ERCP or MRCP allows for evaluation according to the Cambridge-classification, which is at present still the only broadly accepted classification-system. However, an ERCP or MRCP is not mandatory, and if surgery is indicated should be omitted because of the risk of pancreatitis and secondary infections. The advantage of CT is the better visualization of parenchymal calcifications. In fact, it is a difficult task to diagnose cancer in a chronically inflamed pancreatic head. Thus, as indicated by a recent review the indication for surgery for a pancreatic mass should not be based on preoperative tissue diagnosis because of frequent false negative results due to sampling problems. We believe that patients with cancer as differential diagnosis should undergo surgical exploration and resection.

Since ethanol abuse is the most common cause of chronic pancreatitis in the Western world, active alcoholism needs to be ruled out before a surgical procedure is performed.

Most of the patients with chronic pancreatitis who are transferred to a surgeon have been treated for intractable pain for many years before and are often dependent on their pain medication. Thus, close perioperative and postoperative follow-up and an individualized pain management must be available.

If a pancreatic malignancy is suspected, a partial pancreatoduodenectomy (PD) should be performed and DPPHR should be omitted, since the DPPHR are not oncologic operations since lymphnodes and adjacent organs are not resected.

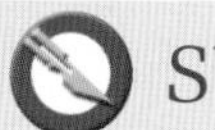

## SURGERY

Patients are positioned on the back in a straight position; the right arm extended (90 degrees) in the shoulder to allow access to the right arm.

A midline laparotomy is performed in most patients, while in adipose patients a transverse incision is preferred by us. After a systematic exploration of the abdomen and after a malignancy (liver metastasis, peritoneal carcinosis) has been ruled out, the pancreas is explored by opening the lesser sac through the gastrocolic ligament and by the Kocher maneuver. Due to the chronic inflammation and especially in case of portal hypertension, these steps might be more difficult than in pancreatic cancer cases. To get access to the complete pancreatic head, the gastroepiploic vessels need to be divided and the right colon flexure should be mobilized into the lower abdomen.

In contrast to an oncologic lymph node dissection, the hepatoduodenal ligament does not need to be dissected and the anatomical structures do not need to be explored. The gallbladder is removed in the typical fashion.

# Beger Procedure

The Beger procedure represents the first DPPHR described and has been the most frequently used technique in Europe in the past.

### Resection

Similar to PD the pancreas is divided at the level of the portal vein (Fig. 10.2A). However, in contrast to PD, the pancreatic head is excavated with preservation of the duodenum and a layer of pancreatic tissue.

The division of the pancreatic neck is performed with a scalpel and bleeding from the resection margin stopped with sutures (e.g., 5-0 prolene). Adequate drainage of the pancreatic duct has to be verified by probing.

Before the excavation of the pancreatic head with a scalpel, sutures are fixed around the complete ventral part of the pancreatic head. These sutures help to reduce the bleeding during the excavation and ease the handling of the pancreatic head. In addition, the left hand of the surgeon can control the blood inflow to the pancreatic head by pressure as well. The aim of this step is to remove the fibrotic and inflamed tissue of the pancreatic head, leaving a thin layer of periduodenal pancreatic tissue (Fig. 10.2A). Any bleeding is stopped by non-resorbable sutures (e.g., 5-0 prolene) and coagulation is avoided.

In case of cholestasis or bile duct stenosis, the bile duct needs to be opened completely. The resection needs to remove all the fibrotic tissue around the proximal bile duct and an internal anastomosis (single stitches) guarantees the outflow of bile.

### Reconstruction

The reconstruction is performed by two anastomoses with a jejunal loop to drain the pancreatic left remnant and to cover and drain the excavation of the pancreatic head (Fig. 10.2B).

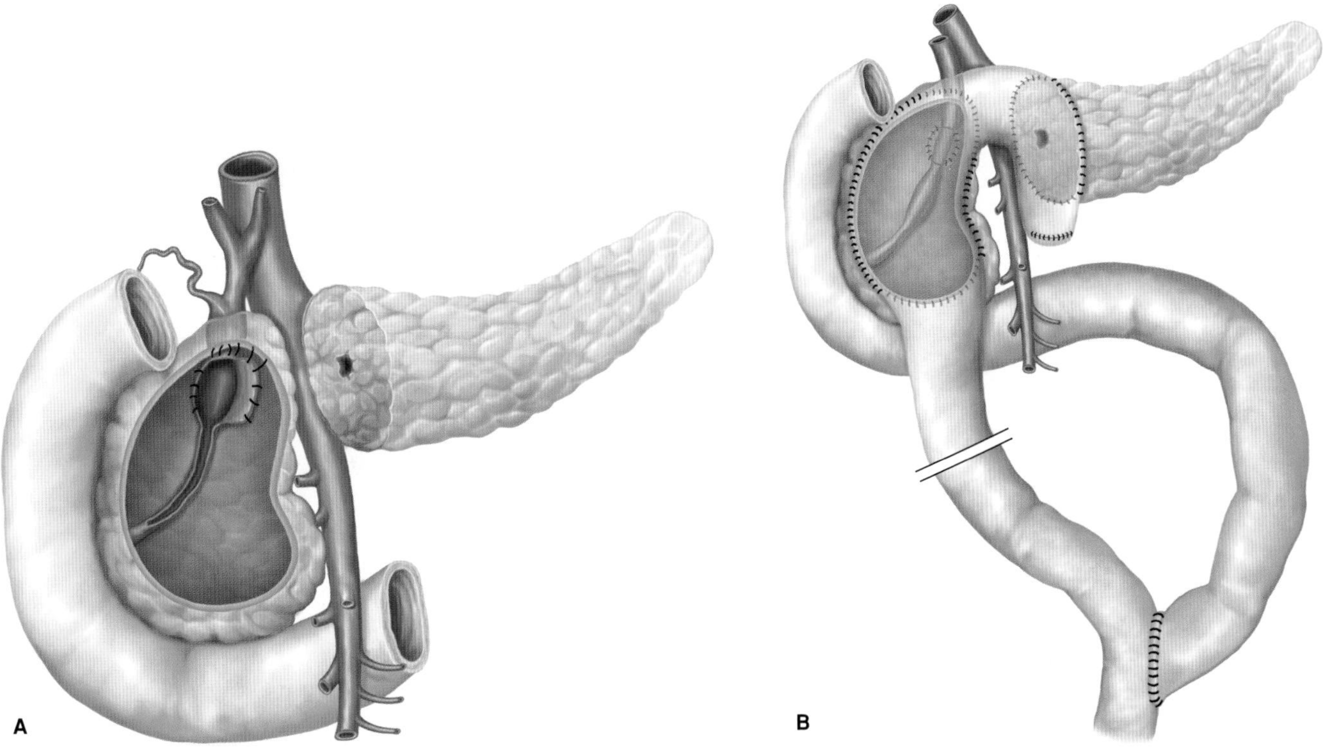


Figure 10.2 Beger procedure. **A:** The pancreas is dissected on the level of the portal vein. The pancreatic head is excavated and the duodenum is preserved with a thin layer of pancreatic tissue. If the bile duct is obstructed it can be opened and an internal anastomosis with the excavated pancreatic head can be performed (not shown). **B:** The reconstruction is performed with two anastomoses, of the pancreatic tail remnant and of the excavated pancreatic head with a Roux-en-Y jejunal loop.

A jejununal loop is divided about 30 cm after the ligament of Treitz and moved transmesocolically into the lesser sac.

At first, a pancreaticojejunostomy identical to the anastomosis performed in the Kausch–Whipple procedure is performed. We prefer a two layer single stitch technique with separate pancreatic duct sutures using PDS 5-0.

The second anastomosis is a side-to-side pancreaticojejunostomy using the same jejunal loop. This anastomosis is performed with running sutures using 4-0 PDS. We perform a two layer anastomosis (Fig. 10.2B).

The final step of the reconstruction is the Y-Roux anastomosis. We perform an anastomosis with two running layers using PDS 5-0.

# Frey Procedure

Instead, Frey et al. developed a modification of DPPHR which represents a hybrid technique between the Beger- and Partington–Rochelle or Puestow procedures. Compared to the Beger procedure the resection in the pancreatic head in the Frey modification is smaller and combined with a laterolateral pancreaticojejunostomy to drain the entire pancreatic duct toward the tail (Fig. 10.3A, B). In contrast to the Beger procedure reconstruction can be performed with one single anastomosis. Nevertheless, secondary to the length of the anastomosis, the suturing is quite time consuming. This procedure is not suitable in patients with a large inflammatory mass in the pancreas without stenosis of the left-sided pancreatic duct, as often observed in the European collectives. However, it appears advantageous in patients with less severe inflammation in the head combined with an obstruction in the left-sided pancreatic duct.

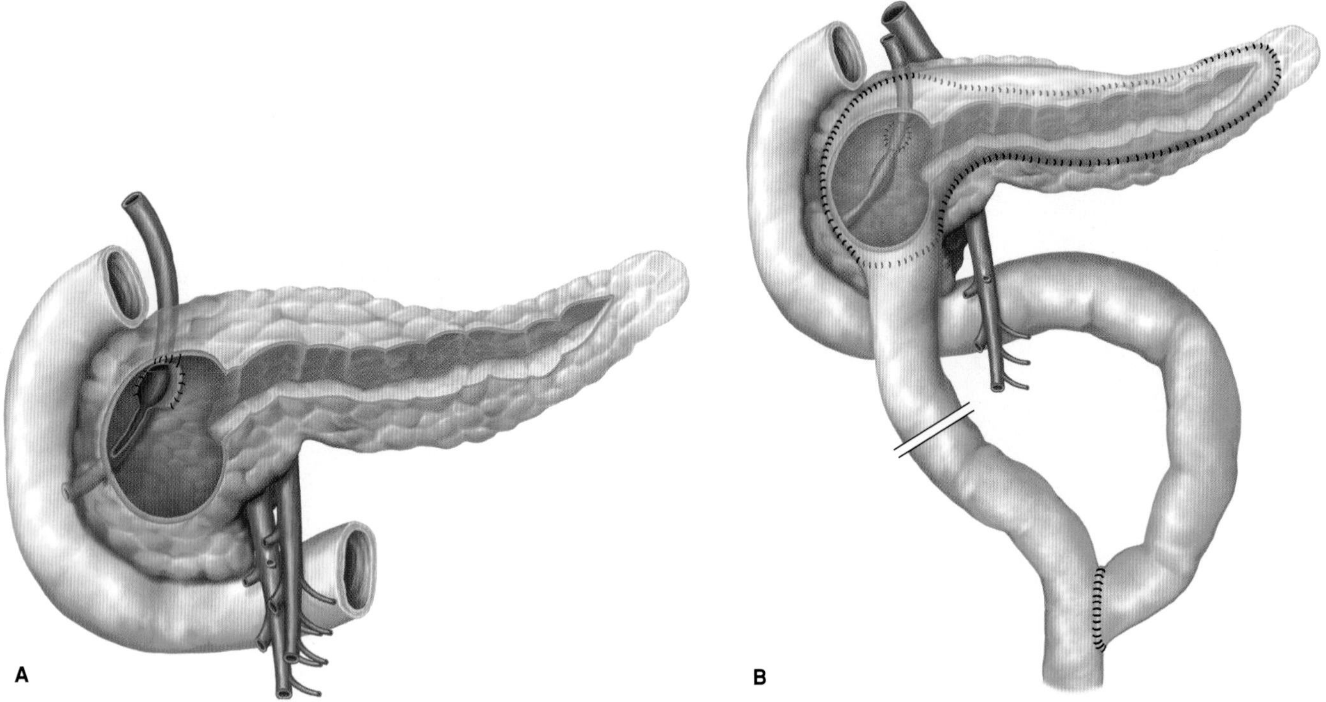


Figure 10.3 Frey procedure. **A:** The Frey procedure combines a circumscript excision in the pancreatic head with longitudinal dissection of the pancreatic duct toward the tail. **B:** Reconstruction is performed with an anastomosis with a Roux-en-Y jejunal loop. Compared to the Beger procedure the extent of resection of the pancreatic head is smaller, however, reconstruction is easier as it only requires one anastomosis to the pancreas.

# Bern Procedure

The Bern operation was introduced about 15 years ago. In contrast to the Beger procedure, the pancreas is not divided over the portal vein, which is especially difficult because of inflammation and portal hypertension and subsequent collaterals (Fig. 10.4A). Thus, only one anastomosis is needed for reconstruction (Fig. 10.4B). The Bern technique is technically easier, the operative time and perioperative blood loss are reduced, while the long-term outcome is identical compared to the Beger procedure. Thus, this modification is now the most widely used DPPHR technique today.

## Resection

The excavation of the pancreatic head can be performed to an identical extent compared to the Beger procedure (Fig. 10.5A). It is important to have a good drainage of the pancreatic neck and tail. This has to be verified by probing of the pancreatic duct toward the left (Fig. 10.5A). If a stenosis is discovered, the resection can be extended toward the left similar to the Frey/Partington–Rochelle procedures until adequate drainage is achieved. However, in our collective this has been necessary in only 2% of cases.

As with the Beger procedure, the bile duct can be opened and drained internally in case of cholestasis or bile duct obstruction (see above).

## Reconstruction

The reconstruction can be performed by one single anastomosis between a jejunal loop and the continuous pancreatic resection rim (Fig. 10.4B). We perform a two layer side-to-side pancreaticojejunostomy with running sutures (PDS 4-0) (Fig. 10.5B, C). The pancreatic duct is separately sutured with three single stitches of the inner layer to guarantee good drainage of the pancreatic duct.

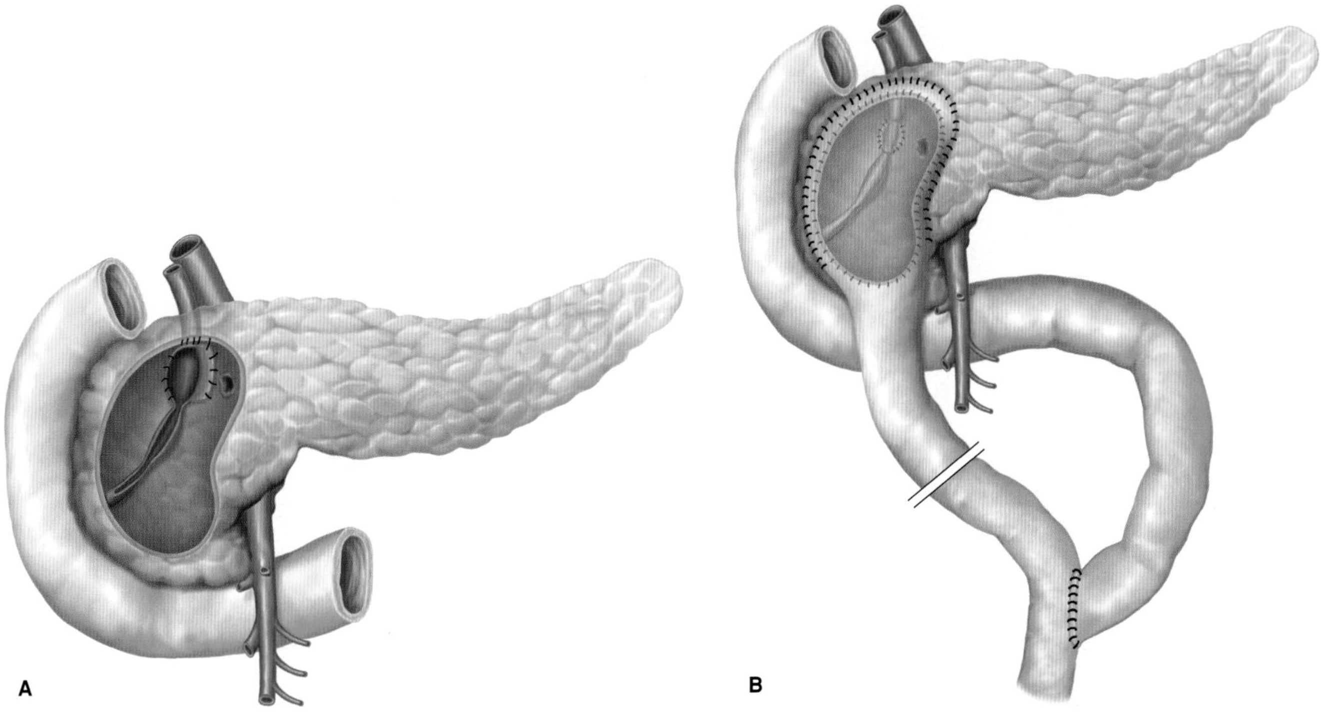


Figure 10.4 Bern procedure. **A:** The Bern modification is a technical simplification of the Beger procedure. The extent of resection of the pancreatic head is comparable to the Beger procedure. However, the pancreas is not dissected on the level of the portal vein. The bile duct can be opened and an internal anstomosis can be performed (as shown). **B:** The reconstruction can be performed with one single anastomosis of the pancreas with a Roux-en-Y jejunal loop. The pancreatic duct toward the tail has to be probed and an internal anastomosis has to be performed to prevent stenosis.

Independent of the technique of DPPHR, an intraoperative frozen section has to be obtained to rule out pancreatic adenocarcinoma. If the frozen section is suspicious for malignancy or if a cancer is suspected already preoperatively, a PD represents the oncologically adequate approach.

## POSTOPERATIVE CARE

Hemodynamically and respiratory stable patients can be transferred to the normal ward after some hours in the recovery room.

Special attention should be taken to the pain management. Since most of the patients have chronic pain, a combination of peridural anesthesia and peripheral pain therapy is helpful for the first postoperative days.

Oral food intake can be started as early as 6 hours after the operation and can quickly be normalized over the first 3 days according to the patient's condition.

Pancreatic enzymes should be taken with all meals and the dosage should be adjusted to the patient's need.

Endocrine insufficiency needs to be reevaluated and therapy adjusted.

A postoperative follow-up should be performed on a regular basis.

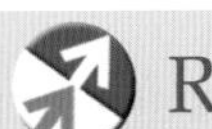

## RESULTS

Irrespective of the technique, if carried out by experienced hands pancreatic head resection is a safe and effective therapy with good short- and long-term results in patients with CP and an inflammatory mass in the head of the pancreas.

The above-mentioned techniques of pancreatic head resection were compared in several randomized-controlled trials (RCTs) (Table 10.2), in which their safety and

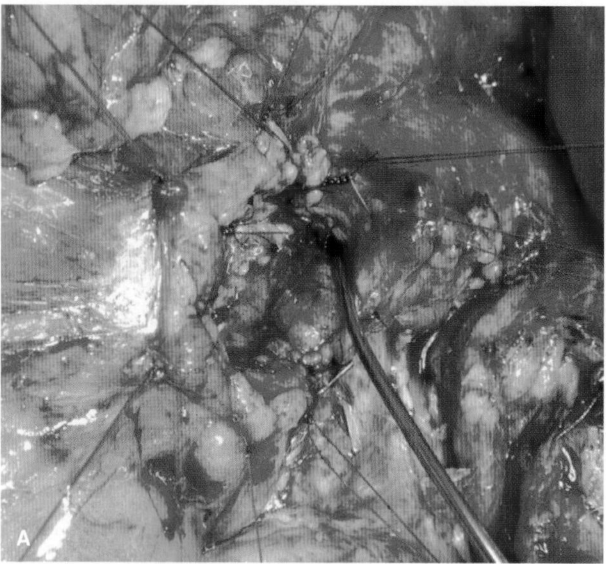

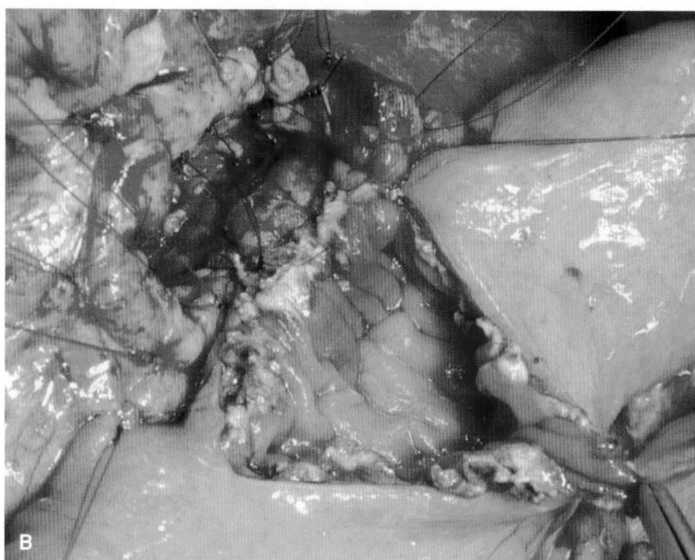

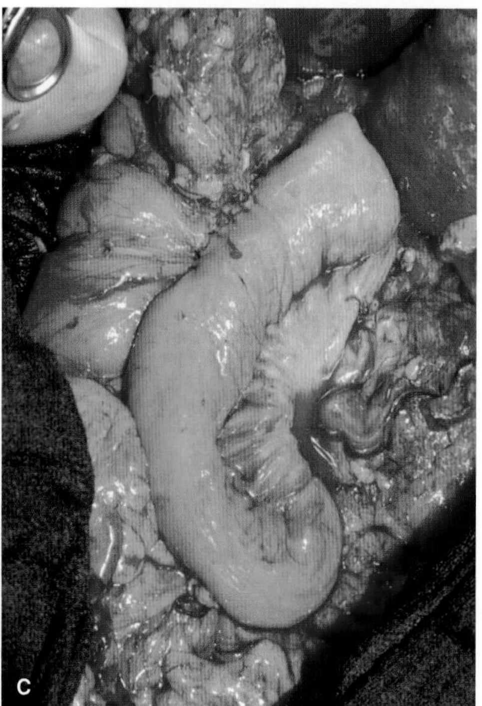

Figure 10.5 Bern procedure. **A:** Excavation of the pancreatic head, pancreatic duct intubated with a probe. **B:** Pancreaticojejunostomy: first layer of the side-to-side anastomosis. **C:** Pancreaticojejunostomy after completion of the anastomosis.

efficacy was confirmed. The RCTs comparing PD and DPPHR as well as a recent metaanalysis demonstrate comparable mortality and efficacy in terms of pain relief as well as endocrine insufficiency; however, the less invasive DPPHR was superior in hospital stay, exocrine insufficiency, weight gain and quality of life in medium-term follow-up. In even more recent studies with long-term follow-up these metabolic advantages appear to be lost over time and long-term results of PD and DPPHR are equal in terms of pain management and quality of life as well as endocrine and exocrine function (results reported in the initial trials and the latest follow-ups in Table 10.2). Of interest, the resection techniques remain effective in terms of pain relief and quality of life but cannot stop the progress of exocrine and endocrine insufficiency on the long term. One explanation may be that resection effectively treats the obstruction and hypertension but does not completely stop continued cellular damage and parenchymal loss. Certainly these observations stress the importance of continued conservative treatment by

**TABLE 10.2 Randomized Controlled Trials Comparing Techniques of Pancreatic Head Resection for CP**

| Author [ref.] (year) | Technique | *N* | Results |
|---|---|---|---|
| ***RCTs comparing PD vs. DPPHR*** | | | |
| Klempa (1995) | Beger<br>ppPD | 21<br>22 | Beger: shorter hospital stay, less exocrine insufficiency, less need of analgesics |
| Büchler (1995) | Beger<br>ppPD | 20<br>20 | Beger: less impaired glucose metabolism, higher gain of weight, more frequent pain relief |
| *Follow-up:* Müller (1997) | Beger<br>ppPD | 10<br>10 | ppPD: more frequent delayed gastric empting, more frequent pathologic secretion of enteral hormones |
| *Follow-up:* Müller (2008) | Beger<br>ppPD | 20<br>20 | equal in pain relief, exocrine & endocrine function equal in QoL |
| Izbicki (1998) | Frey<br>ppPD | 31<br>30 | Frey: lower morbidity, better QoL better professional rehabilitation equal in pain relief |
| *Follow-up:* Strate (2008) | Frey<br>ppPD | (23)<br>(23) | equal in pain relief and QoL, equal in exocrine & endocrine function |
| ***RCTs comparing different techniques of DPPHR*** | | | |
| Izbicki (1995) | Beger<br>Frey | 20<br>22 | comparable in pain relief, QoL, exocrine & endocrine function, management of local complications |
| *Follow-up:* Izbicki (1997) | Beger<br>Frey | 38<br>36 | comparable in pain relief, QoL, professional rehabilitation, exocrine & endocrine function |
| *Follow-up:* Strate (2005) | Beger<br>Frey | 34<br>33 | comparable in pain relief, QoL, exocrine & endocrine function. |
| Köninger (2008) | Beger<br>Bern | 32<br>33 | Bern: shorter operative time & hospital stay<br>Comparable in QoL |

RCT: Randomized-controlled trial, PD: pancreatoduodenectomy, ppPD: pylorus-preserving pancreatoduodenectomy, DPPHR: duodenum-preserving pancreatic head resection, QoL: Quality of life.

reducing etiologic factors, substitution for exocrine and endocrine insufficiency and probably antioxidant therapy.

The RCTs comparing different techniques of DPPHR demonstrate equal outcome in both pain control/quality of life and metabolic parameters after Beger versus Frey and Beger versus Bern technique (Table 10.2). However, the latter trial demonstrated that, with equal outcome, the Bern modification of DPPHR represents a technically simpler alternative, as reflected by a significantly (by 46 minutes) operative time as well as a significantly shorter hospital stay (11 vs. 15 days). Recent reports confirm that the Bern modification of DPPHR can be performed without severe complications or mortality in smaller series. Thus, the Bern technique represents a modification of DPPHR which may find broader acceptance due to technical and economic advantages.

## CONCLUSIONS

The adequate therapy of chronic pancreatitis is adjusted to the symptoms of the patient, the stage of the disease and the morphology of the pathologic changes of the pancreas.

Conservative therapy is the basis of treatment in all patients and has to accompany both interventional and surgical therapy.

Most of the patients with chronic pancreatitis present with an inflammatory mass in the head of the pancreas. These patients are best treated with a pancreatic head resection. The different forms of DPPHR have several advantages compared to the partial pancreaticoduodenectomy with comparable long-term results and should thus be considered the treatment of choice.

The Bern procedure of DPPHR represents a technical variation which is equally effective but technically less demanding. In cases with massive collaterals and portal hypertension, it is the only feasible technique to resect the pancreatic head safely.

Whereas surgical therapy provides effective long-term pain-relief and improvement of quality of life, it does not stop a decrease in both endocrine and exocrine function. Thus, endocrine and exocrine function should currently not be considered to define a successful therapy in CP. Instead, strategies for improvement or maintenance of endocrine and exocrine function remains an interesting field of research.

## Recommended References and Readings

Beger HG, Witte C, Krautzberger W, et al. Experiences with duodenum-sparing pancreas head resection in chronic pancreatitis. Chirurg. 1980;51(5):303–307.

Beger HG, Krautzberger W, Bittner R, et al. Duodenum-preserving resection of the head of the pancreas in patients with severe chronic pancreatitis. *Surgery.* 1985;97(4):467–473.

Beger HG, Büchler M, Bittner RR, et al. Duodenum-preserving resection of the head of the pancreas in severe chronic pancreatitis. Early and late results. *Ann Surg.* 1989;209(3):273–278.

Beger HG, Schlosser W, Friess HM, et al. Duodenum-preserving head resection in chronic pancreatitis changes the natural course of the disease: a single-center 26-year experience. *Ann Surg.* 1999;230(4):512–519; discussion 519–523.

Büchler MW, Friess H, Bittner R, et al. Duodenum-preserving pancreatic head resection: long-term results. *J Gastrointest Surg.* 1997;1(1):13–19.

Buchler MW, Friess H, Muller MW, et al. Randomized trial of duodenum-preserving pancreatic head resection versus pylorus-preserving. *Am J Surg.* 1995;169:65–69.

Buchler MW, Warshaw AL. Resection versus drainage in treatment of chronic pancreatitis. *Gastroenterology.* 2008;134:1605–1607.

Cahen DL, Gouma DJ, Nio Y, et al. Endoscopic versus surgical drainage of the pancreatic duct in chronic pancreatitis. *N Engl J Med.* 2007;356:676–684.

Diener MK, Rahbari NN, Fischer L, et al. Duodenum-preserving pancreatic head resection versus pancreatoduodenectomy for surgical treatment of chronic pancreatitis: a systematic review and meta-analysis. *Ann Surg.* 2008;247:950–961.

Gloor B, Friess H, Uhl W, et al. A modified technique of the Beger and Frey procedure in patients with chronic pancreatitis. *Dig Surg.* 2001;18:21–25.

Hartwig W, Schneider L, Diener MK, et al. Preoperative tissue diagnosis for tumours of the pancreas. *Br J Surg.* 2009;96:5–20.

Izbicki JR, Bloechle C, Knoefel WT, et al. Duodenum-preserving resection of the head of the pancreas in chronic pancreatitis. A prospective, randomized trial. *Ann Surg.* 1995;221:350–358.

Izbicki JR, Bloechle C, Knoefel WT, et al. Drainage versus resection in surgical therapy of chronic pancreatitis of the head of the pancreas: a randomized study. *Chirurg.* 1997;68:369–377.

Izbicki JR, Bloechle C, Broering DC, et al. Extended drainage versus resection in surgery for chronic pancreatitis: a prospective randomized trial comparing the longitudinal pancreaticojejunostomy combined with local pancreatic head excision with the pylorus-preserving pancreatoduodenectomy. *Ann Surg.* 1998;228:771–779.

Klempa I, Spatny M, Menzel J, et al. Pancreatic function and quality of life after resection of the head of the pancreas in chronic pancreatitis. a prospective, randomized comparative study after duodenum preserving resection of the head of the pancreas versus Whipple's operation. *Chirurg.* 1995;66:350–359.

Koninger J, Seiler CM, Sauerland S, et al. Duodenum-preserving pancreatic head resection–a randomized controlled trial comparing the original Beger procedure with the Berne modification (ISRCTN No. 50638764). *Surgery.* 2008;143: 490–498.

Muller MW, Friess H, Leitzbach S, et al. Perioperative and follow-up results after central pancreatic head resection (Berne technique) in a consecutive series of patients with chronic pancreatitis. *Am J Surg.* 2008;196(3):364–372.

Muller MW, Friess H, Martin DJ, et al. Long-term follow-up of a randomized clinical trial comparing Beger with pylorus-preserving Whipple procedure for chronic pancreatitis. *Br J Surg.* 2008; 95:350–356.

Strate T, Taherpour Z, Bloechle C, et al. Long-term follow-up of a randomized trial comparing the beger and frey procedures for patients suffering from chronic pancreatitis. *Ann Surg.* 2005;241: 591–598.

Strate T, Bachmann K, Busch P, et al. Resection vs drainage in treatment of chronic pancreatitis: long-term results of a randomized trial. *Gastroenterology.* 2008;134:1406–1411.

Strobel O, Buchler MW, Werner J. Duodenum-preserving pancreatic head resection : Technique according to Beger, technique according to Frey and Berne modifications. *Chirurg.* 2009;80:22–27.

Warshaw AL, Banks PA, Fernandez-del Castillo C. AGA technical review: treatment of pain in chronic pancreatitis. *Gastroenterology.* 1998;115:765–776.

# 11 Roux-en-Y Lateral Pancreaticojejunostomy for Chronic Pancreatitis

**Charles J. Yeo, Eugene P. Kennedy, and Keith D. Lillemoe**

##  INDICATIONS/CONTRAINDICATIONS

Chronic pancreatitis is a single term applied to a complex spectrum of disease. The essence of this disease process is the progressive destruction of the pancreatic parenchyma and its replacement with fibrotic tissue, which over time, leads to both exocrine and endocrine insufficiency.

The most common etiology of chronic pancreatitis is chronic excessive ethanol consumption, followed by other toxic or metabolic causes such as hypercalcemia, hyperlipidemia, certain medications, and perhaps tobacco. Other well-described etiologic factors for chronic pancreatitis include hereditary pancreatitis, cystic fibrosis, autoimmune disease, prior severe acute pancreatitis with necrosis, and pancreatic ductal obstruction from developmental abnormalities (pancreas divisum), sphincter of Oddi dysfunction, or obstruction from trauma or neoplasm. Patients not fitting one of these diagnostic categories are classified as idiopathic, a group that ranks second to ethanol consumption when etiologies are tallied.

The hallmark symptom is chronic, often disabling pain. The pain is classically located in the epigastric region and presents as a dull ache that radiates to the back. The exact nature of the pain and the timing of its occurrence in relationship to other aspects of the disease can vary greatly between patients. Some patients experience intermittent pain that can last days and be disabling. Fatty foods are often cited as a trigger, but the pain can frequently arise without any obvious trigger. Between episodes, these patients can be symptom free but the severity, duration, and frequency of episodes often increases over time. Other patients experience a more chronic, daily form of pain with intermittent exacerbations. The onset of episodes of chronic pain can vary greatly between patients, with certain patients experiencing pain early in the course of chronic pancreatitis while, less commonly, other patients can exhibit endocrine and exocrine insufficiency and dramatic radiographic evidence of chronic pancreatitis without any significant pain episodes.

The pain associated with chronic pancreatitis is typically the most disabling feature of the disease and the symptom that drives patients to seek frequent medical attention.

Since the pain typically increases over time, patients may become addicted to narcotic pain medications and often require episodic inpatient care. The pain and the side effects of pain medications dramatically impair quality of life and often result in disability and loss of employment. Ultimately, failure of medical approaches to pain management leads patients to surgical intervention for their conditions.

In addition to chronic pain, patients with chronic pancreatitis often present with a combination of other symptoms related to the exocrine and endocrine insufficiency that results from destruction of the gland. Steatorrhea, malabsorption, fat soluble vitamin deficiencies, malnutrition, and weight loss are all common. Diabetes may result from impaired islet cell function. Associated medical problems from long-term ethanol abuse as well as side effects from narcotic pain medications are also common.

The diagnosis of chronic pancreatitis is made via a combination of patient history, the constellation of symptoms, and radiographic findings. Evaluation typically is prompted by a complaint of chronic abdominal pain. Patient history may reveal ethanol use, prior episodes of acute pancreatitis, suspected drug abuse, or a family history or known genetic predisposition. Laboratory evaluation is often not helpful, as patients with chronic pancreatitis can have severe exacerbations with normal serum amylase and lipase levels.

Imaging is a key element in diagnosis. Classically, patients with chronic pancreatitis have dilatation of the pancreatic duct which can be detected on imaging. A "chain of lakes" is often seen from segmental strictures due to the inflammatory process. Calcifications in the pancreatic parenchyma are essentially pathognomonic. The initial imaging study of choice to evaluate the possible diagnosis of chronic pancreatitis is a high quality, multi-detector, contrast enhanced computed tomography (CT) scan (Fig. 11.1). CT is quite accurate for detecting dilatation of the pancreatic duct as well as parenchymal calcifications. With proper contrast enhancement, it also gives an excellent assessment of the pancreatic parenchyma and surrounding vasculature.

When greater resolution of the pancreatic duct is necessary, magnetic resonance cholangiopancreatography (MRCP) provides excellent imaging of the pancreatic duct. Utilizing T2-weighted images, the detailed structure of the pancreatic duct can be seen with high resolution. In our practice, we strongly prefer MRCP over endoscopic retrograde cholangiopancreatography (ERCP), as ERCP, as an invasive procedure, is associated with significant risk of complications, including exacerbation of the pancreatitis. Endoscopic ultrasound (EUS), although not required for most cases, can help evaluate the parenchyma of the pancreas in fine detail, particularly when trying to discern an inflammatory stricture or mass from a subtle neoplasm. In addition, EUS offers the additional advantage of providing a tissue diagnosis via fine needle aspiration when a diagnosis is uncertain from imaging alone.

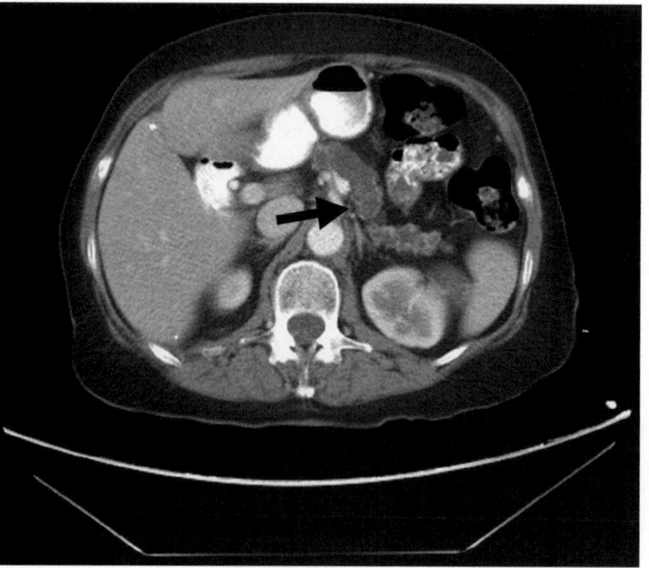

**Figure 11.1** Dilated, irregular pancreatic duct throughout the body and tail of pancreas indicated by *black arrow* in a patient with alcohol associated chronic pancreatitis. The patient was symptomatic with abnormal pain from chronic pancreatitis and had an excellent response to a Roux-en-Y lateral pancreaticojejunostomy.

The treatment of chronic pancreatitis is truly multi-modal and requires cooperation between specialties. Once a diagnosis is made, every effort should be made to identify the etiology of the pancreatitis. If the chronic pancreatitis is due to ethanol abuse, then aggressive steps should be made to assist the patient in ethanol cessation. Simply stopping the consumption of ethanol can lead to improvements in symptoms and decrease the rate of progression of the disease. Similar efforts should be applied toward smoking cessation for patients who abuse tobacco. Metabolic abnormalities that trigger pancreatitis should be treated and any possibly related drugs stopped or changed.

Once triggering factors are removed, treatment focuses on symptom relief. Pain is managed with analgesics and often requires significant doses of narcotics. Collaboration with a chronic pain specialist and careful monitoring of narcotic prescriptions and dosing can help differentiate appropriate management from signs of abuse. Exocrine and endocrine insufficiency is managed with pancreatic enzyme replacement and insulin therapy, respectively. Nutritional support is also initiated when appropriate.

The most common indication to intervene surgically in chronic pancreatitis is unremitting pain that significant interferes with quality of life and cannot be adequately addressed medically. Evidence exists that surgical interventions for chronic pancreatitis can slow the progression of the disease and delay the loss of pancreatic function. However, this in and of itself is not an adequate indication for surgical intervention. Traditionally, it was taught that chronic pancreatitis would "burn itself out" and if surgical intervention was delayed long enough, symptoms would improve. This theory has not held up to scientific scrutiny however, and patients randomized between medical and surgical interventions had significantly less pain over the ensuing 10 years of follow-up if they had undergone surgery. In addition, a recent randomized study comparing endoscopic and surgical interventions for chronic pancreatitis was stopped early due to clear superiority at interim analysis in the surgical arm.

Surgical interventions for chronic pancreatitis can be divided into two broad groups: drainage operations and resectional operations. In 1960, Partington and Rochelle described the side-to-side longitudinal pancreaticojejunostomy that is currently referred to as the Puestow procedure. This procedure remains the standard approach to pancreatic ductal decompression. It is best applied to patients with parenchymal disease and pancreatic ductal dilatation diffusely involving the pancreatic head, neck, body, and tail of the gland. It requires a significant degree of pancreatic ductal dilatation to be technically feasible with a ductal diameter of at least 5 mm.

Segmental pancreatic resection is best applied when parenchymal disease and pancreatic ductal abnormality are primarily confined to one portion of the gland. The same resectional approaches used for neoplasms (pancreaticoduodenectomy, distal pancreatectomy) are utilized as well as total pancreatectomy with islet cell auto-transplant at some centers. When properly applied, these approaches yield acceptable results. Finally, there are also two additional approaches developed more recently that combine aspects of both resectional and drainage approaches. First, the duodenum-preserving pancreatic head resection or Beger procedure addresses the problem of an inflammatory mass in the head of the pancreas. Second, the local resection of the pancreatic head with longitudinal pancreaticojejunostomy or Frey procedure seeks to address the problem that occurs in patients with significant disease in the pancreatic head as well as a "chain of lakes" along the pancreatic duct throughout the body and tail. All of these approaches will be addressed in other chapters of this atlas.

## PREOPERATIVE PLANNING

Preoperative planning for a Roux-en-Y longitudinal pancreaticojejunostomy begins with appropriate patient selection. As mentioned, it is best applied to patients with parenchymal disease and ductal dilatation diffusely involving the pancreatic head, neck, body, and tail of the gland. The degree and distribution of ductal dilatation noted on preoperative imaging is key to patient selection. Although there have been reports of success with lateral pancreaticojejunostomy in patients with small duct disease, this procedure is usually for those patients with a pancreatic duct that measured at least 5 mm in diameter.

In addition to evaluation of pancreatic ductal anatomy, the overall condition of the patient must be assessed prior to operative intervention. A patient's symptoms must be severe enough and disabling enough to justify surgical intervention. Surgical intervention via lateral pancreaticojejunostomy for chronic pancreatitis has essentially one goal, relief of pain. Patients with other sequelae of chronic pancreatitis such as biliary or duodenal obstruction or pseudocyst formation are best served with a different approach. As relief of pain is the primary goal, alcohol and tobacco cessation are a must. In our practice, it is our policy to not offer a surgical intervention for pain to patients who continue to abuse ethanol or to those who smoke cigarettes. Patients demonstrating significant malnutrition (with serum albumin levels less than 3 g/dl) may require nutritional supplementation prior to operative intervention. Other medical conditions such as cardiac disease must be assessed and optimized prior to surgery as well.

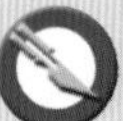

## SURGICAL TECHNIQUE

All patients are admitted as same day surgery patients, having been previously seen in the anesthesia preoperative evaluation clinic. No preoperative bowel preparation is utilized and patients are simply instructed to limit intake to clear liquids on the day before surgery. Necessary cardiac medications including beta blockers and aspirin are continued. Patients receive 5,000 units of heparin subcutaneously in the preoperative holding area and a second generation cephalosporin (or appropriate equivalent if allergic) is administered in the operating room less than 30 minutes prior to incision. Sequential compression devices (SCDs) are utilized. A nasogastric tube and a urinary catheter are placed after the induction of anesthesia. Central venous access is obtained only when deemed necessary by the attending anesthesiologist. Epidural analgesia may be used and can be helpful for postoperative pain management. A preoperative briefing involving all members of the surgical team is performed prior to incision.

A midline incision from the xiphoid to the umbilicus is used for the procedure. A self-retaining retractor system is used to aid with exposure and wet, antibiotic soaked laparotomy pads are used to protect the wound edges. A thorough exploration of the abdomen is performed. If a patient has not yet undergone a cholecystectomy, one is performed in the classic, top-down fashion.

Next, the pancreas is approached by opening the gastrocolic ligament, along the greater curve of the stomach up to the first short gastric vessel, thereby entering the lesser sac. The ligament is divided using Kelly clamps and silk ties or a surgical energy device, being careful to avoid the gastroepiploic vessels. The short gastrics are not divided. Any adhesions between the back wall of the stomach and the ventral surface of the pancreas are divided and the entire ventral surface of the pancreas is exposed. Typically, there is no need to perform a Kocher maneuver to safely complete the procedure.

Once exposed, the pancreas is palpated along its length. This serves two purposes. First, the duct can often be identified as a soft, compressible area running the length of the pancreas. Secondly, additional abnormalities, such as pancreatic duct stones or neoplasms may be identified and further investigated. Once the duct is located by palpation, a 21 gauge needle on a 5 cc syringe is advanced into the duct while aspirating (Fig. 11.2A). The return of clear pancreatic fluid is confirmation of the location of the pancreas duct. The tip of the needle is kept in the duct and the electrocautery is used to cut down on the needle utilizing an incision that runs lengthwise along the ventral surface of the duct. Once the lumen of the duct is visible, the needle is removed and a lacrimal duct probe or #2 or #3 Bakes dilator is used to probe the pancreatic duct. A right angle clamp can then be introduced and used as a guide to open the length of the duct with electrocautery (Fig. 11.2B). The duct should be opened along as much of the

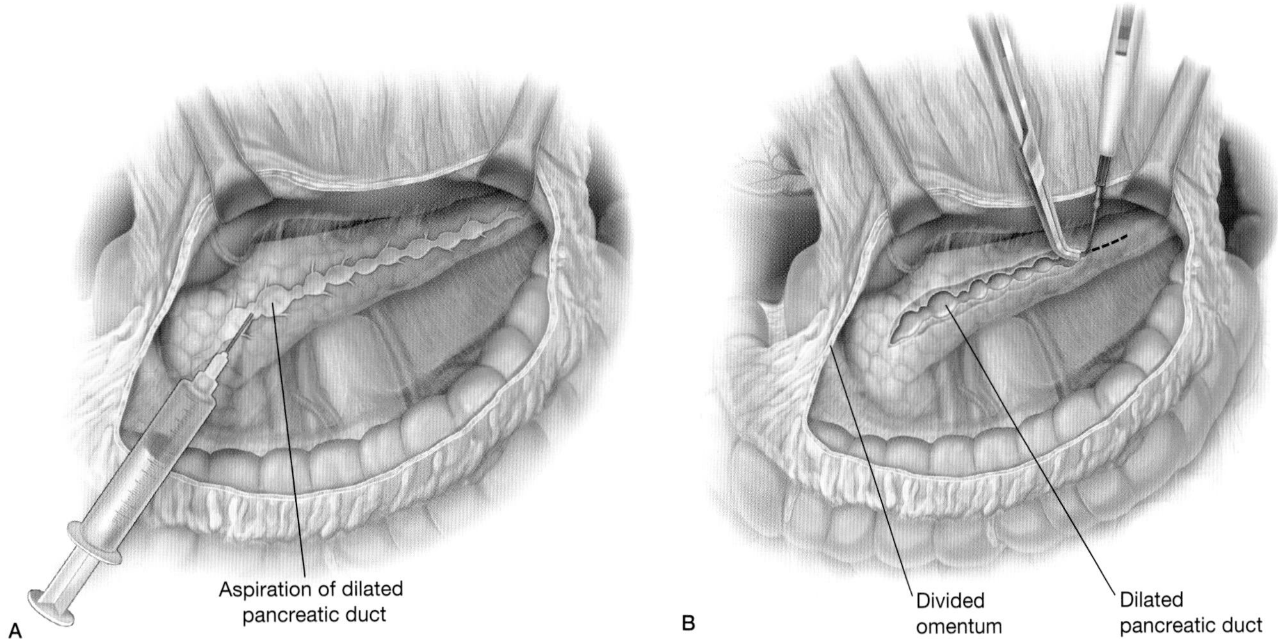


Figure 11.2 **A:** After exposure of the full length of the pancreas, the pancreatic duct is identified by aspiration using a 21 gauge needle on a 5 ml syringe. **B:** The pancreatic duct is then entered using the cautery first by "cutting down" along the needle and for as much of the length of the entire duct from just medial to the gastroduodenal artery through the neck and body and out into the tail of the gland. A right angle clamp may facilitate this maneuver.

ventral surface as is feasible, from just medial to the gastroduodenal artery through the neck and body and out into the tail. We strive to obtain at minimum an 8 cm long pancreatic ductotomy. Once the duct is opened, a biopsy is of the pancreas is typically taken and sent for frozen section evaluation. Ideally, the biopsy is taken from the most proximal area of stricture to evaluate for the possibility of an occult malignancy precipitating or mimicking chronic pancreatitis.

Occasionally, the pancreatic duct cannot be identified by palpation. In this situation, several approaches are available. First, several passes with the needle can be made into the proximal body of the pancreas, to the patients left of the superior mesenteric vein. The approximate location of the duct can often be estimated from preoperative imaging and used as a starting point. If unsuccessful, intraoperative ultrasound is an excellent technique for locating the duct. With the probe along the ventral surface of the pancreas, a needle can be advanced under ultrasound guidance into the duct.

Once the pancreatic duct is opened, attention is turned to preparation of a Roux-en-Y limb. An appropriate place is identified along the small bowel, approximately 20 cm from the ligament of Treitz. The bowel is divided using a gastrointestinal anastomosis (GIA) stapler and the staple line on the downstream side is oversewn with 3-0 silk sutures. The mesentery is divided using silk ties down through the outer vascular arcade. A second appropriate location is identified approximately 50 cm downstream from the place the bowel has been divided, and an end-to-side jejunojejunostomy is fashioned, creating the Roux limb. We utilize a hand sewn technique for this jejunojejunostomy, employing an outer layer of interrupted 3-0 silk sutures and an inner layer of running 3-0 absorbable polyglycolic acid suture. Once the Roux limb has been created, it is brought up into the lesser sac in a retrocolic fashion, traversing a rent in the right side of the transverse mesocolon. We prefer to position the limb in an isoperistaltic direction with respect to the pancreas duct.

Once in position, the lateral pancreaticojejunostomy is fashioned with a single layer of interrupted 3-0 silk sutures. Two corner sutures are first placed between the apices of the opening along the pancreatic duct and the antimesenteric side of the small bowel. These are placed such that the knots will be on the outside of the anastomosis once tied down. The length of small bowel must be carefully assessed as it tends to stretch once opened, and the bowel is opened with the electrocautery

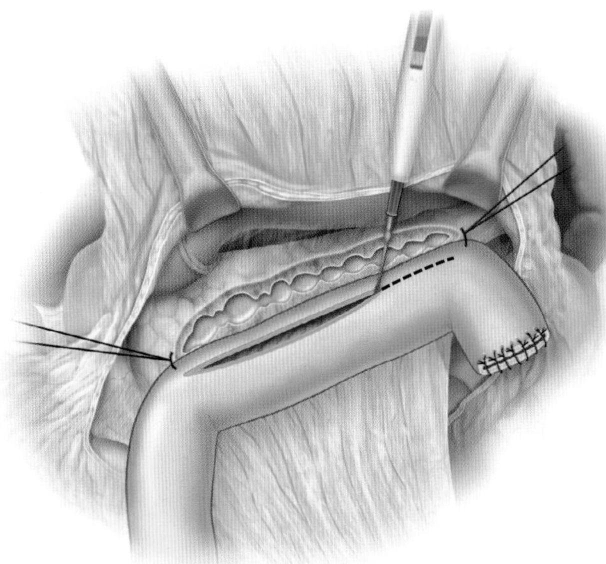

**Figure 11.3** The Roux-en-Y limb is brought alongside the pancreas in an isoperistaltic fashion. The longitudinal pancreatic ductotomy is visible. Two corner stitches are placed between the jejunum and the apices of the ductotomy. An enterotomy is then made lengthwise along the jejunum, in parallel to the pancreatic ductotomy.

(Fig. 11.3). Interrupted silk sutures are then placed between the small bowel and the cut edge of the pancreas, creating the inner aspect of the pancreaticojejunostomy. Careful full thickness bites of the small bowel are first taken followed by a full thickness bite of the transected edge of the pancreas. Care is taken to incorporate both the pancreatic capsule and the duct mucosa when possible. Once all the sutures are appropriately placed along the back wall of the anastomosis, they are tied down. These sutures are placed such that the knots will be on the inside aspect of the anastomosis once tied down (Fig. 11.4).

After all the inferior row sutures are tied down, the sutures (except the ends) are cut. Next, the superior row of the anastomosis is completed. Again, 3-0 silk suture is used and a full thickness bite of jejunum is taken from serosa to mucosa. This is

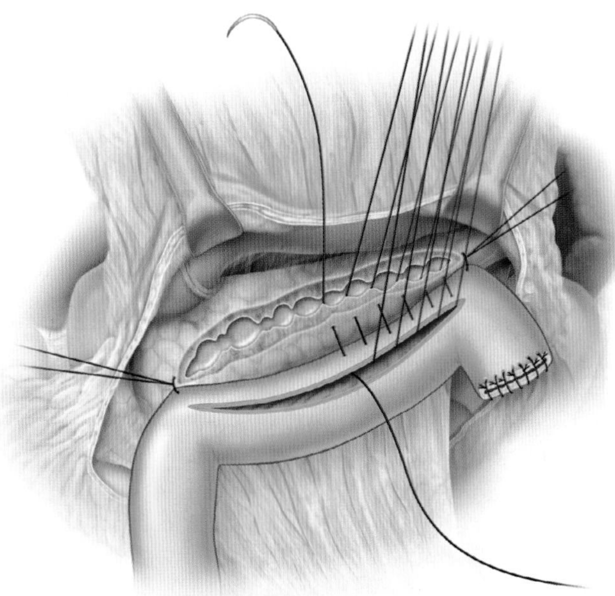

**Figure 11.4** Interrupted 3-0 silk sutures are placed along the inferior row of the pancreaticojejunostomy. Full thickness bites of the small bowel are first taken followed by a full thickness bite of the transected edge of the pancreas. Both the pancreatic capsule and the pancreatic duct mucosa are incorporated in a single suture when possible. Note that these sutures are placed such that the knots will be on the inside aspect of the anastomosis once tied down.

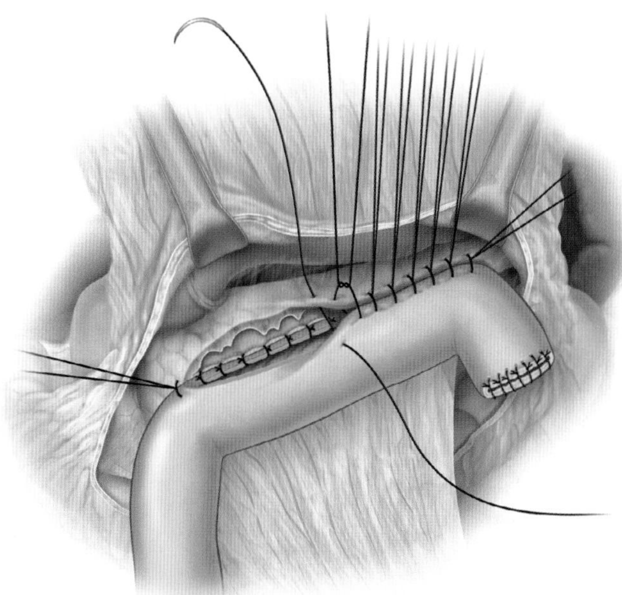

**Figure 11.5** The superior row of the anastomosis is fashioned using 3-0 silk suture, taking a full thickness bite of jejunum from serosa to mucosa. The cut edge of pancreas is then taken with a full thickness bite, incorporating pancreatic duct and then capsule. The knots for this superior row are left on the outside of the anastomosis.

carried through to the cut edge of pancreas where a full thickness bite incorporating duct and then capsule is taken. Once all sutures are placed, they are tied down and trimmed. The knots for this superior row are left on the outside of the anastomosis (Fig. 11.5).

Once the anastomosis is complete, the defect in the transverse mesocolon is closed using interrupted silk suture by tacking the mesocolon to the Roux-en-Y limb (Fig. 11.6). In addition, the defect between the jejunal limbs is closed to avoid a potential space for an internal hernia. A single 3/16 inch Jackson-Pratt drain is placed on the patient's left side with the side holes near the pancreaticojejunostomy. Fascial closure is performed using a running #2 nylon suture, with skin closure per routine.

One valuable adjunct to this procedure is the performance of a celiac plexus neurolysis (alcohol nerve block). This procedure has been shown to decrease pain in the setting of chronic pancreatitis or pancreatic malignancy. It is easily and quickly performed at the time of open surgery and carries minimal risk or expense. The area of the celiac plexus is identified by palpation along the aorta, at the level of the thrill of the celiac artery. A 20 cc syringe is filled with 50% ethanol solution and fitted with a 21 gauge spinal needle. Twenty milliliters of the 50% ethanol are injected along each side of the aorta at the level of the celiac axis.

## 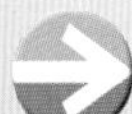 POSTOPERATIVE MANAGEMENT

All patients are cared for postoperatively according to a critical pathway for pancreatic surgery patients. Patients are extubated in the operating room when no contraindication exists and in most cases can be admitted to a standard surgical ward. Electrolyte abnormalities and fluid status are aggressively monitored and corrected. Postoperative analgesia is provided using the epidural catheter of present or with intravenous narcotics via a patient controlled anesthesia (PCA) device. All patients also receive an intravenous proton pump inhibitor (PPI) and a beta-blocker, in addition to subcutaneous daily heparin.

Patients are mobilized in the early morning of the first postoperative day. The nasogastric tube is removed that morning and patients are started on sips of water and

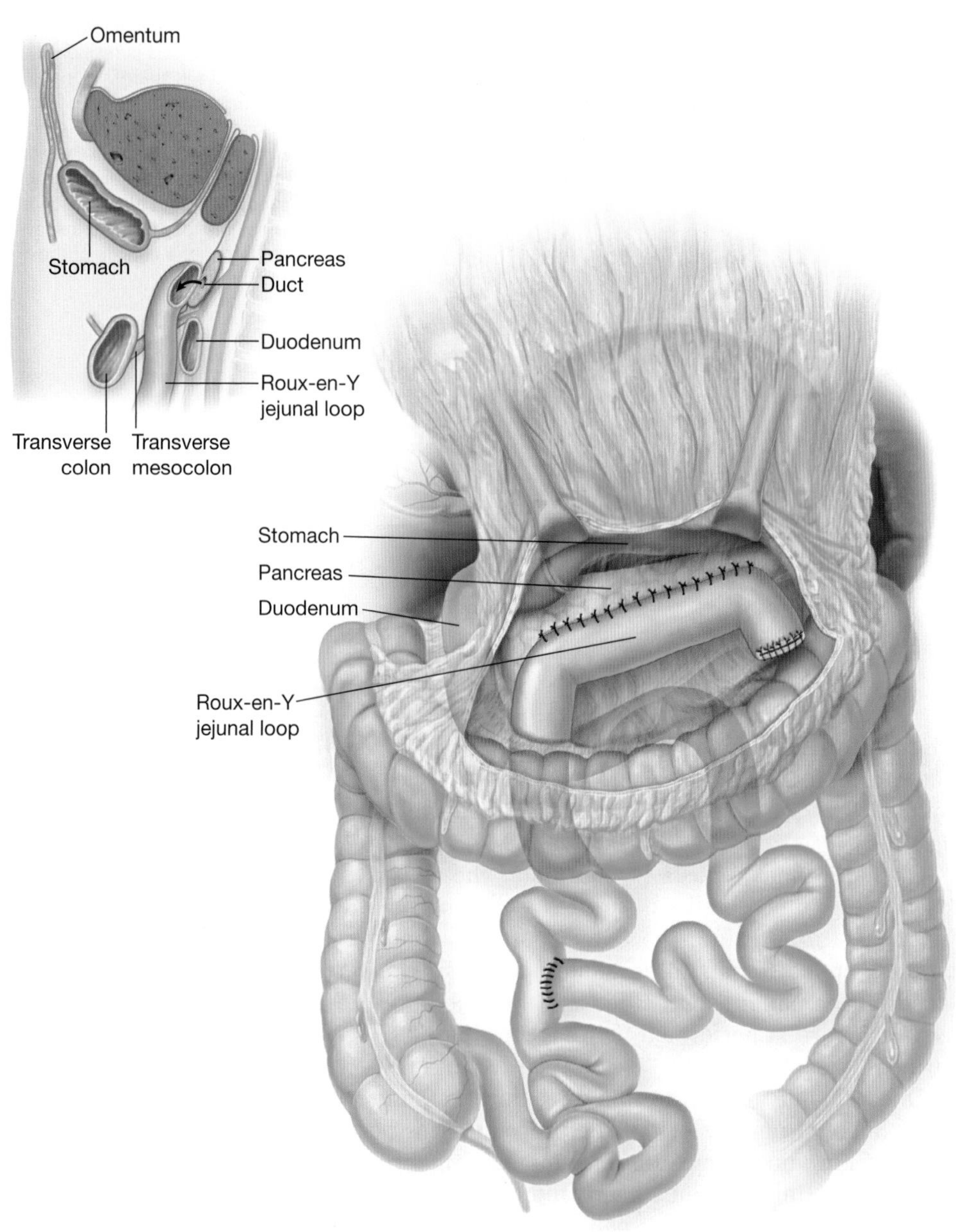


Figure 11.6 A completed Roux-en-Y lateral pancreatojejunostomy.

ice chips (≤30 cc/hour). SCDs are discontinued, while TED stockings, subcutaneous heparin, intravenous beta-blockade, and PPI are continued until hospital discharge.

On postoperative day 2, patients are advanced to an unlimited clear liquid diet. The urinary catheter is removed and patients are assisted in increasing their frequency and duration of ambulation. Fluids are minimized and most patients receive low dose diuretics to aid in the mobilization of the perioperative fluid which was administered intraoperatively and immediately postoperatively. The epidural catheter is removed when appropriate.

In most patients the initiation of a regular diet begins on postoperative day 3, with oral pancreatic enzyme supplementation if required preoperatively. Medications, including beta-blockade and PPI, are continued as intravenous formulations until postoperative day 4 to assure that a diet is tolerated. Intravenous fluids are discontinued on postoperative day 4. The surgical drain is removed on postoperative day 4, if appropriate. Preprinted discharge instructions are distributed to allow time for patients and their families to review and formulate questions prior to discharge. Discharge is targeted for postoperative day 5. A follow-up appointment is scheduled for 4 weeks after discharge.

Typical discharge medications include necessary preoperative medications plus a PPI and analgesics.

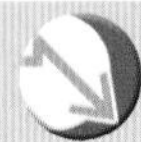

## COMPLICATIONS

Overall, lateral pancreaticojejunostomy can be performed safely, with low operative mortality and morbidity. Large series report operative mortality of less than 2%. As a result of the fibrotic nature of the pancreatic parenchyma, pancreatic fistula rates are low, between 2% and 5%. Typically, these fistulae, when they do occur, heal spontaneously with conservative management (maintenance of the operatively placed drain). Overall complication rates are in the 20% range.

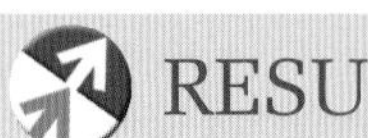

## RESULTS

Published series report overall improvements in pain in between 50% and 90% of patients. The long-term outcomes of lateral pancreaticojejunostomy are, however, a more valid measure of success than pain relief in the immediate postoperative period. Success can be best assessed by a combination of pain scores, quality of life surveys, and return to work. The initial degree of pain relief is high (approaching 90%) across most published studies. Over longer periods of follow-up however, the percentage of patients reporting good or complete pain relief declines to closer to 50%. This is thought to be due to a variety of factors including the slowly progressive nature of the disease. Recurrent pancreatic duct stricture, particularly in the head of the pancreas, is cited as a source of long-term failure for patients undergoing lateral pancreaticojejunostomy. These patients are candidates for subsequent surgical intervention, often with resectional approaches. In addition, the resumption of the abuse of ethanol is strongly correlated with long-term failure of surgical intervention for chronic pancreatitis. Patients should be offered appropriate referral for professional ethanol abuse counseling.

Quality of life, as documented by patient reported surveys, after lateral pancreaticojejunostomy is typically quite good, particularly when compared with preoperative measures. The quality of life scales used across studies have never been standardized, but all studies show improvement. The percentage of patients reporting significant improvement approaches 70% across both physical and mental health domains. Also of importance is the rate of return to work after surgical intervention for chronic pancreatitis. Rates of return to work vary between 40% and 75%, with most studies reporting rates above 60%. Given the disabling nature of chronic pancreatitis, these rates should be considered very successful.

Another outcome to be considered after longitudinal pancreaticojejunostomy is endocrine and exocrine dysfunction. Chronic pancreatitis, if untreated, commonly results in long-term dependence on pancreatic enzyme supplementation and insulin therapy to replace the diminished function of the pancreas. Many patients with chronic pancreatitis experience significant pain and undergo surgical intervention before becoming dependant on pancreatic replacement therapies. Published series of longitudinal pancreaticojejunostomy report a rate of subsequent long-term progression to exocrine and endocrine insufficiency near 30%. One study, published in 1993, comparing patients undergoing surgical intervention for chronic pancreatitis with patients managed more conservatively showed a decrease in the rate of progression to pancreatic insufficiency for surgically treated patients. In addition, a recent study comparing endoscopic therapy with surgical therapy for chronic pancreatitis documented a 15% rate of resolution of exocrine insufficiency in surgical patients at 2-year follow-up. Taken as a whole, the available evidence indicates that lateral pancreaticojejunostomy does not exacerbate exocrine or endocrine insufficiency of the pancreas, and may have some mild beneficial effect.

## Recommended References and Readings

Adams DB, Ford MC, Anderson MC. Outcome after lateral pancreaticojejunostomy for chronic pancreatitis. *Ann Surg.* 1994; 219:481–487.

Andersen DK, Frey CF. The evolution of the surgical treatment of chronic pancreatitis. *Ann Surg.* 2010;251:18–32.

Cahen DL, Gouma DJ, Nio Y, et al. Endoscopic versus surgical drainage of the pancreatic duct in chronic pancreatitis. *N Engl J Med.* 2007;356:676–684.

Greenlee HB, Prinz RA, Aranha GV. Long-term results of side-to-side pancreaticojejunostomy. *World J Surg.* 1990;14:70–76.

Nealon WH, Thompson JC. Progressive loss of pancreatic function in chronic pancreatitis is delayed by main pancreatic duct decompression. A longitudinal prospective analysis of the modified Puestow procedure. *Ann Surg.* 1993;217:458–466.

Nealon WH, Walser E. Duct drainage alone is sufficient in the operative management of pancreatic pseudocysts in patients with chronic pancreatitis. *Ann Surg.* 2003;237:614–620.

Schnelldorfer T, Lewin DN, Adams DB. Operative management of chronic pancreatitis: Longterm results in 372 patients. *J Am Coll Surg.* 2007;204:1039–1045.

Sielezneff I, Malouf A, Salle E, et al. Long terms results of lateral pancreaticojejunostomy for chronic alcoholic pancreatitis. *Eur J Surg.* 2000;166:58–64.

Sohn TA, Campbell KA, Pitt HA, et al. Quality of life and long-term survival after surgery for chronic pancreatitis. *J Gastrointest Surg.* 2000;4:355–364.

# 12 Drainage of Pancreatic Pseudocyst

**Kfir Ben-David and Kevin E. Behrns**

##  INDICATIONS/CONTRAINDICATIONS

Pancreatic pseudocysts arise in the settings of acute and/or chronic pancreatitis and have protean manifestations that may depend on size, location, and underlying pancreatic pathophysiology. Appropriate treatment is dependent on understanding the pathophysiology that led to the formation of the pseudocyst. Pseudocysts that are the result of a bout of acute pancreatitis may require significantly different treatment than those that are a complication of chronic pancreatitis.

Pseudocysts complicate 27% of acute pancreatitis episodes that may be either acute interstitial (edematous) pancreatitis or acute necrotizing pancreatitis. Establishing the type of acute pancreatitis is critical for appropriate management since a pseudocyst that results from acute interstitial pancreatitis, in which the underlying pancreatic duct is essentially normal with the exception of a single site of disruption, is markedly different from a pseudocyst that forms following acute necrotizing pancreatitis that exhibits substantial destruction of the pancreatic parenchyma and surrounding peripancreatic tissue. In addition, pseudocyst formation occurs over time with a maturation process of approximately 6 weeks. A bout of acute pancreatitis that results in ductal disruption produces a localized collection of pancreatic secretions that incite an inflammatory response which is accompanied by deposition of fibrous tissue that serves to localize and wall-off the injurious fluid. Therefore, over this 6 week time period the pseudocyst takes on a relatively spherical shape with a homogenous internal fluid-filled center as the pancreatic and peripancreatic debris is digested. It is imperative that the clinician recognize this maturation process and not quickly treat an ill-defined pancreatic or peripancreatic fluid collection (acute fluid collection) that results from the inflammatory response but is not associated with pancreatic ductal disruption (Fig. 12.1). These acute fluid collections will spontaneously resolve over time and, therefore, treatment of a presumed pseudocyst should generally not occur until the pathophysiologic process has been clearly established.

Chronic pancreatitis is more frequently associated with pseudocyst development than acute pancreatitis. Up to 40% of patients with chronic inflammation will manifest pseudocyst development at some time in the course of disease; however, many of these pseudocysts are small, asymptomatic and, thus, do not require treatment. Chronic

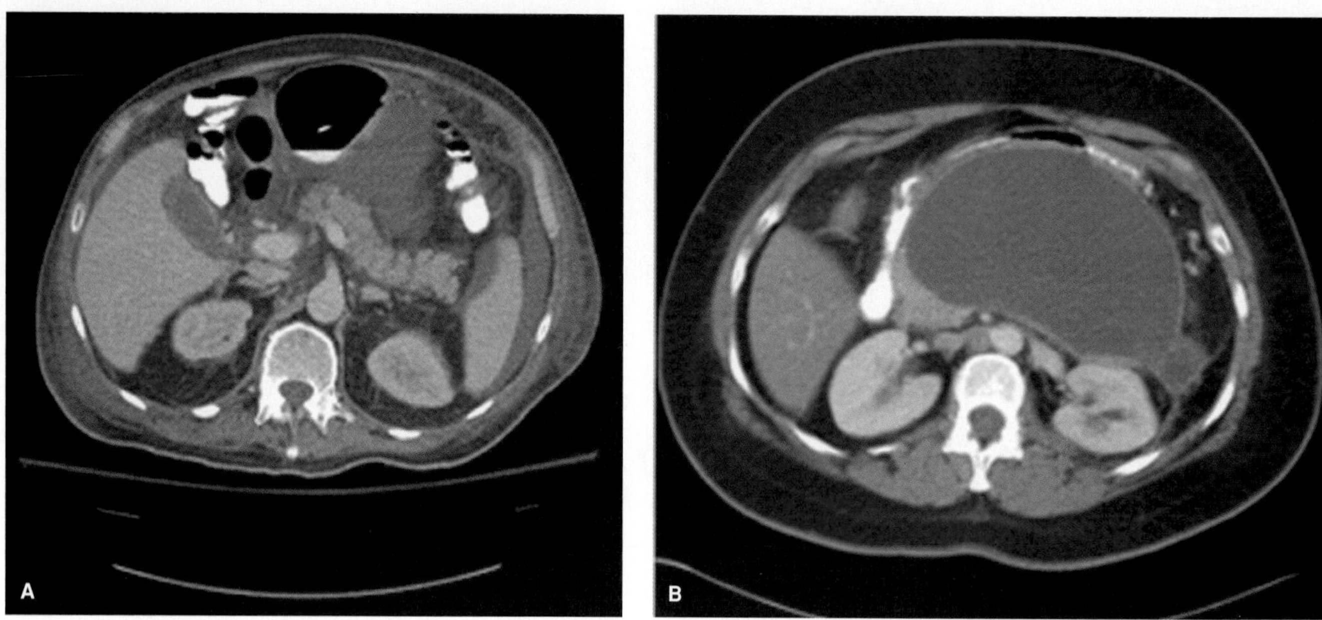


Figure 12.1 **A:** CT scan demonstrating an acute fluid collection associated with acute interstitial pancreatitis. **B:** CT showing a well-circumscribed, large pseudocyst containing homogeneous fluid.

pancreatitis is characterized by fibrosis and acinar cell drop out that over time results in ductal strictures, parenchymal atrophy, and decreased exocrine and endocrine functions. As a result of the fibrotic process, pancreatic strictures and ductal hypertension produce duct disruption with pseudocyst development. Since a permanently stenotic or an occluded pancreatic duct will frequently not improve over time, pseudocysts that arise in this setting and are symptomatic will frequently require treatment.

Although pseudocyst size may be an important determinant of treatment, symptoms that result from pseudocysts are frequently the result of adjacent organ compromise. Pseudocysts located in the head of the pancreas may cause gastroduodenal obstruction and may be associated with the development of nausea, vomiting, or early satiety. Similarly, relatively small but precisely located pseudocysts in the head of the gland

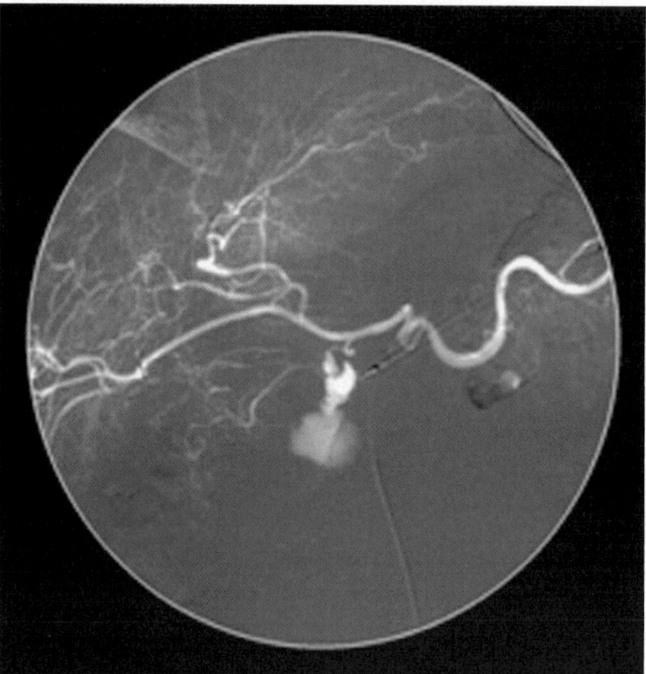

Figure 12.2 Visceral angiogram of celiac access demonstrating bleeding from an arterial pseudoaneurysm that complicated pancreatitis with pseudocyst formation.

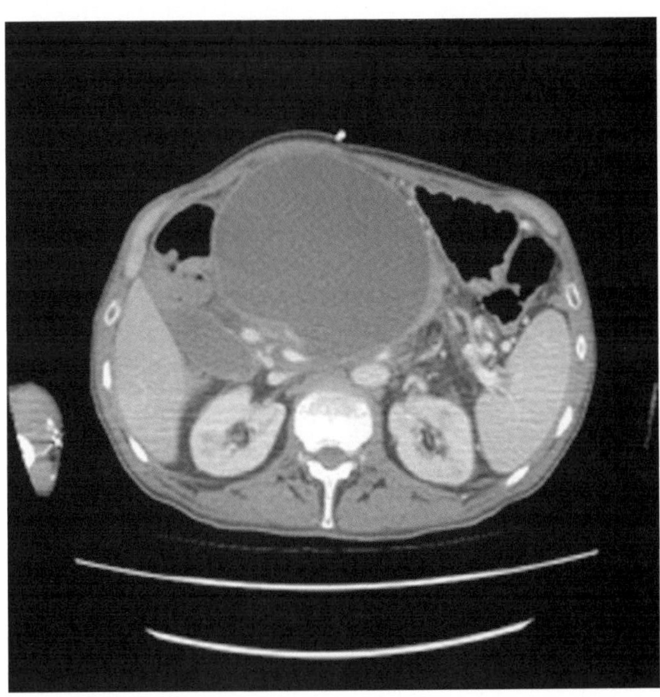

Figure 12.3 CT demonstrating giant (15 × 14 cm) pancreatic pseudocyst occupying the mid-abdomen.

may obstruct the biliary tract and result in jaundice, pruritus, and other symptoms of cholestasis. Importantly, a relatively large pseudocyst in the body and/or tail of the gland may cause few noticeable symptoms but result in compression or thrombosis of the mesenteric, portal, and/or splenic venous systems. The indolent, but potentially devastating consequences, of pseudocyst formation and location on nearby vascular structures, such as arterial pseudoaneurysm formation, must be recognized (Fig. 12.2). In addition, infection of a pancreatic pseudocyst requires prompt treatment to prevent systemic sepsis and rupture of a pancreatic pseudocyst, though rare, requires appropriate recognition and treatment.

Some pancreatic pseudocysts require special consideration including those defined as huge (>15 cm; Fig. 12.3), arising primarily in the spleen (Fig. 12.4), and associated

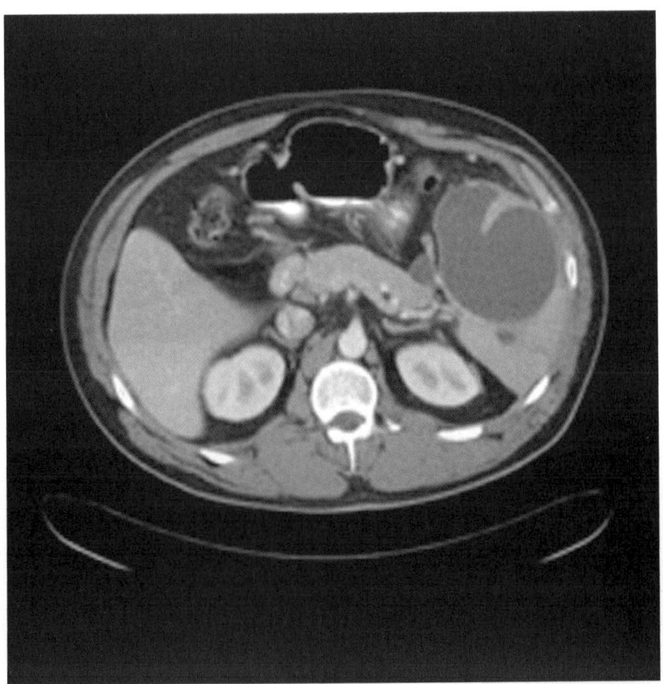

Figure 12.4 CT findings include a tiny pseudocyst in the tail of the pancreas with a large, primarily intrasplenic, pseudocyst.

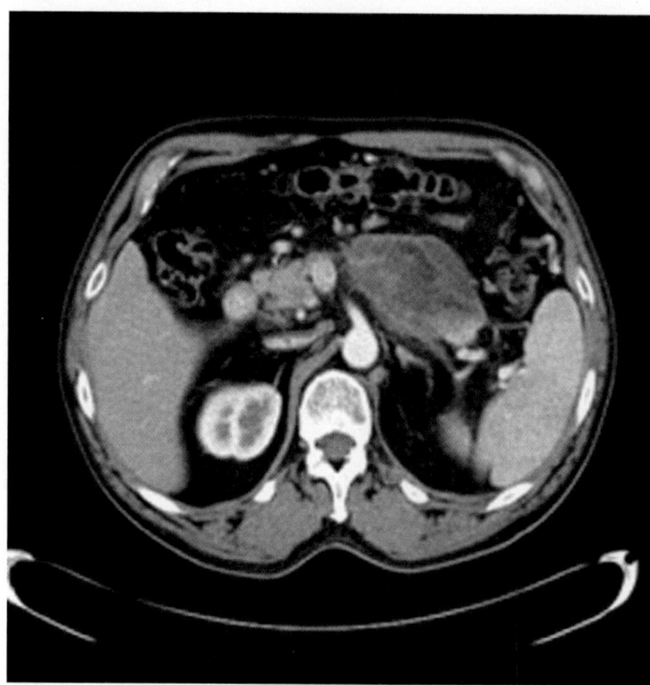

**Figure 12.5** CT showing a disconnected pancreatic duct with a small tail of viable pancreas separated from the body of the gland by an evolving pseudocyst.

with the disconnected pancreatic duct syndrome (Fig. 12.5). Pseudocysts with these features should be recognized and treated appropriately. Treatment of these pseudocysts with special considerations will be detailed later in the chapter.

Perhaps, more important than the pseudocysts that require treatment are those that do not require therapy. Notably, as mentioned previously, acute fluid collections must be distinguished from pseudocysts and these should not be treated as they will resolve spontaneously. Previously, size was an important determinant of treatment; however, recent work suggests that pseudocysts less than 6 cm in size rarely cause complications and treatment is not required. Conversely, pseudocysts greater than 10 cm in size do not necessarily require therapy if they do not cause symptoms. However, pseudocysts this large frequently cause insidious problems and no long-term data with significant numbers of patients document the safety of an observational approach in these patients.

The differential diagnosis of cystic lesions of the pancreas is delineated in Table 12.1.

**TABLE 12.1 Differential Diagnosis of Cystic Lesions of the Pancreas Exclusive of Pancreatic Pseudocysts**

| | Incidence |
|---|---|
| Serous cystadenoma | 30% |
| Mucinous cystic neoplasm | 50% |
| Intraductal papillary mucinous neoplasm | 10% |
| Papillary cystic tumor | |
| Cystic islet cell tumor | |
| Cystic adenocarcinoma | |
| Lymphangioma | |
| Cystic teratoma | 10% combined |
| Hemangioma | |
| Paraganglioma | |
| Benign simple cyst | |

## PREOPERATIVE PLANNING

Preoperative assessment and planning the management of patients with pseudocysts require establishing the cause of pseudocyst formation. Obtaining a careful history is important to determine if a pseudocyst is a consequence of acute pancreatitis that was caused by gallstones, ethanol consumption, or otherwise. Likewise, establishing a diagnosis of alcohol-related chronic pancreatitis is germane to the treatment of pseudocysts since continued use of ethanol may be associated with progressive disease and recurrence. Moreover, the presence of associated symptoms that suggest an alternative diagnosis such as a pancreatic tumor or a long-standing pancreatic disease should be ascertained. These symptoms include weight loss, jaundice, pruritus, acholic stool, dark urine, steatorrhea, the recent onset of diabetes mellitus, or, rarely, skin manifestations.

Because of the deep, retroperitoneal location of the pancreas, physical examination rarely results in palpation of a pseudocyst and only the most gravely ill patients with acute pancreatitis exhibit features of the disease that are evident on examination. In a similar fashion, laboratory evaluation is almost never diagnostic and likely is most useful in suggesting alternative diagnoses such as pancreatic cancer in a patient with a markedly increased CA 19-9 concentration.

Imaging of the pancreas and surrounding structures, however, is of paramount importance. Typically, cross-sectional imaging with thin-slice computed tomography (CT) is the preferred modality for many surgeons. Magnetic resonance imaging (MRI), especially when accompanied by magnetic resonance cholangiopancreatography (MRCP), may also be a useful diagnostic tool that provides valuable information and has some advantages over CT in institutions with specific MRI-related expertise. Regardless, precise imaging of the pancreatic parenchyma and duct, associated pseudocyst, adjacent organs, and surrounding vascular structures is critically important to operative planning. Importantly, when CT is the preferred imaging, a triple phase scan that demonstrates the arterial blood supply and the venous drainage of the pancreas should be critically examined. Needless to say, cross-sectional imaging provides a necessary roadmap for surgical management.

Pancreatography is as important as meticulous cross-sectional imaging in many patients. Essentially, all patients with chronic pancreatitis require endoscopic retrograde cholangiopancreatography (ERCP) to define pancreatic ductal anatomy and to determine the presence of a clinically asymptomatic biliary stricture. Pancreatography may identify pancreatic duct strictures or stenoses, communication with the pseudocyst, and duct cut-offs, all of which are important to recognize prior to surgical treatment. Pancreatic ductal anatomy often determines the operative procedure and the outcome. Though pancreatography is not required for all patients with acute pancreatitis–induced ductal disruptions, it should be contemplated in each patient that requires treatment since a pseudocyst resulting from a disruption in an otherwise normal duct may be treated by transpapillary duct stenting. In addition, ERCP may be helpful to detect otherwise unappreciated ductal changes induced by acute pancreatitis.

The outcome of surgical management is often determined by careful preoperative assessment including a complete history, imaging, and pancreatography. Detailed assessment and preoperative planning is requisite for an optimal outcome.

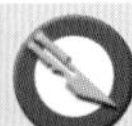

## SURGICAL TECHNIQUE

Management of pseudocysts includes initial observation followed by surveillance, percutaneous treatment, endoscopic therapy, and surgical treatment. The indications and procedures for each of these options will be reviewed.

Many patients with small (≤6 cm) pancreatic pseudocysts can be managed by observation regardless of the cause of pancreatitis or etiology. Multiple studies have demonstrated the safety of this recommendation and most of these small pseudocysts will

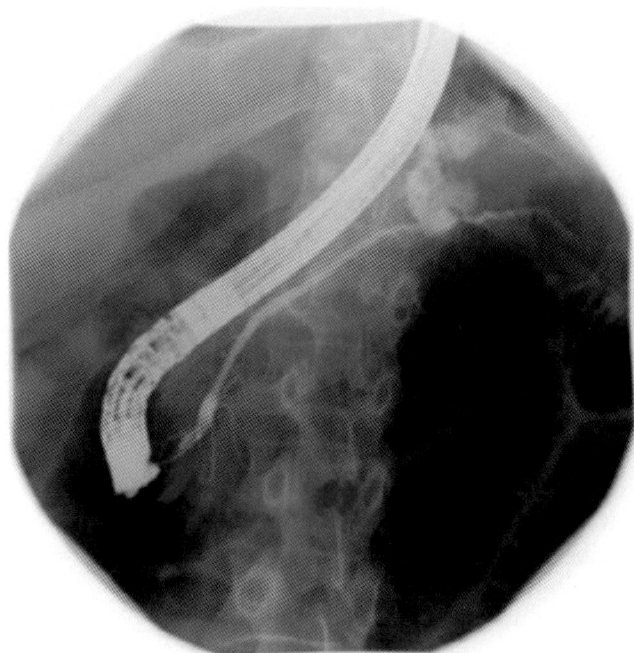

**Figure 12.6** ERCP demonstrating a relatively normal pancreatic duct following an episode of acute pancreatitis. A single duct disruption in the tail of the gland resulted in pseudocyst formation. The pseudocyst was readily treated by transpapillary drainage.

spontaneously resolve over time. However, it is important to follow patients to ensure resolution or at least stability in the size of the pseudocyst.

Percutaneous drainage was once a favored treatment for pseudocysts of all origins; however, long-term follow-up demonstrated that many patients treated by this modality had persistent pseudocysts, required surgical salvage procedures, developed multiple infections, or had a persistent pancreatic fistula. Therefore, percutaneous drainage is currently recommended for patients in whom the co-morbidities preclude endoscopic or surgical therapy and those patients that have an infected pseudocyst, for which percutaneous drainage is first-line treatment.

For many patients, endoscopic therapy is the initial choice of management. Symptomatic pseudocysts that result from acute pancreatitis and in which the pancreatic duct communicates with the pseudocyst may be adequately treated by transpapillary stenting (Fig. 12.6). Alternatively, if a connection between a pseudocyst and the pancreatic duct is not evident on pancreatography and the pseudocyst causes gastrointestinal luminal compression, then transmural endoscopic drainage is an excellent option. This is best accomplished by endoscopic ultrasound-guided treatment which permits visualization of intervening vascular structures, determination of wall thickness (optimally wall thickness should be <1.0 to 1.5 cm) and fine needle aspiration for intracystic fluid assessment (Fig. 12.7). Pseudocysts that complicate chronic pancreatitis may be treated by endoscopic therapy, but careful assessment of the pancreatic duct is necessary since transmural drainage downstream from a duct stricture or of a pancreatic pseudocysts from an isolated pancreatic segment frequently does not result in resolution of the pseudocyst.

The surgical options for management of pancreatic pseudocysts include external drainage, internal drainage including cystogastrostomy, cystoduodenostomy, and cystojejunostomy, pancreatic resection, and combined resection and drainage. Many of these procedures can be performed laparoscopically, one of which will be highlighted below.

Surgically accomplished external drainage should rarely be necessary if appropriate preoperative assessment is performed, especially since this treatment can readily be performed percutaneously. However, if infection or an unexpected large amount of pancreatic necrosis is present then surgical external drainage may be appropriate.

Surgical internal drainage may be indicated for patients who have a retrogastric pseudocyst that produces luminal compression of the stomach, pancreatic head pseudocysts that compromise the duodenal lumen, or giant (>15 cm) pseudocysts in which the most dependent portion of the pseudocyst extends well into the transverse

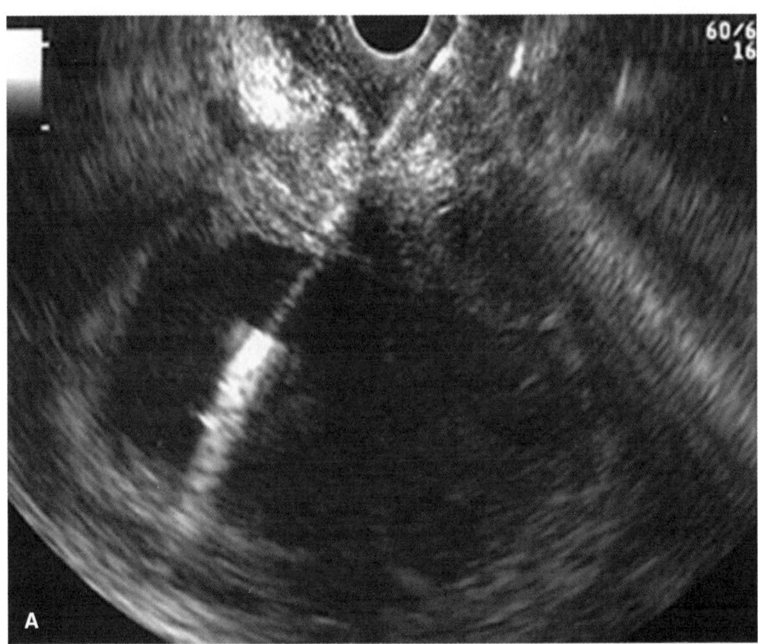

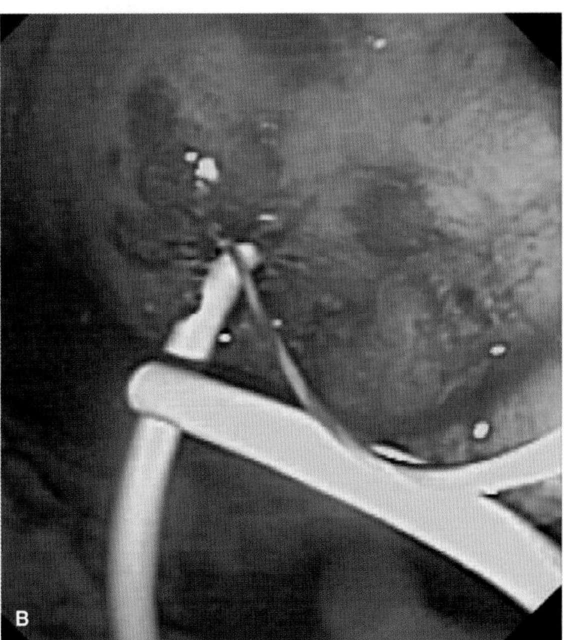

Figure 12.7 **A:** Endoscopic ultrasound showing a pseudocyst with insertion of a fine needle for aspiration. **B:** Endoscopic drainage of a pancreatic pseudocyst by dilatation of a enterocystic communication between the pseudocyst and gastric lumen with placement of a stent.

mesocolon. Cystogastrostomy may be performed for the pseudocyst that is located in the body and/or tail of the pancreas and bulges into the posterior wall of the stomach. Cystogastrostomy was formerly frequently performed for such pseudocysts, but with the development of endoscopic transmural drainage, most of these cysts are now treated endoscopically. However, laparoscopic approaches to these pancreatic pseudocysts are also appropriate and readily accomplished (Fig. 12.8A, B). One such approach is detailed in Figure 12.8C. A recent randomized trial of cystogastrostomy versus endoscopic drainage demonstrated that endoscopic drainage was associated with a decreased length of stay and decreased procedure-related costs.

Cystoduodenostomy is an infrequently performed procedure for pseudocysts located in the head of the pancreas. These pseudocysts may not only cause duodenal obstruction but may also compromise the biliary tract and result in jaundice and cholestasis. Cystoduodenostomy can be accomplished by mobilizing the duodenum and head of the pancreas, performing a lateral, longitudinal duodenostomy and identifying the pseudocyst. The mesenteric wall of the duodenum with the compressive pancreatic pseudocysts can be identified and incised. Needle aspiration of the pseudocyst before incising the mesenteric duodenal wall can confirm the location of the pseudocyst and assess the depth of the pancreatic tissue that must be traversed to enter the pseudocyst. Obviously, care must be taken not to injure the intrapancreatic and intraduodenal bile duct and the pancreatic duct. If the papilla is difficult to identify and the gallbladder is in place, a cholecystectomy can be performed and the cystic and common bile duct traversed with a biliary catheter that will enter the duodenal lumen for identification of the papilla. Once the mesenteric duodenal wall is incised and the pseudocyst entered, a defect of at least 3 cm should be created. The common walls of the duodenum and pseudocyst should be approximated with an absorbable suture (Fig. 12.9). As with all surgical approaches, a biopsy of the pseudocyst wall should confirm the lack of an epithelial surface.

Pseudocysts that extend well into the transverse mesocolon are most appropriately treated by Roux-en-Y cystojejunostomy to the most dependent portion of the pseudocyst. This technique is most appropriate for giant pseudocysts. Cystogastrostomy has not been proven to be a reliable surgical therapy for giant pseudocysts. This operation is readily accomplished by incising the pseudocyst, biopsying the wall, then sewing the Roux limb to it in a single layer with absorbable suture. Alternatively, this can be accomplished laparoscopically by a surgeon skilled in intracorporeal sewing (Fig. 12.8B).

Pancreatic resection for pancreatic pseudocysts is uncommon because preservation of pancreatic parenchyma, especially islet cell mass, is a primary principle of pancreatic surgery for benign disease. However, pseudocysts located in the tail of the gland and associated with a pancreatic duct cut-off may be treated by a limited resection. Furthermore, if the diagnosis of a pseudocyst versus a cystic neoplasm is unclear, then resection may be advisable. Pancreatic resection, especially pancreatoduodenectomy, however, should be one of the last surgical treatment options employed for the treatment of a pseudocyst.

Surgical resection of the pancreatic head parenchyma in combination with a drainage procedure of the distal pancreatic duct is not uncommon in patients with alcohol-induced chronic pancreatitis complicated by a pancreatic head pseudocyst. Unroofing of the pancreatic pseudocysts with resection of an enlarged, indurated pancreatic head can be combined with a longitudinal pancreatojejunostomy to provide complete drainage of the pancreas. This operation can be performed by adequate exposure of the pancreas and an associated pseudocyst through a xiphoid to infraumbilical midline incision, wide exposure of the pancreas through the lesser sac, and a generous Kocher maneuver. Careful exposure of the pancreatic head by separating an inflamed mesentery, identifying the superior mesenteric vein (SMV), and dividing the gastrocolic trunk provide excellent exposure for ample resection of the pancreatic head. Identification and separation of the SMV from the head of the pancreas is important to gain wide exposure of the pancreatic head and uncinate process. The SMV should be cleared anteriorly and laterally up to the inferior border of the pancreas such that its location and course are noted to prevent injury to the vein. However, its course beneath the pancreas need not be exposed because of the risk of venous injury. In addition, the

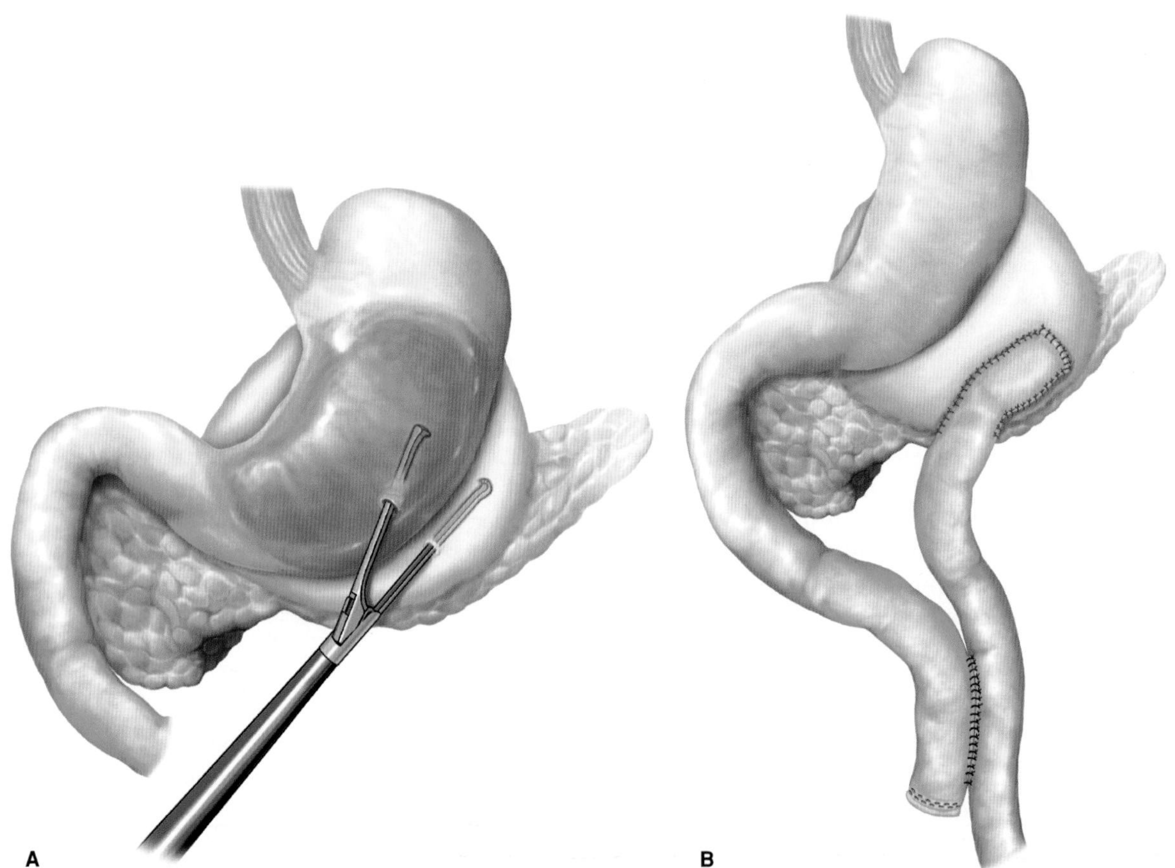


**Figure 12.8 A:** Illustration of a laparoscopic cystogastrostomy. **B:** Illustration of a laparoscopic cystojejunostomy.

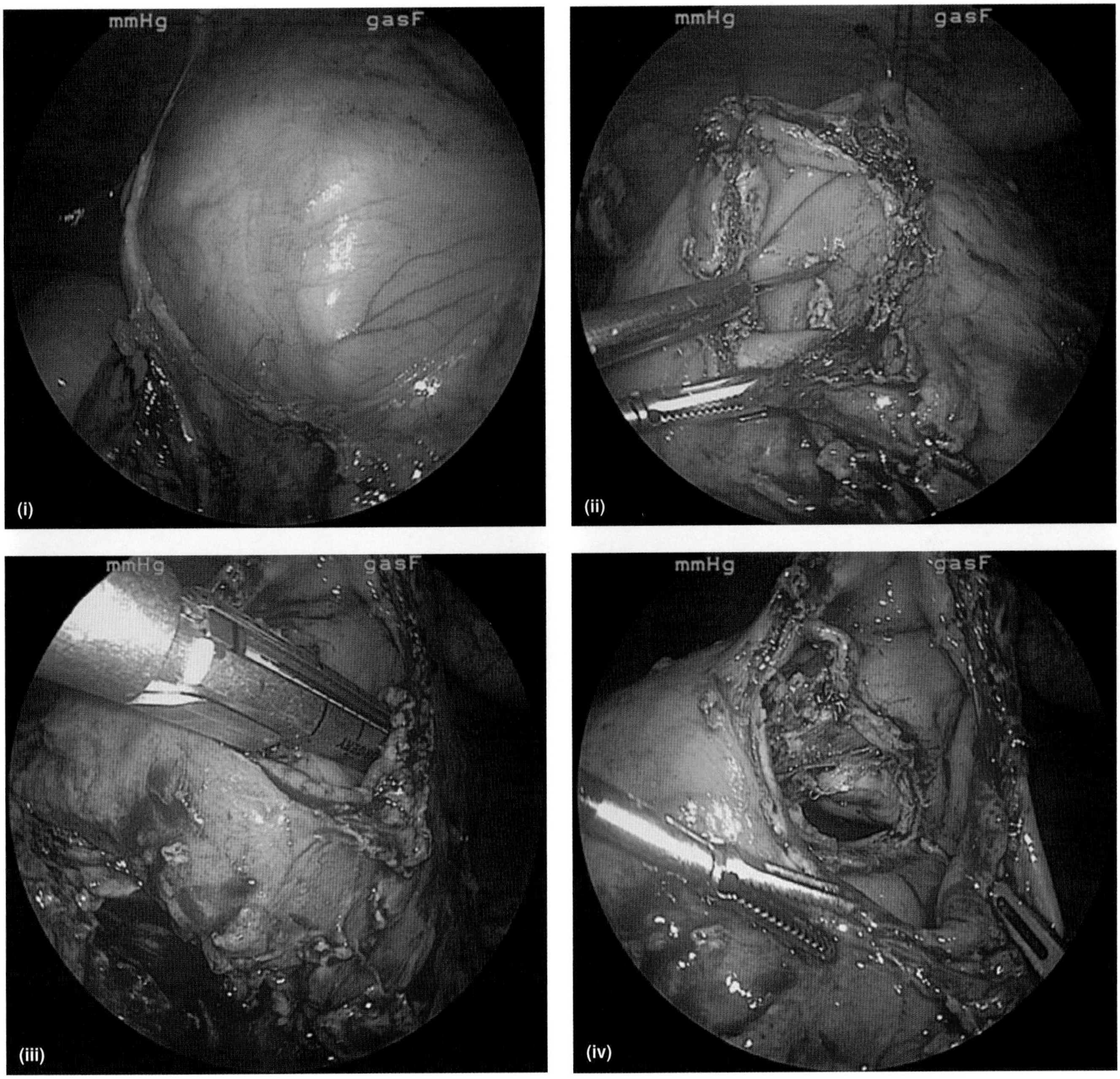

**Figure 12.8** (*Continued*) **C:** Laparoscopic cystogastrostomy via an anterior gastrotomy—images illustrating a large pancreatic pseudocyst bulging underneath the antrum (i), an anterior gastrotomy with aspiration of the pancreatic pseudocyst (ii), stapled cystogastrostomy through the anterior gastrotomy (iii), and a view of the pancreatic cystogastrostomy opening (iv).

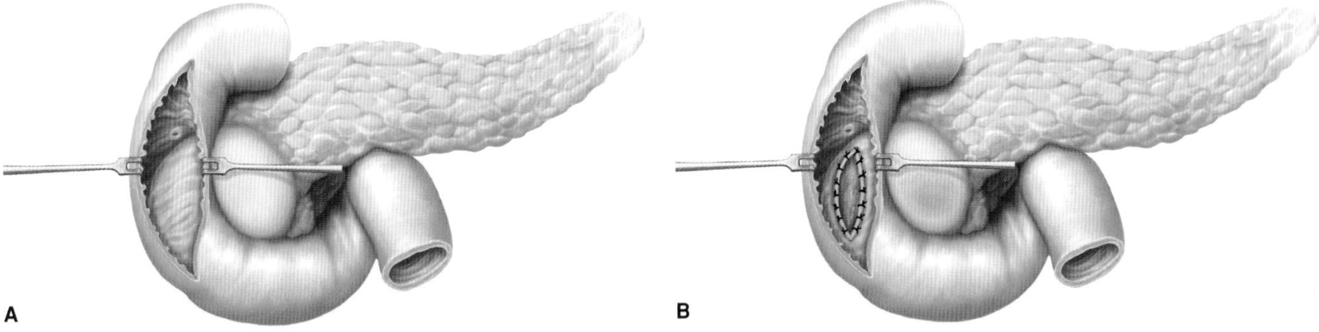


**Figure 12.9** Illustration of creation of a cystoduodenostomy. **A:** The pseudocyst was approached through a lateral, longitudinal duodenotomy. **B:** The pseudocyst was identified by needle aspiration and the medial wall of the duodenum was opened into the pseudocyst. The cyst–duodenal communication was secured with an absorbable suture.

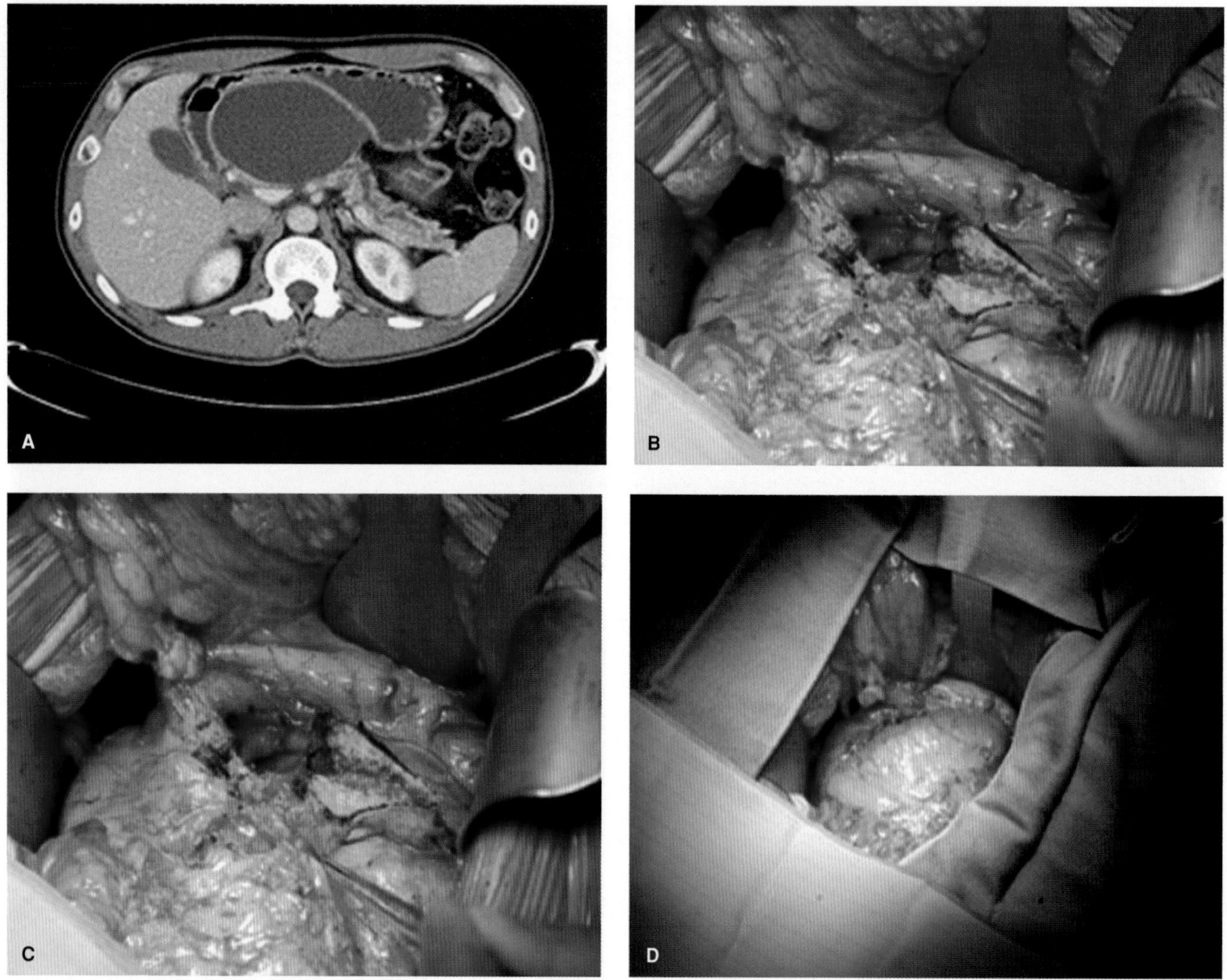

Figure 12.10 **A:** CT demonstrating a large pseudocyst occupying a portion of the pancreatic head and body with obstruction of the pancreatic duct in the body and tail of the gland. **B:** Intraoperative photograph showing unroofing of the pseudocyst with ductotomy in the body and tail of the gland. **C:** Intraoperative photograph demonstrating the open pseudocyst, resected head of the gland, and the intrapancreatic biliary sphincteroplasty. **D:** Intraoperative photograph showing a Roux-en-Y limb of jejunum sewn to the pancreatic head, pseudocyst, and pancreatic tail.

distal stomach and proximal duodenum should be freed from the pancreas and the gastroduodenal artery controlled superior to the pancreas. The remainder of the operation consists of the pancreatic head resection, ductotomy of the neck, body, and tail of the gland, and an intrapancreatic biliary sphincteroplasty as indicated by cholestasis.

The pancreatic head is resected leaving only a thin (3 to 5 mm) rim of pancreas attached to the duodenum (Fig. 12.10). The resection should extend from the medial aspect of the duodenum to the right of the SMV and the pancreatic neck in the transverse direction. Longitudinally, the resection should extend from the entry of the gastroduodenal artery into the pancreas and to the anterior portion of the pancreas as it becomes the uncinate process. A 3 to 5 mm thickness of the gland is all that remains as the posterior surface of the pancreas. Extensive pancreatic head resection is an important component that leads to excellent long-term relief of pancreatic pain. Bleeding during the resection is controlled with precise suture ligation using 5-0 Prolene sutures.

Within the pancreatic head, the pancreatic duct is identified and opened from the duodenum over the neck and onto the body and tail of the gland. All pancreatic stone material is removed. Although the duct need not be opened its entire length, the duct should be widely patent from the duodenum to the tail of the gland.

An intrapancreatic biliary sphincteroplasty can be facilitated by the palpation of a biliary stent. The bile duct is opened longitudinally over the stent, and the stent removed. The bile duct is opened superiorly until it easily accepts a 5 to 7 mm probe. The bile duct is tacked circumferentially to the surrounding pancreas with interrupted 6-0 PDS sutures. This completes the intrapancreatic biliary sphincteroplasty, which provides excellent relief of an associated biliary stricture.

A Roux-en-Y jejunal loop is then sewn in a side-to-side fashion to the edges of the pancreas surrounding the resection and ductotomy. A jejunojejunostomy is created 50 cm distal to the pancreatojejunostomy.

When a pseudocyst is present anteriorly in the head of the pancreas, it should be unroofed prior to the resection of the gland, and a portion of the wall submitted for histopathologic examination. When a posteriorly located pseudocyst is present in the pancreas, the duct should be identified in the body of the gland and opened toward the head until it enters the pseudocyst. The pseudocyst should be unroofed and the head should then be resected.

# Special Considerations

Infrequently, patients with chronic pancreatitis and a stenosis or stricture in the distal pancreatic duct will develop a pseudocyst that is located almost exclusively in the spleen. These intrasplenic pseudocysts may cause pancreatic enzyme–induced digestion of the spleen and destruction of the splenic capsule. Ultimately, rupture of the spleen with massive exsanguination may occur. Therefore, recognition of an intrasplenic pseudocyst should result in prompt splenectomy and treatment of the underlying pancreatic pathology, that is, relief of the duct stricture. Since the chronic inflammation may be severe in these cases, preoperative splenic artery embolization has resulted in decreased intraoperative transfusion.

Patients with acute necrotizing pancreatitis and the disconnected pancreatic duct syndrome, in which the body of the gland has become necrotic but a viable pancreatic juice-secreting tail results in pseudocyst formation, resection of the tail of the gland may be appropriate. Alternatively, if the remnant tail is of reasonable size and contains a dilated pancreatic duct, a drainage procedure may be performed. The senior author, however, has encountered this infrequently. Optimally, the disconnected duct syndrome would be identified during the episode of necrotizing pancreatitis and the necrotic pancreas and viable tail removed at the time of necrosectomy. However, some data suggests that diagnosis of the disconnected pancreatic duct syndrome occurs months after the episode and, therefore, resection of the pancreatic tail remnant at this time may not be obvious.

Since many of the patients undergoing operative intervention for management of pseudocysts have sustained considerable damage to the pancreas, a prophylactic cholecystectomy should be considered in all cases since gallstone-induced pancreatitis may have devastating consequences in these patients.

# POSTOPERATIVE MANAGEMENT

Postoperative management of patients that have treatment of a pseudocyst is generally straightforward and follows standard treatment for postoperative patients. Hospitalization can be as short as 1 to 2 days if endoscopic or laparoscopic procedures are performed in the elective setting or length of stay can be approximately 7 days following a complex, combined resection and drainage procedure. Regardless of the procedure performed, cross-sectional imaging about 4 weeks following the procedure should document a marked diminution in size or absence of the pseudocyst.

In patients with chronic pancreatitis, it is important to ensure that they have adequate exocrine and endocrine functions or that they receive appropriate medical care for pancreatic enzyme supplementation and/or diabetes mellitus. Though pancreatic

**TABLE 12.2 Complications of Endoscopic and Surgical Treatment of Pseudocysts**

| | Percent |
|---|---|
| **Endoscopic Complications** | |
| Hemorrhage | 1–2% |
| Infection | <5% |
| Stent migration | 5–10% |
| **Surgical Complications**[a] | |
| Bleeding | 5% |
| Infection | 12% |
| Fistula | 3% |
| Persistent pseudocyst | 3% |
| Recurrent pseudocyst | 10% |
| Recurrent pancreatitis | 12% |
| Death | 0% |

[a]From Heider R, Meyer AA, Galanko JA, et al. Percutaneous drainage of pancreatic pseudocysts is associated with a higher failure rate than surgical treatment in unselected patients. *Ann Surg.* 1999;229:781–787; discussion 787–789.

procedures in patients with alcohol-induced chronic pancreatitis should generally be reserved for patients who have abstained from alcohol for some time, occasionally patients will need counseling for alcohol withdrawal and cessation.

## COMPLICATIONS

The complications following endoscopic and surgical treatment are generally few, depending on the complexity of the case. Endoscopic treatment has a complication rate of approximately 5% and includes primarily hemorrhage and infection. Hemorrhagic complications have decreased markedly since the adoption of procedures that use dilatation rather than cutting to establish the alimentary tract–cyst communication. Infection occurs when an unexpected amount of pancreatic or peripancreatic necrosis is associated with the pseudocyst. Although not a complication *per se,* the inability to obtain definitive histology during endoscopic treatment may lead to an inappropriately treated cystic lesion. Finally, though infrequent, when surgical salvage procedures are required for failed endoscopic therapy, the mortality and morbidity of these procedures is increased significantly compared to primary surgical procedures.

Surgical treatment of pancreatic pseudocysts is associated with a mortality rate of 1% or less and the complication rate is 20% to 25%. Surgical morbidity is typically related to complications associated with any major operative procedure and includes bleeding and infection, especially pulmonary-related infections.

See Table 12.2 for a more complete list of complications.

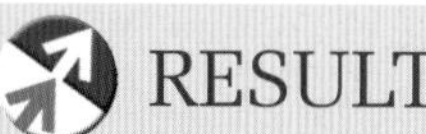

## RESULTS

The results of pseudocyst drainage depend greatly on the underlying cause. Generally, the recurrence rates for pseudocyst formation are 15% for endoscopic therapy and 5% for surgically treated pseudocysts. The recurrence rate is highly dependent on choosing the appropriate therapy for the underlying condition. It must be recognized that the long-term patency of an endoscopic or surgically created cyst–enteric communication by either stent placement or surgical approximation will be zero since the cyst does not contain an epithelial lining and, therefore, the establishment of a long duration communication is not possible. For pseudocysts that arise from acute pancreatitis with an underlying normal pancreatic duct, a long-term communication between the pseudocyst and the gastrointestinal tract is not necessary and the results are excellent. However, in patients with chronic pancreatitis and underlying parenchymal and ductal pathology, more definitive treatment is often required and a simple endoscopic drainage or surgical drainage of a pseudocyst may have time-limited value. For these patients, more durable operations that correct the underlying pathologic disturbance should be considered.

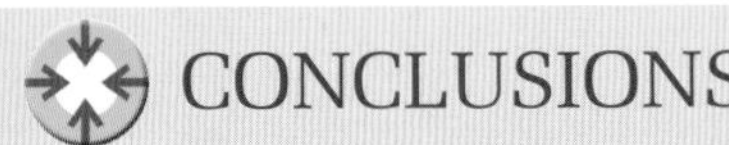

## CONCLUSIONS

The management of pseudocysts depends significantly on the underlying pancreatic parenchymal and ductal pathology. Appropriate identification of either acute or chronic pancreatitis through history, cross-sectional imaging, and/or ductal imaging may be required to securely establish the diagnosis and plan appropriate therapy. Endoscopic therapy is first-line for many patients with pseudocysts, but surgical treatment may be more appropriate for patients with chronic pancreatitis and underlying pathologic perturbations. Nonetheless, both treatments can provide excellent long-term relief. Care of patients with pseudocysts requires a multidisciplinary, communicative approach to ensure high-quality care.

## Recommended References and Readings


Barthet M, Lamblin G, Gasmi M, et al. Clinical usefulness of a treatment algorithm for pancreatic pseudocysts. *Gastrointest Endosc.* 2008;67:245–252.

Behrns KE, Ben-David K. Surgical therapy of pancreatic pseudocysts. *J Gastrointest Surg.* 2008;12:2231–2239.

Behrns KE. Local resection of the pancreatitic head for pancreatic pseudocysts. *J Gastrointest Surg.* 2008;12:2227–2230.

Behrns KE. Pancreatic Pseudocysts. In: Cameron JL, ed. *Current Surgical Therapy.* 9th ed. Philadelphia, PA: Mosby Elsevier; 2008: 491–493.

Cannon JW, Callery MP, Vollmer CM Jr. Diagnosis and management of pancreatic pseudocysts: what is the evidence? *J Am Coll Surg.* 2009;209:385–393.

Heider R, Behrns KE. Pancreatic pseudocysts complicated by splenic parenchymal involvement: results of operative and percutaneous management. *Pancreas.* 2001;23:20–25.

Heider R, Meyer AA, Galanko JA, et al. Percutaneous drainage of pancreatic pseudocysts is associated with a higher failure rate than surgical treatment in unselected patients. *Ann Surg.* 1999; 229:781–787; discussion 787–789.

Johnson LB, Rattner DW, Warshaw AL. The effect of size of giant pancreatic pseudocysts on the outcome of internal drainage procedures. *Surg Gynecol Obstet.* 1991;173:171–174.

Johnson MD, Walsh RM, Henderson JM, et al. Surgical versus nonsurgical management of pancreatic pseudocysts. *J Clin Gastroenterol.* 2009;43:586–590.

Macari M, Finn ME, Bennett GL, et al. Differentiating pancreatic cystic neoplasms from pancreatic pseudocysts at MR imaging: value of perceived internal debris. *Radiology.* 2009;251: 77–84.

Morton JM, Brown A, Galanko JA, et al. A national comparison of surgical versus percutaneous drainage of pancreatic pseudocysts: 1997–2001. *J Gastrointest Surg.* 2005;9:15–20; discussion 20–21.

Nealon WH, Walser E. Main pancreatic ductal anatomy can direct choice of modality for treating pancreatic pseudocysts (surgery versus percutaneous drainage). *Ann Surg.* 2002;235:751–758.

Pelaez-Luna M, Vege SS, Petersen BT, et al. Disconnected pancreatic duct syndrome in severe acute pancreatitis: clinical and imaging characteristics and outcomes in a cohort of 31 cases. *Gastrointest Endosc.* 2008;68:91–97.

Varadarajulu S, Lopes TL, Wilcox CM, et al. EUS versus surgical cyst-gastrostomy for management of pancreatic pseudocysts. *Gastrointest Endosc.* 2008;68:649–655.

Varadarajulu S. EUS followed by endoscopic pancreatic pseudocyst drainage or all-in-one procedure: a review of basic techniques (with video). *Gastrointest Endosc.* 2009;69:S176–S181.

Vitas GJ, Sarr MG. Selected management of pancreatic pseudocysts: operative versus expectant management. *Surgery.* 1992;111:123–130.

Yekebas EF, Bogoevski D, Honarpisheh H, et al. Long-term follow-up in small duct chronic pancreatitis: A plea for extended drainage by "V-shaped excision" of the anterior aspect of the pancreas. *Ann Surg.* 2006;244:940–946; discussion 946–948.

Yeo CJ, Bastidas JA, Lynch-Nyhan A, et al. The natural history of pancreatic pseudocysts documented by computed tomography. *Surg Gynecol Obstet.* 1990;170:411–417.

# 13 Laparoscopic Cholecystectomy With and Without Laparoscopic Common Bile Duct Exploration

**David B. Renton and W. Scott Melvin**

## Introduction

Revolutions in the realm of surgery have been predicated on advances in technology. From inhaled anesthetics, to electrocautery, to cardiopulmonary bypass, all have been possible due to scientific advances in the understanding of physiology and physics. This is especially true for even truer for laparoscopy. Beginning in the late 1980s, laparoscopy became the standard of care for the treatment of many surgical diseases, none more so that diseases of the gallbladder. The laparoscopic cholecystectomy has become the gold standard for treatment of acute cholecystitis and symptomatic cholelithiasis. In this chapter we will discuss indications and techniques for performing laparoscopic cholecystectomy, intraoperative cholangiogram (IOC), and laparoscopic common bile duct exploration (LCBDE).

## Indications for Laparoscopic Cholecystectomy

**Symptomatic Cholelithiasis** is by far the most common indication for cholecystectomy in modern surgical practices. The symptoms of this process are: crampy abdominal pain, usually centered in the right upper quadrant (RUQ) or epigastric area, pain that is brought on or exacerbated by a fatty meal, and the presence of gallstones on imaging studies. With the acceptance of laparoscopic cholecystectomy in the late 1980s, the threshold for removing the symptomatic gallbladder may have even been has lowered because of the decrease in morbidity associated with the laparoscopic procedure. Careful patient selection is still necessary to optimize results. Other indications for cholecystectomy include gall bladder polyps or porcelain gallbladder.

**Choledocholithiasis** with or without associated pancreatitis is also an indication for cholecystectomy. When available, endoscopic retrograde cholangiopancreatography (ERCP) preoperatively can clear common duct stones and negate the need for operative common duct exploration. Once the duct is cleared, laparoscopic cholecystectomy can be performed after pancreatic enzymes have returned to normal. If ERCP is not performed preoperatively, IOC should be performed. If stones are detected, either LCBDE can be performed, or postoperative ERCP can be used to clear the duct.

**Acute Cholecystitis** has been a controversial area for the performance of laparoscopic cholecystectomy in the past. The argument of timing of the operation, either during the acute stage, or waiting 6 weeks to allow a decrease in the inflammation has raged for several years. The current consensus is that cholecystectomy should be performed during the admission for cholecystitis, usually during the first 72 hours of admission. Conversion to an open procedure is more common when dealing with acute cholecystitis than with uncomplicated symptomatic cholelithiasis, but is still within an acceptable rate. Delay in operation risks a repeat attack of cholecystitis, increased hospital stay times, and an equal or higher conversion rate as those operated on within the first 72 hours of presentation.

# Biliary Dyskinesia

Patients with no evidence of gallstones on imaging studies and laboratory values with persistent RUQ pain may suffer from biliary dyskinesia. This phenomenon occurs due to lack of contraction of the gallbladder when presented with hormonal stimulus. Nuclear imaging, namely the quantitative HIDA scan, is used for confirmation. Meta-analysis has shown that of patients with an ejection fraction less than 35%, up to 85% of these patients receive relief of symptoms after having undergone laparoscopic cholecystectomy.

## Patient Selection

While laparoscopic cholecystectomy should be the first choice in all patients for gallbladder removal, some patients provide special challenges which should be considered before beginning the operation. Morbid obesity is a common condition in patients with gallstones. Initial port placement can be a challenge in the patients and should be considered preoperatively to ensure proper equipment is present in the operating room. These patients should be secured to the bed well, as positioning during the operation can cause shifting on the table. Patients with previous surgery, especially upper abdominal procedures should be counseled preoperatively about the possibility of conversion to an open procedure. However, none of these are contraindications for laparoscopic cholecystectomy, which remains the procedure of choice for almost all patients undergoing cholecystectomy.

# Laparoscopic Cholecystectomy

Since gaining acceptance in the late 1980s, the laparoscopic cholecystectomy technique has not undergone significant change. As with any procedure, there are variations of each step that can be used depending on surgeon preference. The patient is usually positioned supine with arms out. OG tube decompression is recommended to decrease the size of the stomach to ease in visualization. A foley catheter is not necessary in most cases.

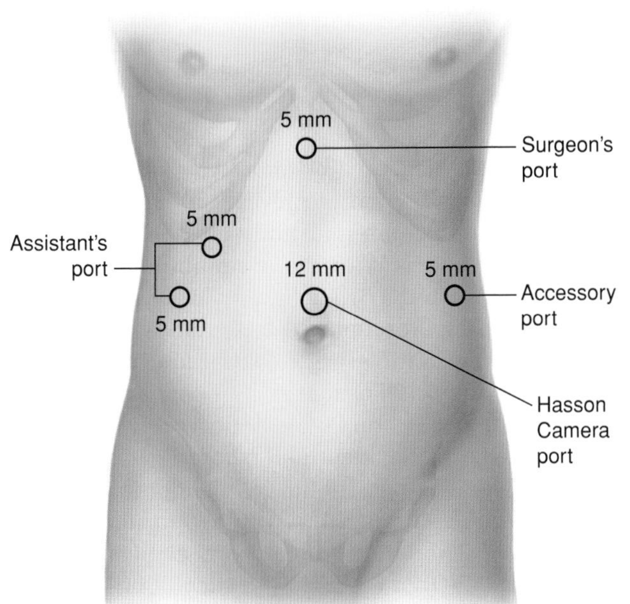


**Figure 13.1** Trocar placement for a laparoscopic cholecystectomy. The surgeon stand on the patient's left. The subxyphoid port is the operating port; the two right upper quadrant ports are for gallbladder retraction. An accessory port can be placed in the left upper quadrant if needed.

## Trocar Placement

The start of any laparoscopic operation begins with safe trocar placement (Fig. 13.1). Placement of the initial trocar aids in successful and safe placement of subsequent trocars. The authors favor a Hasson approach at the umbilicus for initial placement of a 12 mm trocar for a laparoscopic cholecystectomy. The safety of Hasson technique has been well established. Other options are Veress needle access at the umbilicus or off midline or an optical view trocar access. Supra-umbilical placement of the initial trocar allows a global view of the abdomen, and can be used to rule out any other pathology. The placement of a 12 mm trocar will ease removal of the gallbladder later in the case, especially those laden with large stones. When it comes to trocar placement, the technique that the surgeon is most comfortable with and most proficient with is the best choice. In the setting of previous upper abdominal surgery, the cut down Hasson method is the preferred method, as this allows sweeping down of adhesions around the initial trocar. With this trocar placed, RUQ can be surveyed, and secondary trocars placed safely.

Once initial trocar placement has been successfully achieved, the abdomen is insufflated to 15 mm Hg using $CO_2$. Working trocars are then placed. The trocar placement diagramed shows a standard design used to triangulate on the target structure. The retracting trocars are placed subcostally with one in the right midclavicular line and the second in the right anterior axillary line. The working trocar is placed in the subxiphoid position. This design can be varied depending on surgeon preference, the assistance available to the surgeon, and experience level. A fifth trocar is shown in the left lateral area. This trocar can be added if excessive inflammation is present and the need for repeated irrigation and suctioning is necessary. This fifth trocar can also be used to retract organs that may obstruct the view of the gallbladder and cystic structures such as the transverse colon, duodenum, or omentum.

The subject of trocar size should be mentioned at this point. The need for a second 10 mm or greater trocar, usually placed at the subxiphoid position had been necessary for the completion of this operation. This was due to the need to move the 10 mm camera to this position during gallbladder extraction. It was also necessary because all laparoscopic clip appliers only came in a 10 mm size. With the advances made in current laparoscopic equipment, 5 mm clip appliers are readily available and are usually adequate for ligation of the uncomplicated cystic duct and artery. Optics have also made advances, with current 5 mm 30 degree cameras being equal in image quality to their larger 10 mm counterparts. This author uses 5 mm ports for all working and retracting ports on a regular basis.

## Steps of the Operation

The operation begins with cephalad retraction of the gallbladder. Any adhesions can be taken off the underside of the gallbladder at this point to reveal the infundibulum. Care should be taken to avoid injuring the duodenum and transverse colon as these can be adhesed to the underside of the gallbladder. With the infundibulum exposed, it is retracted laterally to the right. This opens up the Triangle of Calot. If needed, the distended gallbladder can be drained using a laparoscopic needle. Blunt dissection is the undertaken to delineate the cystic duct and cystic artery. Electrocautery and other heat sources should be used judiciously during this portion of the operation to avoid inadvertent injury to surrounding undefined structures. A critical view must be obtained to ensure that these structures are correctly identified before ligation can be undertaken. The critical view is achieved when the neck of the gallbladder is dissected off the liver bed giving a clear view of the liver through the window created around the cystic duct and cystic artery (Fig. 13.2). It is vital to obtain this critical view to avoid injury to either the common bile duct (CBD) or the right hepatic duct (Fig. 13.3). With a critical view obtained, the cystic duct and artery can both be ligated. Ligation is done with two clips being placed on the downside of the structures and one clip being placed toward the gallbladder. When unusual or unexpected anatomy is encountered it is important that the surgeon reestablish appropriate landmarks and consider

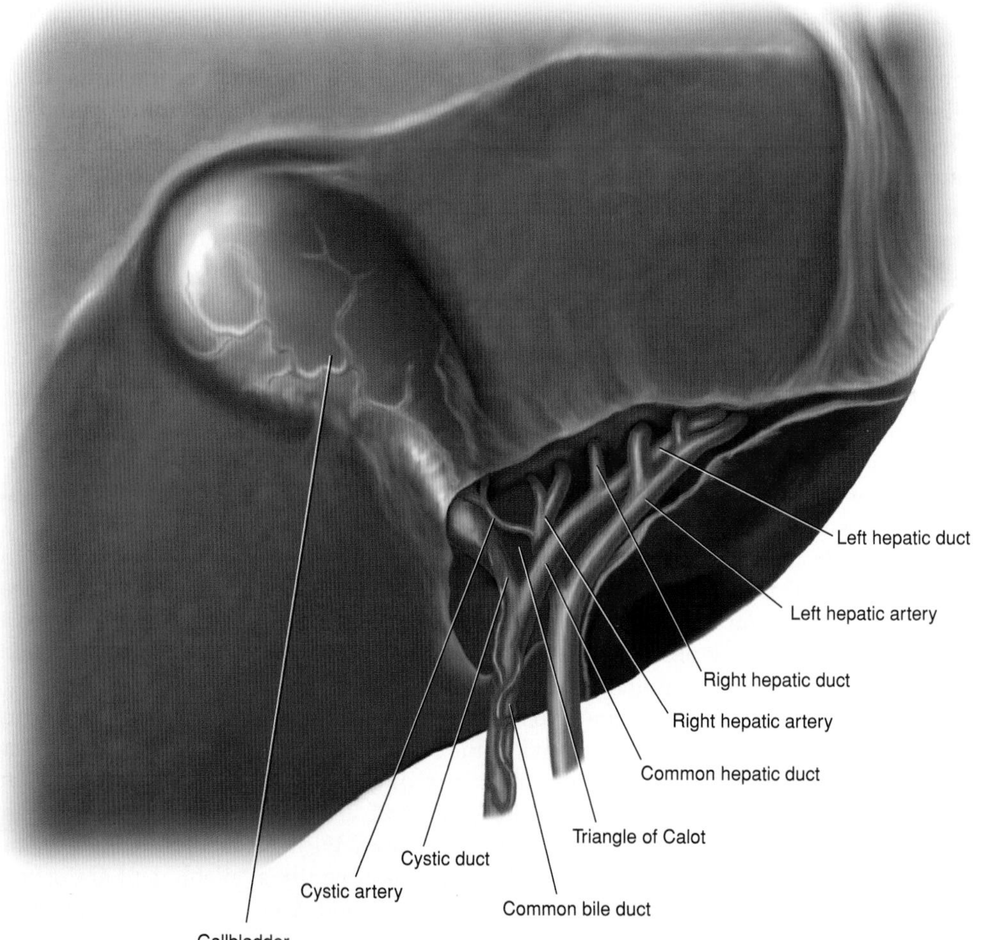


**Figure 13.2** A representation of the critical view needed during laparoscopic cholecystectomy. The area from the infundibulum, to the base of the cystic duct, then to the connection of the gallbladder to the liver bed must be fully dissected.

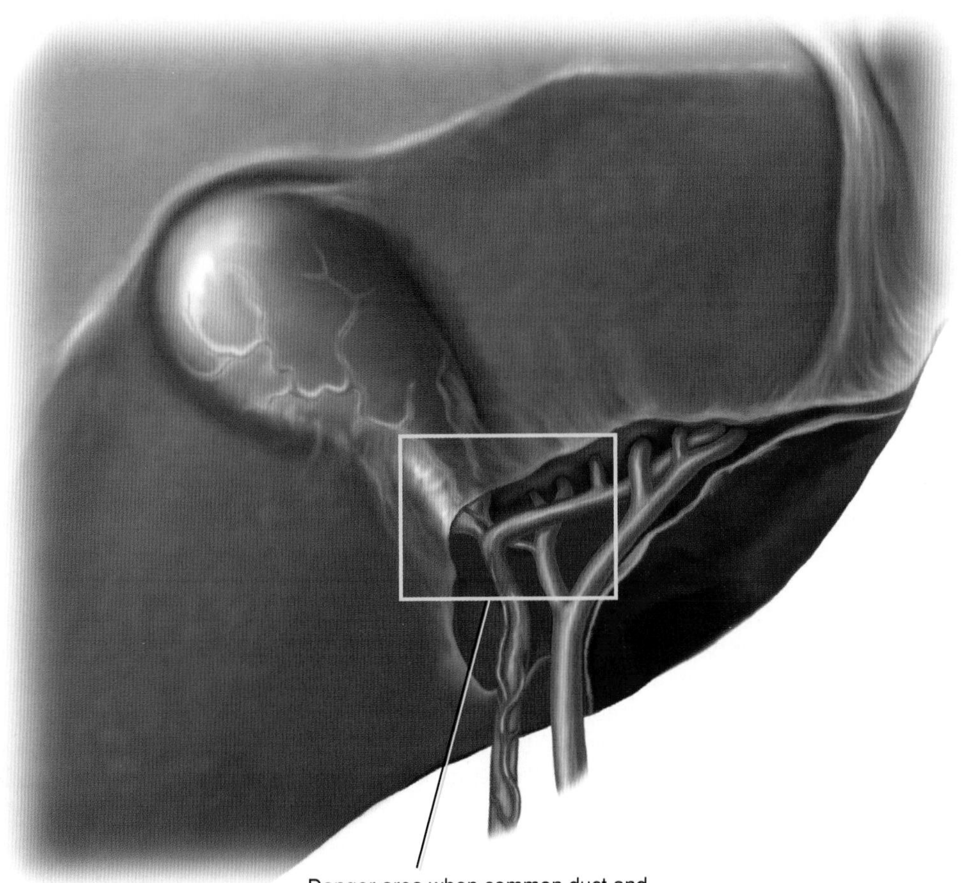

Danger area when common duct and
right hepatic duct are drawn up to
the base of the gallbladder. If a
critical view is not obtained, dissection
can occur too low and injury can occur.


Figure 13.3 A demonstration of an improper critical view. The base of the gallbladder has not been dissected out to the attachment to the liver bed. If there is a short cystic duct, the common duct can be erroneously ligated.



intraoperative consultation, cholangiography, or open conversion. Occasionally a large cystic duct is encountered that can be sutured or tied rather than attempt to close with a clip that is too small.

Once proper identification and ligation of the cystic duct and artery have been completed, the removal of the gallbladder from the gallbladder fossa can begin. This is done with a hook or spatulated cautery. Care must be taken to stay in the plane created by the fusion of the gallbladder to the liver, as this is an avascular plane. Too shallow will puncture the gallbladder and allow spillage of bile, to deep will enter the liver parenchyma and cause bleeding and possible a bile leak. Once the gallbladder has been freed of all attachments, it can be placed in a retrieval bag and removed through the supra-umbilical trocar site. The trocar should be replaced after removal of the specimen to take another look at the operative site to ensure hemostasis and clip placement is adequate. Trocar removal should then be visualized to confirm there is no bleeding from any of the working trocar sites. The fascia is then closed at the supra-umbilical site and skin closure can be performed according to surgeon preference.

Conversion to an open procedure should be considered when proper anatomy cannot be identified, when excessive bleeding is encountered, or when inflammation or adhesions make laparoscopic dissection too difficult. Predisposing factors such as patient age, number of biliary colic attacks, a history of acute cholecystitis, and previous upper abdominal surgery can be risk factors for conversion to an open procedure. Using these risk factors in counseling patients as to their risk of having an open procedure can be useful.

| TABLE 13.1 Equipment Needed for Laparoscopic Intraoperative Cholangiogram |
|---|
| C-arm |
| Drape for C-arm |
| 14 gauge angiocatheter |
| Flexible cholangiogram catheter with metal nonocclusive tip |
| 3 way stop-cock |
| 50 cc syringe of saline |
| 50 cc syringe of water soluble contrast material |
| Lead shielding for yourself and OR staff |

# Intraoperative Cholangiogram

Correct identification of biliary structures is vital during cholecystectomy. IOC uses a useful tool to assist the surgeon in performing a safe operation. Liberal use of IOC is recommended by this author, especially in the cases of unsure anatomy, suspicion of choledocholithiasis, abnormal preoperative liver function tests, or enlargement of biliary structures on preoperative imaging or intraoperative findings of unusual anatomy or a large cystic duct. Evaluation of a clear and patent CBD is always indicated in the setting of abnormal preoperative liver function tests or other indicators of possible obstruction. Performance of an accurate and informative IOC depends on the operative team working together. Radiology should be informed ahead of time if an IOC is to be performed, and all the necessary equipment listed in Table 13.1 should be collected ahead of time to make the procedure run more efficiently. Once the pieces are in place, the IOC can be performed.

With dissection of what is suspected to be the cystic duct complete, a single clip is placed toward the gallbladder side of the cystic duct. A ductotomy is made just below this that is just large enough to allow placement of the cholangiogram catheter within the lumen of the cystic duct (Fig. 13.4). A 14 gauge angiocatheter is then placed through the abdominal wall in the RUQ. The needle portion is removed and the cholangiogram catheter is placed through the plastic sheath. Alternatively a clamp with an aperture for placement of a catheter can be placed via one of the subcostal ports or one of the commercially available disposable cholangiogram catheters can be placed via one of the existing trocars. The tip of the cholangiogram catheter is then threaded into the cystic duct. A clip or the clamp can then be applied to the cystic duct to hold the catheter in place. The use of a catheter with a metal tip will aid in preventing this clip from occluding the catheter lumen. A three way stop-cock is attached to the end of the catheter, with a syringe of saline going on one port and water soluble contrast medium affixing the other. The visualization of air bubbles will be avoided by flushing the catheter, all tubing and the stop-cock with saline before placing in the patient. If difficulty is encountered advancing the catheter into the cystic duct, gentle infusion of saline may help dilate the

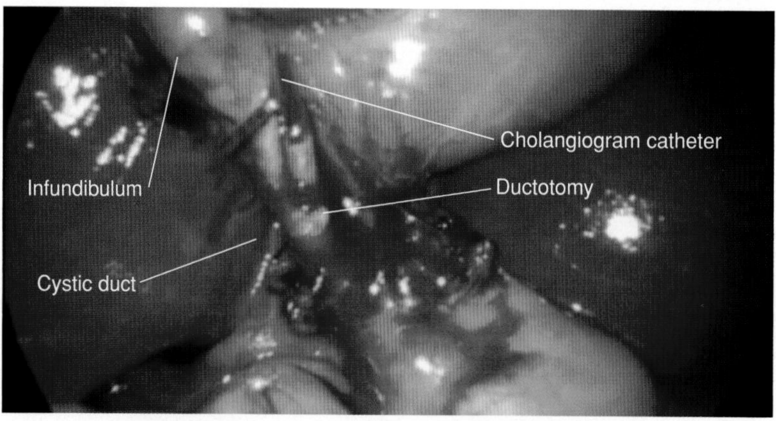


**Figure 13.4** An intraoperative picture of a laparoscopic cholangiogram. The partial ductotomy is made and the cholangiogram catheter is placed and secured.

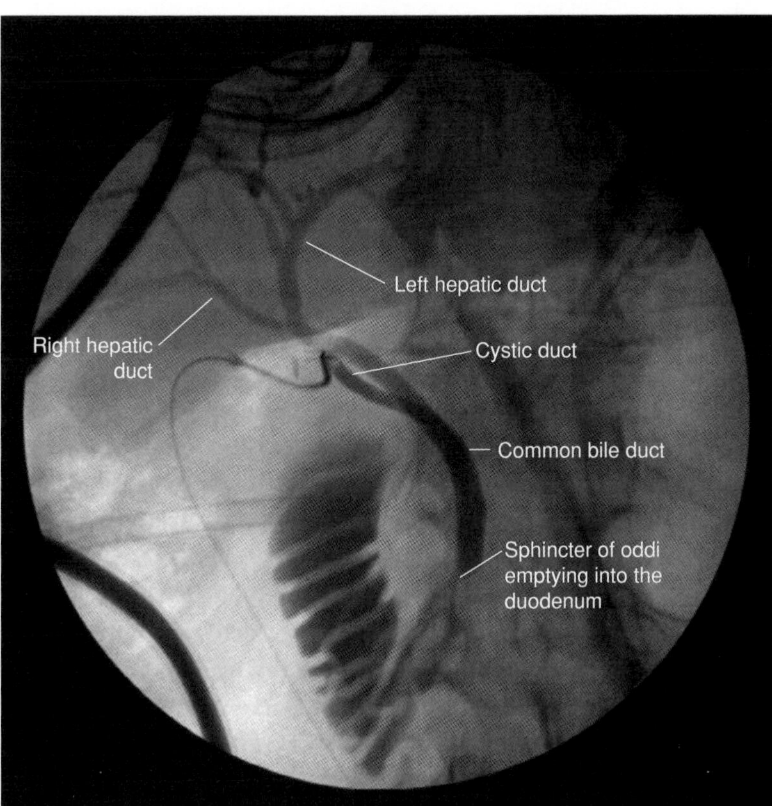


**Figure 13.5** A normal intraoperative cholangiogram with filling of the common duct, left and right hepatic duct, and emptying into the duodenum.

cystic duct. The opening of the cystic duct can also be dilated or gently enlarged distally, however care should be taken to avoid extending the opening into the CBD.

While the above is taking place, the scrub tech can be draping the C-arm with a sterile covering to aid, it is being brought up to the field. Once the cholangiogram catheter is correctly placed, it is flushed using the saline syringe to test patency to assure there is no leakage from the ductotomy. If there is leakage or the catheter is not patent, it must be removed and placed again. If the test is negative, the gallbladder is placed back in its anatomic position and the graspers are removed from the trocars. The laparoscopic camera can be left in place and used as a fixed point on which the surgeon can orient the C-arm. Once the C-arm is in place, real time fluoroscopy is used while the contrast material is injected.

With successful completion of the IOC, the catheter and the clip holding it in place can be removed (Figs. 13.5 and 13.6). The cystic duct is then clipped with two clips below the ductotomy, and the ductotomy is continued to ligate the cystic duct. Care must be taken not to close the ductotomy too close to the CBD and make sure complete closure of the duct is obtained. In some situations the ductotomy should be sutured using a single suture of fine absorbable suture or ligated with a loop in the situation of an enlarged duct or a suspected CBD retained stone when a postoperative ERCP is planned. After cholangiography, the laparoscopic cholecystectomy can then be completed in normal fashion. As with many laparoscopic procedures, the experience of the surgeon and their team will predict the ease at which advanced procedures will be performed. If cholangiogram indicates CBD stones, LCBDE should be undertaken, the steps of which will be discussed later in this chapter.

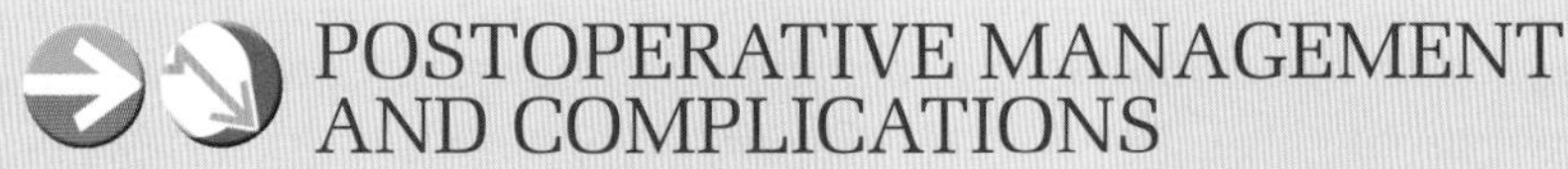

## POSTOPERATIVE MANAGEMENT AND COMPLICATIONS

Laparoscopic management of gallbladder disease has changed the postoperative care of cholecystectomy patients. An open cholecystectomy, which used to require a 2- to 4-day

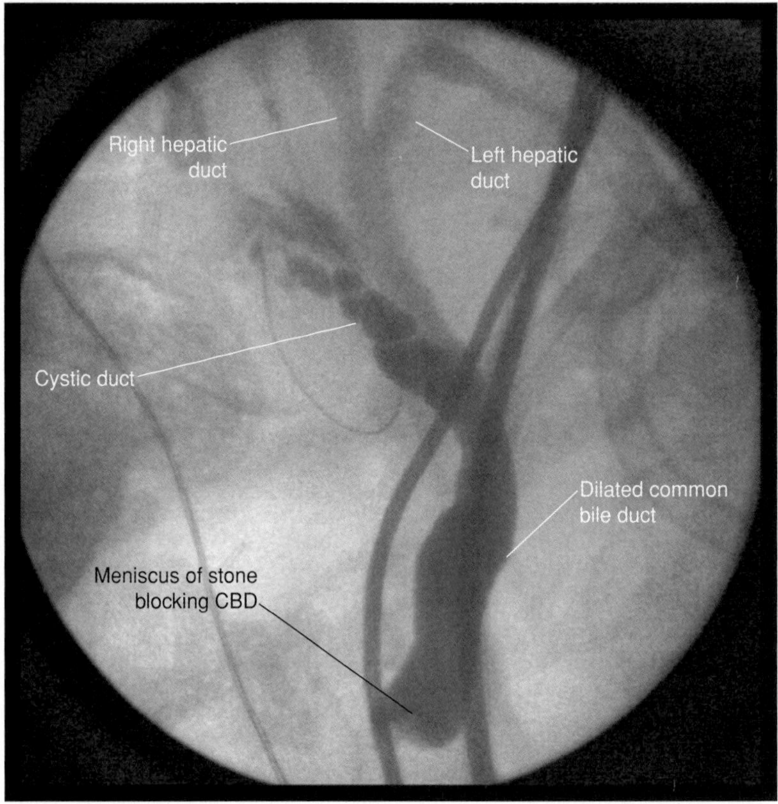


**Figure 13.6** An abnormal cholangiogram showing a dilated common bile duct. The meniscus formed by the top of the stone can be seen at the bottom of the picture.

hospitalization is now performed laparoscopically, typically as an outpatient procedure. Up to 90% of laparoscopic cholecystectomies performed as outpatient procedures do go home on the operative day. Most patients do quite well and return to taking a normal diet and resume normal activity quickly. If they experience excessive postoperative pain or other symptoms, investigative studies should be performed to evaluate for severe postoperative complications. There are several warning signs of complications that the surgeon must be aware of including persistent RUQ pain, jaundice, or persistent nausea and vomiting.

Bile duct injury rates have fallen since the general acceptance of laparoscopic cholecystectomy, and surgeon facility with this procedure has risen. Current rates of bile duct injury range from 0.3% to 1.0%. Up to half of these injuries are not identified at the time of initial operation. The patient returns with complaints of RUQ pain. Liver function tests are usually abnormal, with an elevation in total bilirubin being the most common abnormality. The most common site of injury is to the CBD, just below the insertion of the cystic duct. ERCP is the method of choice for delineating the extent of injury to the common duct. If injury is present, most will require operative reconstruction.

Bile duct leak, either from misplaced or dislodged clips or aberrant anatomy, can present with similar symptoms to a bile duct injury, and carries the same rate of occurrence from 0.2% to 2%. The collections associated with a bile leak may be sterile or infected; in which cases the patient may present with sepsis. CT scan is the preferred method of imaging for suspected bile collections after cholecystectomy. The current treatment for biloma after laparoscopic cholecystectomy is biloma drainage, usually via CT guided drain, and then ERCP with stent placement. The stent allows a path of least resistance for the bile to flow into the small bowel. Drain removal is based on clinical improvement of the patient and quantitative output of the drain. Hematoma in the liver bed after laparoscopic cholecystectomy should be imaged the same way, and drain placement undertaken if the hematoma is sizable or if infection is suspected.

| TABLE 13.2 Equipment Needed for Laparoscopic Transcystic Common Bile Duct Exploration |
|---|
| 14 gauge angiocatheter |
| Flexible J type hydrophilic guide wire |
| Balloon angioplasty catheter |
| Stone retrieval basket catheter |
| Cystic duct dilator with external sheath for choledochoscope |
| Fogarty catheters |

# Laparoscopic Common Bile Duct Exploration

There are two methods for LCBDE. Transcystic CBD exploration is the most common performed, and is the simplest. Laparoscopic choledochotomy is the second technique and is suited for patients with dilated CBDs and for surgeons with advanced laparoscopic skills. Both require specialized equipment that is not commonly used in most operating rooms. It is important that the surgeon inform the OR staff as soon as they have decided to perform CBD exploration so this equipment can be gathered to reduce idle time in the OR. Keeping a dedicated box with the necessary equipment in the OR will facilitate this process. The equipment needed is listed in Table 13.2.

Transcystic CBD exploration begins with clear dissection of the cystic duct, and with confirmation by obtaining a critical view. Once this is accomplished, a clip is applied to the gallbladder side of the cystic duct, and a ductotomy is made. IOC can be performed at this time to confirm position of the CBD stone. On the basis of the anatomic size and location a variety of different techniques can be used to clear the bile duct. Initial attempts with forceful flushing of the bile ducts with administration of glucagon should be utilized, especially in the settings of non obstructive small stones. Fogarty type balloon catheters can be placed distally to the stones and gentle retraction used to retrieve the stones back into the cystic duct.

Guide wires can be placed into the cystic duct, which can be mechanically dilated if needed with small dilating balloons designed for biliary dilation or short angioplasty balloons. Fluoroscopy should be used to confirm correct guide wire and balloon placement during this portion of the procedure. With dilation complete, the next portion of the procedure can be completed either with fluoroscopic guidance or using a choledochoscope. If fluoroscopy is used alone, then a wire basket or biliary balloon catheters can be used for stone extraction. If a choledochoscope is used, direct visualization of the stone is possible. A wire basket can then be used to extract stones under direct visualization, or they can be forced into the small bowel through the sphincter or Oddi if possible. Balloon dilation of the ampulla is acceptable in attempts to get the stones to pass distally if proximal retrieval is deemed to be unlikely. If the surgeon has difficulty passing the choledochoscope into the cystic duct, disposable peel away sheaths are available that accommodate the scope, and can dilate the cystic duct to the correct size. Following removal of CBD stones, completion cholangiogram should be performed to confirm patency of the duct. Drainage of the biliary system or the operative site is usually not necessary.

Laparoscopic Choledochotomy is another method of exploring the CBD. Once the cystic duct has been identified, it is followed down to the common duct, which is cleared for 2 cm on the anterior surface. Once sufficient visualization of the CBD is obtained, a longitudinal incision is made in the CBD (Fig. 13.7). This incision needs to be as large as the largest calculi visualized in the CBD during IOC. Once access to the CBD is obtained, either the fluoroscopic basket retrieval, or choledochoscope assisted stone extraction can be performed as above (Fig. 13.8). Once stone extraction is complete, a T tube is placed for completion cholangiogram. The T tube must be sutured in using absorbable suture. Advanced laparoscopic skills are helpful for this portion of the

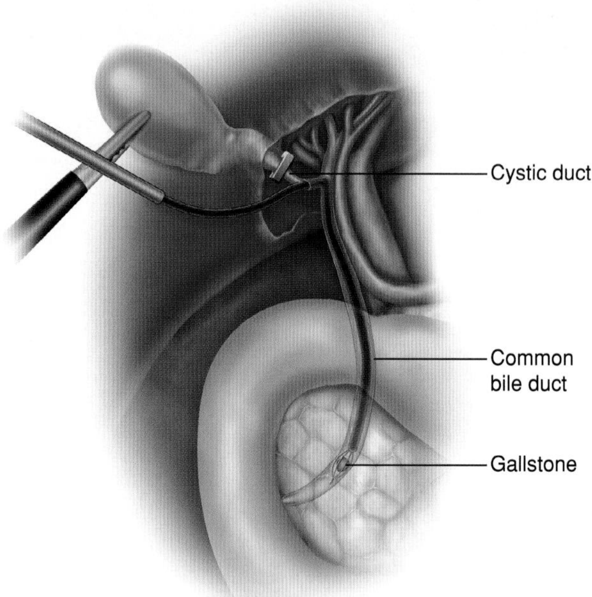


**Figure 13.7** The anatomy during a transcystic common bile duct exploration. The dilator is first placed into the cystic duct to enlarge it, the choledochoscope is introduced into the cystic duct, and the dilator can be drawn back.

procedure. Once the T tube is secured, the gallbladder is removed from the gallbladder fossa in a standard fashion. Drainage of the operative site with a closed suction system is recommended.

LCBDE is a viable option for surgeons to treat choledocholithiasis in one setting. This negates the need for the patient to undergo ERCP, which carries with it its own morbidities. ERCP itself carries a 15% failure rate to cannulate the CBD, even in the best of hands. With proper equipment and OR staff training, these procedures can be performed efficiently and safely with good outcomes. If CBD stones are encountered during laparoscopic cholecystectomy, attempt at their removal should be performed using one of the above techniques.

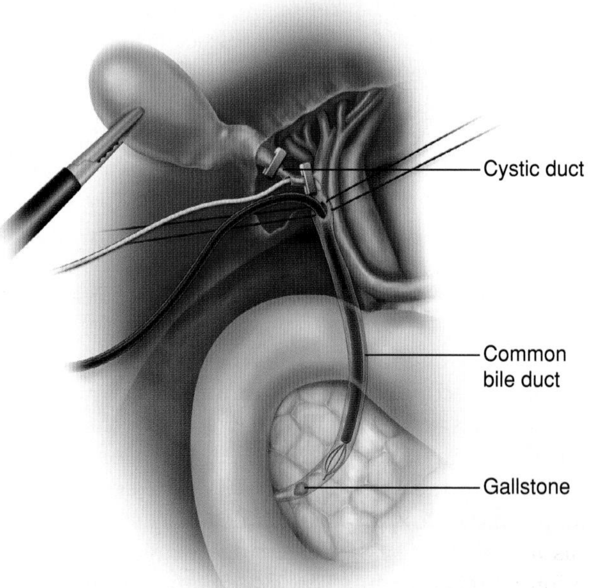


**Figure 13.8** The anatomy during a trans-common duct exploration. The choledochoscope is introduced directly through a ductotomy made vertically in the common bile duct. Stay sutures can be used to hold the common duct open if needed.

## RESULTS

Common duct exploration can be accomplished laparoscopically with excellent outcomes. Multiple studies show success rates ranging from 83% to 96% (Grubnik). For many institutions, laparoscopic extraction of common duct stones has become first line therapy. This requires only one anesthetic for the patient and can reduce hospital stays and morbidity in this patient population (Hanif). Some preoperative factors that are associated with poor outcomes for laparoscopic common duct exploration are:

1. Stones >6 mm
2. Increased patient age
3. Increased serum bilirubin (Noble)

The use of T tubes for common duct exploration has also been studied, with lower rates of short-term biliary complications being seen in the primary closure group versusthe T tube group (Guruysamy). This however did not study for stricture rates over the long term. The treatment of choledocholithiasis through one step laparoscopic cholecystectomy and common duct exploration has become a good choice for patients with this disease.

## Recommended References and Readings


Grubnik VV, Tkachenko AI, Ilyashenko VV. Laparosocpic common bile duct exploration versus open surgery: comparative prospective randomized trial. *Surg Endosc.* 2012 Feb 21. [Epub ahead of print].

Guruysamy KS. Primary closure versus T-tube drainage after open common bile duct exploration. The Cochrane Library Jan 2009. http://www.ncbi.nlm.nih.gov/pubmed/17253566

Hanif F, Ahmed Z, Samie MA, et al. Laparosocpic trancystic bile duct exploration: the treatment of first choice for common bile duct stones. *Surg Endosc.* 2010;24(7):1552–1556.

Noble H, Whitley E, Norton S, et al. A study of preoperative factors associated with a poor outcome following laparoscopic bile duct exploration. *Surg Endosc.* 2011;25(1):130–139.

# 14 Open Cholecystectomy With Choledochotomy and Common Bile Duct Exploration

**Mark P. Callery and Lygia Stewart**

## Open Cholecystectomy

### Indications/Contraindications

In the last 20 years, the clinical indications for cholecystectomy have not changed, but the operative approach has. Biliary colic, acute/chronic cholecystitis, gallstone pancreatitis, and cholangitis, in that order, remain the most common indications. Another important entity is biliary dyskinesia, as diagnosed by HIDA scan. Most agree a gallbladder ejection fraction below 40% supports the diagnosis, especially when pain occurs during cholecystokinin injection. There are however some patients where surgical treatment of asymptomatic gallstones is indicated. These include patients with diabetes mellitus, transplant patients, patients with chronic liver disease, patients undergoing bariatric operations, patients undergoing other gastrointestinal operations, patients with sickle cell anemia or other chronic hemolytic anemia, and patients with a potentially increased risk of gallbladder carcinoma.

Laparoscopic cholecystectomy is our preferred method of removing the gallbladder regardless of the indication. Open cholecystectomy can be performed in conjunction with another open procedure or become the fall-back option particularly in the following scenarios:

- Patients who may not tolerate the physiologic changes associated with the pneumoperitoneum (COPD, CHF) Open cholecystectomy may be lower risk
- Patients with cirrhosis and portal hypertension (relative contraindications)
- Third trimester of pregnancy
- Type II Mirizzi Syndrome (Cholecystobiliary fistula)
- Gallbladder cancer (suspicion or confirmed)

Purulent or gangrenous cholecystitis or previous upper abdominal procedures are no longer absolute indications for an open approach. Surgeons must carefully weigh the feasibility and safety relative to disease severity. Acute cholecystitis in this subset of patients can be effectively managed with percutaneous cholecystostomy as a less invasive but effective alternative. In many cases, elective laparoscopic cholecystectomy can be performed once the severe illness subsides, and the patient is physiologically improved. Recurrent biliary symptoms occur in 9% to 33% of patients who do not have a subsequent cholecystectomy. In some, operation can be entirely avoided.

## Converting to Open Cholecystectomy

Laparoscopic cholecystectomy is not always possible or safe in some patients. Conversion to open cholecystectomy becomes necessary. Biliary injuries are more likely to occur during difficult laparoscopic cholecystectomies, no different than with open operations. When laparoscopic cholecystectomy is performed for acute cholecystitis, biliary injuries occur three times more often than during elective laparoscopic cases, and twice as often compared to open cholecystectomy for acute cholecystitis.

Is conversion as easy as it seems? Perhaps for some, but certainly not all. The reality is that open cholecystectomy has been far less frequently performed over these past 20 years. Trainees during this period presumably received valid instruction and proctoring for laparoscopic cholecystectomy, but rarely for open cases. Established surgeons needed to command the laparoscopic operation to compete, all the while potentially diluting their comfort with the open variant. Finally, there is the pressure and patient expectation for rapid recovery. Two very different operations lead to two scenarios which, though not proven, could subtly account in part for static biliary injury rates. Because of inexperience, the surgeon ignores or resists the sensible default option to convert, does not and incurs injury. In other instances, the surgeon overextends laparoscopic experience when disease severity warrants conversion, and incurs injury. *Is open cholecystectomy becoming a specialty operation?* No. The anatomical considerations of cholecystectomy are constant regardless of open or laparoscopic approach, and a talented surgeon has these to abide by for safety.

## Technical Principles of Open Cholecystectomy

### Preoperative Planning and Positioning

During informed consent, every patient should understand that conversion from laparoscopic to open cholecystectomy may occur. Patients are positioned supine with their right arm tucked. If you anticipate an open procedure, alert the anesthesia team, request the scrub team to have open case instruments available if not open, and make your trocar stab incisions deliberately along a predrawn right subcostal incision line. Unless you need to control bleeding, enter the RUQ deliberately and not stressed by your decision to convert. Make sure everyone is ready for what lay ahead, and clear that it will not be much if at all easier.

### Technique and Pertinent Anatomy

- Some favor a right subcostal incision with careful entry across the fascia below the ribs (1 to 2 cm) to insure durable closure. Some prefer an upper midline incision.
- Whatever your choice of retractor, be certain the right ribs can be elevated, and deep partitioning of the RUQ can be achieved with packs and retractors. The liver can be brought down with packs above its right lobe. Segment IV can be elevated to reveal the porta hepatis. The hepatic flexure of the colon can be partitioned inferiorly. The stomach can be retracted medially. Unless you need explore the common bile duct (CBD), you can forego kocherizing the duodenum.

  Now exposed, how should you tackle the gallbladder? Assuming you will, you may decompress it via a trocar and suction.
- A Kelly clamp can be placed on the fundus for lateral/up retraction. Another Kelly is carefully placed lower on the infundibulum for lateral/down retraction to create an angle between the cystic duct and CBD (Fig. 14.1).

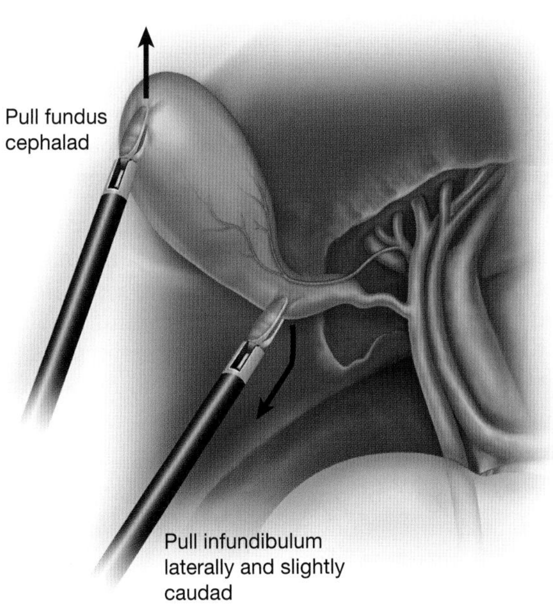


Figure 14.1 Cholecystectomy Retraction to open up the Triangle of Calot.

- An antegrade/top-down or retrograde/infundibulum-up technique is surgeon choice, but often determined by the anatomy and disease conditions.
- There must be positive identification of the cystic duct and artery as they join the gallbladder infundibulum before they can be divided.
- From the technique standpoint, how is this achieved? As with laparoscopic cholecystectomy, some advocate intraoperative cholangiography (IOC), the infundibular technique, and the critical view technique. We recommend the *critical view technique* of Strasberg. It is dictated by porta hepatis/gallbladder anatomy, and not access technique of the operation. It fully applies to open cholecystectomy.
- *Critical View Technique*—consists of tentative identification of the cystic structures by dissection in the anterior and posterior aspects of Calot's triangle, followed by dissection of the gallbladder well off the liver bed. The surgeon achieves conclusive identification of the cystic structures as the only two structures entering the gallbladder, eliminating the possibility of misidentification (Fig. 14.2).
- It is not necessary or recommended to see the CBD. "Tenting injury" of the CBD in fact can occur especially if there is a parallel junction of the cystic duct with the CBD.

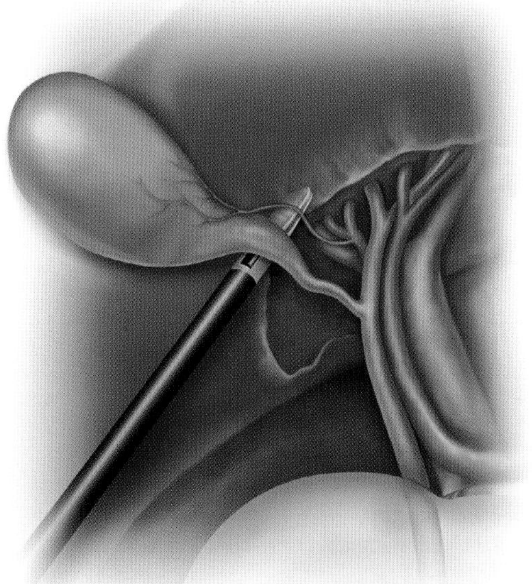

Figure 14.2 The critical view anatomy for cholecystectomy.

Some argue that this critical view technique requires more dissection, and so the opportunity for injury still exists. Once the critical view is attained, however, the cystic structures can be occluded and divided, as they have been positively identified.
- Failure to achieve this critical view warrants cholangiography to define ductal anatomy.
- Surgeons should indicate in dictated operative notes for both open and laparoscopic cholecystectomy precisely how they identified the cystic structures for division.

Advocates of routine cholangiography at open cholecystectomy argue that they identify unsuspected CBD calculi and clarify biliary anatomy. Opponents point out that routine cholangiography leads to unnecessary common bile duct explorations (CBDEs) because of false-positive results and only adds time and cost to the procedure. Cholangiography can also cause direct injury to the bile duct or surrounding structures unless performed properly. There are no large prospective randomized trials that answer the question definitively, so most practicing surgeons perform IOC selectively.

- After an arduous dissection in Calot's triangle, a surgeon may rush the gallbladder removal from the liver, but beware. Avoidance of ductal injury in the liver bed depends upon staying in the correct plane of dissection, and patience combined with meticulous technique and experience will ensure safety.
- In some cases of acute cholecystitis, the gallbladder "shells out" relatively easily from its edematous intrahepatic bed. In other cases, and especially in chronic cholecystitis, the dissection of the gallbladder out of the liver bed can be tedious, frustrating, and quite bloody. Hemostasis can take some time, and many tricks (argon beam, cautery, packing, hemostatics) to achieve, but one must do so. Subtotal cholecystectomy (leaving the hepatic side gallbladder wall) is always a valid option (Fig. 14.3).
- We use postoperative drains selectively but liberally. Conclude by cleaning up the RUQ, re-assuring hemostasis, and closing the incision and skin.
- We use perioperative antibiotic prophylaxis for open, but not laparoscopic, cholecystectomy. Any NG Tubes are removed.
- When dictating the operative note, specify the circumstances of conversion to open cholecystectomy, stressing safety and surgical judgment.

#### Postoperative Management

Typically, recovery from open cholecystectomy is more rapid than other open abdominal procedures. Awareness of complications is paramount, but with none, limited size

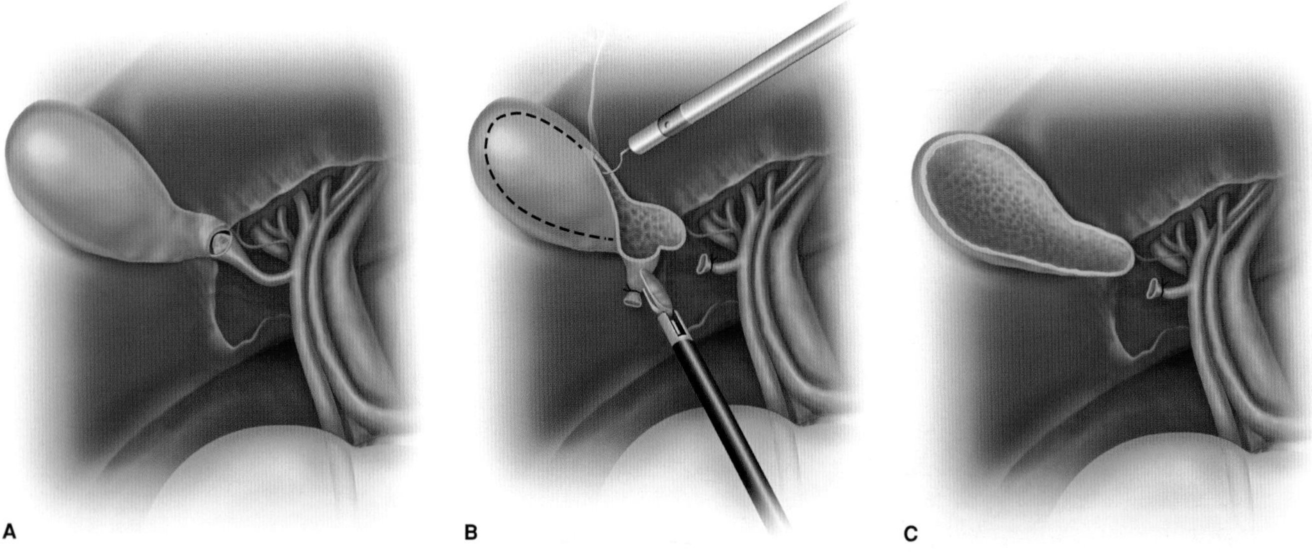


Figure 14.3 **A:** Diseased gallbladder is opened and stones removed. **B:** Gallbladder wall is removed with electrocautery. Common wall to liver is left in place, and its mucosa is cauterized. **C:** Cystic duct is identified from within gallbladder infundibulum and oversewn closed.

incisions heal well, diets can be advanced within 1 to 2 days, and discharge by 3 to 4 days. Full activity is resumed gradually over ensuing weeks, with restricted weight lifting for 6 weeks.

### Complications

Hemorrhage, intra-abdominal abscess and the full-spectrum of bile duct injuries are the most significant postoperative complications of open cholecystectomy. Other less frequent complications include retained bile duct stones, bowel obstruction, hepatic dysfunction, pancreatitis, gastrointestinal bleeding, and the need for reintervention (<1% of patients).

Sources of intraoperative bleeding include the liver bed, hepatic artery and its branches, a replaced right hepatic artery (which courses to the right of the CBD), and the portal vein as well. Most hemorrhage sources are controlled intraoperatively. Rarely postoperative bleeding may result in a self-contained subhepatic hematoma or serious hemoperitoneum with shock.

Injuries to the CBD are the most morbid complication associated with cholecystectomy. Biliary injury during any type of cholecystectomy can result in long-term morbidity, can be fatal, increases costs, and often results in litigation. No discussion of cholecystectomy is complete without considering the technical maneuvers that are key to a safe operation. First, the surgeon must consider the risk factors for injury: improper equipment, improper technique, disease severity, and variable anatomy. Experience alone helps but does not prevent biliary or vascular injury. Avoiding misidentification injuries of the cystic structures is the most important factor in preventing biliary injury.

Surgical site infections, both deep and superficial, will occur with open cholecystectomy. A surgeon should think ahead and obtain bile cultures at operation, as resistant organisms are not uncommon. This helps guide antibiotic therapy. Deep perihepatic abscesses can usually be managed by percutaneous drain placement. Subcutaneous infections can be managed by wound opening and drainage. Whether at a midline or right subcostal incision location, wound infections will increase morbidity significantly, and will certainly drive incisional hernia rates higher. Subcostal incisional hernias can be especially difficult to correct, especially in the obese, elderly and infirmed.

# Open Common Bile Duct Exploration

## Indications/Contraindications and Preoperative Planning

The 1974 introduction of endoscopic retrograde cholangiopancreatography (ERCP) with endoscopic sphincterotomy changed the treatment of CBD stones. Today, most clinicians request ERCP and stone clearance in cases with preoperative evidence of CBD stones. Some surgeons will leave CBD stones discovered intraoperatively for postoperative ERCP clearance. Most clinical data indicate these strategies are safe. In fact, they now prevail almost to the point of many overlooking the inherent short-term and long-term complications of ERCP with endoscopic sphincterotomy. One undeniable casualty for surgeons has been inadequate exposure to and training of open CBD exploration.

Open and laparoscopic IOC can successfully be completed in most patients by most surgeons. IOC can be performed through the direct insertion of contrast medium into the gallbladder or more often by intubating the cystic duct. Plain radiographs have largely been replaced by digital fluoroscopic imaging. IOC is common, and most surgeons receive sufficient training to perform it. When IOC reveals CBD stones, they can readily be removed during cholecystectomy or through postoperative ERCP.

Before the spread of LC, open bile duct surgery was clearly superior to ERCP regarding the bile duct stone clearance and was associated with many fewer procedures. However open choledochotomy to allow cholangioscopy, flushing, forcep and balloon clearance and T-tube placement is less commonly performed or taught today. Instead, laparoscopic common bile duct exploration (LCBDE) has evolved as an efficient, well accepted and broadly utilized technique. It has been shown to be as efficient as preoperative or postoperative ERCP in terms of stone clearance, morbidity and mortality, short hospital stay and is thus recommended for surgeons with appropriate skills.

There are still certain clinical scenarios where open bile duct exploration is indicated, however, there are several issues that need to be considered before proceeding with CBDE with choledochotomy. In many cases, open CBDE using a choledochotomy is *not* the correct choice for the removal of CBD stones, even in patients undergoing an open cholecystectomy or biliary procedure. Depending on the patient characteristics, an open trans-cystic CBDE, or a drainage procedure (transduodenal sphincteroplasty, end-to-side choledochoduodenostomy or other choledochoenterostomy) is the correct surgical choice rather than open CBDE utilizing a choledochotomy (see discussion below).

## Open Transcystic CBDE

Transcystic CBDE should be utilized as a first-line strategy in most cases including: *all cases* where CBD stones are thought to originate from the gallbladder, patients with a small (<6 mm) CBD (choledochotomy carries an increased risk of biliary stricture in this group), and cases with small and/or few CBD stones. Using a transcystic CBDE approach allows clearance of the CBD without the need for a choledochotomy. This decreases biliary complications and patient morbidity, and there are no considerations of a T-tube.

Use of transcystic CBDE also increases surgeon's experience with this approach. CBDE is currently an uncommon procedure for many surgeons. The open transcystic CBDE is easier to perform than the laparoscopic approach. This may well help a surgeon to learn best both open and laparoscopic CBDE anatomy.

Drainage procedures (transduodenal sphincteroplasty, end-to-side choledochoduodenostomy, other choledochoenterostomy, or ERCP)

In some cases open CBDE should be combined with a drainage procedure. The surgeon should consider whether any aspect of the patient's clinical picture warrants the addition of a drainage procedure. Possible indications for a drainage procedure include:

- Primary CBD stones
  - Recurrent primary CBD stones
  - Recurrent CBD stones following ERCP/sphincterotomy
  - Pigment stone caste of CBD or hepatic ducts
- Intrahepatic duct stones
- Caroli's disease
- Periampullary duodenal diverticulum (strong association with primary CBD stones)
- CBD size >13 mm
- Distal biliary stricture (nonmalignant)
- CBD stone impacted in ampulla
  - Intraoperative lithotripsy can be utilized to facilitate stone removal
  - Transduodenal sphincteroplasty can be utilized to remove the CBD stone
- Transduodenal sphincteroplasty is a good option for CBDE in cases with a nondilated CBD

## Open CBDE with Choledochotomy

Once the above considerations have been met, open CBDE may be indicated in a small subset of patients. The possible indications include:

- Open cholecystectomy procedure (planned or conversion from laparoscopic)
- Other open abdominal procedure in a patient with choledocholithiasis
- Unsuccessful CBD clearance using transcystic CBDE or preoperative ERCP
- Surgeon's preference for CBDE utilizing choledochotomy
- Lack of endoscopic expertise locally

There are several contraindications to open CBDE (utilizing choledochotomy). The most common are cases requiring another procedure (e.g., drainage procedure) or cases with a small or normal-sized CBD. Performance of CBDE utilizing a choledochotomy in patients with small CBD is associated with an increased risk of biliary stricture.

Transcystic CBDE or transduodenal sphincteroplasty should be utilized in these cases. A final contraindication to open CBDE with choledochotomy is surgeon inexperience, which is a genuine consideration in the current climate. The same issues discussed in choosing open versus laparoscopic cholecystectomy are accentuated when CBDE itself is considered. Today, many trainees complete residency without ever having performed an open CBDE. Their ability to succeed with laparoscopic CBDE is quite variable, as many train with a default dependence on ERCP.

In summary contraindications to open CBDE with choledochotomy include:

- Small or normal-sized (<6 mm) CBD
- Indications for drainage procedure (see above)
- Surgeon inexperience

## Technical Principles of Open CBDE

We recommend a technique for open CBDE that can be combined with CBD stone removal when a drainage procedure is planned or cases approached using an open transcystic CBDE.

- Perform a cholangiogram to verify need for CBDE, identify gallstone location, rule out distal biliary stricture
- Perform a complete Kocher maneuver
- Gently palpate the common duct to detect the location of any CBD stones (Fig. 14.4)
- Dissect out the CBD, removing areolar tissue anterior to the CBD
- Place two stay sutures into the CBD, inferior to the cystic duct take-off, using fine monofilament absorbable suture (PDS or Maxon)
- Putting gentle traction on the stay sutures—to elevate the anterior wall of the CBD—make a small longitudinal choledochotomy between the stay sutures, using an #11 blade; then enlarge the opening longitudinally using Potts scissors (Fig. 14.5)
- Gently milk any stones into the choledochotomy using the thumb and forefingers; do this superior and inferiorly to the choledochotomy, bring gallstones into the choledochotomy
- Place a small Red-Robinson catheter into the choledochotomy, pass it superiorly and inferiorly into the CBD, irrigating with saline. This will often irrigate floating stones through the choledochotomy (Fig. 14.6)

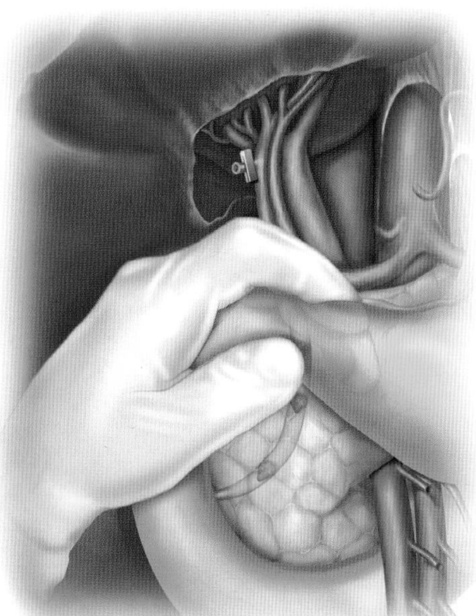

Figure 14.4 Palpation of the common duct to detect the location of any CBD stones.

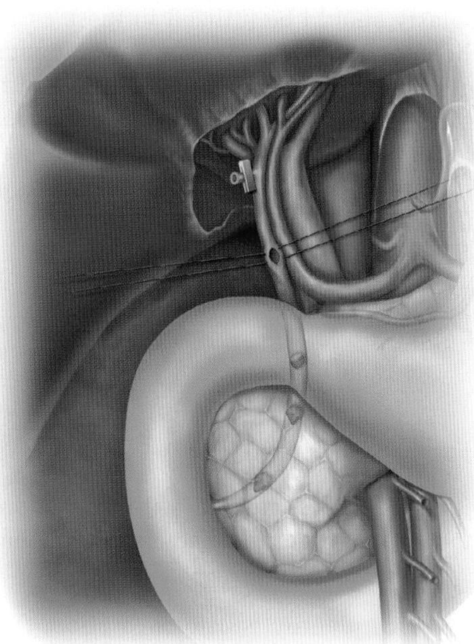

Figure 14.5 Creation of a small longitudinal choledochotomy and enlarging the opening.

- Pass a biliary fogarty catheter distal to any detected CBD stones, inflate it and gently pull back on the catheter, bringing the CBD stones into the choledochotomy; pass this inferiorly and superiorly as needed. This can be repeated as needed
- If the above maneuvers are unsuccessful in removing all the CBD stones, a Randall stone forcep or a pituitary scoop can be gently passed into the CBD to retrieve the stones (Fig. 14.7)
  - Remember that the CBD is not straight, it contours medially as it enters the pancreas and duodenum
  - Care has to be taken, during instrumentation of the CBD, not to create a false passage; the contours of the CBD need to be followed gently
  - It is crucial to hold these instruments gently in the hand so they can move with the contours of the CBD, never use force when inserting these instruments into the CBD. A light touch is crucial to prevent CBD injury or creation of a false passage
- Perform Choledochoscopy using a flexible choledochoscope (Fig. 14.8)

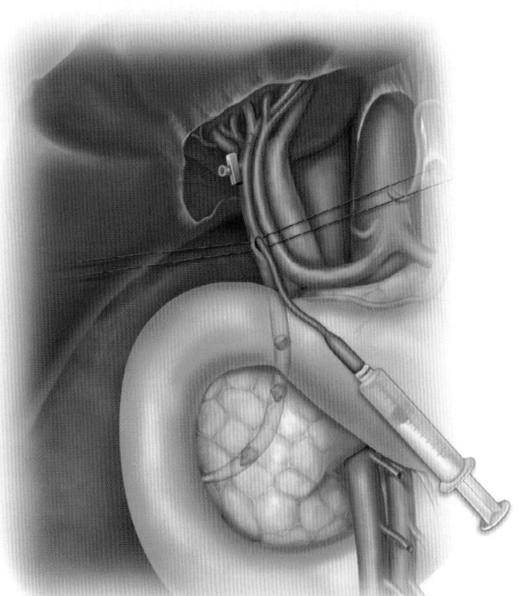

Figure 14.6 Irrigating the CBD with saline.

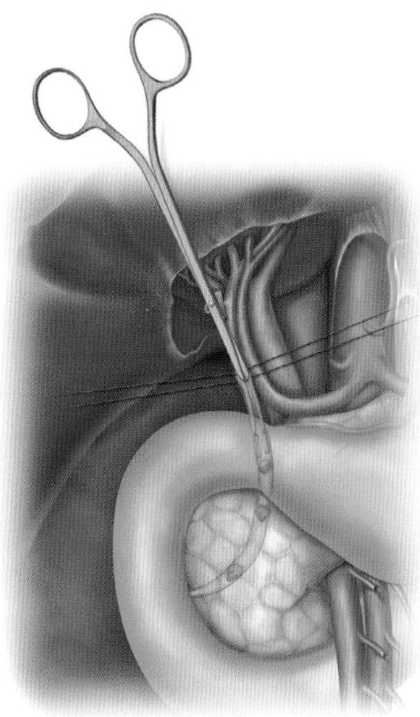

Figure 14.7 A Randall stone forcep or a pituitary scoop can be gently passed into the CBD to retrieve any remaining stones.

- This is crucial to ensure complete removal of all gallstones (Fig. 14.9)
- The choledochoscope should be passed superiorly into the hepatic duct, right, and left hepatic ducts; and inferiorly going through the ampulla into the duodenum and then retracted back through the distal CBD
- In patients with multiple CBD stones, a Dormier basket can be placed down the working port of the choledochoscope and individual CBD stones removed under direct vision. The Fogarty balloon can also be passed under choledochoscopy to facilitate stone removal
- Choledochoscopy should continue until the entire extrahepatic biliary tree is clearly seen to be free of gallstones

- The choledochotomy can be closed with insertion of a T-tube or it can be closed primarily without a T-tube; considerations regarding the risk of retained stones and

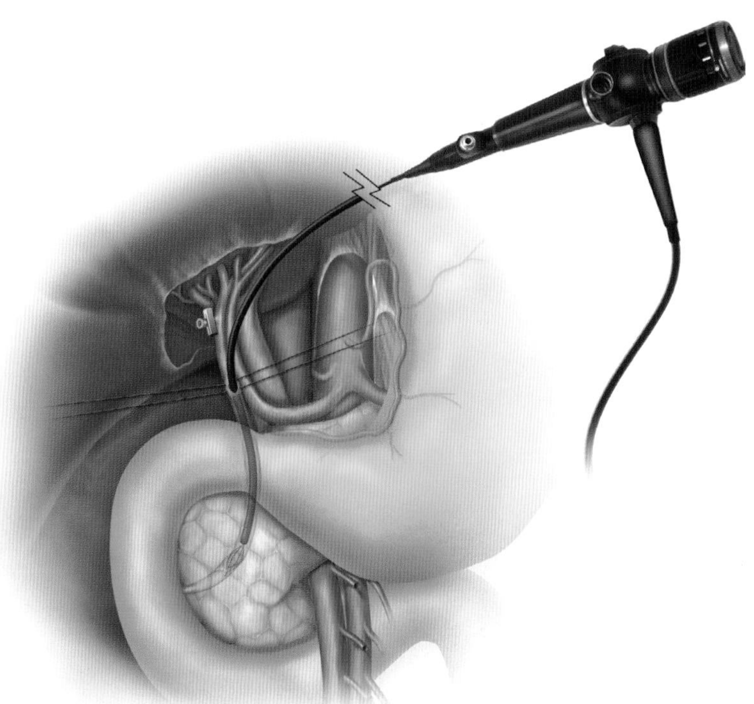

Figure 14.8 Choledochoscopy using a flexible choledochoscope.

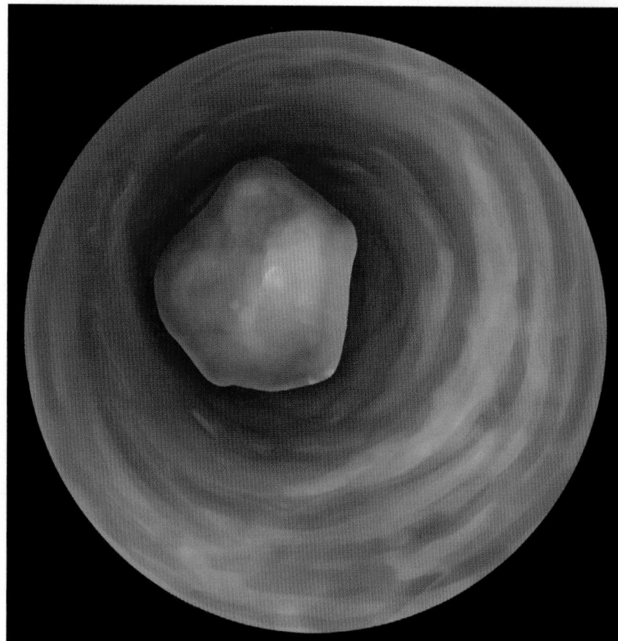

**Figure 14.9** Illustration of a typical endoscopic view of a CBD stone through a choledochoscope.

local endoscopic expertise should guide the choice. T-tube insertion is *not* needed to prevent biliary fistula or stricture. Numerous studies have demonstrated no differences in outcomes for primary closure of the CBD versus T-tube drainage after open CBD exploration.

- Choledochotomy closure without T-tube insertion (Fig. 14.10)
  - Use a fine monofilament absorbable suture (PDS or Maxon); choose the size based on the size of the CBD
  - For larger ducts the choledochotomy can be closed utilizing a running suture
  - For smaller ducts, place interrupted sutures in the choledochotomy; tie the sutures after all sutures have been placed
  - Place a closed suction drain near the choledochotomy and bring it out through a separate stab incision

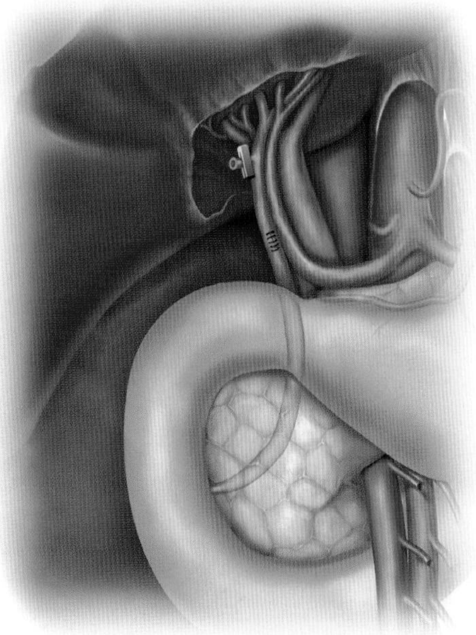

**Figure 14.10** Choledochotomy closure without T-tube insertion.

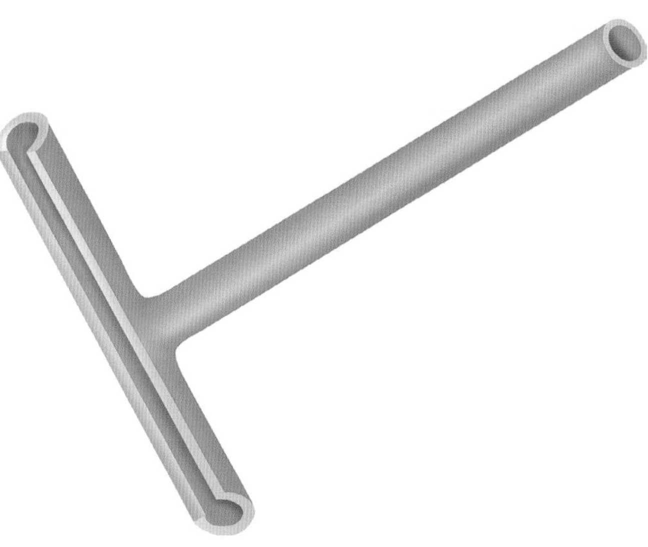

**Figure 14.11** Modification of the T-tube to facilitate insertion.

- Choledochotomy closure with T-tube insertion
  - Use a Whelan-Ross T-tube
- This T-tube has a stem that is 4 Fr larger than the cross bar
- The larger stem facilitates removal of any retained stones, while the smaller cross-bar fits better into the CBD
  - Use a Whelan-Ross T-tube that has a minimum of a 16 Fr stem, use a larger T-tube for larger ducts
  - Cut off half the circumference of the T-tube cross bar longitudinally—creating a channel—and bevel the ends of the T-tube as this facilitates insertion (Fig. 14.11)
  - Close the choledochotomy around the T-tube using a running stitch of fine monofilament absorbable suture (PDS or Maxon) to create a water-tight closure
  - Irrigate the T-tube with saline to ensure that it is water tight
  - Perform a T-tube cholangiogram
  - Bring the T-tube through a stab incision in the abdominal wall using the following parameters
- The T-tube path should be relatively straight
- Allow some slack on the T-tube so that when the patient stands the tube will not be pulled out with the movement of their abdominal wall
- The T-tube should be brought above a Kocher incision or in the upper abdomen in cases with a midline incision
  - Be certain that the T-tube is not positioned in a part of the abdomen that has a large pannus or an area that will move significantly when the patient changes position
- Secure the T-tube to the abdominal wall with two sutures (2-0 nylon) and then tape it as well in two areas using cloth tape with a mesentery. Once secured, pull gently on the T-tube to be certain that it is secure
  - Place and secure a closed suction drain near the choledochotomy and bring it out through a separate stab incision

## Postoperative Management

If no complications, open CBDE patients should recover as swiftly as their cholecystectomy counterparts, especially when safe primary closure of a choledochotomy (*see later*) or even intestinal drainage procedure are used. Today, T-tubes are still commonly placed after completion cholangiography confirms stone clearance. If so, leave T-tubes open to passive drainage bags until a day or two before planned discharge, then cap them without further in-hospital study. We instruct patients on how, why, and when to reopen the tube to passive drainage, and notify us. Typically, we see patients back in 2 to 3 weeks after a same-day out-patient cholangiogram, and if negative, simply slide the tube out, and bandage the site. The tube tract heals down and closes quickly.

If completion cholangiogram reveals retained stones, the T-tube is left open to passive drainage. Several weeks typically pass before out-patient techniques for stone retrieval (ERCP, mature T-tube tract and/or percutaneous transhepatic instrumentation) are begun.

### Complications

Complications following open CBDE, with choledochotomy, include: biliary fistula, dislodgment of the T-tube with biliary fistula, bile peritonitis, surgical site infection, abscess, retained gallstones, recurrent gallstones, sepsis, cardiorespiratory complications, and biliary stricture. Reported complication rates range from 3.4% to 46%; mortality rates range from 0% to 2%. A long-term study of CBDE reported that the number of CBDEs performed annually decreased from 47,000 to 7,700 per year. Correspondingly, the complication rates increased from 3.4% to 17.4% over the same period. Overall perioperative mortality decreased during this period. A recent meta-analysis using Cochran methodology reported significantly increased complications following CBDE utilizing a T-tube compared to those with primary biliary closure. Biliary complications, wound infections and residual stones were all significantly greater in cases utilizing a T-tube. So, if a choledochotomy is required during CBDE, the surgeon should preferentially close the choledochotomy primarily without using a T-tube unless patient characteristics or local expertise (ERCP expertise not available) dictate otherwise.

### Results

Open CBDE remains a safe therapeutic procedure historically achieving the highest success rate (>90%) among all available stone extraction modalities. Today with the integration of minimal invasive techniques both in and out of the operating room, open CBDE has been reserved for patients requiring an open cholecystectomy for other indications or for patients who have failed to achieve laparoscopic or endoscopic bile duct stone clearance.

Before the laparoscopic era, the one stage procedure for open cholecystectomy and CBDE was significantly superior in terms of morbidity, CBD clearance and number of procedures required than ERCP for CBD stones. Classic RCTs reported open CBDE morbidity ranging from 11% to 14% and mortality ranging from 0.6% to 1% with a percentage of retained stones estimated in 1% to 3%. However open choledochotomy, flushing, forcep, and balloon clearance and T-tube placement is rarely performed or taught today. An outcome analysis based on US national discharge data from 1993 to 2001 reported a significant increase in the morbidity rates for open CBDE (from 3.4% to 17.4%). Many believe that this reflects today's decline in both training and volume for Open CBDE.

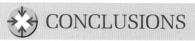

## CONCLUSIONS

Open cholecystectomy with or without open CBDE via choledochotomy reveals the finesse and technical ability of any surgeon. Once very common procedures, today they are notably infrequent owing to the superiority of laparoscopic approaches in most patients, and the dependence on ERCP for CBD stone management. When they are needed, a surgeon must be prepared. Predictably, the case will be complicated, difficult and unsettling. These commonplace procedures of yesterday have become real tests for today's general surgeon.

## Recommended References and Readings

Callery MP. Avoiding biliary injury during laparoscopic cholecystectomy: technical considerations. *Surg Endosc.* 2006;20(11):1654–1658.

Festi D, Reggiani MLB, Attili AF, et al. Natural history of gallstone disease: expectant management or active treatment? Results from a population-based cohort study. *J Gastroent Hepatol.* 2010;25:719–724.

Gurusamy KS, Samraj K. Early versus delayed laparoscopic cholecystectomy for acute cholecystitis. *Cochrane Database Syst Rev* 2006;4:CD005440.

Ishizaki Y, Miwa K, Yoshimoto J, et al. Conversion of elective laparoscopic to open cholecystectomy between 1993 and 2004. *Br J Surg.* 2006;93(8):987–991

Jenkins PJ, Paterson HM, Parks RW, et al. Open Cholecystectomy in the Laparoscopic Era. *Br J Surg.* 2007;94(11):1382–1385.

Keus F, de Jong JAF, Gooszen HG, et al. Laparoscopic versus open cholecystectomy for patients with symptomatic cholecystolithiasis. *Cochrane Database Syst Rev.* 2006;(Issue 4): CD006231. DOI: 10.1002/14651858.CD006231.

Khan MH, Howard TJ, Fogel EL, et al. Frequency of biliary complications after laparoscopic cholecystectomy detected by ERCP: experience at a large tertiary referral center. *Gastrointest Endosc.* 2007;65:247–252.

Livingston EH, Rege RV. technical complications are rising as common duct exploration is becoming rare. *J Am Coll Surg.* 2005;201:426–433.

Pitt HA. Role of open choledochotomy in the treatment of choledocholithiasis. *Am J Surg.* 1993;165:483–486.

Ratych RE, Sitzmann JV, Lillemoe KD, et al. Transduodenal exploration of the common bile duct in patients with nondilated ducts. *Surg Gynecol Obstet.* 1991;173(1):49–53.

Schulman CI, Levi J, Sleeman D, et al. Are we training our residents to perform open gallbladder and common bile duct operations? *J Surg Res.* 2007;142(2):246–249.

Shojaiefard A, Esmaeilzadeh M, Ghafouri A, et al. Various techniques for the surgical treatment of common bile duct stones: a meta review. *Gastroenterol Res Pract.* 2009;2009:840208.

Stewart L, Hunter JG, Wetter A, et al. Operative reports: form and function. *Arch Surg.* 2010;145(9):865–871.

Way LW, Stewart L, Gantert W, et al. Causes and prevention of laparoscopic bile duct injuries: an analysis of 252 cases from a human factors and cognitive psychology perspective. *Ann Surg.* 2003;237(4):460–469.

Wolf AS, Nijsse BA, Sokal SM, et al. Surgical outcomes of open cholecystectomy in the laparoscopic era. *Am J Surg.* 2009;197(6):781–784.

Zhu QD, Tao CL, Zhou MT, et al. Primary closure versus T-tube drainage after common bile duct exploration for choledocholithiasis. *Langenbecks Arch Surg.* 2011;396:53–62.

# 15 Sphincteroplasty of Biliary and Pancreatic Ducts

**Thomas J. Howard**

##  INDICATIONS/CONTRAINDICATIONS

Transduodenal sphincteroplasty (TS) for abnormalities of the biliary and pancreatic duct sphincters is an operation that has generated a great deal of study and interest by both gastrointestinal endoscopists and surgeons. The reason for this attraction is that if true, these syndromes validate a fundamental pathophysiologic concept related to restrictions of flow in a secretory organ. For the pancreas, this involves either a developmental malformation resulting in an inadequately sized sphincter (pancreas divisum), or an acquired sphincter stenosis due to passage of gallstones and/or inflammation [sphincter of Oddi dysfunction (SOD)] both leading to pancreatic-type pain or recurrent episodes of acute pancreatitis. For the liver, the acquired sphincter stenosis, presumably again from passage of gallstones and debris, results in biliary-type pain and liver function test elevations. In both of these situations, the secretory organ somehow ascertains this flow restriction and responds with inflammation (pancreatitis, hepatitis) and symptoms experienced in the organism as pain. Sphincter enlargement of the pancreatic or biliary orifice, or both, either through endoscopic sphincterotomy (ES) or transduodenal sphincteroplasty (TS) should alleviate this flow restriction and its attendant organ response leading to pain relief. Despite this appealing theory, the level of scientific evidence to support either TS or ES for abnormalities of the biliopancreatic sphincters remains meager at best (Level C, Level II-3), certainly not sufficient to establish a causal relationship between stenosis and symptoms. Unfortunately, both medical and surgical data on this topic consist almost exclusively of small case series containing fundamental methodologic flaws including referral bias, lack of blinding, absence of a control group, and short clinical follow-up. As there are no animal models of spontaneously occurring sphincter dysfunction to investigate, all data is derived from humans, which to date, has been carried out without a proper placebo-controlled population. Despite these limitations, there still exists a substantial body of literature reporting decreasing pain scores, reduction in episodes of acute pancreatitis, and reduction in recurrent hospitalizations, in approximately three-quarters of selected patients treated by either

ES or TS, a level of success that cannot be easily be ignored. Perhaps the key word in the above sentence is "selected" as it is clear that there are substantial overlap between symptoms of patients with hypertensive pancreatic or biliary sphincters and those with chronic pancreatitis, alcohol or narcotic addiction, or visceral hypersensitivity syndromes.

Historically, early operative series of TS reported encouraging results in effective symptom control with low associated morbidity and mortality rates. Advances in endoscopic imaging and instrumentation promoted the development of ES, a minimally invasive technique that has supplanted operative TS in the majority of patients with pancreatic or biliary sphincter abnormalities. The ability to manometrically measure biliary and pancreatic duct sphincter pressures endoscopically has brought about the convergence of both diagnosis and treatment within one procedure such that most patients with SOD or pancreas divisum are now treated by ES at the time of their initial diagnosis. This synchronous diagnostic-therapeutic endeavor, while efficient, discourages collaboration and randomization possibly contributing to the slow progress in this field. As another consequence of this efficiency, only a small percentage of patients are now considered candidates for operative TS: Those who have failed one or more prior ESs or those with anatomic abnormalities limiting the endoscopic access to their major or minor papilla (post-bariatric or gastric surgery). From a surgeon's perspective, this results in the paradox that while the total number of patients having TS has declined, the complexity level of each operation (reoperative field, prior gastric surgery, strictured ES) has increased. In this situation, both experience and sound clinical judgment are paramount in achieving optimal therapeutic outcomes. As a byproduct of this endoscopic selection bias and declining referral patterns, the surgical literature over the last decade has focused on improving the indications and patient selection criteria for TS in an effort to maximize long-term benefits. For the purpose of our discussion in this chapter, there are currently three solid indications for TS:

- Impacted gallstone unable to be extracted by endoscopic methods
- Sphincter of Oddi dysfunction
- Pancreas divisum with dominant dorsal duct anatomy

## Impacted Gallstone Unable to be Extracted by Endoscopic Methods

As touched on in the introduction, improved functionality of endoscopic retrograde cholangiopancreatography (ERCP) coupled with extracoporeal shock wave lithotripsy (ESWL) for stone fragmentation, has made an impacted gallstone at the ampulla of Vater a rare indication for TS.

## Sphincter of Oddi Dysfunction

SOD is defined as a benign, noncalculus obstructive disorder occurring at the level of the sphincter of Oddi which, depending on the dominant manifestation, can produce either biliary or pancreas predominant symptoms although significant abnormal manometric findings in both sphincters exist (Fig. 15.1). Encompassed by this nebulous definition is a wide variety of abnormalities running the gamut from mechanical fibrotic stricturing secondary to the passage of gallstones to dysmotility conditions caused by a defective neuronal or hormonal milieu. Pancreas or biliary-type pain syndromes, cholestasis, and recurrent episodes of acute pancreas without another etiology are all contained under this large umbrella of clinical manifestations which are believed to be due to a hypertensive sphincter segment which fails to relax normally under the influence of CCK, other gastrointestinal hormones, and cholinergic neural factors during a meal. This physiologic obstruction acts as a deterrent to the flow of bile and pancreatic juice into the intestine during a meal. A large number of indirect clinical tests have been evaluated (radionucleotide, ultrasonography, magnetic resonance imaging, morphine–neostigmine) in an effort to quantify this "functional obstruction" and identify patients

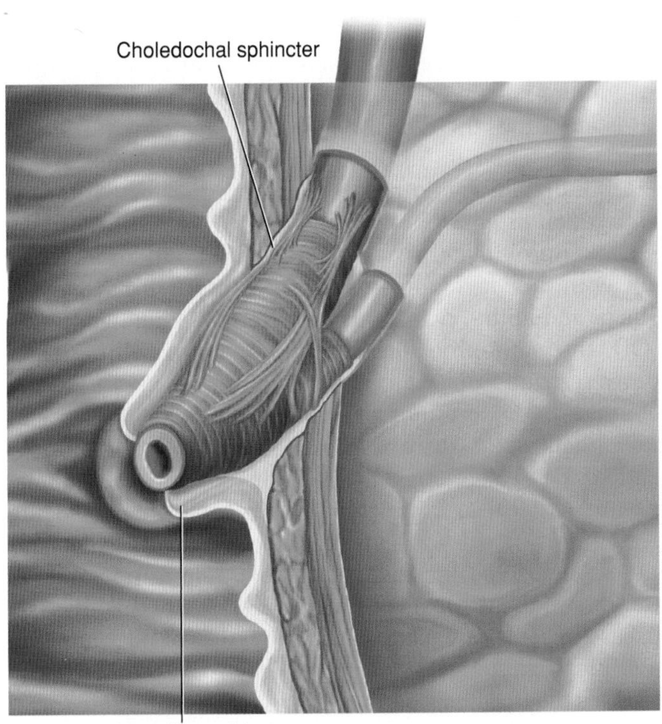


**Figure 15.1** Anatomic and functional zones of the sphincter of Oddi.

with this disease. Endoscopic sphincter of Oddi manometry (ESOM), which directly measures sphincter pressures in real time, remains the *only* objective measure to accurately predict beneficial outcomes from either ES or TS. Manometric studies of normal human subjects reveal a basal sphincter pressure of approximately 10 mm Hg over which are superimposed episodic contractions with a frequency of 2 to 6/minute and an amplitude of 50 to 140 mm Hg above duodenal pressure. The complexity of these recordings makes the interpretation of pathophysiologic derangements challenging due to multiple potential abnormalities including elevated basal sphincter pressure, lack of superimposed contractions, or absence of sphincter relaxation. Given our present level of understanding, the most objective information on which to base a decision for operation in patients with SOD is finding an *elevated basal sphincter pressure greater than 40 mm Hg*. Large clinical experience from the endoscopy groups in both Wisconsin and Indiana have facilitated the grouping of patients with either predominate biliary-type pain or pancreatic-type pain and their associated clinical and manometric findings into a classification system useful for predicting their response to ES (Table 15.1).

**TABLE 15.1 Modified Milwaukee Classification System with Criteria for Both Biliary and Pancreatic Sphincter of Oddi Dysfunction**

| Type | Biliary | Pancreatic |
|---|---|---|
| I | 1. Biliary-type pain (lasting 30 min occurring at least once per year)<br>2. Elevated AST/ALT on two occasions<br>3. Dilated CBD (>10 mm) | 1. Recurrent pancreatitis or pain suspected of pancreatic origin<br>2. Elevated serum amylase or lipase level on at least one occasion<br>3. Dilated pancreatic duct (>6 mm in the head or >5 mm in the body) |
| II | Biliary-type pain but only one additional criteria listed above | Pancreatic-type pain but only one additional criteria listed above |
| III | Biliary-type pain *only* | Pancreatic-type pain *only* |

## Pancreas Divisum

Pancreas divisum is an embryologic abnormality where the dorsal and ventral duct segments during their complex counter-clockwise rotation around the GI tract fail to fuse during embryogenesis. In this situation, the dorsal pancreatic duct which drains a large portion of pancreatic parenchyma (anterior head, body, and tail segments) drains into the duodenum through the minor pancreatic duct sphincter (duct of Santorini) (Fig. 15.2). This particular developmental abnormality is common based on autopsy studies, and is estimated to occur in approximately 8% of the general population. Interestingly, only a subset of patients with this developmental abnormality will have either episodes of recurrent pancreatitis or abdominal pain syndromes felt to be related to this altered anatomy. Similar to SOD, the pathophysiologic basis for these symptoms is presumed to be a relative outflow restriction/obstruction caused by pancreatic secretions traveling through a congenitally narrow minor pancreatic sphincter rather than the more patulous major pancreatic sphincter (duct of Wirsung). This relative outflow tract obstruction causes pancreatic ductal hypertension, which, in susceptible patients, produces acute recurrent pancreatitis (ARP) and pancreatic pain syndromes. Despite this appealing hypothesis, direct supporting evidence for this theory remains vague and indirect, implying that other as yet identified factors (i.e., genetic, environmental, or psychological) may play a crucial role in the ultimate clinical expression of this disease. Because of this variability in disease expression, accurate identification of patients who will benefit from TS remains a clinical challenge, bordering more on art than science.

ERCP is the reference standard for the diagnosis of pancreas divisum and other dorsal duct variants although recent improvements in image acquisition and resolution has allowed several noninvasive techniques such as: Endoscopic ultrasound (EUS), magnetic resonance cholangiopancreatography (MRCP) with secretin stimulation, and multi-detector row CT (MDCT) with post-processing reformations to approximate the accuracy of ERCP in making this diagnosis. In patients with PD, the ventral pancreatic duct is typically from 1 to 4 cm in length and is formed by finely tapered normal ducts servicing the anatomic distribution of the posterior pancreatic head and uncinate process (remnant ventral pancreatic bud). This ductal morphology appears normal up to the point of prompt duct termination, always found on the right side of the midline. When this anatomic relationship is recognized during ERCP, it is essential that cannulation of the minor papilla be pursued to demonstrate the presence of dominant dorsal duct anatomy and exclude the possible secondary causes of ductal obstruction such as tumor (*pseudo divisum*) or chronic pancreatitis (*false pancreas divisum*). EUS is a useful tool not only to identify this anatomy but also to evaluate the pancreatic parenchyma for small focal parenchymal abnormalities that could explain the ductal changes seen. It seems prudent in the contemporary evaluations of these patients to include both ductography (ERCP, EUS, MRCP) and a method of parenchymal evaluation (EUS, MRCP, CT) to fully characterize the disease process and discern whether or not operative intervention is appropriate.

In a patient with PD and recurrent pancreatitis or pancreatic pain syndromes, identification of a dominant dorsal duct system is a necessary but not sufficient finding to establish their candidacy for accessory papilla therapy. As previously mentioned, while 8% of the general population has PD, it is only in those patients with outflow tract obstruction due to accessory papillary stenosis where endoscopic or surgical sphincteroplasty has a high likelihood of success. The dorsal pancreatic duct in most patients with PD has a normal, nondilated appearance, making the demonstration of outflow tract obstruction demanding. Of those tests which have been studies, simple endoscopic assessment of accessory papilla size, degree of difficulty encountered during endoscopic cannulation (indirect assessment of patency), as well as direct manometric measurements of sphincter pressures have all proven *unreliable* in predicting the response of patients to sphincterotomy. Direct evidence of outflow obstruction, identified by duct imaging techniques utilizing either EUS or MRCP, both before and after an intravenous bolus of secretin to stimulate pancreatic secretions, has been advanced as a provocative test to identify patients with PD who will benefit from dorsal duct therapy. Stenosis of the minor papilla causing outflow obstruction is defined utilizing secretin-stimulated

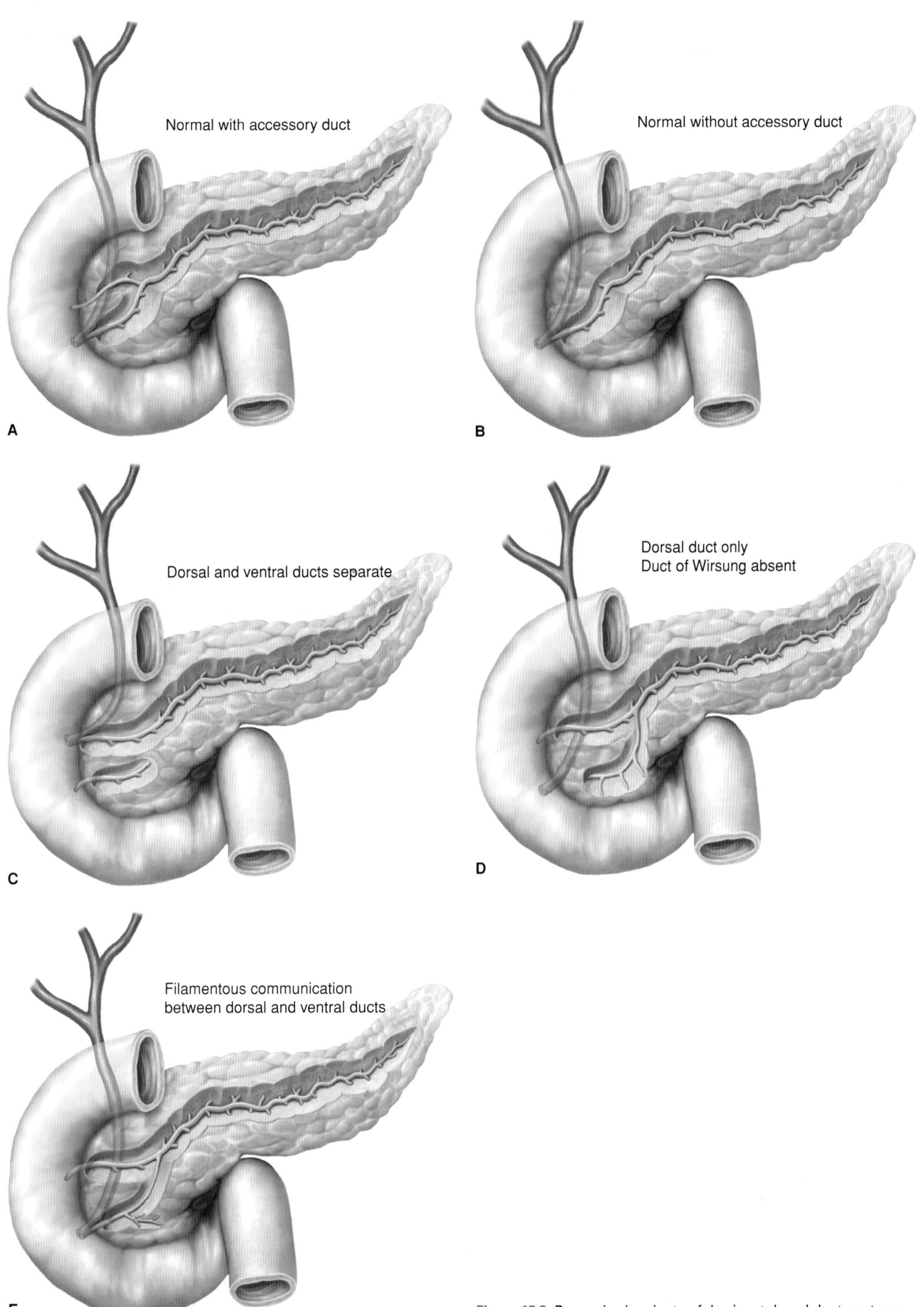


**Figure 15.2** Recognized variants of dominant dorsal duct anatomy.

MRCP as a persistent dilatation (>3 mm above baseline) of the dorsal pancreatic duct 10 minutes after secretin injection in patients younger than 60 years of age. A Santorinicele is defined as a cystic dilatation of the distal dorsal pancreatic duct just proximal to the minor papilla which becomes more prominent during secretin stimulation. Speculation as to its etiology centers on a combination of both dorsal duct obstruction plus a weakness of the distal pancreatic duct wall leading to a circumscribed ductal dilatation or bulge. In a small series of mostly elderly patients (mean age 70 years), identification of a Santorinicele during secretin-stimulated MRCP predicted a good response following endoscopic sphincterotomy. Despite this positive report, questions remain regarding the prevalence of Santorinicele in patients with PD, its association with the elderly, and whether or not it represents a congenital or acquired ductal abnormality. While a single structural mechanism (e.g., outflow obstruction) causing ARP in patients with PD is appealing, a recent paper has identified abnormalities of the cystic transmembrane conductance regulator (CFTR) fibrosis gene in 22% patients with PD and idiopathic pancreatitis implying a more complex disease phenotype than simple obstruction.

## PREOPERATIVE PLANNING

Patients evaluated for transduodenal sphincteroplasty of the biliary and pancreatic ducts should be appropriate surgical candidates for an open upper abdominal operation and meet the following clinical and laboratory criteria based on a careful preoperative assessment.

### Sphincter of Oddi Dysfunction

- ARP or typical pancreatobiliary-type pain
- Abnormal liver function tests (AST and alkaline phosphatase >2× the upper limit of normal) for biliary SOD or altered pancreatic enzymes (amylase or lipase >2× the upper limits of normal) for pancreatic SOD
- Dilated common bile duct (>10 mm), or dilated pancreatic duct (>6 mm in the pancreatic head or >5 mm in the pancreatic body)
- Absence of alcohol or narcotic dependence

SOD is subdivided into Type I through Type III disease based on the number of established criteria present in each individual patient. In patients with all the three criteria (Type I SOD), sphincterotomy has a high chance of success whether or not they have a manometrically abnormal pancreatic sphincter (Table 15.2). In contrast, patients with pancreatobiliary-type pain and one of the two remaining criteria (Type II SOD) have a high chance of postoperative success *only* if they have evidence of a manometrically abnormal sphincter. In those patients who only have pancreatobiliary pain (Type III SOD), sphincterotomy has a low chance of success regardless of the results of pancreatic or biliary sphincter manometry. In patients with SOD and imaging evidence

**TABLE 15.2 Likelihood of Pain Relief from Endoscopic Sphincterotomy (ES) in Different Subtypes of Patients with Biliary SOD Depending on Whether They Have a Normal or Abnormal Endoscopic Sphincter of Oddi Manometry Test**

| SOD Subtype | Presenting Characteristics | ESOM Abnormal | ESOM Normal |
|---|---|---|---|
| I | Pancreatobiliary pain<br>Abnormal liver function tests[a]<br>Dilated common bile duct[b] | High | High |
| II | Pancreatobiliary pain and one additional criteria above | High | Low |
| III | Pancreatobiliary pain only | Moderate | Very low |

Original classification system included delayed drainage of contrast greater than 45 minutes from the biliary tree on ERCP.
[a]Abnormal liver function tests = aspartate aminotransferase (AST) and alkaline phosphatase greater than 2 × the upper limit of normal on two separate occasions.
[b]Dilated common bile duct = >10 mm.

of chronic pancreatitis, sphincterotomy is *not indicated,* and these patients are best managed by either formal pancreatic resection or drainage operations.

### Pancreas Divisum

It should be emphasized that most series of TS for patients with pancreas divisum are limited to patients with ARP or pancreatic-type pain without evidence of chronic pancreatitis In patients with PD with evidence of chronic pancreatitis based on imaging studies, are best managed surgically by a duodenal-preserving pancreatic head resection.

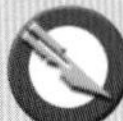

## SURGICAL TECHNIQUE

Operative intervention for Type I biliary or pancreatic SOD is by far the most straightforward. In biliary SOD, biliary sphincteroplasty and cholecystectomy is the operation of choice whereas in pancreatic SOD, both biliary sphincteroplasty and concomitant pancreatic septectomy is the optimal operative procedure. In Patients with Type I PD, a dual sphincteroplasty of both the major (Wirsung) and minor (Santorini) papilla to include a septoplasty of the major pancreatic duct is the treatment of choice. Intervention in patients with Type II or III biliary or pancreatic SOD represents a heterogeneous group of disorders with longstanding controversy over the exact pathophysiology, natural history, and response to treatment; therefore, these patients should be approached cautiously when surgery is contemplated.

### Pertinent Anatomy

The surgeon who endeavors to perform transduodenal sphincteroplasty should be quite familiar with the right upper quadrant anatomy including the head of the pancreas, stomach and duodenum, extrahepatic biliary system, and the associated vascular supply to the duodenum and liver. In addition, altered anatomy from prior gastric operations such as Roux-en-y gastric bypass, duodenal switch, or Billroth II gastrectomy has become common and should not dissuade the surgeon from carrying out TS in an appropriately selected patient. The duct system of the pancreas and biliary tree and the variants of dorsal duct anatomy based on foregut embryology should be completely understood (Fig. 15.2). High-quality hepatopancreatobiliary imaging preoperatively (MRI/MRCP, computed tomography, ERCP, transhepatic cholangiography), intraoperatively (cholangiography and pancreatography), and postoperatively, are essential for proper patient selection and appropriate clinical follow-up.

### Positioning, Mobilization, Identification

The patient is placed in a supine position, deeply anesthetized with appropriate monitoring. A nasogastric tube, a Foley catheter, lower extremity sequential compression devices (SCDs), systemic antibiotics, and an appropriate deep venous thrombosis (DVT) prophylaxis are inserted, applied, and administered. Chlorhexidine scrub is utilized for skin preparation after the clipping of hair from the incision site. A time out is done confirming the patient, the diagnosis, the operation, and the patient's known drug allergies prior to beginning the operative procedure; all personnel in the room should be in agreement. An upper midline incision is made and taken down to the fascia where the abdomen is entered. The falciform ligament is ligated and divided, or divided using an energy device (e.g., Ligasure) to open up the right upper quadrant. A Bookwalter retractor is placed to maintain exposure by retracting the anterior abdominal wall and associated viscera. In those patients with a gallbladder, a cholecystectomy is routinely performed. Sharp division of the hepatocolic ligament with cautery and mobilization of the right colon inferiorly exposes the head of the pancreas and duodenum. An extensive Kocher maneuver is done from the caudate lobe of the liver to the third portion of the duodenum in a superior to inferior orientation, and from Gerota's fascia to the aorta in the lateral to medial direction. Mobilization of the omentum off the transverse mesocolon, entering the lesser sac, and extending this dissection

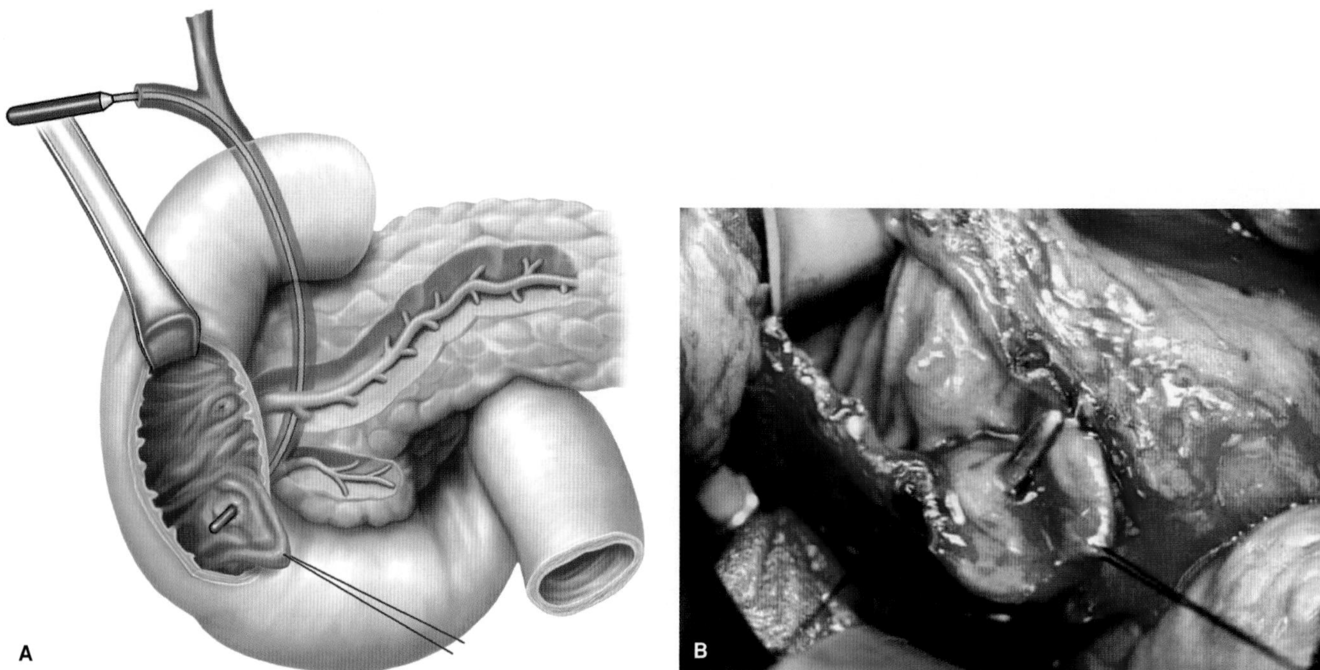


Figure 15.3 **A:** Bakes dilator in the cystic duct to facilitate identification of the ampulla of Vater. **B:** Intraoperative photo showing ampullary identification with a Bakes dilator.

laterally to the right is necessary to release the hepatic flexure of the colon and allow mesocolon lengthening and retraction inferiorly to allow access to the third portion of the duodenum. This extensive mobilization will pay off in visualization during the remaining portions of the procedure. Inability to obtain this level of mobilization should alert the surgeon to the possibility of chronic pancreatitis which can be confirmed by intraoperative ultrasonography. Stay sutures of 2-0 silk are placed superiorly (first portion) and inferiorly (third portion) on the antimesenteric border of the duodenum and the entire head of the pancreas and duodenum are rotated 90 degree clockwise until the duodenum lies superficially in the wound with the lateral duodenal wall positioned anteriorly. Gentle palpation, intraoperative ultrasonography, or passing a metal probe or biliary Fogarty catheter through the cystic duct down into the duodenum will allow localization of the ampulla of Vater and a longitudinal duodenal incision is centered over this area (Fig. 15.3A, B). Additional 2-0 silks can be used to hold the duodenal walls open for exposure. Once the major papilla is identified, the minor papilla is typically located 1 cm superior and 1 cm medial to the major papilla (Fig. 15.4). Intraoperative ultrasonography can also aid in the identification of both the major and the minor pancreatic duct in patients with complex anatomy. In difficult cases of identification of the pancreatic sphincters, SecreFlo™, an intravenous injection of secretin (0.2 mcg/kg patient body weight by intravenous injection over 1 minute) can be given to facilitate pancreatic juice flow to identify a miniscule or scarred and stenotic minor pancreatic duct sphincter. A set of lacrimal duct probes and Bakes dilators should be available on the operative field as they are essential instruments for TS.

#### Transduodenal Sphincteroplasty—Sphincter of Oddi Dysfunction

The ampulla of Vater is identified and both the distal common bile duct and the pancreatic duct orifice are identified. The pancreatic duct is intubated with a metallic probe (lacrimal duct probe or Bakes dilator) to prevent pancreatic ductal occlusion during biliary sphincteroplasty. Electrocautery is used to divide the mucosa and muscle making up the ampulla of Vater toward the 11 o'clock position to create a biliary sphincterotomy. Once the sphincterotomy is of adequate size, the biliary and duodenal mucosa are approximated with 5-0 monofilament absorbable sutures starting at the apex and extending down both side walls of the bile duct (Fig. 15.5). Next the pancreatic duct orifice is opened by a septotomy incising the overhanging tissue present on a small Bakes dilator with an 11 blade. If technically possible, the edges of the pancreatic duct

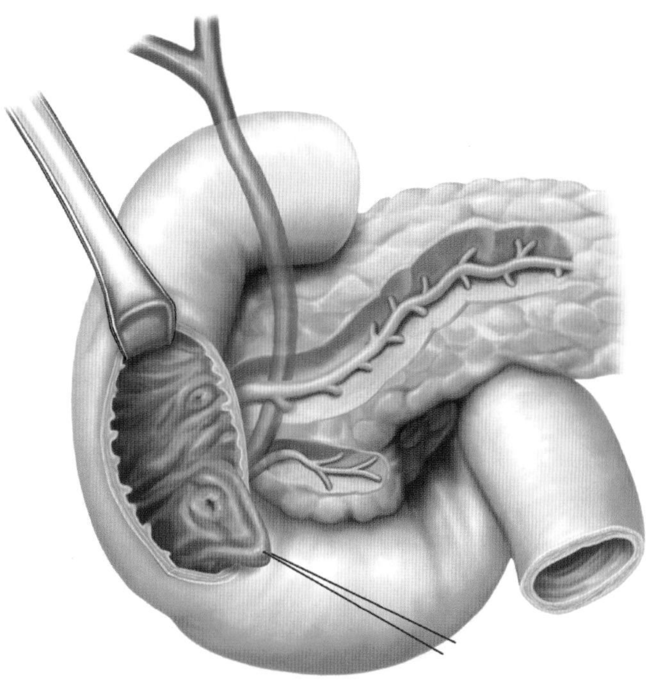

**Figure 15.4** Identification of the major (Wirsung) and minor (Santorini) sphincter in a patient with pancreas divisum.

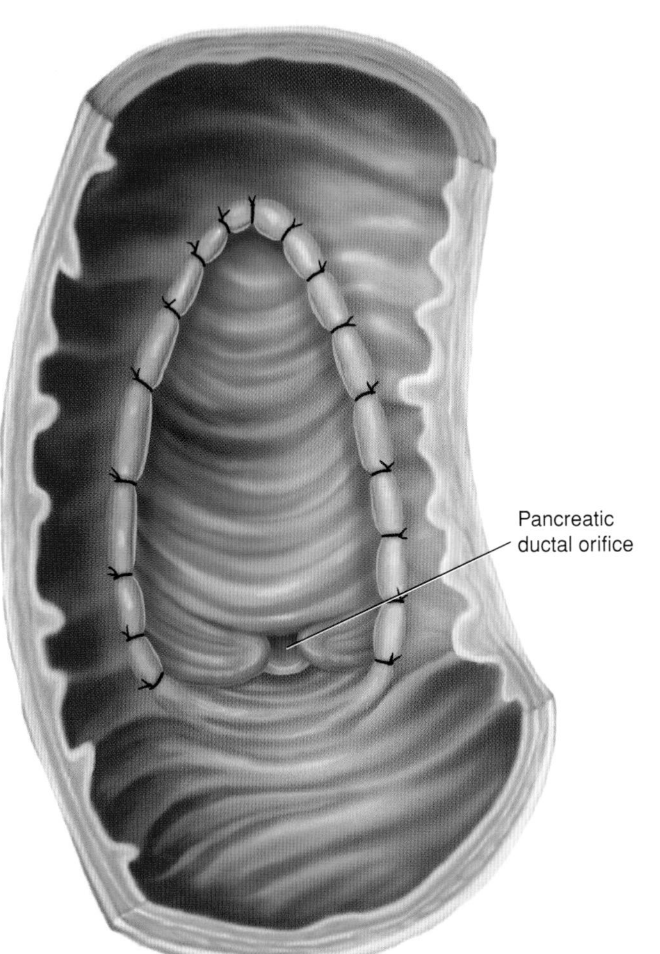


**Figure 15.5** Bile duct to duodenal mucosa approximation in transduodenal sphincteroplasty.

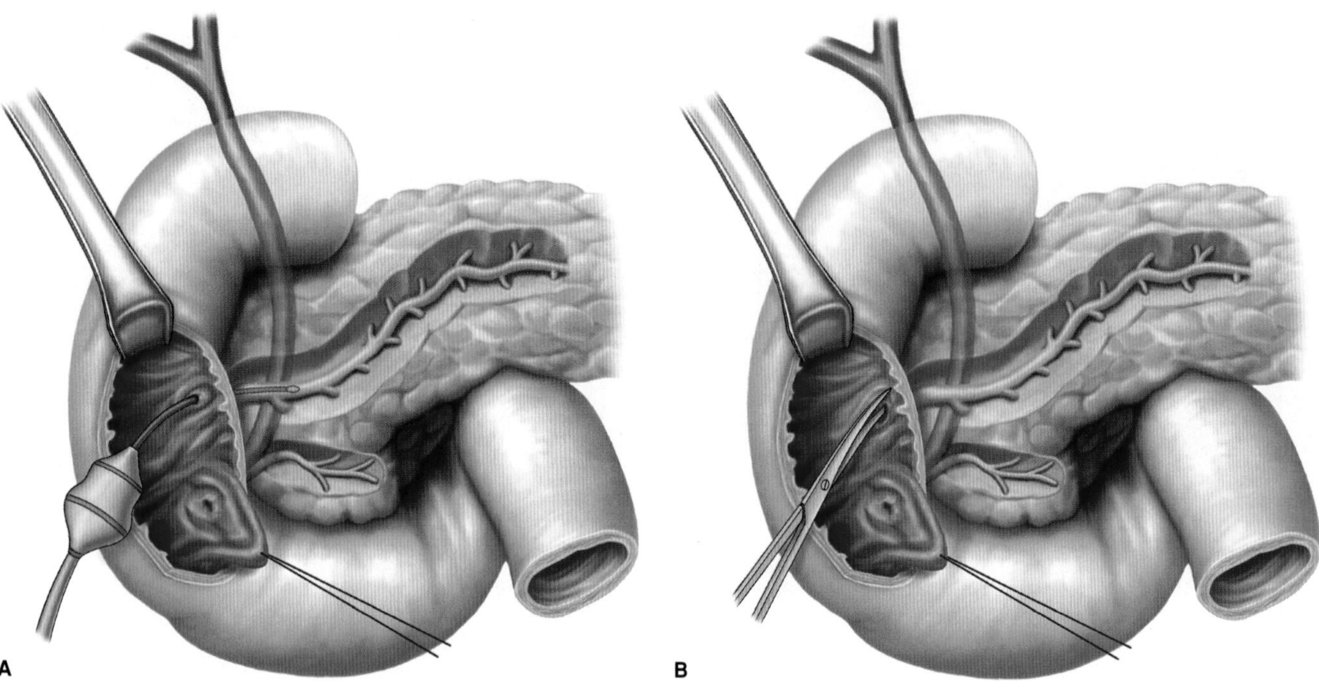


**Figure 15.6** **A:** Lacrimal duct probe identification of a stenotic accessory pancreatic duct sphincter in a patient with pancreas divisum. **B:** Use of tenotomy scissors for accessory duct sphincterotomy in a patient with pancreas divisum.

mucosa are approximated to the biliary mucosa using 6-0 monofilament absorbable sutures (pancreatic duct septoplasty).

#### Transduodenal Dual Sphincteroplasty—Pancreas Divisum

In patients with pancreas divisum, usually both the major and minor pancreatic duct sphincters require sphincteroplasty; thus a "dual sphincteroplasty" is routinely carried out. A biliary sphincteroplasty as described in the preceding paragraph is performed. Following this, the accessory papilla is localized 1 cm superior and 1 cm medial to the major papilla and intubated with a lacrimal duct probe (Fig. 15.6). This accessory pancreatic duct is opened in a medial and cephalad direction using electrocautery and the cut edges of the sphincterotomy are approximated to the duodenal mucosa with 5-0 monofilament absorbable sutures. In certain circumstances, particularly patients with multiple prior ES and significant scarring of their accessory papilla, a 2 cm, 5-F Geenen stent can be positioned in the minor ductal orifice following sphincteroplasty to facilitate healing without recurrent stricture formation. This temporary stent can then be removed endoscopically 4 to 6 weeks postoperatively. After completion of sphincteroplasties, the area is carefully assessed for bleeding. Occasionally, small duodenal arterioles are severed in the duodenal submucosa and these can cause troubling bleeding in the early postoperative period. Careful attention to hemostasis using interrupted 6-0 monofilament suture at this point is essential. After completion of sphincteroplasties, the duodenotomy is reapproximated longitudinally using a single layer of continuous running 3-0 absorbable suture and the duodenum is placed back in its normal position in the retroperitoneum and covered by the hepatic flexure of the colon. In the absence of duodenal wall inflammation, scarring, or a technical concern with the duodenal closure, routine closed suction (Jackson-Pratt) postoperative drainage is unnecessary (Fig. 15.7).

##  POSTOPERATIVE MANAGEMENT

Patients should be admitted to the postoperative recovery area and then the general surgical floor if they exhibit normal vital signs, oxygen saturation, urine output, and pain control. In patients with tolerance to narcotic analgesics, we often supplement these with

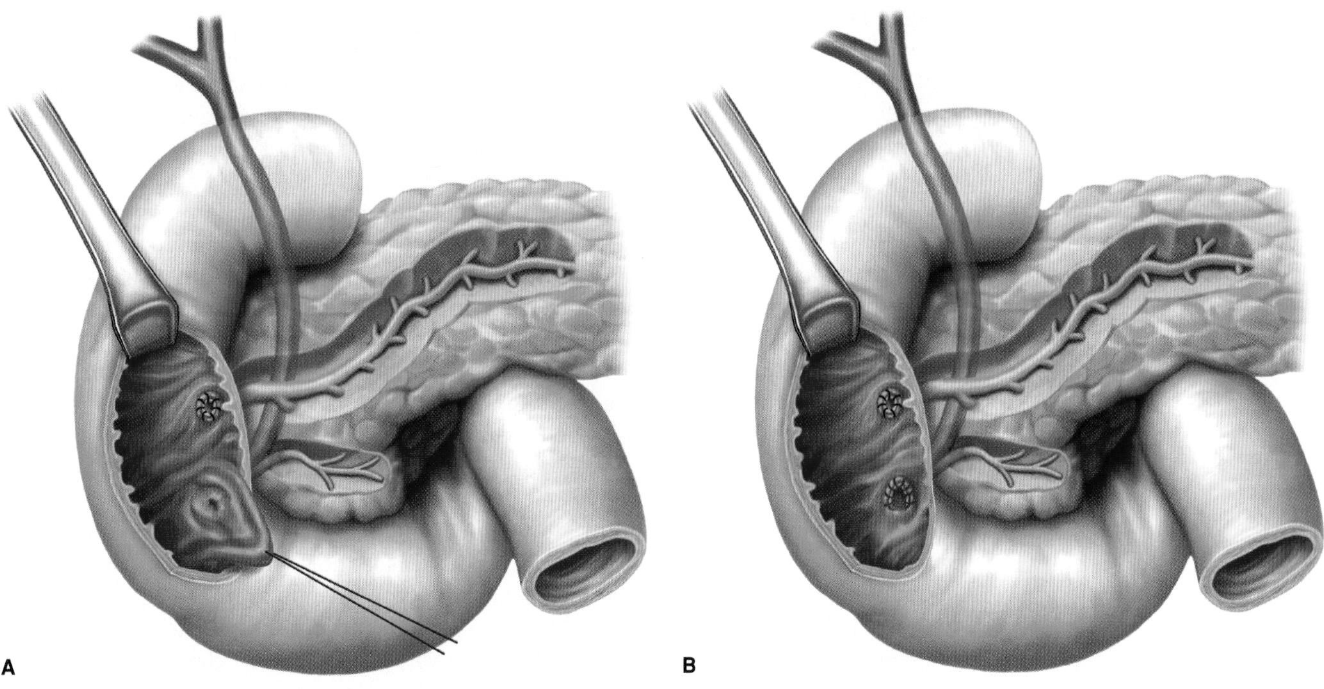


Figure 15.7 Completed dual sphincteroplasty in a patient with pancreas divisum.

nonsteroidal anti-inflammatory medications to provide dual mechanism for pain relief. In patients following a normal postoperative course, their nasogastric tube and Foley catheter are removed on the first postoperative day. DVT and ulcer prophylaxis are routinely provided and perioperative antibiotics are limited to two doses postoperatively (<24 hours). Early ambulation and incentive spirometry are encouraged. Routine laboratory investigations including a CBC, liver function tests, and serum amylase levels are obtained on the first postoperative day. These data help to reassure the surgeon that the sphincteroplasties freely open into the duodenum and are draining properly. Patients who require additional intravenous fluid above maintenance requirements in the first 24 hours postoperatively (supplemental intravenous fluid boluses, persistent tachycardia, oliguria, or severe abdominal pain) should alert the surgeon to the possibility of postoperative pancreatitis or an early duodenal leak (see Complications below). On postoperative day #3, patients are advanced to a clear liquid diet, and if this is tolerated, a soft diet is given on postoperative day #4. Abdominal distension, early satiety, or heartburn are frequently signs of poor gastric emptying and should prompt the de-escalation of oral intake and consideration of NG tube replacement. Those patients who vomit after initiating oral intake should have their NG tube reinserted. Wounds are carefully assessed daily for signs of infection. When taking adequate oral intake of a soft diet, pain medications are transitioned from intravenous to oral analgesics. In patients who follow an uncomplicated postoperative course, discharge to home on postoperative day 4 to 5 should be anticipated.

## COMPLICATIONS

The most common early postoperative complications following TS are as follows.

- Acute pancreatitis—this complication can run the gamut from a mild biochemical hyperamylasemia with abdominal pain (common) to an episode of severe acute pancreatitis with organ failure and necrosis (rare). Prompt identification and aggressive treatment of patients with severe acute pancreatitis is essential. Any patient with postoperative acute pancreatitis should be transferred to an intensive care unit setting with careful monitoring of organ system function and provided adequate volume resuscitation, supplemental oxygen, and pain control.

- Postoperative bleeding—usually localized to the site of the sphincteroplasty. Can respond to transfusion and correction of any identified coagulation abnormalities. If it does not, early re-exploration is indicated with direct suture control of the site. Because of the small duodenal submucosal arterioles commonly responsible for this type of bleeding, angiographic embolization is not usually helpful in its control.
- Delayed gastric emptying—edema at the duodenotomy closure is common producing delayed gastric emptying and prolonged resumption of adequate oral intake. Some patients develop profound gastric distension with associated nausea and vomiting and will require NG tube reinsertion and nasogastric decompression. A careful investigation for occult duodenal leak should be undertaken. In these patients, serum electrolytes should be monitored and replaced with careful attention to volume deficits which require replacement. Intravenous prokinetic agents are judiciously used particularly in patients suspected of having corresponding gastric dysmotility (diabetics).
- Infectious—urinary tract, surgical site, intra-abdominal fluid collections, intravenous lines, cholangitis. Appropriately timed and selected prophylactic antibiotics should minimize surgical site infections in this cohort to less than 10%. Intra-abdominal fluid collections can be treated by percutaneous drainage and culture. A leak from the duodenotomy should be suspected and carefully searched for using cross-sectional imaging (CT scanning), contrast fluoroscopy, or drain tract sinography in those patients with an intra-abdominal fluid collection or bilious output from their operatively placed drains. If a duodenal leak is identified, we institute NG tube decompression and begin total parenteral nutrition to carefully maintain fistula control. With adequate nasogastric decompression and percutaneous drainage, reoperation is rarely required. Patients who develop cholangitis require urgent percutaneous transhepatic cholangiography and transhepatic tube placement both to provide adequate decompression of their biliary system and to provide access for assessing technical problems at the anastomosis. Endoscopic evaluation should be done exceedingly rarely in the setting of a fresh duodenotomy as the likelihood of suture line disruption is high.

## RESULTS

The collective experience of surgeons suggests that in carefully selected patients, excellent to good results should be obtained in approximately 74%. The results from the four largest English language surgical series are given in Table 15.3. The caveats from these experiences are that patients whose indication for operation is ARP have the highest success rate and patients with established chronic pancreatitis have the lowest. Patients with SOD operated on for recurrent abdominal pain have outcome results that parallel those reported following ES where best results are obtained in patients with abnormal sphincter pressures and one or more manifestations of obstruction (altered liver function tests or dilated common bile duct) (Table 15.2).

**TABLE 15.3 Results of Transduodenal Sphincteroplasty from the Largest Surgical Series Reported in the English Language Literature Between 1983 and 2008**

| | | | | Procedure Related | | | |
|---|---|---|---|---|---|---|---|
| First Author | Pts. | SOD/PD | Improved SOD/PD | Restenosis | Major Complications | Death | FU |
| Moody | 92 | 92/0 | 76%/NA | NA | 23 | 0.8 | NA |
| Warshaw | 100 | 0/100 | NA/70% | 7% | 1% | 0 | 53 |
| Madura | 446 | 372/74 | 87%/63% | NA | 15 | 0.2 | NA |
| Morgan | 68 | 51/17 | 66%/54% | 28% | NA | 0 | 42 |

## CONCLUSIONS

Transduodenal sphincteroplasty of the biliary and pancreatic ducts are infrequent operations that require careful and meticulous preoperative investigation and categorization of patients into clinical subtypes which predict their response to treatment. A dedicated team of gastrointestinal endoscopists and pancreatobiliary surgeons well versed in the nuances of these challenging disorders should work collaboratively to obtain optimal results.

## Recommended References and Readings


Cotton PB. Congenital anomaly of pancreas divisum as a cause of obstructive pain and pancreatitis. *Gut.* 1980;21:105–114.

Eversman D, Fogel EL, Rusche M, et al. Frequency of abnormal pancreatic and biliary sphincter manometry compared with clinical suspicion of sphincter of Oddi dysfunction. *Gastrointest Endosc.* 1999;50:637–641.

Fogel EL, Toth TG, Lehman GA, et al. Does endoscopic therapy favorable affect the outcome of patients who have recurrent acute pancreatitis and pancreas divisum? *Pancreas.* 2007;34:21–45.

Gark PK, Khajuria R, Kaba M, et al. Association of SPINK1 gene mutation and CFTR gene polymorphisms in patients with pancreas divisum presenting with idiopathic pancreatitis. *J Clin Gastroenterol.* 2009;43:848–852.

Geenen JE, Hogan WJ, Dodds WJ, et al. The efficacy of endoscopic sphincterotomy after cholecystectomy in patients with sphincter of Oddi dysfunction. *N Engl J Med.* 1989;320:82–87.

Klein SD, Affronti JP. Pancreas divisum, an evidence-based review: part II, patient selection and treatment. *Gastrointest Endosc.* 2004;60:585–589.

Lehman GA, Sherman S. Sphincter of Oddi dysfunction. *Int J Pancreatol.* 1996;20:11–25.

Madura JA, Madura JA II, Sherman S, et al. Surgical sphincteroplasty in 446 patients. *Arch Surg.* 2005;140:504–511.

Moody FG, Becker JM, Potts JR. Transduodenal sphincteroplasty and transampullary septectomy for postcholecystectomy pain. *Ann Surg.* 1983;197:627–636.

Morgan KA, Romagnuolo J, Adams DB. Transduodenal sphincteroplasty in the management of sphincter of Oddi dysfunction and pancreas divisum in the modern era. *J Am Coll Surg.* 2008;206:908–917.

Nardi GL, Acosta JM. Papillitis as a cause of pancreatitis and abdominal pain: role of evocative test, operative pancreatography and histologic evaluation. *Ann Surg.* 1966;164:611–621.

Rios GA, Adams DB. Outcome of surgical treatment of chronic pancreatitis associated with sphincter of Oddi dysfunction. *Am Surg.* 2001;67:462–466.

Schlosser W, Rau BM, Poch B, et al. Surgical treatment of pancreas divisum causing chronic pancreatitis: the outcome benefits of duodenum-preserving pancreatic head resection. *J Gastrointest Surg.* 2005;9:710–715.

Toouli J. Sphincter of Oddi: function, dysfunction, and its management. *J Gastroenterol Hepatol.* 2009;24:(suppl 3):S57–S62.

Warshaw AL, Simeone JF, Shapiro RH, et al. Evaluation and treatment of the dominant dorsal duct syndrome (pancreas divisum redefined). *Am J Surg.* 1990;159:59–64.

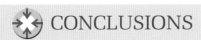

# 16 Transduodenal Resection of Ampullary Tumor: Pancreas-preserving Duodenal Resection

**Kristy L. Rialon and Theodore N. Pappas**

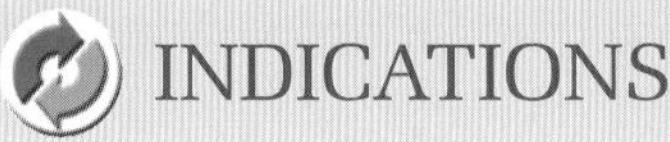



## Indications for Surgical Ampullectomy

The first ampullary resection was performed by Halsted in 1897 by resecting part of the ampulla and reimplanting the common bile duct and pancreatic duct back in the duodenum. Tumors of the ampulla of Vater are rare lesions that comprise less than 10% of pancreatic and periampullary cancers. Benign tumors include lipomas, hamartomas, lymphangiomas, hemangiomas, leiomyofibromas, and neurogenic tumors. Most malignant tumors are adenocarcinomas but adenosquamous carcinoma, leiomyosarcoma, fibrosarcoma, neuroendocrine carcinomas are also found. Patients typically present at an earlier stage than tumors of the pancreatic head or tail or the distal common bile duct. The most common symptom is jaundice, though this is more frequently seen in adenocarcinoma than adenomas. Other common symptoms include fever, weight loss, nausea, pruritus, pancreatitis (more common in adenomas), abdominal pain, and anemia secondary to bleeding.

Controversy exists regarding the procedure of choice for ampullary masses. Surgical options for treating ampullary tumors include endoscopic removal, transduodenal ampullectomy, or pancreaticoduodenectomy (PD). In patients with sporadic ampullary polyps, all should undergo attempts at resection when medically possible. Endoscopic removal is an alternative to surgery that has become technically more feasible. Most ampullary neoplasms that are 2 cm or less and are confined to the superficial layers of the duodenum can be resected endoscopically by experienced practioners. Relative contraindications to endoscopic resection, and indications for surgical resection, include large lesions, recurrence after endoscopic resection, lesions in a duodenal diverticulum, penetration into the duodenal wall or along the bile duct, inability to access the duodenum endoscopically, and multiple polyps.

TABLE 16.1 Spigelman Classification of Duodenal Polyposis

| | Number of points | | |
|---|---|---|---|
| | 1 | 2 | 3 |
| Polyp number | 1–4 | 5–20 | >20 |
| Polyp size | 1–4 mm | 5–10 mm | >10 mm |
| Histologic type | Tubular polyp, hyperplasia, inflammation | Tubulovillous | Villous |
| Dysplasia | Mild | Moderate | Severe |

Stage 0: 0 points; Stage I: 1–4 points; Stage II: 5–6 points; Stage III: 7–8 points; Stage IV: 9–12 points.
Adapted from Spigelman et al., *Lancet* 1989.

Several authors have recommended surgical ampullectomies for benign lesions less than 3 cm, small neuroendocrine tumors, and T1 carcinomas of the ampulla. Surgical ampullectomy is contraindicated in those with lesions so large and irregular that reconstruction is not possible. If frozen section is free of cancer, but carcinoma is found on final pathologic examination, the patient should be considered for interval pancreaticoduodenectomy. Pancreaticoduodenectomy is performed when (1) invasive carcinoma is found on preoperative biopsy, (2) margins are not safely obtainable, (3) frozen section shows carcinoma, and (4) histologic confirmation of cancer is not possible on selected patients with ampullary obstruction.

## Indications for Pancreas-preserving Duodenectomy

The first case of duodenal carcinoma was described by Hamburger in 1746. Duodenal carcinoma represents about 0.3% of all malignant neoplasms of the gastrointestinal tract and 25% to 45% of malignant neoplasms of the small intestine. Patients may present with obstructive symptoms, jaundice, abdominal pain, anorexia, or bleeding. Most duodenal cancers are preceded by premalignant polyps in the duodenum. Adenomatous tissue has been found within duodenal cancer, suggesting the existence of an adenoma–carcinoma sequence in the duodenum. Polyps may be sporadic or in conjunction with polyposis syndromes, such as familial adenomatous polyposis (FAP), Gardner's, and Peutz-Jeghers. These patients are at increased risk for duodenal cancer. After colectomy, this accounts for the majority of cancer-related deaths. Duodenal polyposis is staged according to polyp number, polyp size, histologic type, and dysplasia (Table 16.1).Although 95% of polyposis patients have adenomatous polyps in the duodenum, only 10% have severe or stage IV duodenal polyposis, and only 5% go on to develop cancer. These patients should undergo regular endoscopic examinations. Those who are unable to undergo surveillance, or whom have rapid polyp growth or severe dysplasia, should undergo either pancreaticoduodenectomy or pancreas-sparing duodenectomy (PSD) since the entire duodenal mucosa is at risk. Pancreaticoduodenectomy, however, carries a morbidity and mortality that are too high for dealing with a premalignant condition. In patients with FAP or other polyposis syndromes, endoscopic removal is impractical, as there are typically multiple polyps, most are sessile, and they frequently cluster around the ampulla of Vater. Local excision of polyps is not sufficient surgical treatment, as morbidity is high and recurrence is expected. Contraindications to pancreas-preserving duodenectomy include invasive cancer in the duodenum or neoplasm that tracks up the bile duct outside the confines of the duodenum.

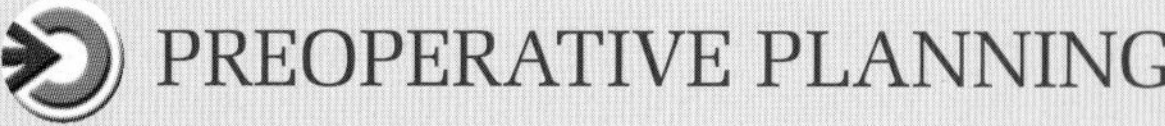

# PREOPERATIVE PLANNING

## Laboratory Values

Serum bilirubin, alkaline phosphatase, transaminases, and pancreatic enzymes should be checked as these can be elevated in cases of biliary obstruction and pancreatitis. The prothrombin time may be elevated secondary to malabsorption of vitamin K. Those who present with bleeding need to be followed with serial hematocrits and hemoglobins.

## Imaging

The presentation of symptoms described above leads to further evaluation by abdominal ultrasonography (US), computed tomography (CT), endoscopic ultrasound (EUS), magnetic resonance cholangiopancreatography (MRCP), and endoscopic retrograde cholangiopancreatography (ERCP). On ultrasound, the lesion is seen as a lump echo in the ampullary region of the common bile duct and there may be distention of the intrahepatic and extrahepatic ducts. CT is a common imaging modality that is useful in detection of diseases of the abdominal cavity and will show ductal dilatation and hepatic metastases, but can miss small tumors.

Prior to both operations, one must obtain either EUS, MRCP, or ERCP to be certain the tumors are not growing through the duodenal wall (which would suggest invasive disease), to determine the location of the minor ampulla, and to know if divisum anatomy is present. EUS provides high-resolution images of the duodenum, ampulla, bile and pancreatic duct walls, pancreatic head, local lymph nodes, and neighboring blood vessels. Tumor extension into the wall of the duodenum or head of the pancreas, as well as lymph node involvement, can be demonstrated by EUS. However, EUS cannot differentiate early malignant tumors from benign ones and inflammatory lymph nodes from malignant ones, demonstrate distant metastases, or identify the margins of large tumors, due to its 2 to 4 cm depth of view.

ERCP is helpful in identifying the extent, size, and gross appearance of the tumor. If cannulation of the ampulla is possible, biliary or pancreatic ductal dilatation can be demonstrated as well as the specific termination of the ducts. If the major pancreatic duct drains into the minor papilla, preoperative stenting of the minor papilla will facilitate its reimplantation. ERCP is more invasive than other modalities and several noteworthy complications can occur, including pancreatitis, perforation, hemorrhage, and infectious and cardiopulmonary complications. This modality is not useful for staging purposes, as it cannot detect infiltration into the surrounding lymph tissue or other organs. MRCP can detect obstruction and dilatation of the biliary system, but it can be difficult to discern small masses at the ampulla. In a comparison of studies, EUS is more accurate than US or CT at detecting ampullary tumors and lymph node metastases. ERCP has similar sensitivity (95%) in detection of ampullary tumors. EUS was found to be superior to CT and US and equivalent to magnetic resonance imaging (MRI) for tumor detection and T and N staging of ampullary tumors.

## Preoperative Biopsies and Frozen Sections

Preoperative biopsy of ampullary tumors can be done in two stages. Sphincterotomy is performed and increases visualization of the tumor and permits biopsy to be performed. Biopsies have been found to be more reliable when obtained 10 days or more after sphincterotomy. Biopsies done at the time of sphincterotomy may be difficult to obtain because of frequent bleeding or hyperperistaltic duodenum. Inaccurate biopsy results due to sampling errors occur in 15% to 40% of cases. In biopsies of villous tumors of the duodenum, the diagnosis of malignancy is missed 40% to 60% of the time. Brush cytology was found to be up to 40% falsely negative for adenocarcinoma. Biopsies should not be done at the ulcer base but rather at the nodular edges. Intraoperative frozen section examination can be useful in deciding whether to perform pancreaticoduodenectomy on patients whose preoperative biopsies were benign. In one study, frozen sections accurately predicted the final histology in all patients undergoing ampullary resection.

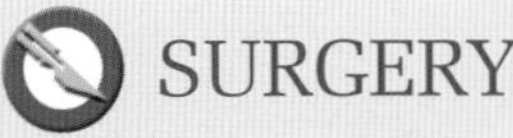

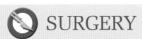

# SURGERY

## Transduodenal Resection of the Ampulla of Vater (Adapted from Barnum et al.)

With the patient in the supine position, a subcostal or midline incision is made. A Kocher maneuver is performed to expose the duodenum. The mass can usually be

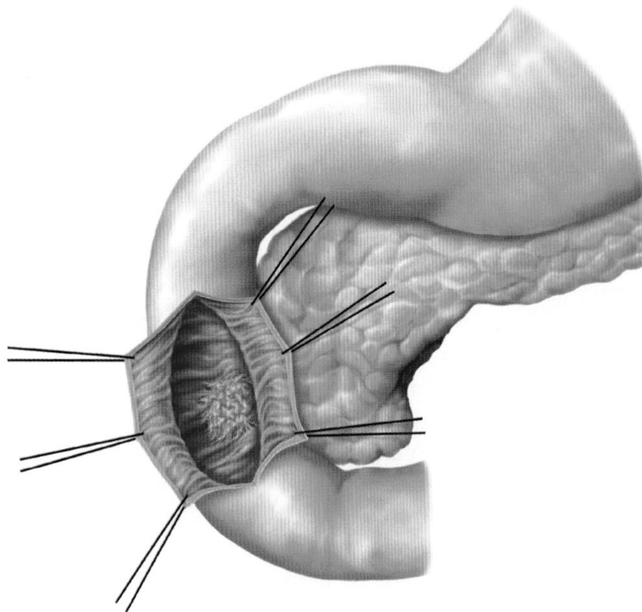

**Figure 16.1** A generous Kocher maneuver is performed to the fourth portion of the duodenum and posteriorly to the vena cava. A duodenotomy is performed after palpation of the tumor or stent or both and extended to yield adequate exposure of the ampulla and surrounding mucosa. Stay sutures are placed circumferentially and secured.

palpated through the duodenal wall. Endoscopic stents can be placed preoperatively to help delineate the duct. A small incision is made over the lesion and the duodenectomy is then extended proximally and distally for improved exposure (Fig. 16.1). Stay sutures are placed in the duodenal wall circumferentially and secured. The bile duct, pancreatic duct, and ampulla are then identified and can be marked by biliary or lacrimal duct probes. In order to identify the exact position of the ducts for probe placement, one may need to resect a portion of the tumor (Fig. 16.2). Once the duct has been identified, the tumor is circumferentially excised with needle-tip electrocautery, set on moderately low setting (to avoid excessive cautery artifact on the excised specimen) at a depth necessary for complete removal (Fig. 16.3). Frozen sections can be utilized at this point to ensure negative margins. If clear margins cannot be obtained or the entire tumor cannot be removed, pancreaticoduodenectomy should be performed.

Once the tumor is removed, the bile and pancreatic ducts are then reconstructed by approximating the pancreatic and bile duct to form a common channel (Fig. 16.4).

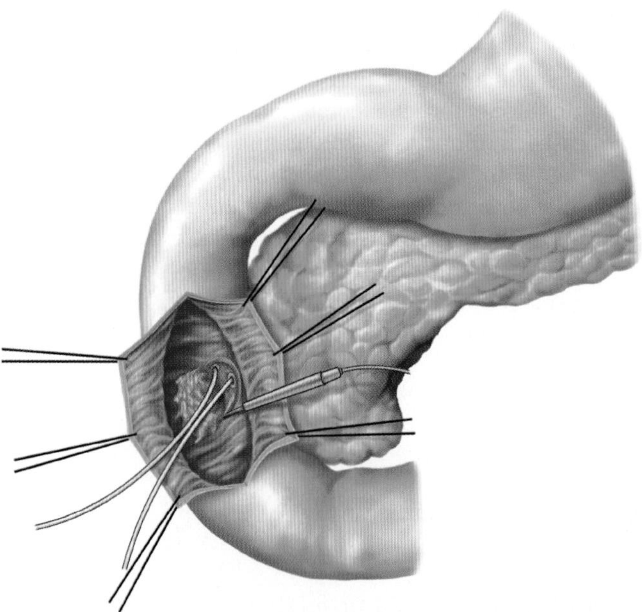

**Figure 16.2** The position of the bile and pancreatic ducts is determined by cannulation using small biliary or lacrimal duct probes. It may be necessary to begin elevation of the duodenal mucosa to be able to identify the orifices of the ducts at the 11 o'clock and 2 o'clock positions. This identification is critical to accurate reconstruction and duct patency.

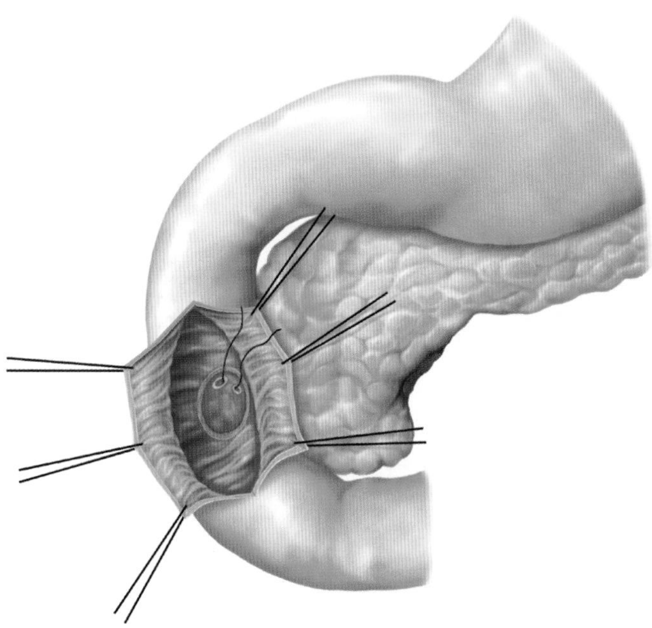

**Figure 16.3** The tumor is excised to whatever depth is necessary for complete removal using needle electrocautery. Depending on tumor size and ductal anatomy (dual or common channel), the bile and pancreatic ducts with be transected at right angles (as in the figure) or spatulated along their anterior surfaces. In either case, the adjacent walls are coapted to begin the reconstruction.

The duodenal mucosa is then reapproximated to this common channel with absorbable monofilament sutures. Patency and appropriate size is demonstrated by using biliary dilators. Assuming that scarring will reduce the diameter of each duct by 50%, the diameter should be 6 to 8 mm for the bile duct and 4 to 5 mm for the pancreatic duct at the completion of the reimplantation. Once adequate patency has been obtained, the duodenum is then closed transversely with sutures or a stapling device (Fig. 16.5). A closed suction drain is placed in the right upper quadrant.

## Pancreas-preserving Duodenectomy (Adapted from Kalady et al.)

The patient is placed on the operating room table in the supine position. A midline or right subcostal incision is made. The duodenum is mobilized using the Kocher maneuver. The gastrointestinal tract is divided at the pylorus. In the first portion of the duodenum, a dissection plane is made between the duodenum and the pancreas, taking care to identify and divide the small blood vessels between the two organs.

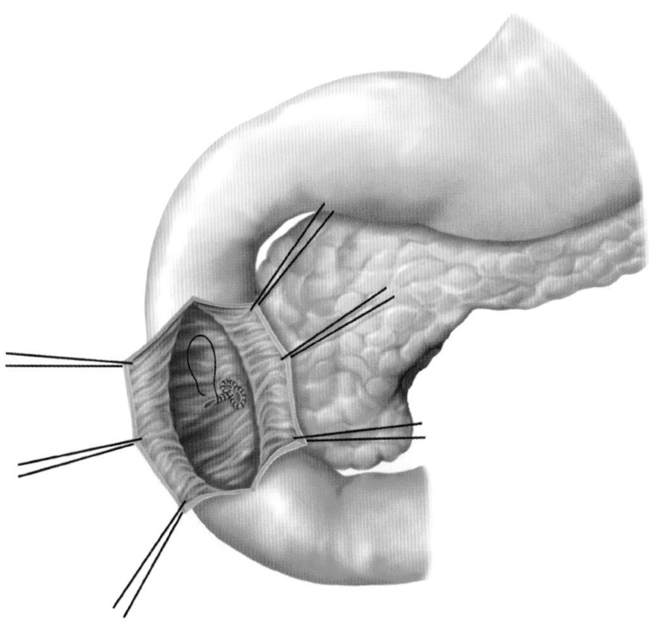

**Figure 16.4** After the common walls of the bile and pancreatic ducts are approximated, duct mucosa is anastomosed circumferentially to duodenal mucosa using absorbable monofilament suture. There often will be a segment of residual duodenal mucosa to close separately.

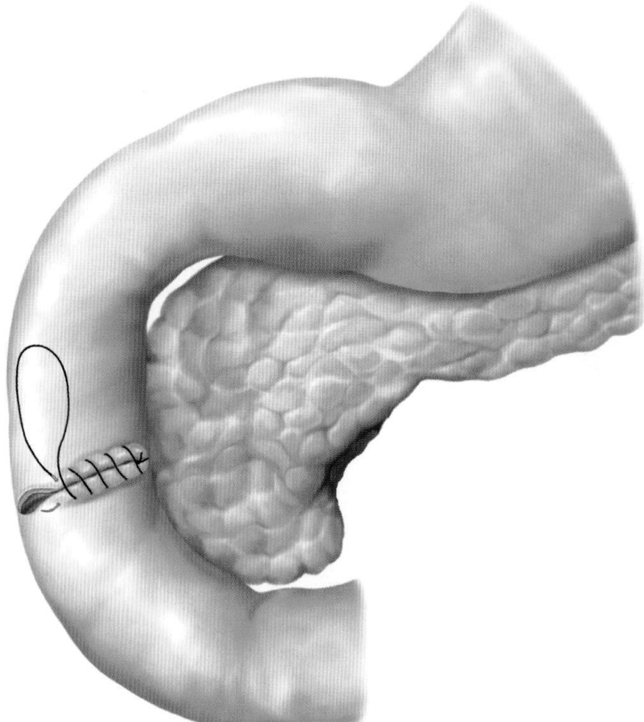

**Figure 16.5** Once adequate patency of the bile and pancreatic ducts has been ensured using biliary dilators, the duodenum is closed transversely with sutures or a TA 55 stapler.

Preoperatively, pancreatic divisum anatomy must be understood by either ERCP or MRCP so reconstruction can be planned accordingly. If the main pancreatic duct is patent, the accessory duct may be safely ligated. The duodenum is then excised from the orifice of the pancreatic duct/bile duct confluence and the cuts ends of both ducts are left for later reconstruction. The remainder of the dissection is completed to the fourth portion of the duodenum and the ligament of Treitz is divided with a stapling device (Fig. 16.6). The bile and main pancreatic ducts are sutured together to form a

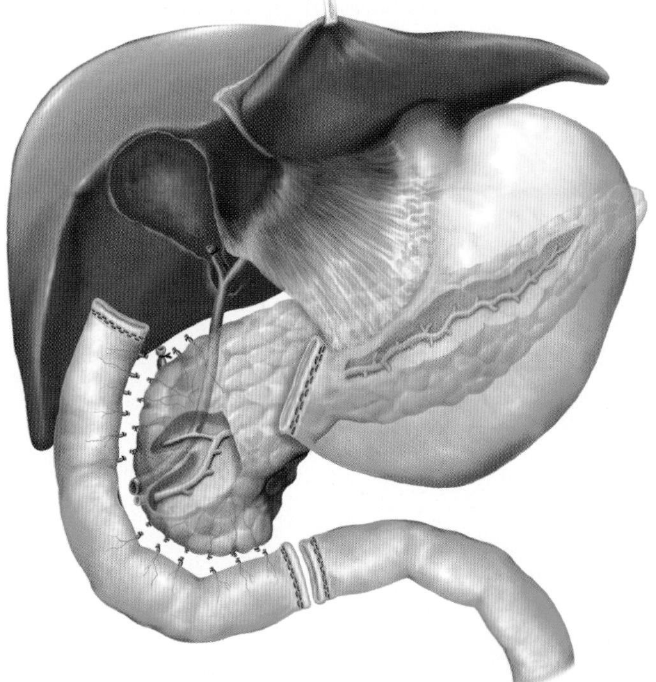

**Figure 16.6** Planes of dissection between the pancreas and duodenum, and boundaries of resection.

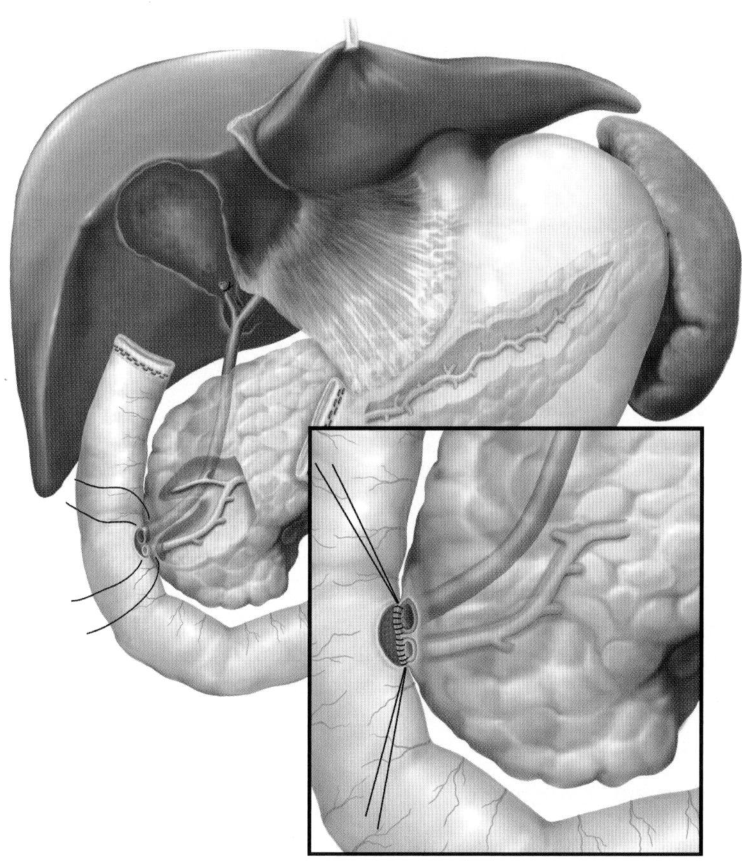

**Figure 16.7** The distal common bile duct and main pancreatic duct are sutured together and reimplanted as a single anastomosis to the jejunum.

common channel, which is then anastomosed to the jejunum (Fig. 16.7). If pancreatic divisum is present, two separate anastomoses are performed for the minor pancreatic duct and the bile duct/main pancreatic duct. Reconstruction of the gastrointestinal tract is accomplished by creating a loop gastrojejunostomy (Fig. 16.8). Closed suction drains are placed around the anastomoses.

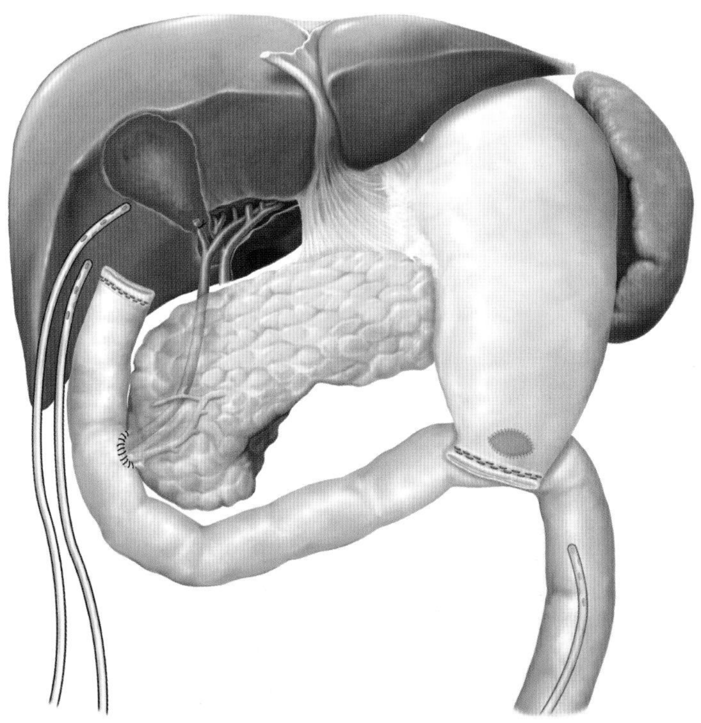

**Figure 16.8** Completed resection with ductal anastomosis, loop gastrojejunostomy, and drains.

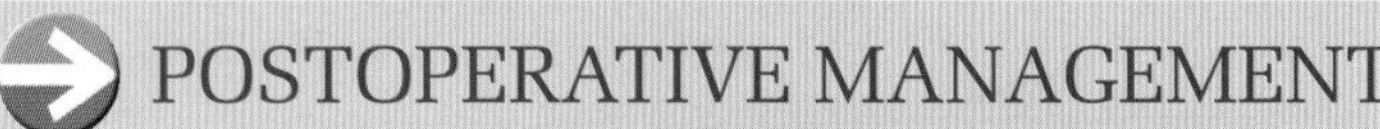

## POSTOPERATIVE MANAGEMENT

### Transduodenal Resection and Pancreas-preserving Duodenectomy

Patients have a nasogastric tube placed intraoperatively, which is usually left in one day following the procedure. Once the patient's bowel function returns, their diet is advanced from clear liquids, to regular diet. The drain is removed when output is minimal. It is common that the patient experiences early satiety during the first month after surgery and therefore may require multiple small meals per day.

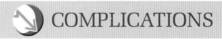

## COMPLICATIONS

### Transduodenal Resection

The complication rate after ampullectomy has been reported as anywhere between 19% and 45%. Complications include wound infection, bowel obstruction, gastric outlet obstruction, pancreatitis, ascending cholangitis from retrograde infection of the biliary tree, common bile duct stricture, intraabdominal abscess, and anastomotic leak. Mortality rates following the procedure are low.

### Pancreas-preserving Duodenectomy

Complications following this procedure have been documented as high as 60%, and include wound infection, biliary and ampullary leak, pancreatic fistula, pancreatitis, gastric outlet obstruction, and delayed gastric emptying. Mortality rates are also low when compared to pancreaticoduodenectomy.

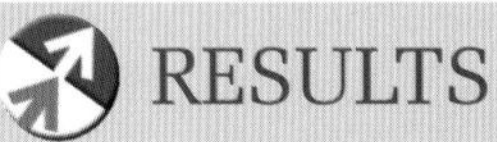

## RESULTS

### Transduodenal Resection

It is difficult to compare transduodenal resection and pancreaticoduodenectomy because of the small number of patients and selection bias, though in several small series, local resection had a lower morbidity and mortality than PD. Recurrence rates have been reported from 10% to 46%. The average length of stay is around 9 to 10 days. Mean operative time in one series was 169 minutes with a mean blood loss of 192 ml. Previous studies examining local resection for adenocarcinoma in patients who were poor candidates, refused pancreaticoduodenectomy, or in whom cancer was discovered only on permanent pathologic section, found an overall 5-year survival rate of 40%. Unless there are unique circumstances, ampullectomy, or pancreas-preserving duodenectomy should not be offered for patients with cancer. Pancreaticoduodenectomy for ampullary cancer is associated with a 5-year survival rates of 32% to 63% in several series.

### Pancreas-preserving Duodenectomy

Patients with polyposis syndromes that undergo pancreas-preserving duodenectomy have a low rate of recurrence of polyps in other parts of the small intestine. The mean operative time has been reported from 279 to 370 minutes. The average length of stay was 11 to 18 days. Comparisons between this procedure and pancreaticoduodenectomy are difficult as studies with sufficient numbers of patients have yet to be performed.

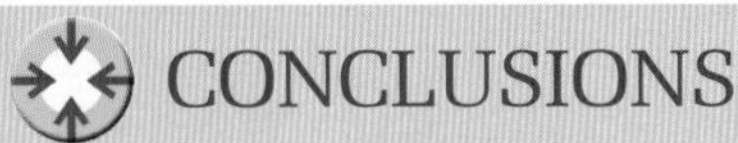


In patients who cannot undergo endoscopic resection for sporadic ampullary adenomas, transduodenal resection is the procedure of choice for benign ampullary lesions. Patients with polyposis syndromes and evidence of rapid polyp grown or severe dysplasia are candidates for pancreas-preserving duodenectomy. Pancreaticoduodenectomy should be performed in those with ampullary cancer who are fit for the operation.

## Recommended References and Readings


Branum GD, Pappas TN, Meyers WC. The management of tumors of the ampulla of Vater by local resection. *Ann Surg.* 1996;224(5): 621–627.

Chen CH, Tseng LJ, Yang CC, et al. The accuracy of endoscopic ultrasound, endoscopic retrograde cholangiopancreatography, computed tomography, and transabdominal ultrasound in the detection and staging of primary ampullary tumors. *Hepatogastroenterology.* 2001;48(42):1750–1753.

Chung RS, Church JM, vanStolk R. Pancreas-sparing duodenectomy: indications, surgical technique, and results. *Surgery.* 1995;117(3):254–259.

Clary BM, Tyler DS, Dematos P, et al. Local ampullary resection with careful intraoperative frozen section evaluation for presumed benign ampullary neoplasms. *Surgery.* 2000;127(6):628–633.

Halsted WS. Contributions to the surgery of the bile duct passages, especially of the common bile duct. *Boston Medic Surg J.* 1899; 141:645–654.

Jones BA, Langer B, Taylor BR, et al. Periampullary tumors: which ones should be resected? *Am J Surg.* 1985;149(1):46–52.

Kalady MF, Clary BM, Tyler DS, et al. Pancreas-preserving duodenectomy in the management of duodenal familial adenomatous polyposis. *J Gastrointest Surg.* 2002;6(1):82–87.

Neoptolemos JP, Talbot IC, Carr-Locke DL, et al. Treatment and outcome in 52 consecutive cases of ampullary carcinoma. *Br J Surg.* 1987;74(10):957–961.

Ponchon T, Berger F, Chavaillon A, et al. Contribution of endoscopy to diagnosis and treatment of tumors of the ampulla of Vater. *Cancer.* 1989;64(1):161–167.

Rattner DW, Fernanzdez-del Castillo C, Brugge WR, et al. Defining the criteria for local resection of ampullary neoplasms. *Arch Surg.* 1996;131(4):366–371.

Sarmiento JM, Thompson GB, Nagorney DM, et al. Pancreas-sparing duodenectomy for duodenal polyposis. *Arch Surg.* 2002;137(5): 557–562.

Spigelman AD, Talbot IC, Penna C, et al. Evidence for adenoma-carcinoma sequence in the duodenum of patients with familial adenomatous polyposis. The Leeds Castle Polyposis Group (Upper Gastrointestinal Committee). *J Clin Pathol.* 1994;47(8):709–710.

Spigelman AD, Williams CB, Talbot IC, et al. Upper gastrointestinal cancer in patients with familial adenomatous polyposis. *Lancet.* 1989;2(8666):783–785.

# 17 Repair of Bile Duct Stricture/Injury and Techniques for Accessing the Proximal Biliary Tree

**Chad G. Ball, James J. Mezhir, William R. Jarnagin, and Keith D. Lillemoe**

##  INDICATIONS/CONTRAINDICATIONS

Bile duct injuries are the most serious complication associated with cholecystectomy. The incidence of biliary injury has increased substantially in the era of laparoscopic cholecystectomy. Currently, data from large surveys of patients undergoing laparoscopic cholecystectomy suggest an incidence of 0.4% to 0.6%. Management of these injuries requires a multidisciplinary approach involving interventional radiology and endoscopy combined with experienced hepatobiliary surgeons. Although mortality is uncommon, these injuries remain a major source of patient morbidity and major hospital costs and negativity affect patients' short-term quality of life.

Less than one-third of iatrogenic bile duct injuries are actually detected at the time of the cholecystectomy. The majority are therefore identified postoperatively, and in general, present in one of two forms: biliary leak with biloma formation or complete biliary obstruction. Most commonly, the hepatic duct has been transected and incompletely clipped resulting in bile leakage into the peritoneal cavity. These patients usually present 24 to 72 hours after cholecystectomy with increasing abdominal pain, distension, nausea, and evidence of early sepsis. Patients in whom the common hepatic duct has been completely clipped will present days to weeks after cholecystectomy with pain and jaundice, or less commonly pain and fever indicative of cholangitis. Any such atypical course from the routine recovery for a laparoscopic cholecystectomy should prompt an immediate evaluation for possible biliary injury.

The precise indications and contraindications for operative therapy of a bile duct injury/stricture are based on (1) the mode of injury, (2) the interval between the injury and its diagnosis, (3) the clinical condition of the patient, and (4) the local conditions inherent within the operative field.

The general strategy for managing the injury however involves avoiding immediate operative intervention to attempt definitive repair. If early laparotomy is performed in the face of sepsis continued uncontrolled bile leak or following complete transection of the common bile duct, marked inflammation in the operative field will obscure the area and make identification of the biliary system difficult. Biliary reconstruction under these circumstances is therefore a relative contraindication because it will be technically challenging and frequently end in long-term failure in the form of an anastomotic leak or biliary stricture. To avoid this outcome, early management involves less invasive measures to first define the anatomy of the injury, and then to control biliary sepsis or the ongoing bile leak. Definitive repair is carefully planned and undertaken weeks following the initial injury, well after periportal inflammation has been allowed to resolve. Delaying definitive repair also has the substantial advantage of allowing the clinician time to investigate for concurrent hepatic arterial vascular injury using arterial phase computed tomography (CTA). If there has been a concurrent arterial injury however, a delay will also allow the delineation of both the zone and level of ischemia. Early bile duct repair in the setting of an unrecognized hepatic arterial injury leads to a significantly higher stricture rate.

In cases in which the injury is actually recognized at the time of the cholecystectomy, an attempt at immediate repair is often warranted. The first step in this repair is an intraoperative cholangiogram, which will confirm and better define the injury and will help determine the most appropriate surgical management. If a small segmental duct (<3 mm in diameter) has been injured and cholangiography demonstrates segmental or subsegmental drainage by the injured system, simple ligation of the injured duct will be adequate treatment. If the injured duct is larger (4 mm in diameter) or provides sectoral or lobar drainage as demonstrated by the cholangiogram, surgical repair is required. If the injured segment of the bile duct is short (<1 cm) and two resultant viable ends can be opposed without tension, an end-to-end primary anastomosis is a reasonable strategy, recognizing, however, that late stricture rates are not insignificant. In this case, a generous Kocher maneuver will mobilize the duodenum out of the retroperitoneum and alleviate tension at the repair. The injured ends of the bile duct are debrided to healthy mucosa and a spatulated end-to-end repair is made using interrupted 5-0 monofilament absorbable suture. A T-tube should be placed below and not through the anastomosis (Fig. 17.1). For proximal injuries near the hepatic duct bifurcation or if the injured segment of the bile duct is longer than 1 cm, an end-to-end primary biliary anastomosis will result in excessive tension and should always be avoided in favor of a Roux-en-Y reconstruction.

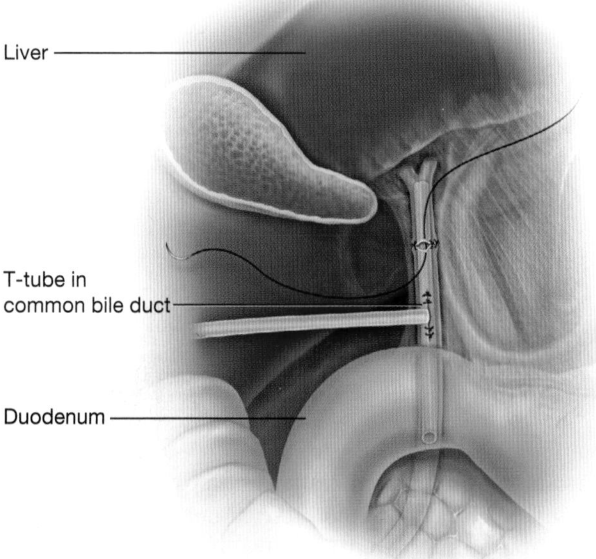


**Figure 17.1** A completed end-to-end biliary repair of a bile duct injury. The T-tube should be placed below and not through the repair.

Finally, if the circumstances of the procedure or the experience of the surgeon are such that an optimal repair is not possible, adequate drainage and transfer to a tertiary care biliary surgeon is advised.

## PREOPERATIVE PLANNING

Preoperative investigation and planning are of paramount importance to ensure a successful and durable bile duct repair. High quality cross-sectional imaging, typically a triple phase contrast-enhanced CT, is critical and will provide much of the necessary information regarding the extent of the problem, including areas of bile collection requiring drainage, the level of biliary obstruction, and associated vascular injuries. In addition, in patients with a complex history or a protracted course, imaging may show evidence of lobar atrophy (see Chapter 26) or cirrhosis. The former is more likely to arise in the setting of a combined biliary and vascular injury and has important technical implications for repair, related to rotational distortion of the porta hepatis structures (Fig. 17.2). Hepatic fibrosis or cirrhosis can result from prolonged biliary obstruction and is typically encountered in patients with multiple failed attempts at repair over a prolonged period. While uncommon, cirrhosis is an ominous finding, usually an end stage event, and attempts at repair in this setting are associated with very high mortality rates.

In patients presenting early following cholecystectomy, the most common mode of presentation will be a bile leak. Significant right upper quadrant pain and fever will be evident days after the procedure (direct hyperbilirubinemia and leukocytosis). The diagnosis of bile leak is made by either CT or ultrasound. Every attempt is then made to first control the associated sepsis via nonoperative means and delay surgical intervention. Once the biloma is identified, it is drained percutaneously. Broad spectrum antibiotics with adequate biliary penetration are started and tailored to culture results. In most cases, simple drainage is adequate to control the infection. Unresolved sepsis should, however, prompt imaging assessment to ensure that the drain or drains are positioned adequately; in some cases multiple drainage catheters will be necessary, or in rare cases, percutaneous biliary drainage may be required to divert bile flow away from the area of injury.

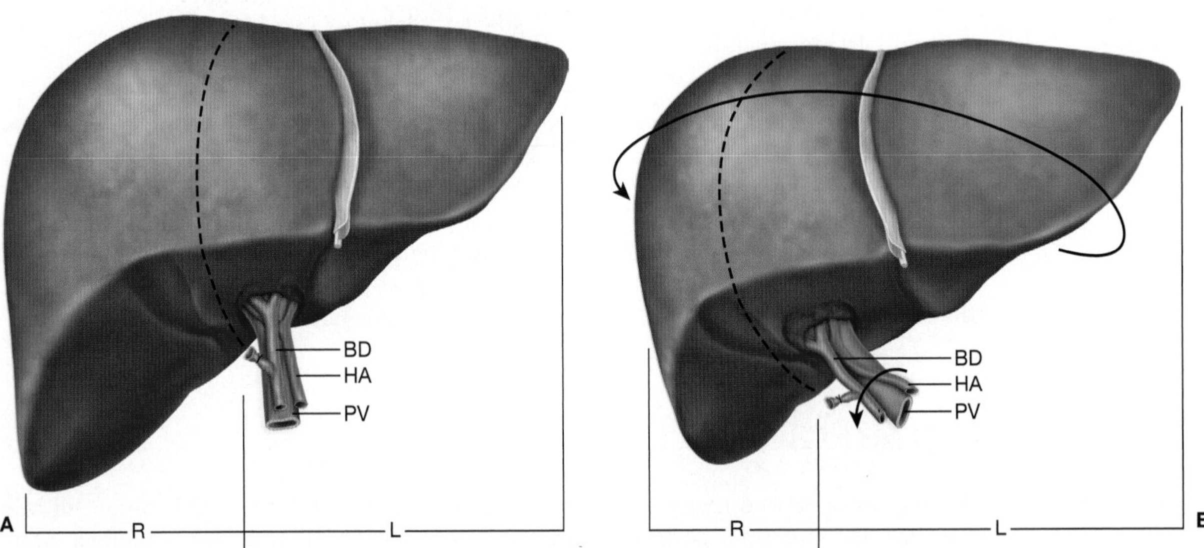


**Figure 17.2** **A:** Standard relationship of the porta hepatis structures, with the bile duct (*BD*) anterior to the hepatic artery (*HA*) and portal vein (*PV*). **B:** With atrophy of the right liver, the compensatory hypertrophy of the left liver leads to counter-clockwise rotation of the porta hepatis structures. In extreme cases, the bile duct may come to lie posterior and lateral to the portal vein. The principal resection plane (IE, Cantlie's line) separating the right (*R*) and left (*L*) hemi-livers is indicated by the *dotted line.*

Once adequate drainage is established, the next preoperative phase is defining the location of the leak (minor injury (an open cystic duct stump or open biliary radical in the gallbladder fossa (duct of Lushka)) versus major injury (right hepatic or common hepatic duct laceration)). Endoscopic retrograde cholangiogram (ERC) has the advantage of being less invasive than percutaneous cholangiography and, in the case of a minor leak, can provide definitive therapy. On the other hand, ERC will not define the proximal biliary tree when there has been transection of the bile duct. For cystic duct stump leaks and duct of Lushka leaks, a transampullary stent may facilitate biliary drainage through the sphincter of Oddi and may be enough to allow the patient to heal the leak, although the added benefit of this procedure above and beyond drainage of the biloma has not been shown. Major lacerations or complete transections to the common hepatic duct or right hepatic duct will not be amenable to endoscopic therapy and will ultimately require biliary-enteric anastomosis. Since ERC will usually identify the site of the injury but will not adequately define the proximal biliary anatomy, as clips are usually obstructing retrograde filling, a complete cholangiogram must be obtained with either MRC or percutaneous cholangiography. Obtaining a detailed outline of the proximal anatomy prior to definitive reconstruction is of paramount importance for preoperative planning.

Although the preoperative placement of a percutaneous biliary drain is controversial, many authors utilize this technique. These drains may (1) aid in the manual palpation/identification of the common bile duct at the time of exploration, and (2) simplify the placement of transhepatic catheters. If this approach is used, at least one small (7 to 10 French) biliary drain is placed as close to the site of the injury as possible. If the biliary injury is above the bifurcation of the bile ducts and definitive repair will require a double barrel reconstruction, two biliary drains should be placed: one in the left system and one in the right biliary system. The timing of the biliary drain placement is dictated by the degree of sepsis at presentation. If the sepsis or the ongoing leak can be controlled with subhepatic drains, percutaneous biliary drain placement is not required at the time of presentation and will only add risk of preoperative biliary sepsis. An MRC may be used to define the anatomy and the biliary drain is placed immediately prior the definitive repair. If subhepatic drains do not control the biliary sepsis or the bile leak, the biliary drainage catheters may be required at the time of presentation.

As a result, comprehensive preoperative planning for major bile duct injuries requires:

- Complete control/evacuation of peritoneal sepsis and bile
- Accurate definition of the site of the injury (ERC)
- Complete identification of the proximal biliary anatomy (MRC or PTC)
- Placement of percutaneous biliary catheter/drain(s) (PTD) in selected patients

In patients who present with biliary stricture or complete obstruction of some element of the biliary system days to weeks after cholecystectomy, the overall strategy is similar. For patients with a stricture and symptoms of cholangitis, biliary decompression should be performed and is usually best accomplished with by transhepatic percutaneous catheter placement. In selected cases, endoscopic biliary stents can be places to decompress the proximal biliary system. In these situations nonoperative balloon dilation with long-term stenting is an option for management.

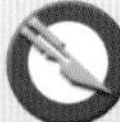

## SURGICAL TECHNIQUE

The goal of operative management for any biliary injury is the reestablishment of bile flow into the proximal gastrointestinal tract in a manner that prevents sludge, stone formation, cholangitis, stricture and cirrhosis related to prolonged biliary obstruction. Invariably, there is loss of bile duct length as a result of periductal fibrosis associated with the injury, and simple excision of a bile duct stricture with end-to-end ductal anastomosis or repair is rarely technically feasible and frequently unsuccessful even if

possible. Consequently, principles for a successful biliary-enteric (Roux-en-Y hepatico-jejunostomy) reconstruction include:

- Exposure of healthy proximal bile duct that provides drainage of the entire liver
- Preparation of a suitable section of intestine that can be anastomosed without tension
- Creation of a biliary-enteric anastomosis that approximates healthy biliary mucosa to enteric mucosa

## Positioning and Incision

A midline upper abdominal or extended right subcortal incision in a supine patient provides adequate access. A fixed upper abdominal retraction system (i.e., Thompson) is utilized (see Figs. 18.7, 19.3 and 21.5).

## Dissection Technique

Following a complete Kocher maneuver, the porta hepatis structures are carefully dissected using a combination of electrocautery, careful sharp dissection and digital palpation. Scarring in this area can be extensive even 6 weeks post injury and the close proximity between the bile duct and portal vein places the portal vein at risk. If a biliary catheter has been placed, it may help to identify the common hepatic duct. In this dissection, the duct is carefully separated from the portal vein and transected at a point above the level of the stricture (Fig. 17.3). The bile duct proximal to the injury is carefully dissected circumferentially in a cephalad direction for a distance of approximately 5 mm. Excessive dissection should be avoided to prevent vascular compromise to this segment of the duct. The inside of the duct is inspected and the presence of healthy appearing biliary mucosa confirmed. Ensuring that the mucosa at the level of the reconstruction is healthy is probably the most important step in the reconstruction to prevent late stricturing at the biliary anastomosis. In our operative approach, the end of the proximal dissection is ultimately determined by the appearance of the mucosa inside the bile duct. If the mucosa at the site of initial transaction is not normal, further dissection is undertaken to clear the proximal bile duct from surrounding scar and the bile duct debrided until healthy mucosa is evident. An intraoperative cholangiogram may be helpful if the biliary anatomy is not clear.

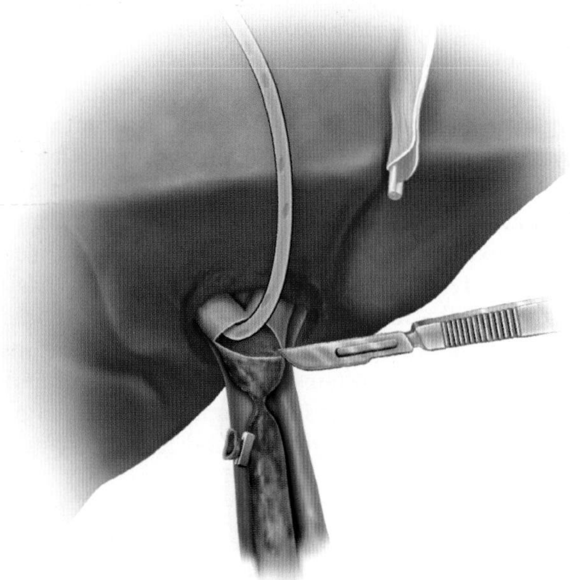

**Figure 17.3** Dissection in the porta hepatis with isolation of the bile duct, which is prepared for transection above the level of the injury.

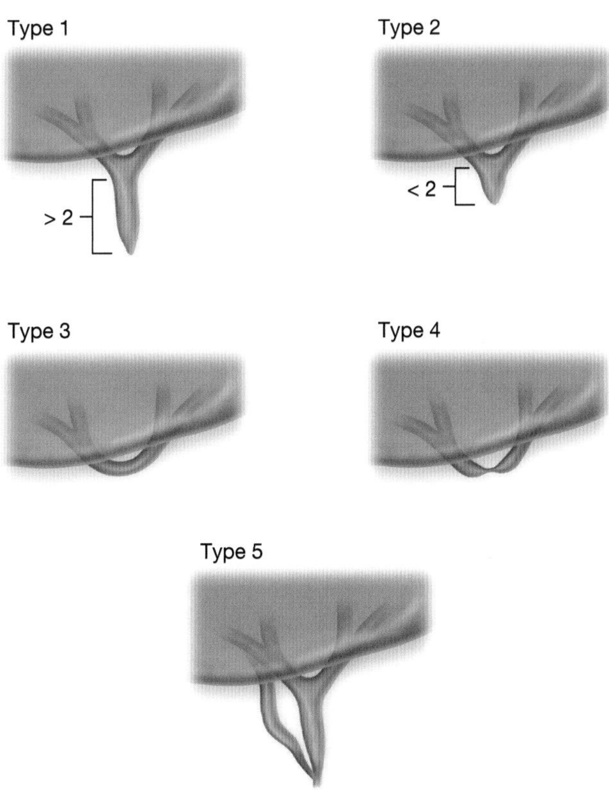


**Figure 17.4** The Bismuth classification of biliary strictures. Type 1—common hepatic duct injury at least 2 cm below the level of the biliary confluence; Type 2—common hepatic duct injury less than 2 cm below the biliary confluence; Type 3—injury extends to but does not involve the biliary confluence (ie, right and left biliary systems communicate); Type 4—injury involves the biliary confluence (ie, right and left systems do not communicate); Type 5—low entry right sectoral hepatic duct injury (see also Fig. 17.9).

## Technical and Anatomical Considerations for Proximal Biliary Tree Injuries

The details of exposure of the bile duct above the area of injury and the reconstruction technique may vary depending on the particular anatomic features of the stricture/injury, its location, as well as the hepatic anatomy itself. When there is greater than 2 cm length of healthy common hepatic duct reserved below the stricture (Bismuth I) (Fig. 17.4) and the scarring in the porta hepatis is not prohibitive, exposure followed by a simple end-to-side biliary-enteric anastomosis may be straightforward and will suffice. In these situations, particularly when the duct is dilated, the surgeon may use a variety of anastomotic techniques; however, in the setting of a decompressed proximal biliary tree, a technique that employs fine, interrupted, absorbable sutures is recommended.

In many cases, identification of the bile duct within a densely scarred porta hepatis is difficult and dangerous. Moreover, for more proximal injuries (Bismuth II and III), such dissection is unnecessary, since the distal bile duct cannot be used for anastomosis. The safest and most reliable approach is to first expose the left hepatic duct by lowering the hilar plate at the base of segment IV (Fig. 17.5A and B). The left hepatic duct has a constant and long extrahepatic course along the undersurface of segment IV to the umbilical fissure (Fig. 17.6). In addition, this area usually has not been disturbed and often is free of dense adhesions. With the left hepatic duct identified, dissection toward the right exposes the biliary confluence. Exposure is improved by dividing the bridge of hepatic parenchyma that often connects segments III and IV at the base of the umbilical fissure (Fig. 17.7). Strictures that completely separate the right and left systems (Bismuth IV) may require separate right and left biliary-enteric anastomoses (see Fig. 17.15).

When a suitable healthy duct length outside the hepatic parenchyma cannot be obtained, exposure of the intrahepatic biliary system is required. Intraoperative ultrasound may be helpful in this setting. The right biliary system may be accessed after

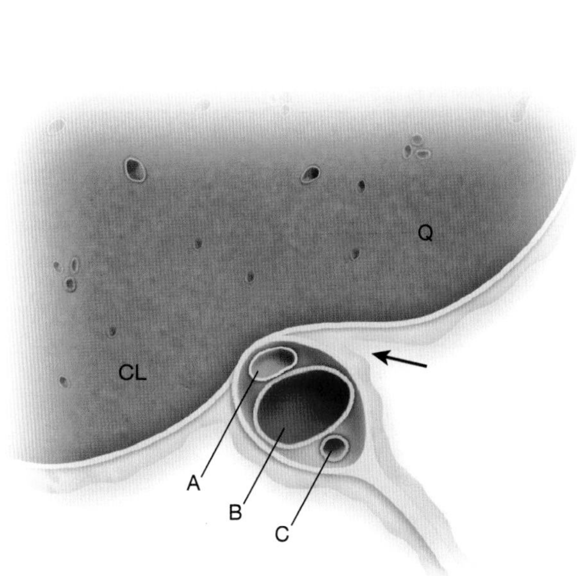


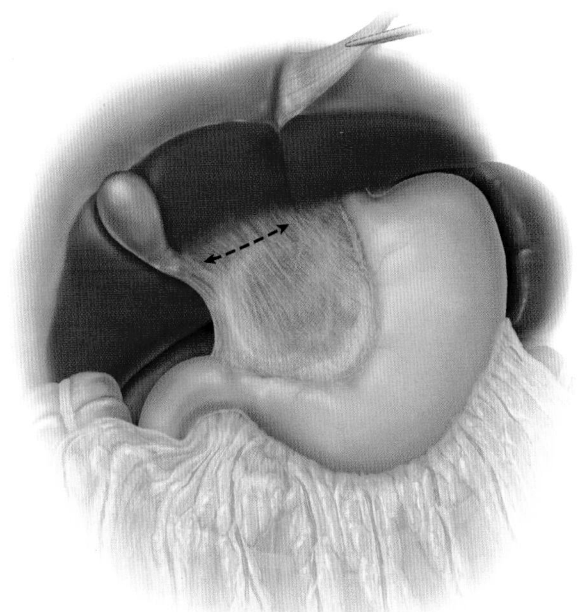

A

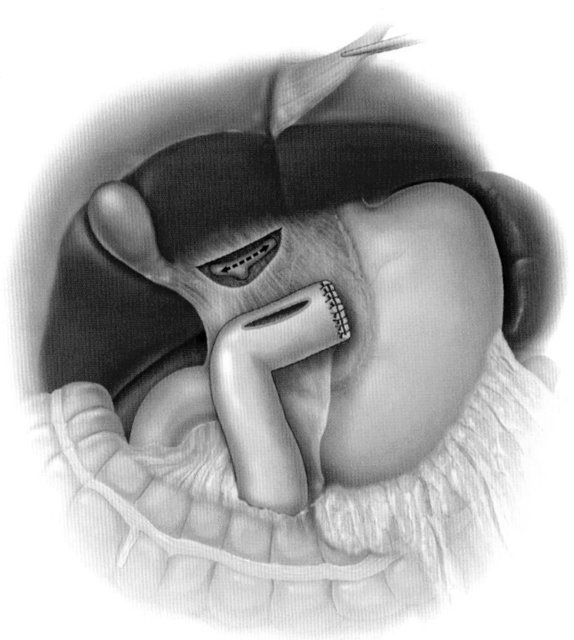

B

Figure 17.5 **A:** Left—sagittal view showing the relationship of the left hepatic duct (*A*), left portal vein (*B*), and hepatic artery (*C*) at the base of the quadrate lobe (i.e., segment IVB (*Q*). CL—caudate lobe. dissection at the base of segment IV, as indicated by the *arrow,* lowers the hilar plate and allows exposure of the left hepatic duct. Right—with the liver is elevated upward, the hilar plate is lowered by dissection along the base of segment IV (*dotted arrow*). Note that the round ligament, which enters the liver at the umbilical fissure, has been divided and is held upward with a clamp. **B:** After lowering the hilar plate, the left hepatic duct is exposed below at the base of segment IV. Careful dissection to the patient's left allows full exposure of the duct to its entry into the umbilical fissure, while dissection toward the patient's right provides access to the biliary confluence and the right hepatic duct.

performing a small hepatotomy in the plane of the gallbladder fossa, which allows access to the right anterior sectoral hepatic duct as a possible anastomotic target (Fig. 17.8). This approach is technically demanding and is further complicated by the more variable anatomy of the right biliary system (Fig. 17.9).A much more reliable intrahepatic target is the segment III duct, which is exposed by first dividing the hepatic parenchymal bridge of variable thickness connecting segments II and III at the base of the umbilical fissure (17.10A; see also Fig. 17.7). The segment III duct is then approached after incising the liver parenchyma just to the left of the falciform ligament (17.10A) and separating it from the hepatic artery and portal vein within the segment III pedicle (Fig. 17.10B, C).

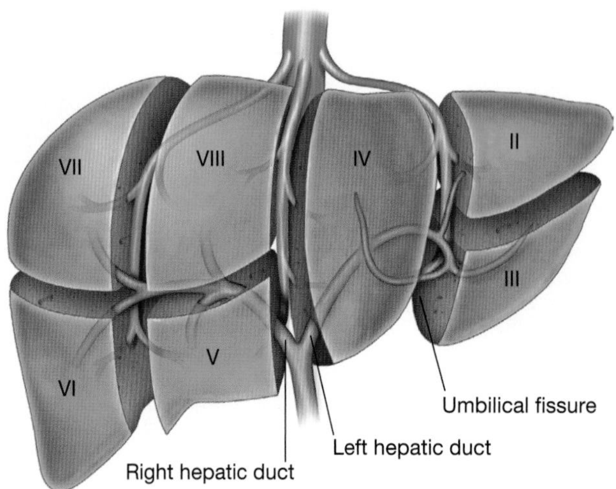


**Figure 17.6** Exploded view of the liver segmental anatomy illustrating the typical long extrahepatic course of the left hepatic duct.

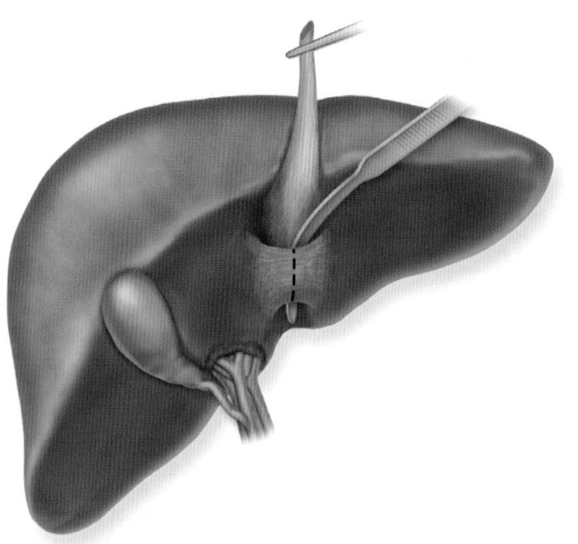

**Figure 17.7** The bridge of tissue connecting segments II and III is divided to expose the base of the umbilical fissure. In some patients, this connection is a well-developed bridge of liver parenchyma, while in others it is merely a fibrotic band.

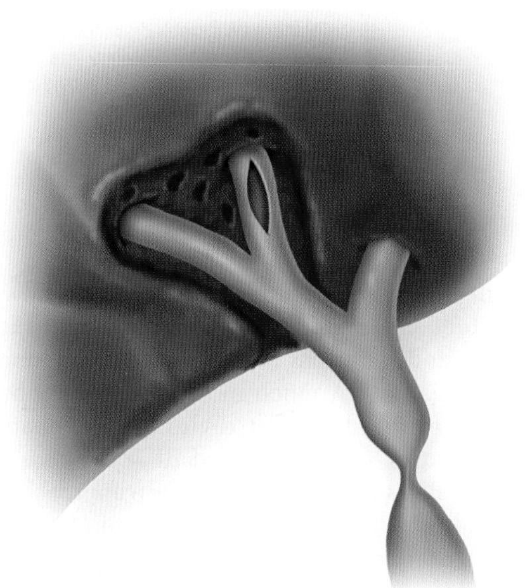

**Figure 17.8** A hepatotomy in the plane of the gallbladder fossa has been made to expose the intrahepatic portion of the right hepatic duct and its anterior and posterior sectoral branches. In this illustration, an incision has been made in the anterior sectoral hepatic duct in preparation for anastomosis to a Roux-en-Y jejunal loop.

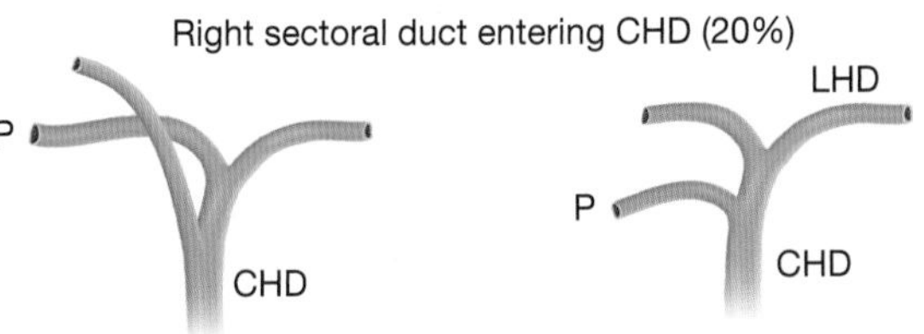


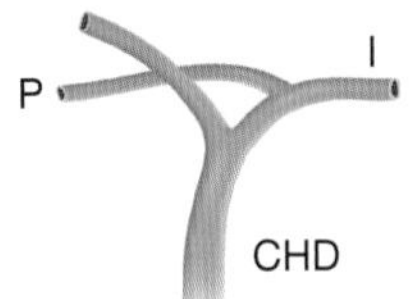


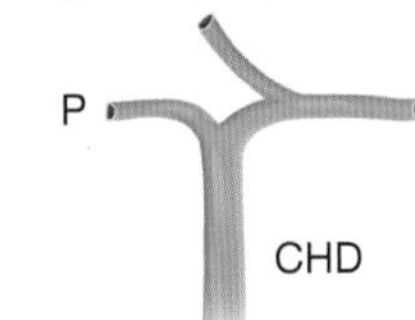


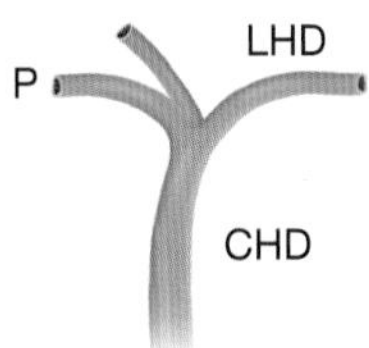


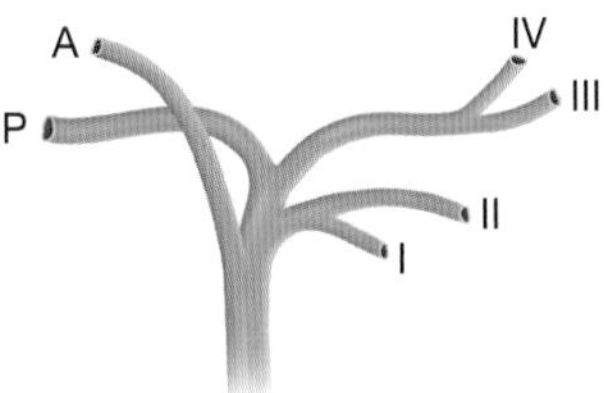


**Figure 17.9** The most common variations in proximal biliary anatomy, which most frequently involve the right biliary system. CHD, common hepatic duct; LHD, left hepatic duct; P, right posterior sectoral hepatic duct; A, right anterior sectoral hepatic duct; I, segment I (caudate) duct; II, segment II duct; III, segment III duct; IV, segment IV duct.

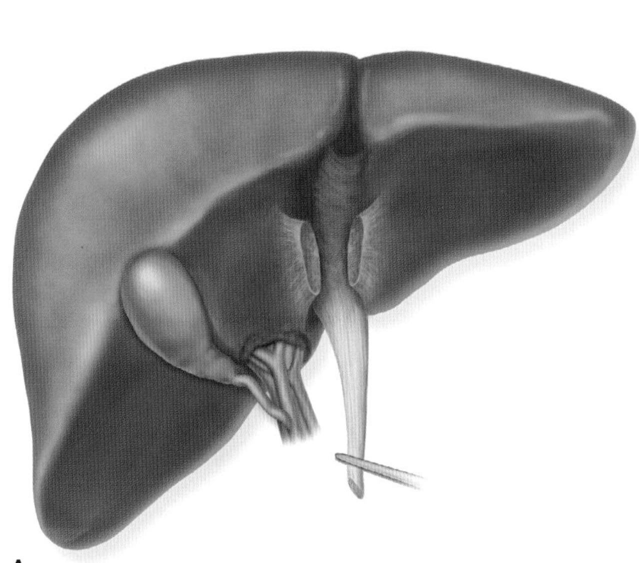


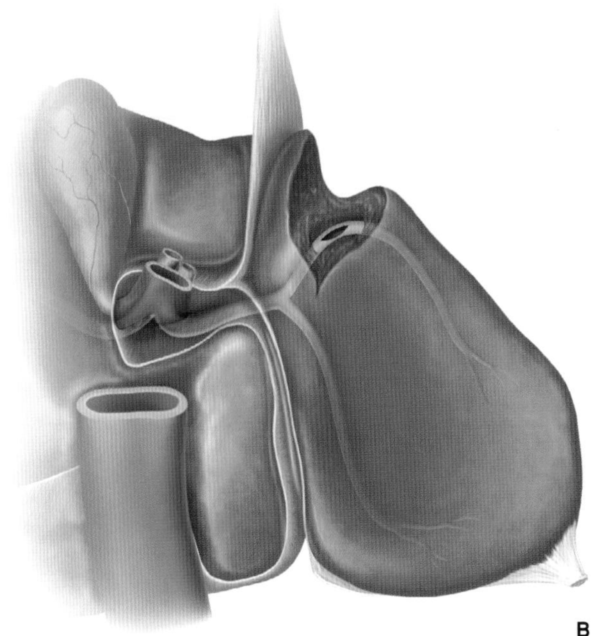


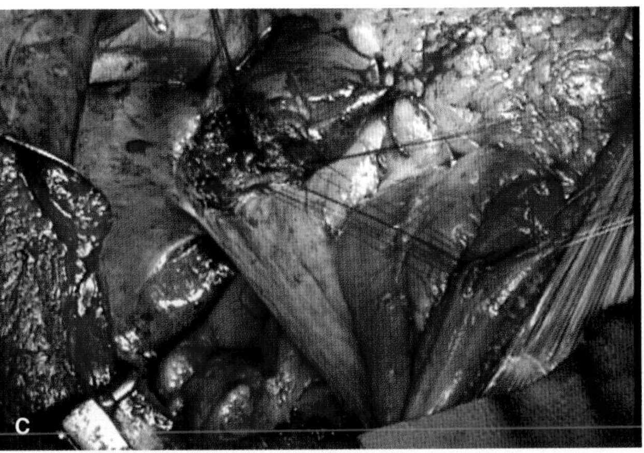


**Figure 17.10** **A:** The round ligament is retracted downward and the parenchymal bridge attaching segments II and III has been divided. The segment III duct can be exposed by incising the liver parenchyma just to the left of the round and falciform ligaments, along the hashed line A. **B:** After incising the liver parenchyma, the segment III duct is identified within the segment III pedicle and prepared for anastomosis to a Roux-en-Y jejunal loop. **C:** Intraoperative view show ing exposure of the segment III duct through a hepatotomy to the left of the falciform ligament. Sutures have been placed in preparation for anastomosis (see Fig. 17.13).

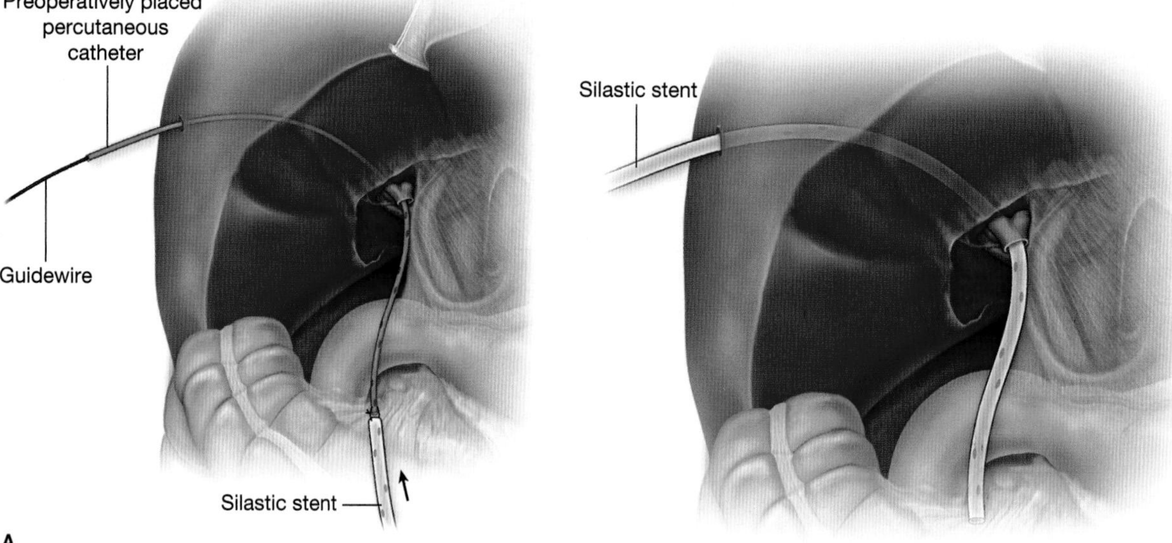


Figure 17.11 Roux-en-Y hepaticojejunostomy performed in the presence of a transhepatic/transanastomotic stent. The biliary stent (placed preoperatively) is cannulated with a guidewire **(A)** and exchanged for a silastic catheter **(B)**. Care must be taken to ensure that the sideholes are positioned to reside within the liver parenchyma or the Roux-en-Y loop of jejunum.

## Anastomosis and Biliary Stent Technique

An end-to-side Roux-en-Y hepaticojejunostomy is preferred by all authors. First, the distal end of the bile duct must be oversewn with nonabsorbable monofilament. When a transhepatic/trans-anastomotic stent is utilized, the percutaneous biliary drain is exchanged for a transhepatic silastic catheter before constructing the anastomosis. It is sized to be as large as the bile duct will allow (14 to 16 French). The sideholes (along 40% of the catheter) are left to reside within the intrahepatic biliary tree and the portion of the Roux-en-Y jejunal limb used for the biliary anastomosis (Fig. 17.11A, B). The end of the stent without the sideholes exits through the hepatic parenchyma and is brought out through a stab wound in the upper anterior abdominal wall. More specifically, once the bile duct is opened proximal to the site of the injury and the preoperative biliary catheter(s) identified, a radiologic guide wire is placed into the catheter(s). A series of progressively larger Coude catheters may then be passed over the guidewire(s) to dilate the biliary system and appropriately large soft silastic stents are then placed over the guidewires. After the stents have been placed, a 50 cm Roux-en-Y limb is prepared and the posterior row of the hepaticojejunostomy constructed. The distal end of the catheter is then fed down the roux limb and the anterior row of the anastomosis completed. The anastomosis is completed as an end-to-side hepaticojejunostomy with interrupted 4-0 or 5-0 absorbable monofilament suture (Fig. 17.12A–D). Closed suction drains are placed behind the anastomosis.

Repairs performed high at the bifurcation and/or to intrahepatic ducts (segment III or anterior sectoral duct) are best completed using a technique described by Blumgart and Kelley, as it allows precise placement of all sutures without steric hindrance from the bowel. This technique first requires interrupted insertion of the anterior row of the anastomosis on the bile duct side (4-0 or 5-0 absorbable sutures) (Fig. 17.13A). This suture line is then retracted superiorly while the posterior row of interrupted stitches is placed (Fig. 17.13B). Once the intestine is parachuted down and the posterior row of sutures is secured, the previously placed anterior wall sutures are then passed through the intestine and serially tied (Fig. 17.13C). Fig. 17.14 shows intraoperative views of the anastomosis at various stages of completion. This technique can be adapted to situations that require anastomosis to multiple ducts (Fig. 17.15). Closed suction drains are again placed dependently to the anastomosis. The abdomen is closed in a standard fashion and the patient is returned to the postanesthesia care unit.

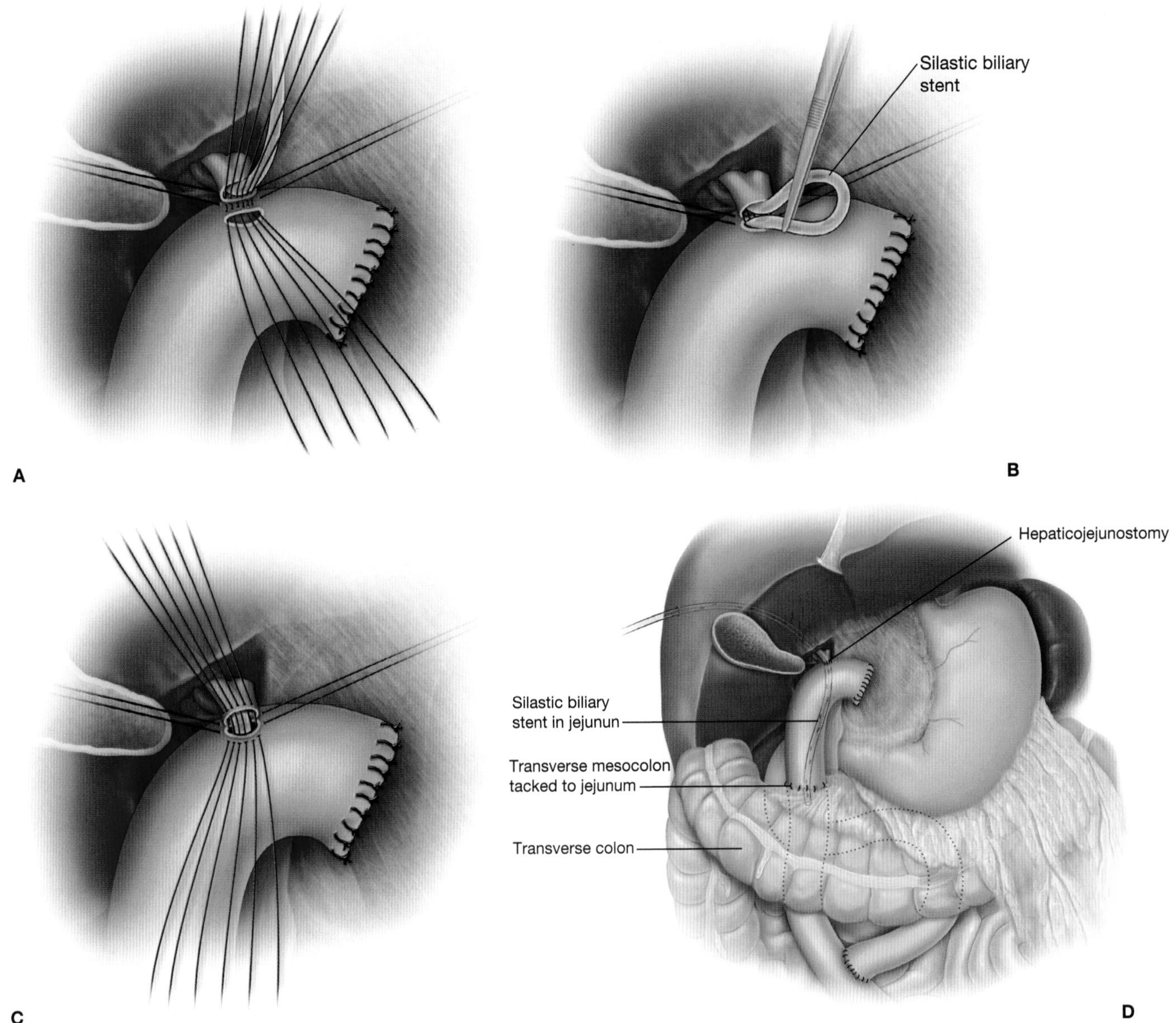


Figure 17.12 Completion of the anastomosis in the presence of a transhepatic/transanastomotic stent. **A:** The posterior row of fine, interrupted, absorbable sutures is placed from the bile duct to the jejunum; **B:** After securing the posterior row, the distal portion of the stent is passed into the lumen of the bowel with a forceps; **C:** The anterior row of interrupted sutures is then placed and serially tied; **D:** The completed anastomosis; the upper end of the silastic catheter is brought out through the skin.

## POSTOPERATIVE MANAGEMENT

The patients initial postoperative stay is often best suited for a monitored bed with one-on-one nursing. Hemodynamic monitoring and fluid management is often not challenging and the complexity of care is often associated with management of multiple stents and drains. Postoperatively, if silastic stents are used they are left to gravity drainage for 3 to 4 days. A postoperative cholangiogram is then performed and, if that study is demonstrates no extravasation of contrast, the stents are internalized, drains removed and the diet advanced. The stents are generally left in place for 3 to 6 months to allow for follow-up cholangiography and to prevent stricturing as healing occurs.

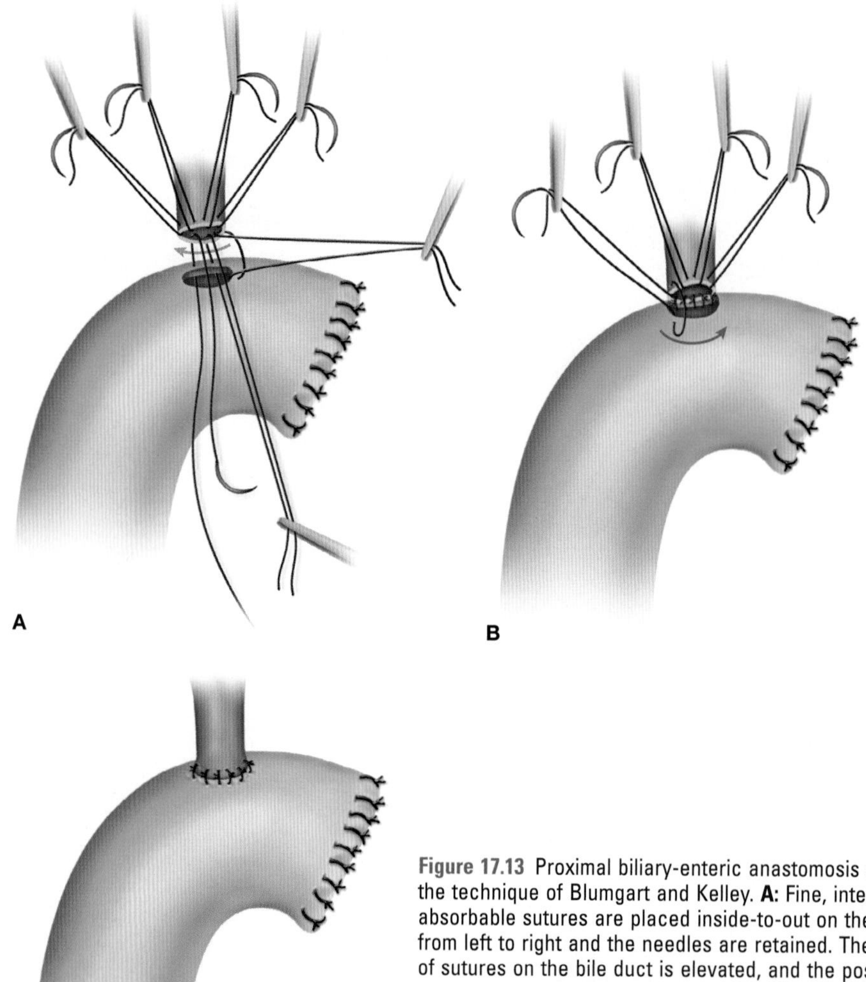


C

Figure 17.13 Proximal biliary-enteric anastomosis according to the technique of Blumgart and Kelley. **A:** Fine, interrupted, absorbable sutures are placed inside-to-out on the bile duct, from left to right and the needles are retained. The anterior row of sutures on the bile duct is elevated, and the posterior row is then placed from the jejunum to the bile duct, again from left to right. **B:** The jejunum is then parachuted down, and the posterior row is secured; the previously placed anterior sutures are then serially passed through the jejunal wall, from right to left. **C:** These sutures are then tied to complete the anastomosis.

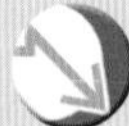

## COMPLICATIONS

In the large series from the Johns Hopkins Hospital, the rate of postoperative complications was 43%. The most common complications included wound infections (8%), cholangitis (5.7%), and intra-abdominal abscess (2.9%). The postoperative mortality rate was 1.7%. Early postoperative cholangiography revealed an anastomotic leak in 4.6% and extravasation at the liver dome-stent site in 10.3% of patients. None of the patients required reexploration postoperatively. Postoperative intervention included percutaneous abscess drainage in nine patients (5.1%) and stent replacement in four patients (2.3%).

## RESULTS

The largest prospective series examining long-term outcomes following surgery for post cholecystectomy stricture is a report of the senior author's experience at the Johns Hopkins Hospital during the decade of the 1990s. In that experience, 60 out of 156

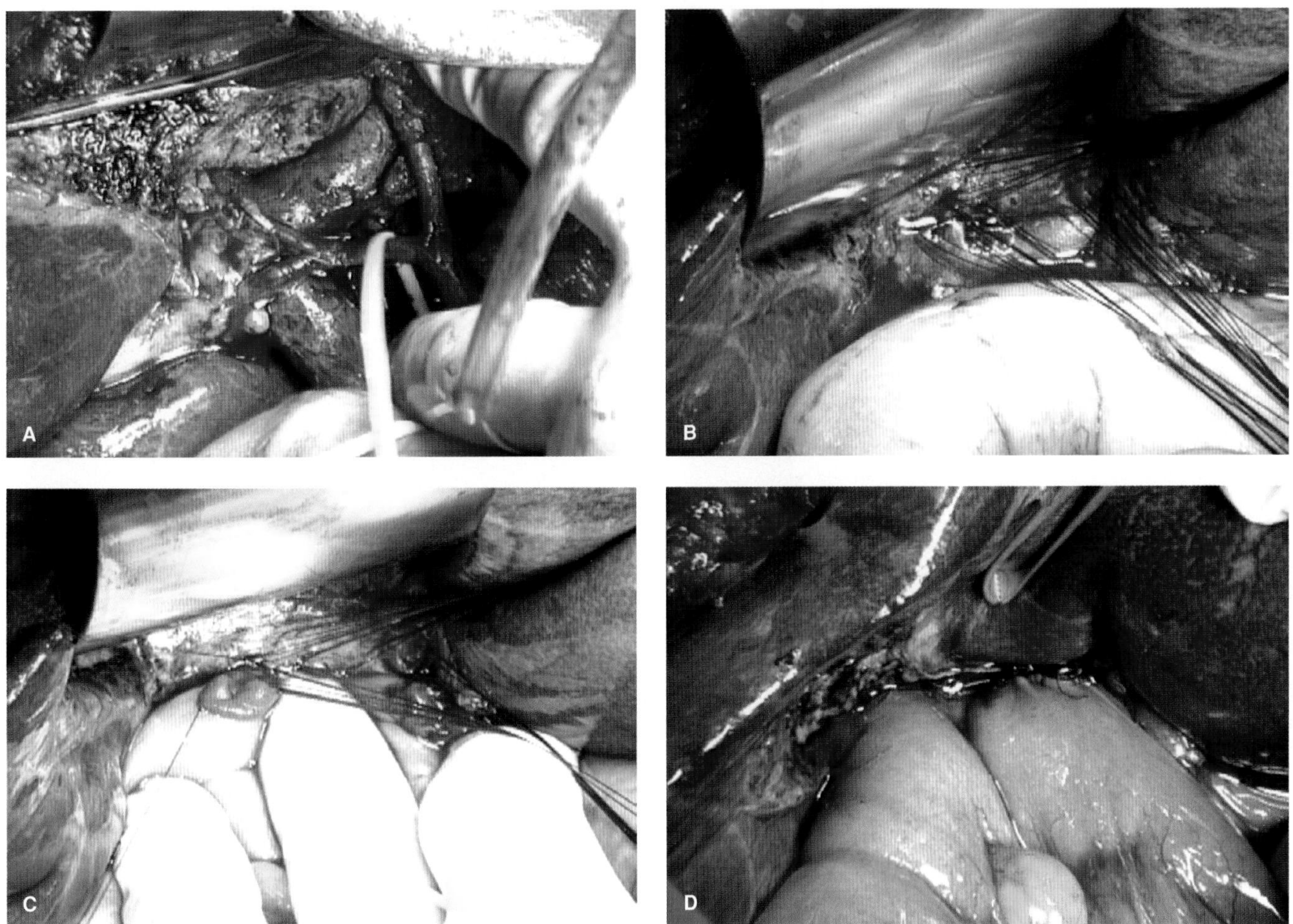


**Figure 17.14** Intraoperative views of the anastomotic technique. **A**: The transected bile duct is readied for anastomosis; note that a loop has been passed around the hepatic artery; **B**: the anterior and posterior row of sutures have been placed, as above; **C**: The jejunum has been parachuted down the posterior row, and the sutures secured; **D**: The completed anastomosis.

patients had undergone a previous attempt at repair. Eight patients had undergone more than one prior attempt at repair. The mean follow-up in this series was 57.5 months. One hundred and forty-two patients had completed treatment and were available for evaluation. Of those, only 13 patients (9.2%) had recurrent stricture. The success rate associated with the surgical repair for biliary injury incurred during laparoscopic cholecystectomy in particular was in excess of 94% and was significantly better than the results for repair of strictures following other operations or trauma. Each of those that failed underwent either surgical revision or balloon dilation. Only three patients continued to require long-term biliary stents to prevent symptoms of biliary obstruction and/or cholangitis. Therefore of the 142 patients who completed therapy, including subsequent interventional procedures, a successful outcome without stents was ultimately achieved in 139 (98%).

Most studies also demonstrate complete return of the individual to functional health following their operative repair. One such comparison was performed in patients from the Johns Hopkins series who had undergone successful surgical reconstruction of a bile duct injury to age-matched healthy controls and to age-matched individuals who had undergone recent prior uncomplicated laparoscopic cholecystectomy. The findings demonstrate that the patients having successful bile duct reconstruction are not statistically different from controls in the assessment of their quality of life in physical and social functional domains but that they score less well in the psychological domains of the assessment tool.

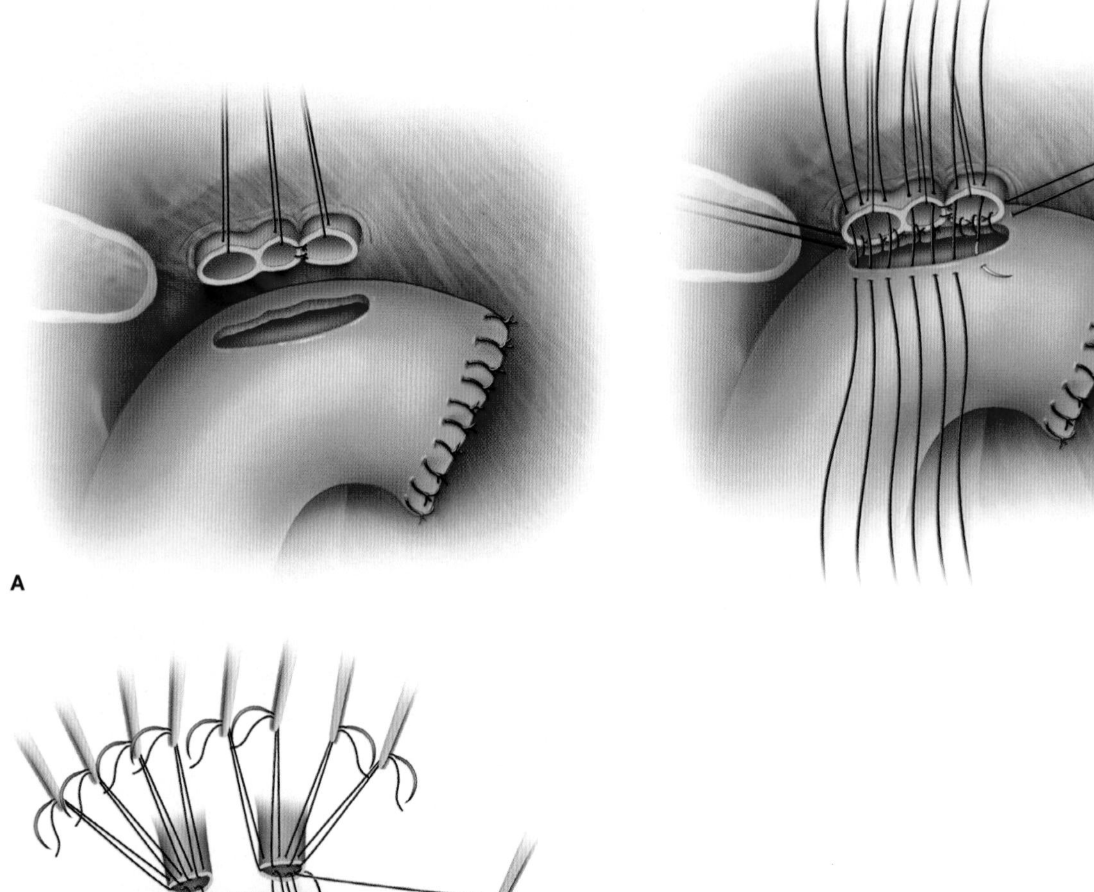


**Figure 17.15** Adaptation of the anastomotic technique to multiple hepatic ducts. **A:** When multiple ducts are in close proximity, they are approximated with sutures, and the anastomosis created to a single jejunal orifice, as outlined above. **B:** When a single common channel not possible, the separated ducts are treated as if single, rather than attempting the usually very difficult, if not impossible, approach of completing one anastomosis followed by the other. The anterior row of sutures is placed to all exposed ducts, and the posterior sutures are placed and tied; the anterior row is then completed, as described above.

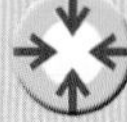

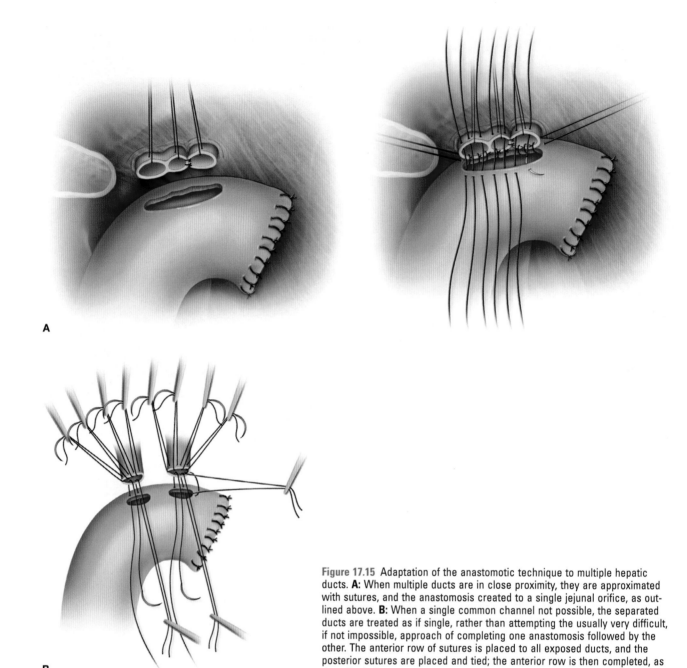

## CONCLUSIONS

Successful repairs for bile duct injuries require a careful and complete preoperative diagnostic and nonoperative therapeutic work-up that includes (1) complete control/evacuation of peritoneal sepsis and bile, (2) accurate definition of the site of the injury (ERC), (3) complete identification of the proximal biliary anatomy (MRC or PTC) and (4) placement of percutaneous intrabiliary catheter(s) (PTD). A durable repair can then be obtained in the setting of an experienced hepatobiliary surgeon and strict adherence to the basic principles of (1) exposure of healthy proximal bile duct that provides drainage of the entire liver, (2) preparation of a suitable section of intestine that can be anastomosed without tension, and (3) creation of a biliary-enteric anastomosis that approximates healthy biliary mucosa to enteric mucosa.

## Recommended References and Readings


Blumgart LH. Hilar and intrahepatic biliary anastomosis. *Surg Clin North Am.* 1994;74:845–863.

Branum G, Schmitt C, Baillie J, et al. Management of major biliary complications after laparoscopic cholecystectomy. *Ann Surg.* 1993;17:532.

Hall JG, Pappas TN. Current management of biliary strictures. *J Gastrointest Surg.* 2004;8:1098.

Lillemoe KD, Melton GB, Cameron JL, et al. Postoperative bile duct strictures: management and outcome in the 1990s. *Ann Surg.* 2000;232:430.

Melton GB, Lillemoe KD, Cameron JL, et al. Major bile duct injuries associated with laparoscopic cholecystectomy: Effect on quality of life. *Ann Surg.* 2002;235:888.

Mercado MA, Chan C, Orozco H, et al. Acute bile duct injury. The need for a high repair. *Surg Endosc.* 2003;17:1351–1355.

Sicklick JK, Camp MS, Lillemoe KD, et al. Surgical management of bile duct injuries sustained during laparoscopic cholecystectomy: Perioperative results in 200 patients. *Ann Surg.* 2005;241: 786.

Silva MA, Coldham C, Mayer AD, et al. Specialist outreach service for on-table repair of iatrogenic bile duct injuries - a new kind of “traveling surgeon”. *Ann R Coll Surg Engl.* 2008;90:243–246.

Stewart L, Way LW. Bile duct injuries during laparoscopic cholecystectomy. *Arch Surg.* 1995;130:1123.

Strasberg SM, Helton WS. An analytical review of vasculobiliary injury in laparoscopic and open cholecystectomy. *HPB.* 2010;13:1–14.

# 18 Hepatic Resection: General Considerations

Jean-Nicolas Vauthey and Junichi Shindoh

## Introduction

Resection is the first-line treatment in selected patients with primary or metastatic hepatic malignancies. In recent decades, refinements in surgical techniques and in perioperative patient care have improved the safety of liver resection; however, the most important factor influencing outcomes after liver resection is the surgeon's knowledge of the basic surgical principles pertaining to the procedure. Postoperative morbidity and mortality rates can be reduced by proper patient selection, attention to liver anatomy and volumetry, and use of the optimal approach and technique for resection. At large-volume centers, the 90-day mortality rates after liver resection are now less than 5%, and the rate of complete resections with negative margins is approaching 90%. These rates are not likely to be substantially further improved, especially as the limits of resectability are continually being pushed; therefore low morbidity rates and early recovery will have to be considered as the new primary endpoints. In this chapter, we report the general principles pertaining to the safe and complete resection of liver tumors.

## Preoperative Assessment

In recent years, the eligibility criteria for liver resection have been expanded to include patients not previously deemed to be surgical candidates, such as those with multiple bilobar liver metastases from colorectal cancer and those with large or multinodular hepatocellular carcinoma (HCC). However, the current definition of resectability still requires that the surgeon be able to completely remove the tumor while preserving a sufficient remnant of healthy liver tissue to limit the risk of postoperative liver dysfunction. This oncosurgical definition necessitates attention to (1) the extent of the tumor and (2) the quality and volume of the anticipated remnant liver after negative margins are achieved.

### Evaluating Tumor Extent

In recent years, advances in imaging technology have made the preoperative evaluation of liver tumors more precise, contributing to both the improvement and safety of liver resection.

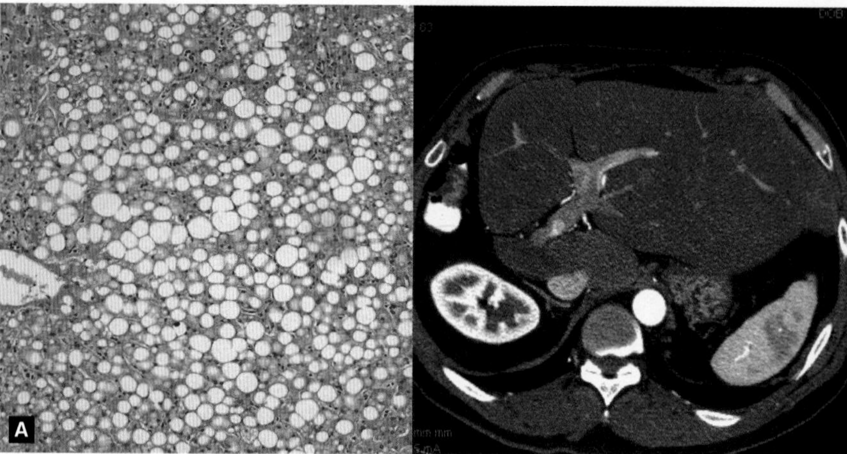


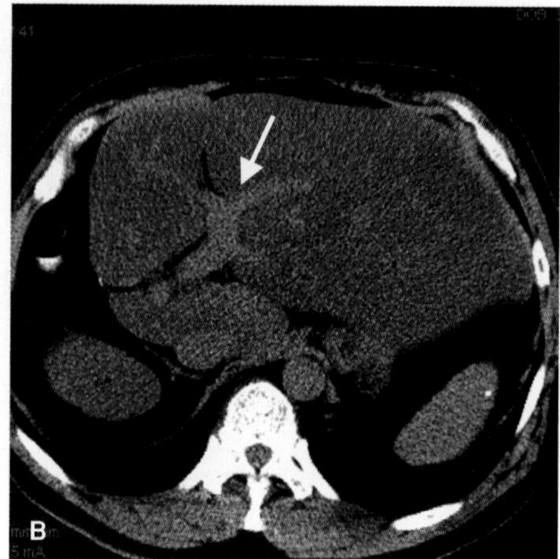


Figure 18.1 Hepatic steatosis or fatty liver. **A:** Severe macrovesicular steatosis, histologic appearance **(left)** and features on contrast-enhanced CT imaging **(right)**. Note the perfusion differences between the liver and spleen. **B:** Unenhanced CT is considered more reliable for assessing the degree of steatosis. This scan shows severe (grade 3) macrovesicular steatosis. Note that the unenhanced vessels are higher in attenuation than the surrounding liver parenchyma.

Helical computed tomography (CT) with a liver protocol (quadruple phase with rapid injection of 150 ml of intravenous contrast material and slice thickness of 2.5 to 5.0 mm through the liver) can accurately evaluate the extent of the tumor or tumors in the liver and each tumor's relationship with the biliary tract and vascular structures. Three-dimensional reconstruction of CT images can be used to better assess the liver's segmental anatomy and volumetry. Chest CT has replaced chest x-ray as the preferred modality for identifying lung metastases in patients with liver tumors. The routine use of enhanced magnetic resonance imaging (MRI) has generally not been recommended because MRI has not been demonstrated to be more accurate than CT for most patients and because it is less reliable for detecting extrahepatic disease, particularly in the chest or peritoneum. However, MRI should be performed for further characterization of presumably benign or atypical liver tumors or when the contrast agents used for CT are contraindicated. In addition, new MRI contrast agents are potentially very useful for delineating hepatic disease extent, particularly in the setting of hepatic steatosis (Figs. 18.1, 18.2).

Because of the improvements in image resolution mentioned above, laparoscopy is less frequently indicated to assess the extent of liver tumors, although additional hepatic disease may well be identified and is still used in selected patients to evaluate for extrahepatic disease, chronic liver disease, or hepatic injury associated with extended chemotherapy.

Although recommended by some surgeons as part of preoperative evaluation, positron emission tomography (PET) is not used routinely for primary liver cancer or liver metastases at all centers. Importantly, PET-CT should not replace high-quality CT imaging combined with interpretation by a radiologist with hepatobiliary expertise. PET-CT is not useful in patients who have received preoperative chemotherapy for colorectal cancer liver metastases because the response to chemotherapy is associated with decreased PET sensitivity.

## Evaluating Determinants of Postoperative Liver Function

Liver function after liver resection depends on the quality of the liver parenchyma, the volume of the future liver remnant (FLR), and the regenerative capacity of the liver. The risk of postoperative liver failure remains high after major or extended liver resection. This risk should be estimated preoperatively to determine whether resection is safe and to optimize the postoperative outcome.

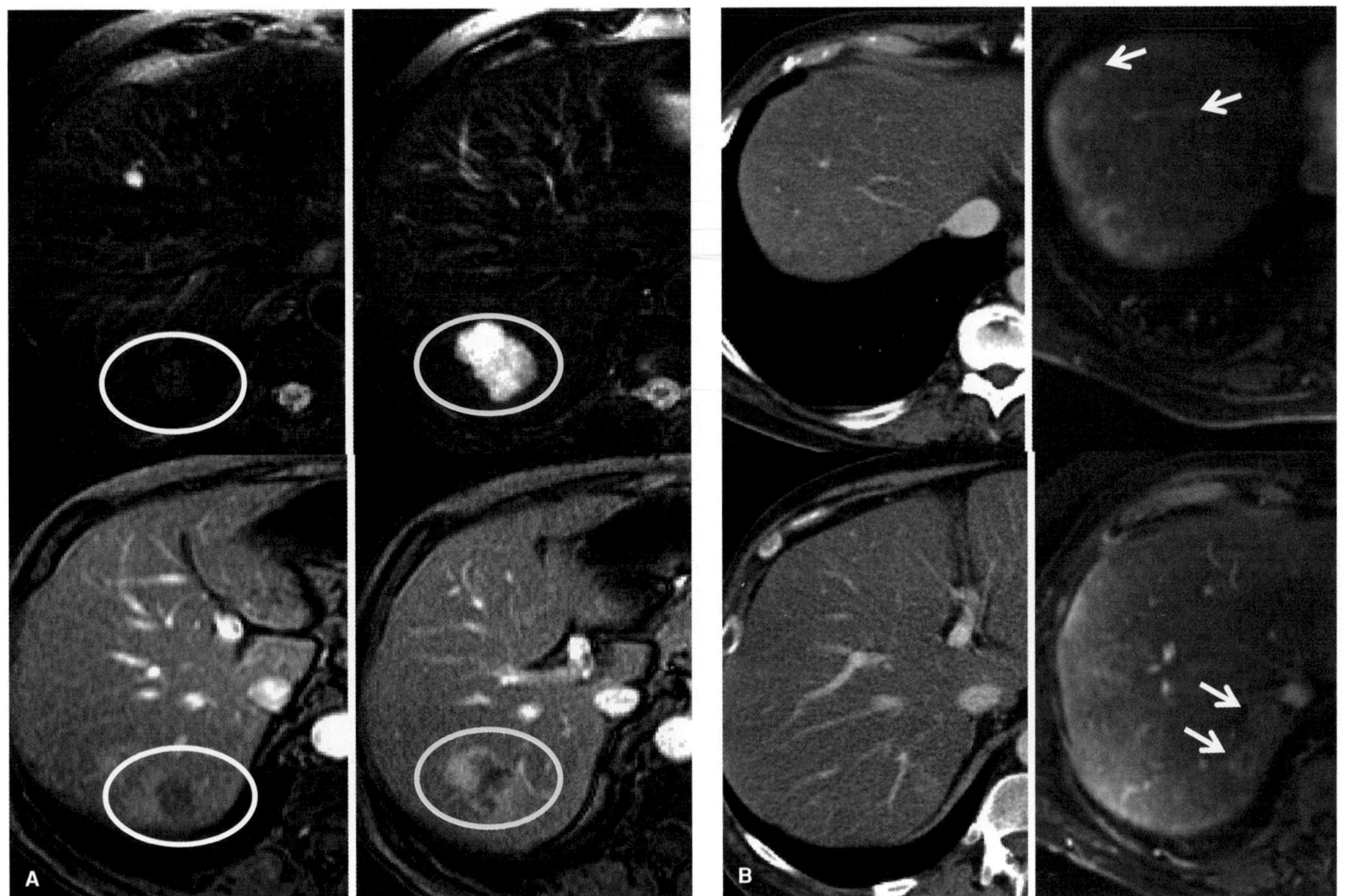


Figure 18.2 **A:** MRI scan illustrating its utility in differentiating benign from malignant liver tumors. T2 weighted **(top)** and post-gadolinium **(bottom)** showing differential imaging features between a contiguous metastatic tumor (**left,** *white circle*) and a hemangioma (**right,** *yellow circle*). Note the bright appearance on T2 and the peripheral nodular enhancement pattern that are characteristic of hemangiomata. **B:** Contrast-enhanced CT **(left)** and MRI **(right)** images of a patient with hepatic colorectal metastases. Fatty infiltration of the liver (steatosis) is apparent on the CT. Multiple liver tumors seen on MRI (*arrows*) were poorly delineated on CT.



In patients with chronic liver disease, the functional reserve of the liver is assessed using composite scoring systems that include biologic data, such as the Child–Pugh classification system for liver disease (Table 18.1). Usually, only patients with Child–Pugh class A disease are considered eligible for liver resection because postoperative mortality rates are higher for patients with higher Child–Pugh class, approaching 50% for those with Child–Pugh class C disease. Since the presence of undiagnosed subclinical portal hypertension can considerably increase the risk associated with surgery, patients should be screened preoperatively for clinical signs of portal hypertension (for ascites, collateral venous circulation), biologic assessment (for platelet count <100,000) and imaging (for evidence of venous collaterals or splenomegaly).

**TABLE 18.1 Child–Pugh Score for Hepatic Functional Reserve**

| | Points | | |
|---|---|---|---|
| **Parameter** | **0** | **1** | **2** |
| Albumin (g/dL) | >3.5 | 2.8–3.5 | <2.8 |
| Bilirubin (mg/dL) | <2 | 2–3 | >3 |
| PT (sec > normal) | <4 | 4–6 | >6 |
| Ascites | None | Mild | Moderate |
| Encephalopathy (grade) | 0 | I–II | III–IV |

Child–Pugh class A = 5–6 points, B = 7–9 points, C = 10–15 points.

A biopsy of the nontumorous liver parenchyma can be used to evaluate for evidence of underlying liver disease. However, this approach has two main limitations. First, the distribution of liver diseases such as fibrosis, steatosis, or chemotherapy-associated liver injury is heterogeneous and the severity of chronic liver disease may not be accurately assessed. Second, histopathologic findings do not accurately reflect liver function and the regenerative capacity of the liver that is pivotal for liver regeneration after major resection.

Indocyanine green (ICG) clearance can also be used to assess liver function. The ICG retention rate at 15 minutes has been adopted in Asia to evaluate liver function in patients with chronic liver disease before resection. However, ICG R15 is a test of global liver function, and it is valuable after minor (limited) resection but may not be as useful as in patients undergoing major resection.

Evaluating the FLR's volume is currently the most reliable approach to predict outcomes for patients who are candidates for major liver resection. Several methods for such evaluation have been described. At The University of Texas M. D. Anderson Cancer Center, we calculate the estimated total liver volume (TLV) using a formula that relies on the linear correlation between the TLV and body surface area (BSA): TLV (in $cm^3$) = −794.41 + 1,267.28 × BSA (in $m^2$). The standardized FLR is then calculated as the ratio of the FLR volume to the estimated TLV. Therefore, the standardized FLR is the FLR as a percentage of the TLV estimated using the above mentioned formula. In a series of 301 patients without chronic liver disease or hepatic injury undergoing extended right hepatectomy for liver tumors, we found that a standardized FLR of equal to or less than 20% was a risk factor for postoperative liver insufficiency and 90-day postoperative mortality.

In patients with small FLRs, portal vein embolization (PVE) can be used to promote hypertrophy of the FLR, making curative resection possible for a subset of patients previously deemed to have borderline or unresectable disease. PVE is recommended for resection that would leave a remnant liver less than or equal to 20% in patients with normal liver, less than or equal to 30% in patients with hepatic injury, such as those who have received extensive chemotherapy (>3 months), and for resection leaving a remnant liver less than or equal to 40% in patients with fibrosis or cirrhosis (Fig. 18.3). PVE is usually performed under fluoroscopic guidance and involves the cannulation of the ipsilateral branch of the portal vein and the embolization, using microparticles followed by coils or absolute ethanol, of the entire portal vein tree to be resected (Fig. 18.4). PVE induces atrophy (apoptosis) of the embolized liver segments and compensatory hypertrophy (regeneration) of the contralateral liver segments. Furthermore, the magnitude of the hypertrophy reflects the liver's regenerative capacity. The rate of volume increase, or degree of hypertrophy (post-PVE FLR minus pre-PVE FLR), appears to correlate with patient outcome after resection. In a series of 112 consecutive patients undergoing PVE before liver resection, we found that the rates of major postoperative complications and 90-day postoperative mortality were higher for patients with a degree of hypertrophy of less than 5% than for patients with higher degrees of hypertrophy (Fig. 18.5).

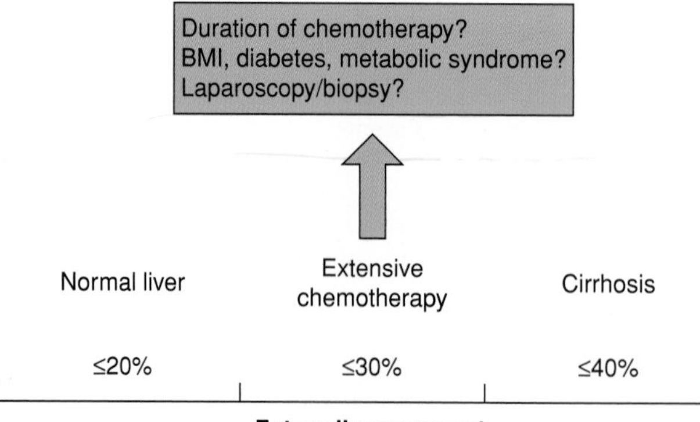


**Figure 18.3** Indications for PVE. There is consensus that, in patients treated with aggressive preoperative chemotherapy, the remnant liver volume should be at least 30% of the TLV to avoid a high risk of complications following hepatic resection. BMI, body mass index. Adapted from Zorzi D et al. *Br J Surg* 2007;94:274–286, with permission.

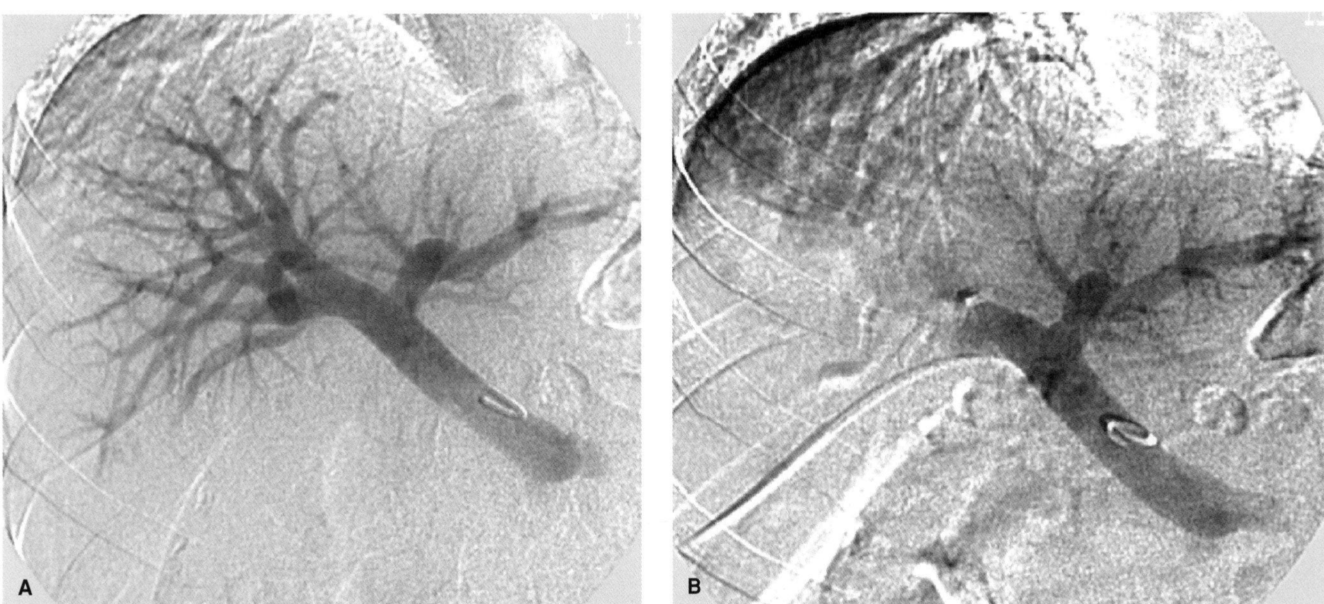

Figure 18.4 Technique of right PVE. **A:** Portogram performed via percutaneous puncture of the right portal system. **B:** Portogram performed after ipsilateral embolization of the right portal vein and its distal branches.



## Timing of Surgery

The treatment of hepatic malignancies, particularly in patients with colorectal cancer liver metastases, requires a multidisciplinary approach that includes not only the surgeon but also the medical oncologist. Currently, most patients with liver metastases have received one or more forms of therapy before being evaluated for surgery. In patients with HCC, regional therapies like transarterial chemoembolization or transarterial embolization do not seem to adversely affect the outcome of liver resection, provided that resection is performed after the recovery of liver function as indicated by liver function tests. However, extended preoperative chemotherapy can adversely affect the outcome of liver resection. In patients with colorectal cancer liver metastases,

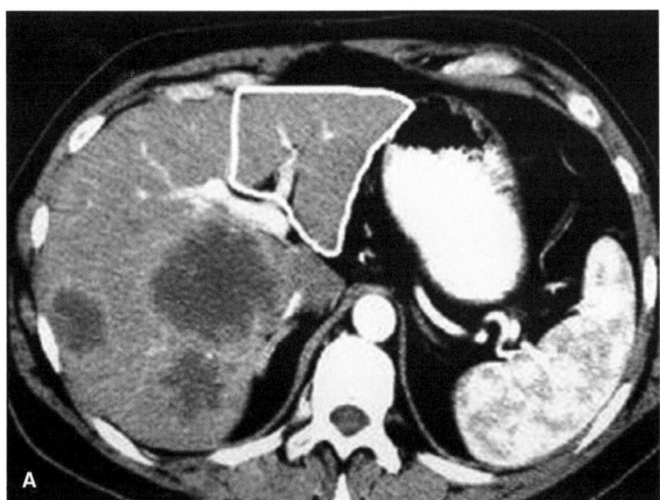

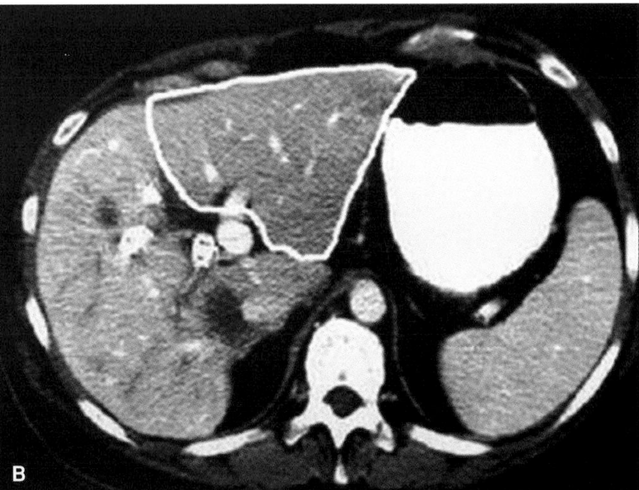

Figure 18.5 A patient with multiple large metastases who required extended right hepatectomy. **A:** The measured volume of the FLR(bisegments II and III, outlined in white) was 291 $cm^3$, and the standardized FLR was calculated as 17% of the estimated TLV. To downsize metastases and induce hypertrophy of the FLR before hepatectomy, chemotherapy was administered, followed by right PVE extended to segment IV. **B:** This led to an increase in the FLR volume to 510 $cm^3$ and in standardized FLR to 30% of the estimated TLV. Adapted from Chun YS and Vauthey JN. *Eur J Surg Oncol* 2007;33:S52–S58, with permission.

chemotherapy-associated liver injuries, including chemotherapy-associated steatohepatitis and sinusoidal injury, can be associated with increased rates of morbidity and mortality after liver resection. The occurrence of chemotherapy-associated liver injuries generally cannot be accurately predicted, but two factors are known to correlate with the occurrence of chemotherapy-associated complications: the duration of preoperative chemotherapy and the time interval between the cessation of chemotherapy and surgery. Thus, we recommend avoiding extended preoperative chemotherapy in patients with potentially resectable liver metastases and operating as soon as the disease becomes resectable in patients whose disease was unresectable prior to treatment. At the university of Texas M.D. Anderson Cancer Center patients with resectable colorectal cancer liver metastases receive 2 to 3 months of chemotherapy before resection. The widespread use of targeted agents like bevacizumab, which may be associated with wound healing complications, has raised new concerns about how long the interval should be between the administration of chemotherapy and surgery. In patients who received bevacizumab, no increase in complications has been reported after liver resection—even after major resection—provided there is an interval of 5 weeks between the last dose of bevacizumab and surgery.

## SURGICAL TECHNIQUE FOR LIVER RESECTION

### Type of Resection

The type of resection performed on a particular patient depends on the type (benign tumor, primary malignant liver tumors, or metastasis) and the extent of the disease. Briefly, liver resections can be classified as major or minor. Major liver resection is generally defined as the removal of three or more contiguous liver segments. Extended resection is defined as resection of a hemiliver with extension to include one or more segments of the contralateral liver. Liver resections can also be stratified as anatomic (removing one or several liver segments) or atypical (wedge) resections (Fig. 18.6).

The influence of the type of resection on oncologic outcomes has been evaluated for HCC and colorectal cancer liver metastases. In patients with HCC, anatomic resection is recommended because of the risks of microscopic portal venous invasion and intrahepatic metastases associated with this disease. Anatomically based resections may also be associated with less intraoperative blood loss and a lower incidence of tumor-involved margins. While small, superficial lesions, particularly metastatic tumors, may be resected with non-anatomical or wedge resections, larger and/or multiple lesions typically require major resections. Regardless of the approach used for resection, tumor-free resection margins should be achieved, not only for primary hepatic malignancies but also for liver metastases, even though the prognostic significance of surgical margins for patients who received preoperative chemotherapy for colorectal cancer liver metastases is a matter of debate.

### Exposure

Incision and exposure are key components of the quality of exploration of the liver and the safety of hepatectomy. Different incisions, including the inverted-T (Mercedes) incision, the bilateral subcostal (chevron) incision, and the right/left subcostal (Kocher/Kehr) incisions or the Makuuchi incision (J incision) are used to achieve these objectives. We have used the inverted L incision in a series of 137 which contribute to excellent exposure of the liver with low rate of wound infection and complication (Fig. 18.7) (see also Figs. 19.3 and 21.5). The inverted L achieves a superb en face view of critical structures, including the hepatocaval junction and the esophageal hiatus, but does not divide the intercostal muscles, thus reducing muscle atrophy and postoperative pain. This incision, previously reported as Rio Branco incision, is particularly useful in patients with large right-sided liver tumors where traditional incisions may not provide optimal exposure for large or recurrent right upper quadrant tumors. The strategic placement of the retractors

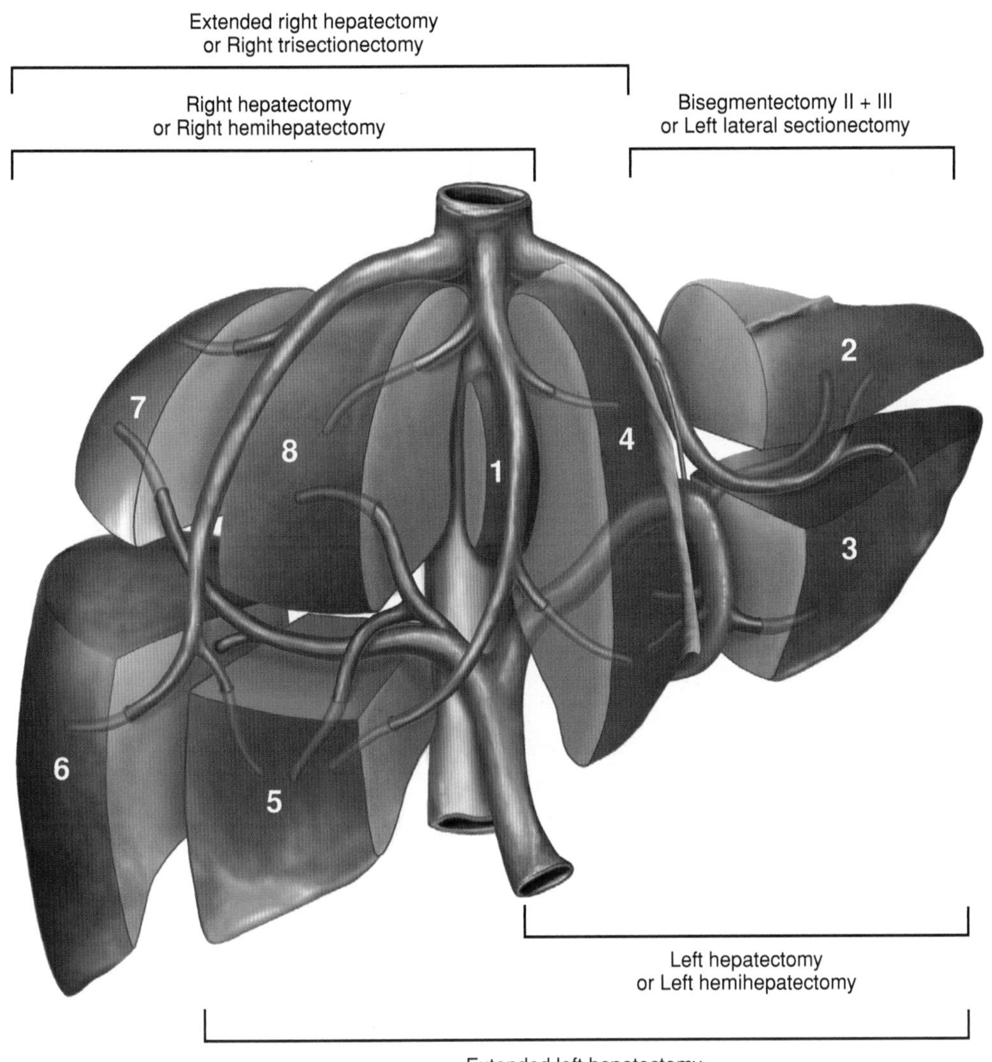


Figure 18.6 Brisbane 2000 terminology for liver resection. Adapted from Abdalla EK, et al. *Surgery* 2004;135:404–410, with permission.



facilitates safe exposure of the right hepatic vein, inferior vena cava, right adrenal gland, and right kidney (Fig. 18.8).

## Principles of Parenchymal Transection

The routine use of intraoperative ultrasonography (IOUS) has contributed to major improvements in liver resection techniques. IOUS confirms the preoperative imaging findings and helps define the extent of the tumor and its relationship with major vascular and biliary structures (Fig. 18.9). IOUS can be used to define the plane of transection while indicating the location and direction of the hepatic veins. Indeed, the surgical plane of major liver resection should follow the plane of the main hepatic veins.

Multiple techniques and devices can be used to perform parenchymal transection. The many tools available to liver surgeons include clamps, staplers, jet cutters, ultrasonic aspirators (CUSA), saline-linked cautery (TissueLink), bipolar electrocoagulation devices, radiofrequency transection devices, harmonic scalpels, and microwave coagulators. To date, none of these devices has been shown to be better than the others. However, we do not recommend the use of radiofrequency or microwave devices or stapling for parenchymal transection because these techniques do not allow the appropriate visualization of important anatomic structures, including the main portal and hepatic veins and biliary radicles, that is required for adequate hemostasis and result in increased blood loss.

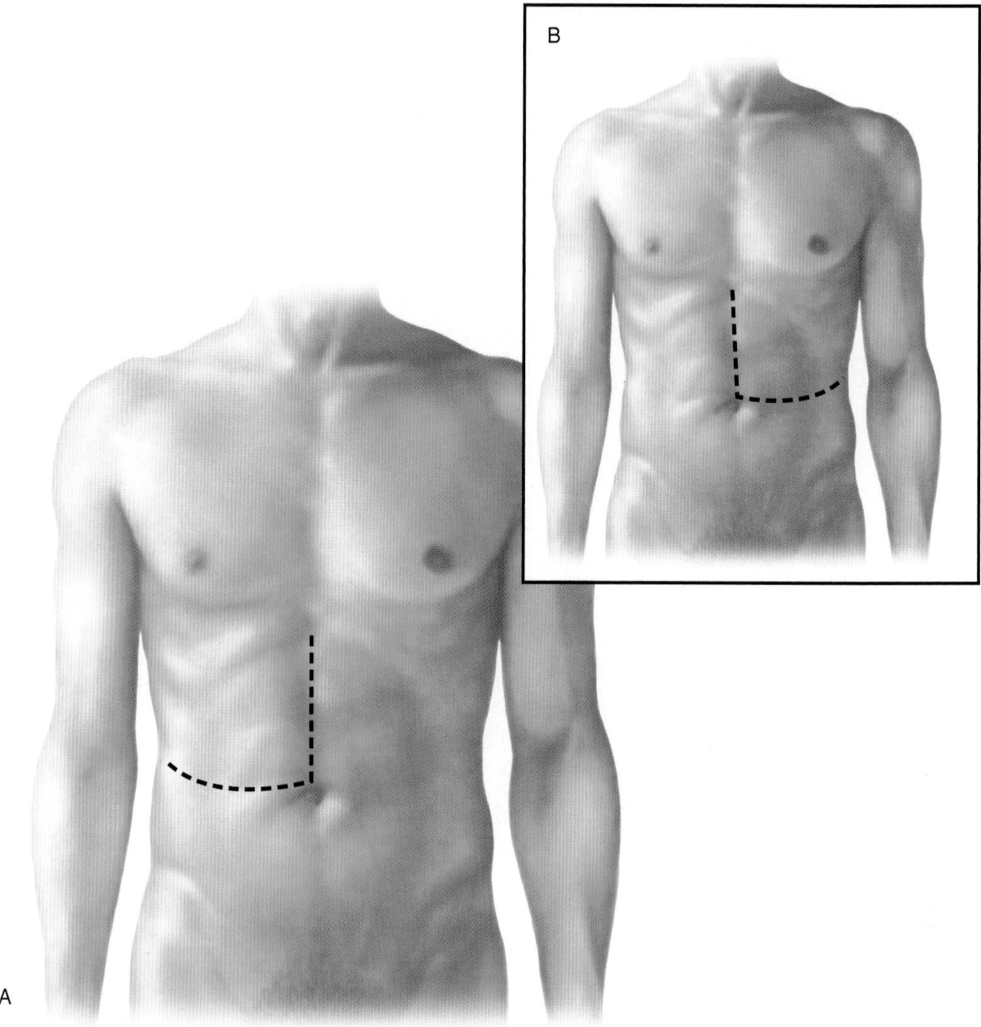


Figure 18.7 The inverted L incision **(A)**. The incision begins cephalad to the xiphoid, extends to 1 cm above the umbilicus, and then extends 4 cm laterally to the right. The L incision **(B)** is used for gastric, pancreatic, and left-sided abdominal surgery. This incision is a mirror image of the modified Makuuchi incision. Adapted from Chang SB et al. *Arch Surg* 2010;145:281–284, with permission.

At M. D. Anderson Cancer Center, we have used a two-surgeon technique combining the use of saline-linked cautery and ultrasonic dissection for parenchymal transection. With this technique, the tasks of parenchymal dissection and hemostasis are divided between the two surgeons (Fig. 18.10). In our experience with 1,557 consecutive liver resections, we have shown that this technique was associated with lower rates of intraoperative blood loss and blood transfusions. This approach also minimizes the passing of instruments because the two surgeons simultaneously perform the two major technical components of parenchymal transection—dissection and hemostasis—thereby allowing the transection to be completed rapidly.

## Prevention and Control of Bleeding

A number of measures can be applied to prevent bleeding during parenchymal transection, including the two-surgeon technique and the use of IOUS to follow the hepatic veins. A strong correlation between the mean vena caval pressure, which reflects the blood pressure in hepatic veins, and blood loss has been demonstrated. A low central venous pressure, with monitoring by anesthesiologists during transection, is used to

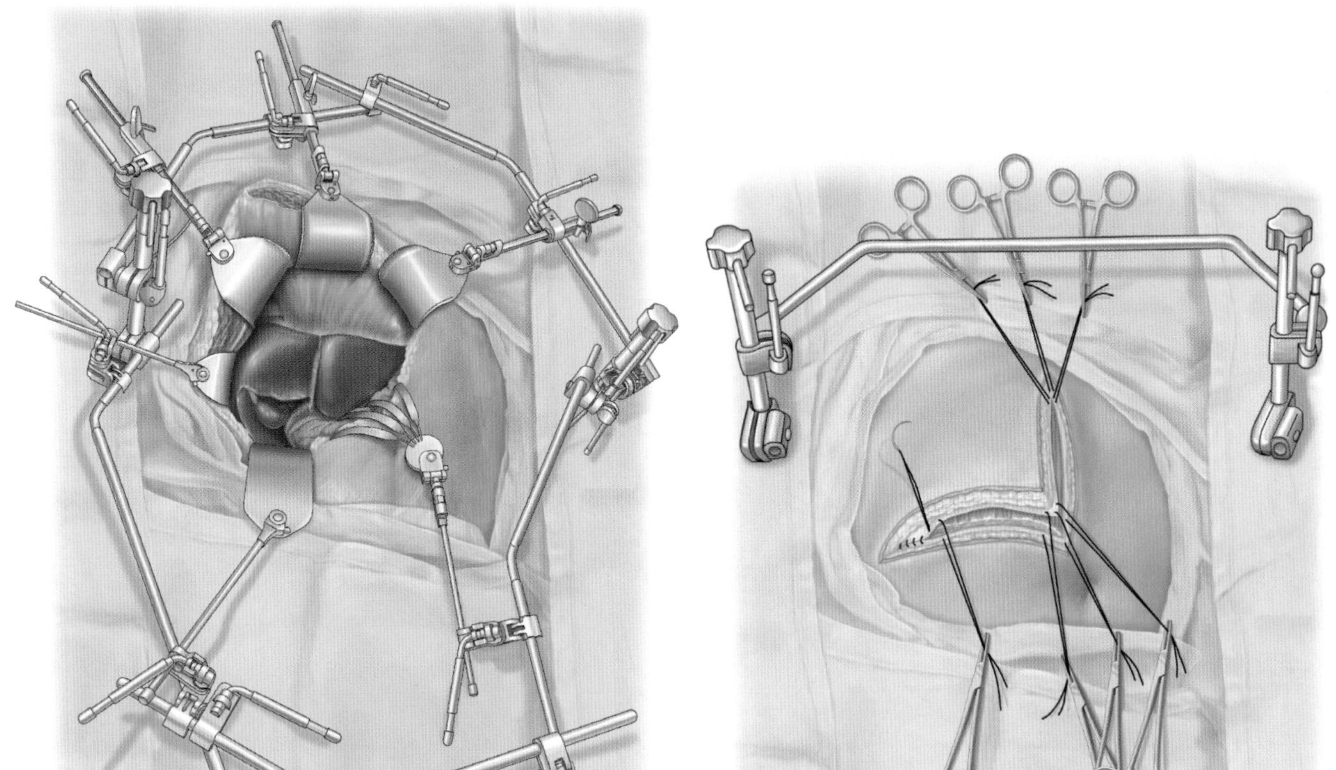

Figure 18.8 Strategic placement of retractors for liver surgery optimizing visualization. Adapted from Chang SB et al. *Arch Surg* 2010;145:281–284, with permission.



decrease the back-bleeding from the hepatic veins. A central venous pressure of less than 5 mm Hg, with urine output maintained at greater than or equal to 0.5 mg/kg/h, is desirable during parenchymal transection.

Using these measures, liver transection can be performed in most patients with vascular inflow occlusion (Pringle maneuver) but without the need for total vascular isolation or exclusion techniques. In patients with chronic liver disease, an intermittent

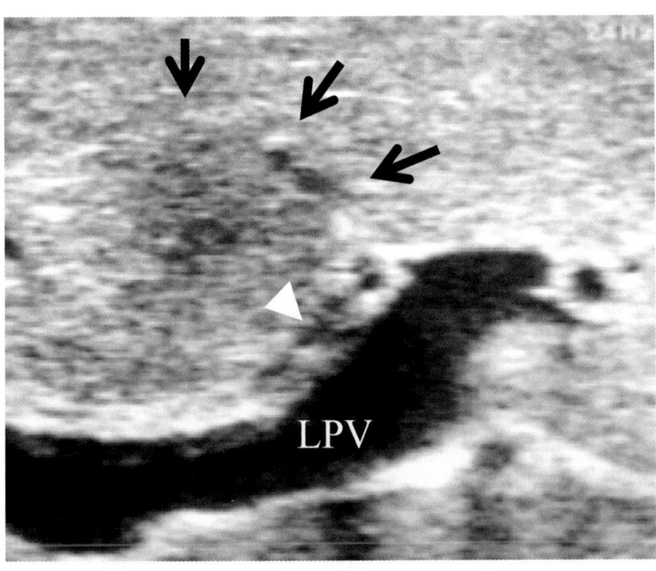


Figure 18.9 Intraoperative ultrasound view showing metastatic tumor at the base of segment IVB, just anterior to the left portal pedicle. The tumor (*dark arrows*) has begun to exert mass effect on the left hepatic duct (*white arrowhead*), which is slightly dilated; this was not apparent on the preoperative CT scan.

Figure 18.10 Two-surgeon technique for hepatic parenchymal transection. Using the ultrasonic dissection device, the primary surgeon directs the dissection from the patient's left side. Simultaneously, the secondary surgeon operates the saline-linked cautery. Adapted from Aloia T et al. *Ann Surg* 2005;242:172–177, with permission.

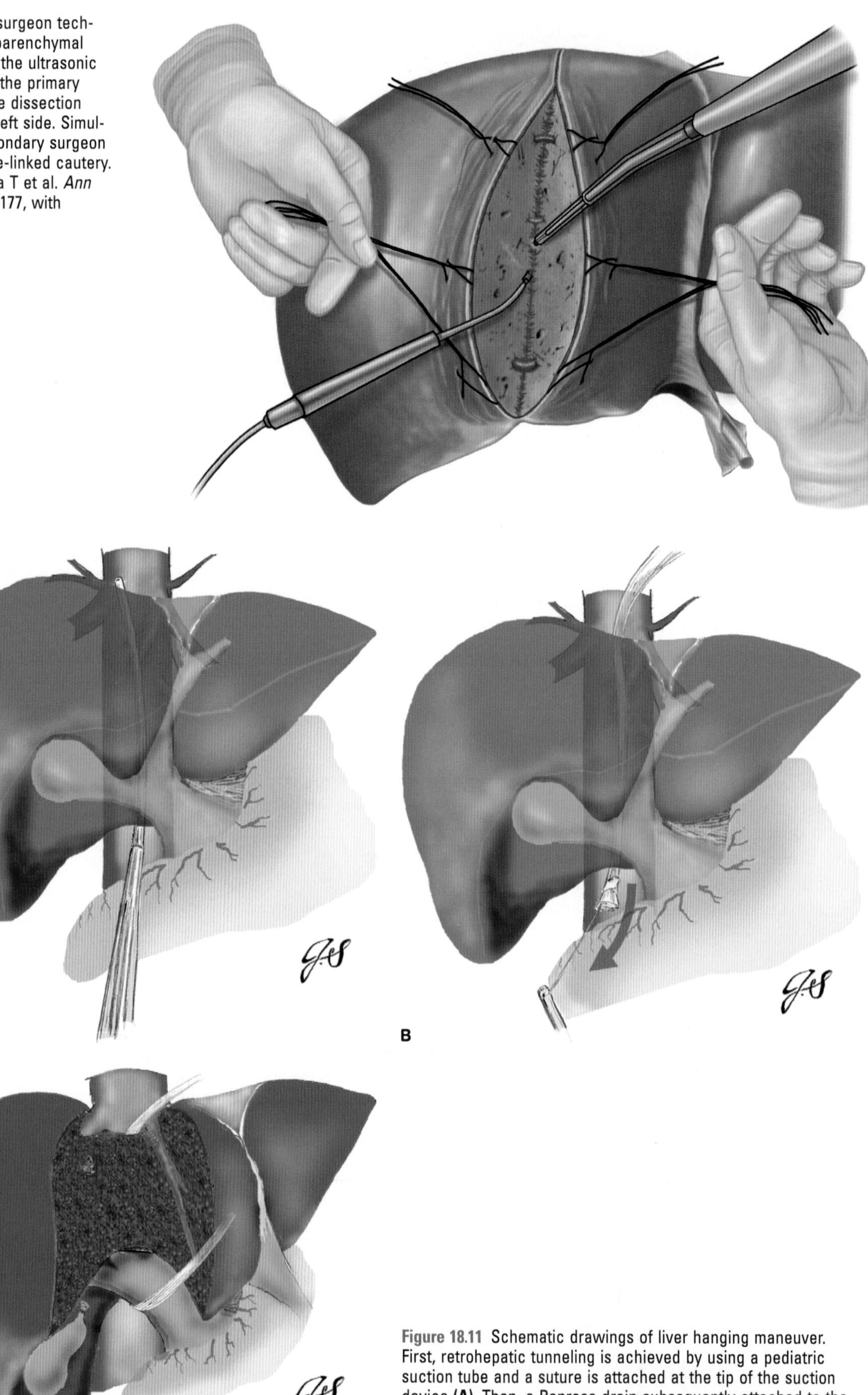


Figure 18.11 Schematic drawings of liver hanging maneuver. First, retrohepatic tunneling is achieved by using a pediatric suction tube and a suture is attached at the tip of the suction device **(A)**. Then, a Penrose drain subsequently attached to the suture is passed behind the liver by pulling back the suture **(B)**. Hepatic parenchymal transaction is performed with hanging the deeper transaction plane liver with the Penrose drain **(C)**.

Pringle maneuver (15 minutes of occlusion alternating with 5 minutes of liver revascularization) has been shown to be safer than continuous occlusion of blood and should be the procedure of choice. The use of total vascular exclusion of the liver is limited to liver resections involving the junction between the hepatic veins and the vena cava.

An anterior approach without prior mobilization of the liver may be indicated in patients with large, right-sided liver tumors invading the diaphragm. The liver hanging maneuver has been proposed in combination with the anterior approach to control bleeding in the deeper part of the transection (Fig. 18.11). This maneuver involves dissecting the retrohepatic space between the middle and right hepatic veins and placing a tape in the avascular space between the vena cava and the liver. Traction on the tape may reduce deep parenchymal bleeding.

# Prevention and Treatment of Common Postoperative Complications

## Postoperative Bleeding

Severe postoperative bleeding after liver resection is uncommon except in the context of severe liver failure, and the hemoglobin levels routinely decline during the first 5 days after resection. Thus, blood transfusion may be avoided in otherwise stable patients when there is no evidence of active bleeding or hemodynamic instability. Low preoperative hemoglobin levels are associated with increased postoperative transfusion requirements. To date, there is no recommendation regarding the minimum hemoglobin level required before or after surgery.



## Postoperative Liver Dysfunction

The risk of postoperative hepatic insufficiency is closely related to the volume and function of the FLR. Postoperative hepatic insufficiency, which is manifested by nonobstructive jaundice, fluid retention/ascites, coagulopathy, and increased susceptibility to septic complications, is best managed by prevention rather than treatment. Predictive factors for postoperative hepatic insufficiency include variables related to the patient (age and body mass index), to the liver (standardized FLR ≤20%) in a normal liver, and to the surgeon (blood loss and the requirement for intraoperative blood transfusions). Some of these factors, like patient age or body mass index, cannot be modified preoperatively, but it is possible to decrease the risk of postoperative hepatic insufficiency by increasing the volume of the FLR with PVE and by limiting intraoperative blood loss to reduce the risk of transfusion. Postoperative hepatic insufficiency is defined as a serum bilirubin peak greater than 7 mg/dL, which is also predictive for postoperative liver-related death (which occurs in >30% of patients with a postoperative serum bilirubin peak greater than 7 mg/dL). The occurrence of postoperative liver dysfunction should be detected early in the postoperative period, and associated complications such as fluid collections and infections should be treated aggressively in order to prevent progression to liver failure. In patients with postoperative serum bilirubin peaks greater than 7 mg/dL, early biliary imaging can be useful to exclude a biliary stricture.

## Perihepatic Fluid Collections and Bile Leaks

Postoperative fluid collections may be related to infections or bile leaks. In most cases, postoperative fluid collections are asymptomatic; however, in some cases, they are associated with fever, abdominal pain, upper gastrointestinal tract symptoms, or pleural effusion. Fluid collections are diagnosed by imaging (CT or ultrasonography) and may be treated by percutaneous drainage (Fig. 18.12). Another major complication after liver resection is bile leak. Despite improvements in postoperative management, bile leaks are

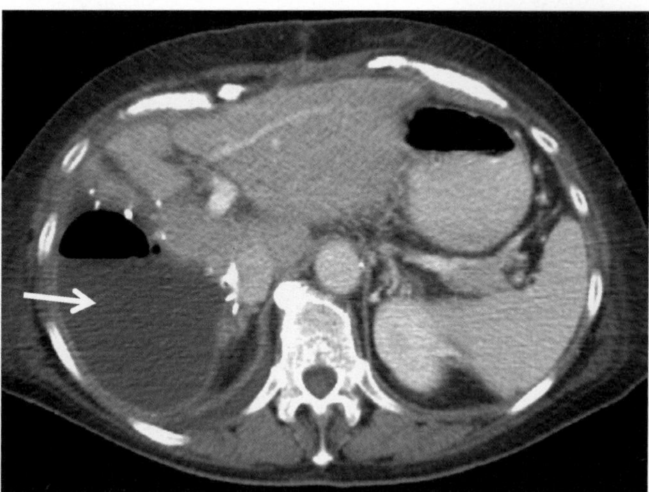

Figure 18.12 CT scan showing a postoperative fluid collection (*white arrow*) after right hepatectomy.

reported in up to 8% of patients who have undergone liver resection. Most bile leaks appear to arise from injured major ductal branches or biliary-enteric anastomoses in cases of combined liver and biliary tract resections, while a few are caused by peripheral biliary radicals. Various intraoperative bile leakage tests have been developed, including the transcystic injection of isotonic saline solution or methylene blue; however, none of these tests has demonstrated a significant benefit for the detection of bile leaks. At M. D. Anderson Cancer Center, we perform a transcystic injection of air into the biliary system to test the patency of the biliary tract and to detect any air leak from the major ducts or the parenchymal transection surface. Although the routine use of intraoperative cholangiography is not recommended, in rare cases it may be indicated to exclude a bile duct injury.

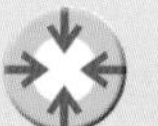

## CONCLUSION

Over the past several years, hepatic resectional surgery has evolved into a safe and effective therapy for a wide range of benign and malignant diseases. Postoperative complications may be related to patient factors, anatomic factors associated with resection extent, or technical factors that result in major intraoperative bleeding. Most patient-related factors (age, Child–Pugh class, and body mass index) cannot not be modified preoperatively. The FLR volume and the degree of hypertrophy after PVE are important predictors of outcome and can help optimize patient selection for major liver resection. Bleeding can be minimized with proper surgical and anesthetic management techniques and using anatomically based resections.

## Recommended References and Readings


Abdalla EK, Denys A, Chevalier P, et al. Total and segmental liver volume variations: implications for liver surgery. *Surgery.* 2004;135:404–410.

Aloia TA, Zorzi D, Abdalla EK, et al. Two-surgeon technique for hepatic parenchymal transection of the noncirrhotic liver using saline-linked cautery and ultrasonic dissection. *Ann Surg.* 2005; 242:172–177.

Belghiti J, Guevara OA, Noun R, et al. Liver hanging maneuver: a safe approach to right hepatectomy without liver mobilization. *J Am Coll Surg.* 2001;193:109–111.

Jarnagin WR, Gonen M, Fong Y, et al. Improvement in perioperative outcome after hepatic resection: analysis of 1,803 consecutive cases over the past decade. *Ann Surg.* 2002;236: 397–406.

Johnson M, Mannar R, Wu AV. Correlation between blood loss and inferior vena caval pressure during liver resection. *Br J Surg.* 1998;85:188–190.

Katz SC, Shia J, Liau KH, et al. Operative blood loss independently predicts recurrence and survival after resection of hepatocellular carcinoma. *Ann Surg.* 2009;249:617–623.

Kishi Y, Abdalla EK, Chun YS, et al. Three hundred and one consecutive extended right hepatectomies: evaluation of outcome based on systematic liver volumetry. *Ann Surg.* 2009;250(4): 540–548.

Kopetz S, Vauthey JN. Perioperative chemotherapy for resectable hepatic metastases. *Lancet.* 2008;371:963–965.

Madoff DC, Hicks ME, Abdalla EK, et al. Portal vein embolization with polyvinyl alcohol particles and coils in preparation for major liver resection for hepatobiliary malignancy: safety and effectiveness—study in 26 patients. *Radiology.* 2003;227:251–260.

Mullen JT, Ribero D, Reddy SK, et al. Hepatic insufficiency and mortality in 1,059 noncirrhotic patients undergoing major hepatectomy. *J Am Coll Surg.* 2007;204:854–862.

Nordlinger B; Sorbye H, Glimelius B, et al. Perioperative chemotherapy with FOLFOX4 and surgery versus surgery alone for resectable liver metastases from colorectal cancer (EORTC

Intergroup trial 40983): a randomised controlled trial. *Lancet.* 2008;371:1007–1016.

Palavecino M, Kishi Y, Chun YS, et al. Two-surgeon technique of parenchymal transection contributes to reduced transfusion rate in patients undergoing major hepatectomy: analysis of 1,557 consecutive liver resections. *Surgery.* 2009;147:40–48.

Pawlik TM, Scoggins CR, Zorzi D, et al. Effect of surgical margin status on survival and site of recurrence after hepatic resection for colorectal metastases. *Ann Surg.* 2005;241:715–724.

Ribero D, Abdalla EK, Madoff DC, et al. Portal vein embolization before major hepatectomy and its effects on regeneration, resectability and outcome. *Br J Surg.* 2007;94:1386–1394.

Strasberg SM, International Hepato-Pancreato-Biliary Association Terminology Committee Survey. The Brisbane 2000 Terminology of Liver Anatomy and Resections. *HPB Surg.* 2000;2:333–339.

Torzilli G, Gambetti A, Del Fabbro D, et al. Techniques for hepatectomies without blood transfusion, focusing on interpretation of postoperative anemia. *Arch Surg.* 2004;139:1061–1065.

Torzilli G, Makuuchi M, Inoue K, et al. No-mortality liver resection for hepatocellular carcinoma in cirrhotic and noncirrhotic patients: is there a way? A prospective analysis of our approach. *Arch Surg.* 1999;134:984–992.

Vauthey JN, Pawlik TM, Abdalla EK, et al. Is extended hepatectomy for hepatobiliary malignancy justified? *Ann Surg.* 2004;239:722–730.

Vauthey JN, Pawlik TM, Ribero D, et al. Chemotherapy regimen predicts steatohepatitis and an increase in 90-day mortality after surgery for hepatic colorectal metastases. *J Clin Oncol.* 2006;24:2065–2072.

Vauthey JN, Rousseau DL Jr. Liver imaging. A surgeon's perspective. *Clin Liver Dis.* 2002;6:271–295.

# 19 Right and Extended Right Hepatectomy

**Michael I. D'Angelica**

##  INDICATIONS/CONTRAINDICATIONS

A right (segments V–VIII) or extended right (segments IV–VIII) hepatectomy (see Chapter 18 and Fig. 18.6) is most commonly indicated for primary liver or biliary malignancies (see Chapter 26) or for metastatic tumors, particularly metastatic colorectal cancer. Less frequently, this operation is indicated for large, symptomatic benign tumors or for large retroperitoneal tumors involving the right liver (see Fig. 23.3B). Rarely, liver or biliary infectious processes or bile duct injuries are an indication for a right or extended hepatectomy. Hepatic resections for live donor transplantation procedures are beyond the scope of this section and are not discussed.

Tumors involving the main inflow pedicle and/or outflow venous drainage to the right liver typically require right hepatectomy for removal. Similarly, this procedure is required for diffuse tumors involving most of the parenchyma or all segments of the right liver. It is important to recognize that the right liver accounts for a much larger proportion of the total liver volume compared to the left. Given that the volume of resected hepatic parenchyma, and therefore, the volume of the residual liver or the future liver remnant (FLR), closely correlates with postoperative morbidity, right and extended right hepatectomy are associated with a higher potential risk of postoperative hepatic failure compared to left or even extended left hepatectomy (see Chapter 18). More limited resections should, therefore, always be considered as an alternative approach (see Chapters 23 and 24). However, if such parenchymal-sparing resections are not possible, the surgeon must consider carefully the volume and quality of the FLR and consider preoperative portal vein embolization (PVE) of the right liver (see below and Chapter 18).

##  PREOPERATIVE PLANNING

Patients with malignant tumors should have a complete extent of disease evaluation, with high-quality contrast-enhanced cross-sectional imaging (computed tomography or magnetic resonance imaging) of the abdomen and pelvis. A chest CT is generally indicated to rule out metastatic disease. In patients with primary liver cancer, a liver protocol CT is the best means of assessing for multifocal hepatic disease (see Chapter 18), while CT angiography is most helpful for patients with biliary tract cancer, particularly hilar cholangiocarcinoma (see Chapter 26). In patients with metastatic cancer treated with preoperative chemotherapy, particularly hepatic colorectal metastases, hepatic steatosis is common, and CT may underestimate the hepatic disease extent. In such patients, MRI may be much more useful (see Chapter 18). Relevant tumor markers should be assessed to serve as a baseline and help monitor for recurrence after complete resection. Although beyond the scope of this chapter and dependent on the specific disease, other imaging such as $^{18}$FDG positron emission tomography or complete colonoscopy should be considered.

High-quality imaging of the liver and its vascular and biliary anatomy are essential for planning operations. Triphasic scans including arterial, portal, and mixed phases provide information on the anatomy of the hepatic arterial system, portal venous system, and the hepatic veins. Information on the relevant anatomic relationships of tumors to these structures can help one plan the resection to avoid positive or close margins. In addition, vascular anomalies such as aberrant branches of the hepatic artery, portal vein, and hepatic veins can be assessed and anticipated at operation. Magnetic resonance cholangiopancreatography, although not mandatory, can be helpful in assessing biliary anatomy.

Assessment of hepatic function is critical and especially relevant for patients with chronic liver disease. Typically, an assessment of the Child–Pugh classification suffices, and in general, only Child–Pugh grade A patients are candidates for a right hepatectomy (see Table 18.1). The possibility of portal hypertension must be considered in patients with underlying liver disease and should be assessed since its presence portends prohibitive morbidity. Portal hypertension can manifest as a history of ascites or variceal hemorrhage, but more subtly, as splenomegaly and thrombocytopenia with a platelet count of less than 100,000/mcl. Contrast-enhanced imaging can also demonstrate portal hypertension with findings such as a patent umbilical vein or gastro-esophageal varices (Fig. 19.1). If there is doubt as to the diagnosis of portal hypertension, a hepatic vein wedge pressure can be obtained. In general, patients with normal liver function, Child–Pugh grade A function, and without portal hypertension are candidates for a right hepatectomy.

Right and extended right hepatectomy are large volume resections and each case should be considered for preoperative right PVE. Volumetric studies are useful to

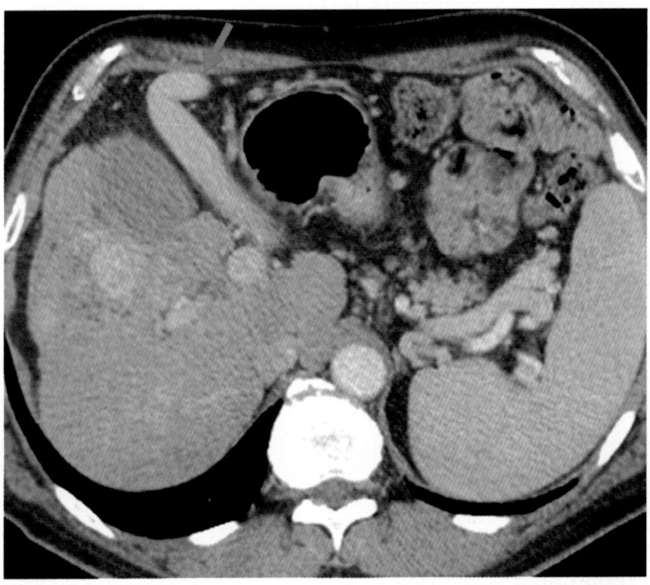

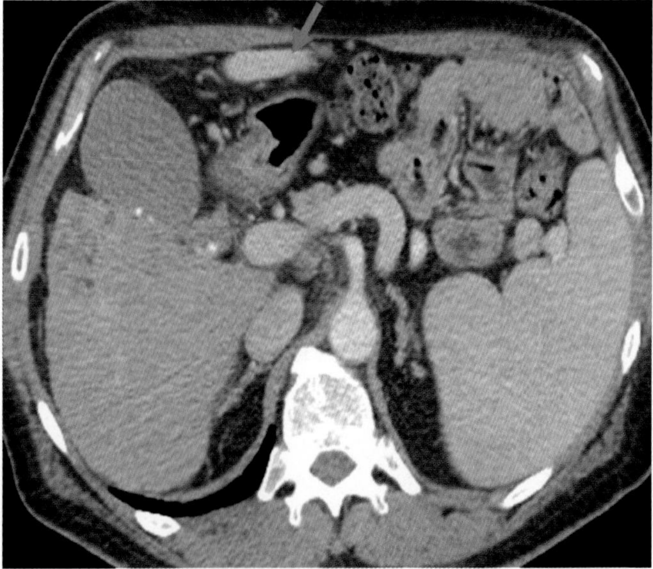

**Figure 19.1** A computed tomography scan illustrating portal hypertension manifested as a patent umbilical vein. Arrows indicate the patent umbilical vein.

determine the relative volume of the FLR. If the FLR volume is under 25% to 30% in a normal liver, preoperative PVE should be considered. Patients with chronic liver disease should probably be considered for PVE at larger FLR volumes. Patients must be assessed for their medical and physical fitness to tolerate a major abdominal operation and its potential complications. Particular attention should be paid to physical fitness, performance status, and cardiopulmonary co-morbidities.

## SURGERY

### Pertinent Anatomy

- Hepatic artery: The right hepatic artery typically runs in the porta hepatis from left to right, posterior to the common hepatic duct, but in about 10% of cases is found anterior to the bile duct. Replaced or accessory right hepatic artery branches are common, originating from the superior mesenteric artery and generally coursing posteriorly in the portacaval space.
- Portal vein: The right portal vein typically has a short extrahepatic course and branches into anterior and posterior sectoral branches. Sometimes there is no common right portal vein but rather a trifurcation of the main portal vein into right posterior, right anterior, and left branches. The right anterior portal vein branch can also arise separately from the left portal vein (Fig. 19.2). The right portal vein almost always gives off a small branch to the caudate process before entering the substance of the right liver, and this branch should be controlled if the right vein is to be divided extrahepatically.
- Bile ducts: Typically a short right hepatic duct divides into anterior and posterior sectoral branches. These sectoral ducts (most commonly the posterior sectoral duct) can be found to drain into the left bile duct. The right sectoral ducts can also exit the liver and join the common hepatic or bile duct inferiorly in the porta hepatis.



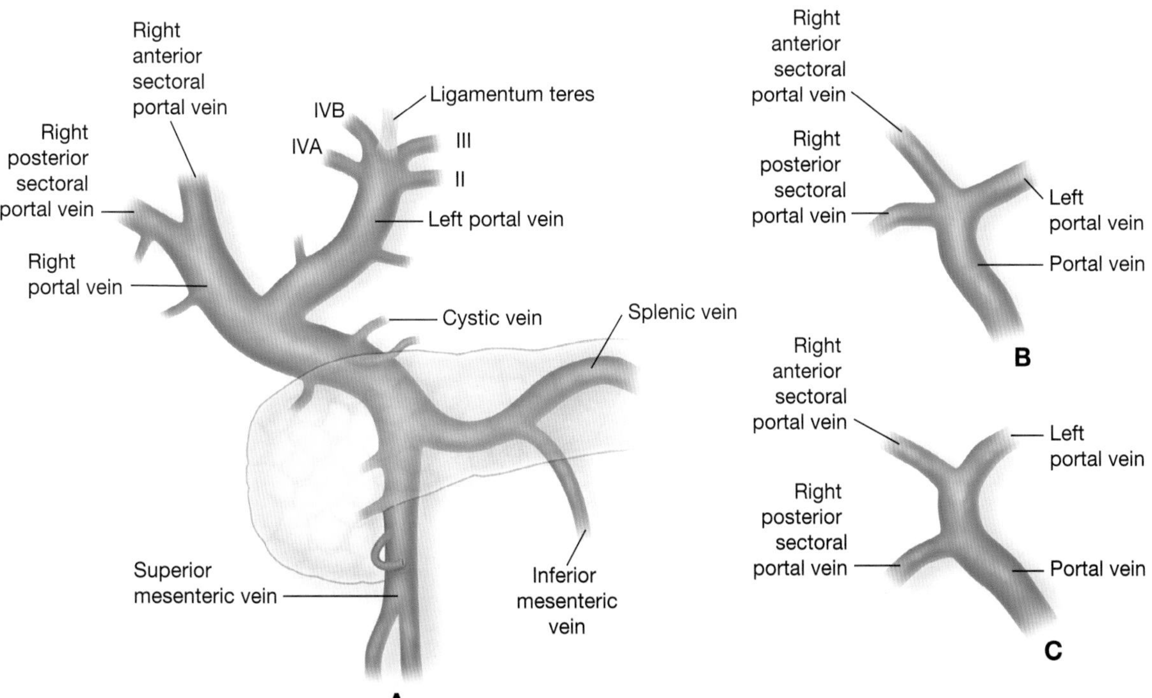


**Figure 19.2** An illustration of a typical portal vein anatomy **(A)** and the most common variations. A trifurcation of the main portal vein into right posterior, right anterior, and left portal vein branches is shown in **(B)** and the right anterior sectoral branch arising from the left portal vein is illustrated in **(C)**.

The surgeon should recognize that variability in the biliary anatomy is more commonly associated with the right hepatic duct.

- Hepatic veins: Large accessory right hepatic veins are relatively common and are encountered early in the caval dissection. When these are present, branches from the right adrenal vein are occasionally found draining into the accessory right hepatic vein. A large vein draining segment VIII typically drains medially into the middle hepatic vein, and is a common source of bleeding deep in the parenchymal dissection.

## Positioning, Incisions, and Retractors

The patient is positioned supine with the arms extended out at right angles allowing for easy peripheral vascular access and monitoring. There are numerous incisions that allow access to the right liver. A bilateral subcostal incision is commonly used and can be extended to the xiphoid in the midline. In our experience, this "Mercedes"-type incision is usually not necessary and results in a high ventral hernia rate. We typically use a right subcostal incision with midline vertical extension to the xiphoid ("hockey stick" incision). Some surgeons use a thoracoabdominal incision with entry into the right chest and division of the diaphragm. While we find this to be rarely necessary, it can be helpful when there is severe right-sided atrophy or when exposure of the suprahepatic vena cava is difficult due to a large mass. The thoracoabdominal incision can be a simple J-type incision or an extension of the "Mercedes" or "hockey stick" incision into the chest (Fig. 19.3). The key issue for exposure is cephalad retraction of the costal margin at approximately a 45 degree angle. Any number of retractor systems can provide this retraction combined with lateral retraction of the right chest wall and inferior retraction of the lower abdominal viscera (see Fig. 18.8).

## Anesthetic Considerations

The most common source of bleeding from the hepatic parenchyma is from the hepatic veins. Maintaining a low central venous pressure (CVP) during resection is invaluable in limiting blood loss (see Chapter 18). While some anesthesiologists place central venous catheters for CVP monitoring, it is quite simple for the surgeon to visualize the vena cava during the operation to assess it and communicate with the anesthesiologist.

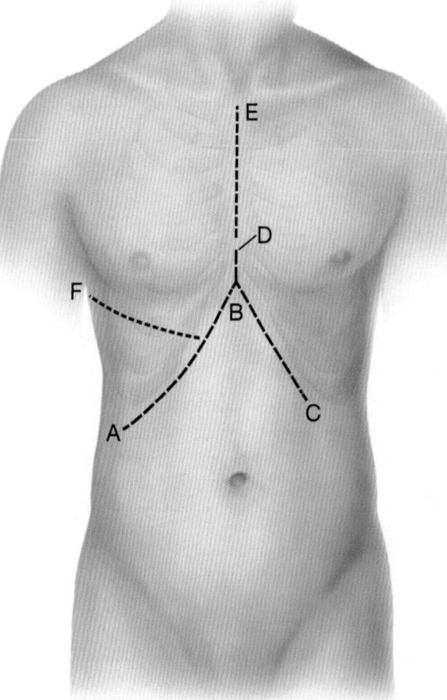


**Figure 19.3** Multiple incisions for exposure of the liver are illustrated. *ABC* illustrates a typical bilateral subcostal incision which can be extended vertically in the midline (*D*) as a "Mercedes" incision. We most commonly use a "hockey stick" incision (*ABD*). Extension into the right chest (*F*) or through a sternotomy (*E*) is rarely necessary.

The vena cava should not appear bulging or "full" but rather should have respiratory variation and be somewhat "collapsing". Mild Trendelenburg position, limitation of intravenous fluids, and pharmacologic management with venodilators are helpful. Once the resection is completed the anesthesiologist should be informed to hydrate the patient. Communication between the surgeon and the anesthesiologist is critical.

## Exploration

- Diagnostic laparoscopy is used selectively based on the risk of occult unresectable disease.
- Thorough open exploration for occult metastatic disease, precluding resection should include bimanual palpation of the liver, as well as inspection/palpation of all peritoneal surfaces and relevant nodal basins.
- Intraoperative hepatic ultrasound is used routinely to identify occult hepatic tumors and assess the details of the tumor and vascular anatomy.

## Mobilization (see also Chapter 23)

- The ligamentum teres is divided and a long tie is left on the liver side as a handle for retraction.
- The falciform ligament is divided with diathermy back to the hepatic veins.
- With sharp dissection, the right hepatic vein and the common trunk of the middle and left hepatic veins are exposed anteriorly. The groove between the right and middle hepatic veins is dissected down to the vena cava.
- The coronary ligaments are divided, exposing the right hepatic veins (Fig. 19.4).
- The liver is turned to the left and the diaphragm is retracted laterally and cephalad. This exposes the peritoneal reflection of the right triangular ligament, which is divided laterally and on the inferior surface of the right liver.
- This dissection is continued lateral to medial, separating the right adrenal gland from the liver and dropping it posteriorly, exposing the lateral wall of the vena cava.
- The right liver is retracted to the left and superiorly, exposing the retrohepatic vena cava. Serial dissection from inferior to superior along the vena cava is commenced. Multiple retrohepatic caval branches are typically encountered (see also Figs. 23.12 and 23.13), serially dissected and divided between clips, ties, or sutures as necessary (Fig. 19.5).
- Large accessory right hepatic veins may be encountered during this dissection and must be divided. Clamping, division, and suturing can be utilized but division with vascular staplers is convenient and effective.
- At the superior end of this caval dissection, a fibrous band of tissue (the vena caval ligament) containing various amounts of hepatic parenchyma will be encountered lateral to the right hepatic vein. This ligament must be encircled with careful dissection lateral to the right hepatic vein, identifying any additional caval branches that may be present. The caval ligament is then divided, exposing the lateral wall of the right hepatic vein. We typically use a vascular stapler, as there may be some vascularized tissue or a small hepatic vein branch that may bleed with sharp division (Fig. 19.6).
- At this stage, we sharply dissect the inferior border of the right hepatic vein and dissect a tunnel between the right and middle hepatic veins. Once this tunnel is finished (usually with dissection from above and below) the right hepatic vein is encircled with a vessel loop.

## Inflow Control (Extrahepatic Dissection)

- A cholecystectomy is performed in the usual manner and a tie is left on the cystic duct stump for retraction.
- The hilar plate is lowered with sharp dissection and division of any small segment IV portal branches. This lowers and protects the left bile duct.
- The right hepatic artery is dissected. In its usual anatomic position posterior to the common hepatic duct, leftward retraction of the cystic duct and common bile duct exposes the underlying artery, which is then encircled, ligated, and divided (Fig. 19.7).

A

B

C

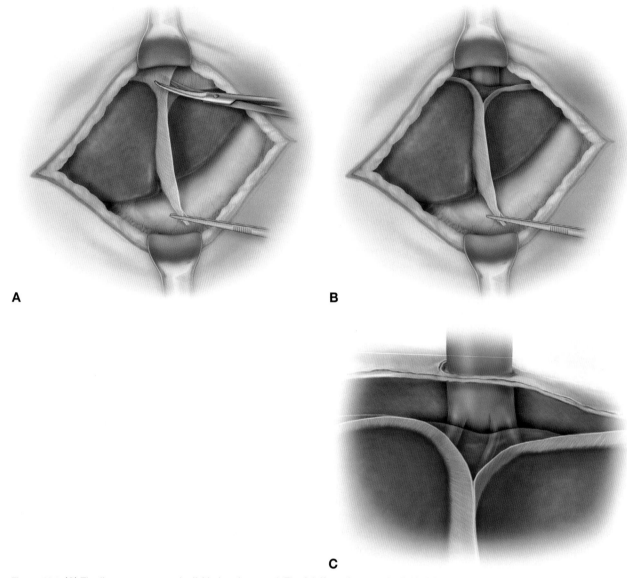

Figure 19.4 **(A)** The ligamentum teres is divided and secured. The falciform ligament is divided back to the coronary ligaments **(B)** which are further divided yielding exposure of the superior and anterior surfaces of the hepatic veins **(C)**.

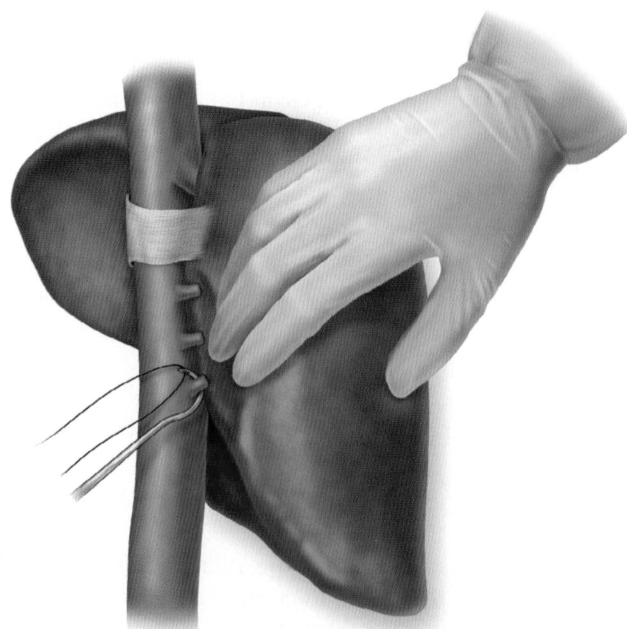

Figure 19.5 The liver is retracted to the left and the vena cava is dissected, serially identifying, securing, and dividing multiple retrohepatic venous branches from the caudate lobe and the right liver. This is necessary for exposure of the right hepatic vein.

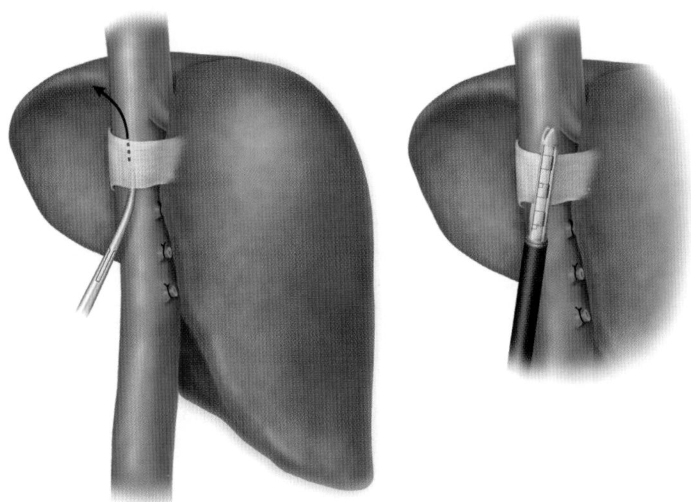

**Figure 19.6** After dissection and clearance of the retrohepatic vena cava, the caval ligament is encountered and dissected along the lateral aspect of the vena cava. For exposure of the lateral aspect of the right hepatic vein the caval ligament must be encircled and then divided.

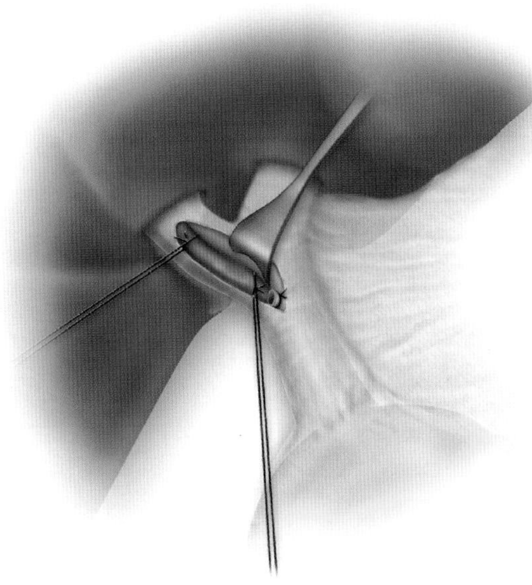

**Figure 19.7** After a cholecystectomy, the cystic duct and/or common bile duct are retracted to the left to expose the underlying right hepatic artery (in its most common location running poster to the bile duct), which can then be ligated and divided.

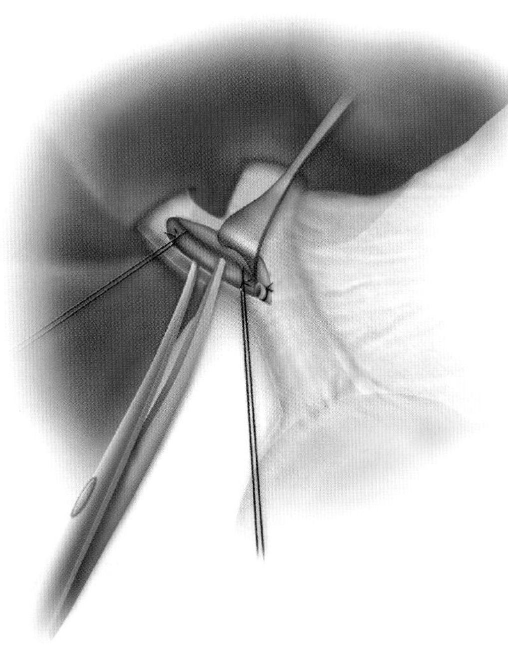

- On occasion the artery will be present anterior to the bile duct or in an accessory/ replaced position in the portacaval space, requiring dissection in these areas.
- It is always prudent to check a pulse in the left hepatic artery at the base of the umbilical fissure with the presumed right hepatic artery clamped to confirm the anatomy.
- In the typical position, the proximal right hepatic artery stump can be used as a sling (retracted by its ligature left long) to retract the biliary tree superiorly and to the left, exposing the underlying portal vein.
- The portal vein anatomy is then dissected sharply. The main, right, and left portal veins should be dissected and visualized in anticipation of any of the anatomic variations mentioned above.
- The right portal vein is then dissected and a relatively constant branch to the caudate process is exposed, encircled, tied, and divided for maximal exposure.
- The right portal vein or its branches (depending on the anatomy) are then encircled. Clamping should demarcate the right liver and a patent left portal vein should be visualized. The right portal vein can then be divided and controlled with ligatures or a vascular stapler (Fig. 19.8).

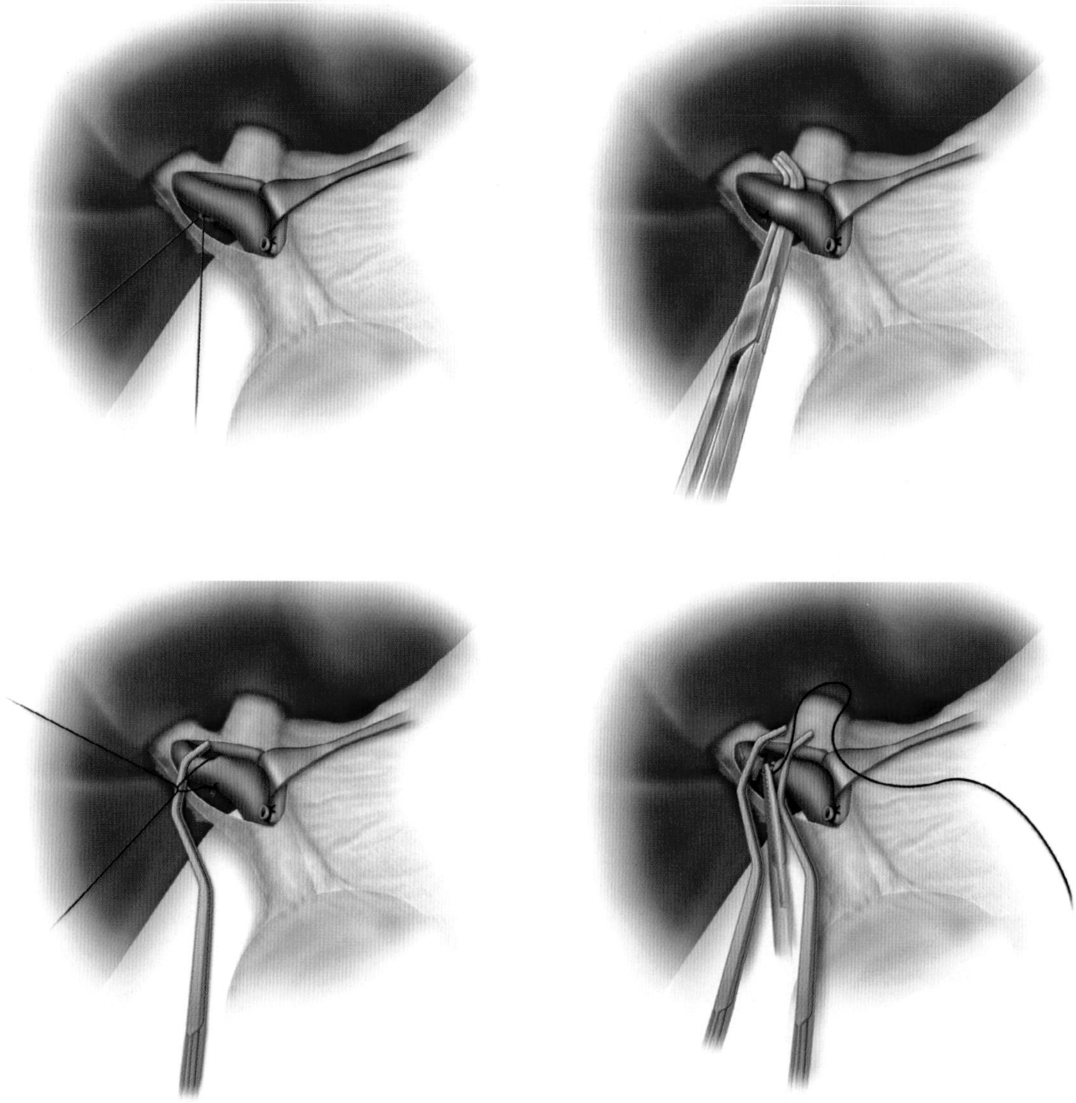

**Figure 19.8** With retraction of the bile duct to the left, the underlying portal vein and its branches are exposed and sharply dissected. A small branch to the caudate process is isolated, ligated, and divided, freeing up the right portal vein. After confirming the anatomy, the right portal vein is isolated, ligated and divided, or sutured and divided. Alternatively, the right portal vein can be divided with a vascular stapler (as shown).

- Unless mandated by tumor proximity, we advocate dividing the right bile duct intrahepatically within its glissonian sheath to minimize the chances of left bile duct injury. If necessary, the usually short extrahepatic right bile duct can be encircled, divided, and oversewn. If there is any concern that the left bile duct has been compromised, a cholangiogram should be obtained.

## Inflow Control (Intrahepatic Approach)

- If tumor proximity does not mandate hilar dissection, the inflow to the liver can be taken intrahepatically as a pedicle within the invaginated glissonian peritoneal sheath. This can be taken as a single main right pedicle or a separate division of the right anterior and posterior pedicles. The right inflow pedicles can be encircled via anterior and posterior hepatotomies or by dividing the parenchyma down to the pedicles. As in the extrahepatic approach, the hilar plate should be lowered to protect the left bile duct (see Figs. 21.14 and 24.4).
- In the hepatotomy approach, incisions are made vertically along the gallbladder fossa and continued transversely along the base of segment IV and separately at the caudate process. The right main pedicle can then be encircled with the thumb and forefinger or with a large right angle clamp. Hepatic parenchyma can be cleared and the right anterior and posterior pedicles can also be separately encircled. One must be wary of inadvertent injury to middle hepatic vein branches. Division of the pedicles can then be carried out with clamping and suturing or with vascular staplers. It is always prudent to clamp and check demarcation and/or flow to the left liver prior to division. Similarly, if there is any concern for compromise of the left hepatic duct, a cholangiogram should be obtained (Fig. 19.9).
- The right pedicles can also be approached by dividing the hepatic parenchyma in the plane of the planned resection down to the anterior portion of the right inflow pedicle. An incision in the caudate process is made and the pedicles encircled, checked, and divided.

## Inflow Control (Segment IV)

Segment IV is part of the left hemi-liver and therefore derives its blood supply and biliary drainage from the left portal inflow. Typically, the left portal structures

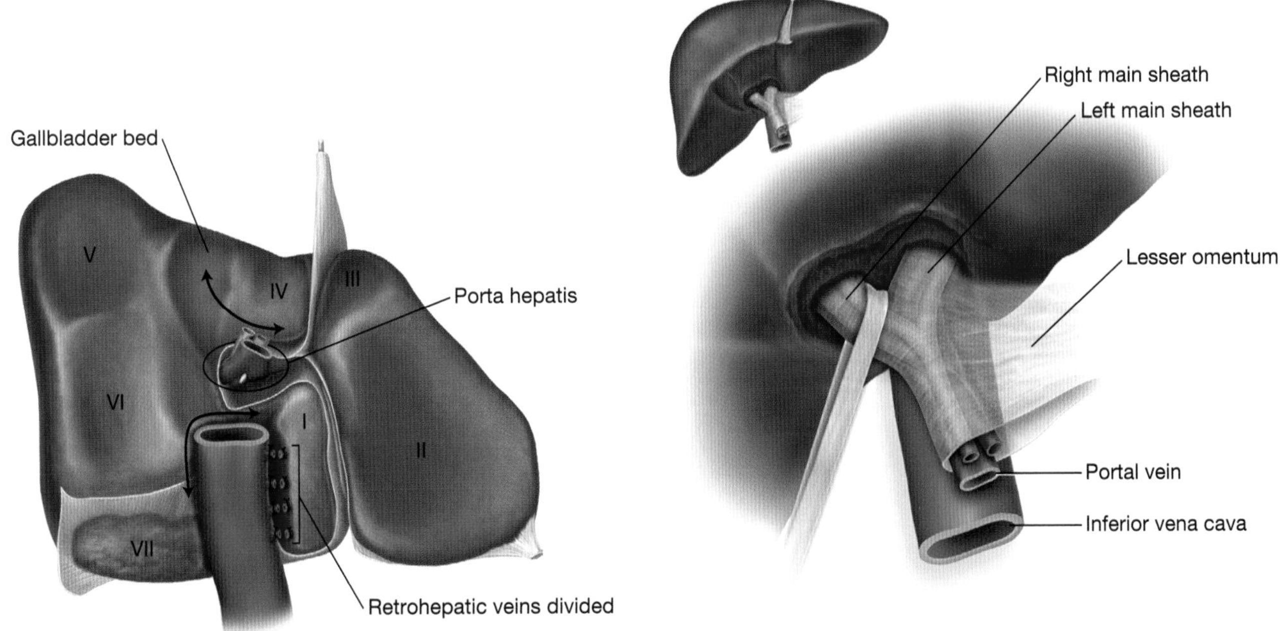


**Figure 19.9** The hepatectomy approach to a right pedicle ligation is illustrated. The caudate process is mobilized off of the vena cava by dividing the short hepatic veins. Incisions are made along the gallbladder fossa and caudate process as demonstrated by the double headed arrows. The right portal pedicle can then be encircled and prepared for division.

Part II: Liver

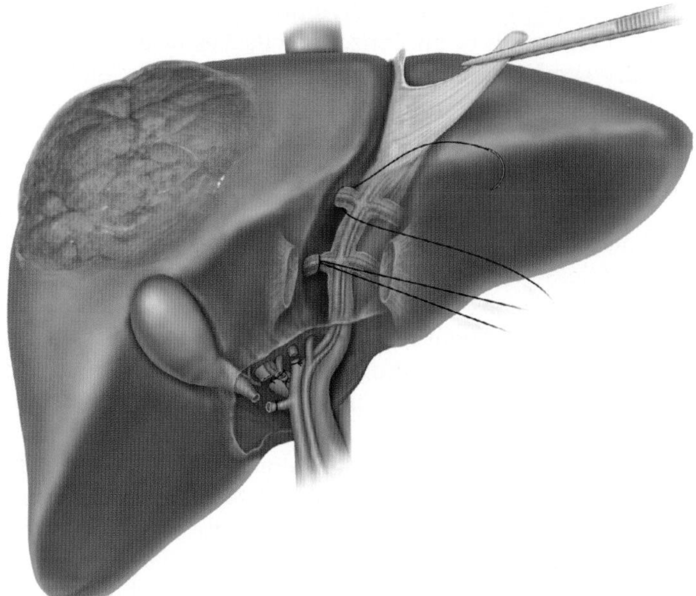

Figure 19.10 The approach to the inflow to segment IV is illustrated. The divided ligamentum teres is drawn to the left and any liver tissue overlying the umbilical fissure is divided with cautery. Multiple pedicle branches to the right of the umbilical fissure can be encircled in the umbilical fissure or within the substance of the liver and dividing, thus depriving, segment IV of its blood supply.

course posteriorly and cephalad into the left liver at the base of the umbilical fissure. The segmental left portal inflow then branches from the umbilical fissure. There are typically multiple branches to segment IV. Although dissection of separate arterial, portal, and biliary branches within the umbilical fissure is possible, it is rarely necessary. For an extended right hepatectomy, the segment IV pedicle branches can most easily be dissected, encircled, and divided within the parenchyma of segment IV to the right of the umbilical fissure. These segment IV inflow pedicles can be encircled through separate hepatotomy or during parenchymal transection (Fig. 19.10) (see also Figs. 21.8–21.10, 24.7 and 27.9).

## Outflow Control

While division of the right hepatic vein can be done intrahepatically, this results in a parenchymal transection to the right of the proper plane for a right hepatectomy. Our practice is to divide the right hepatic vein extrahepatically in most cases. The dissection of the right hepatic vein is done during mobilization as described above (see Fig. 23.18). After division of the right inflow, we typically divide the vein with a vascular stapler, but controlling the vein with vascular clamps followed by division and suturing is reasonable. If the tumor is close or if there is any concern for caval injury, control of the infra- and suprahepatic vena cava is prudent (Fig. 19.11) (see Chapter 30).

The middle hepatic vein runs in the main portal scissura (Cantlie's line). Therefore, a right or extended right hepatectomy may involve resection of a significant length of the middle vein. If the middle hepatic vein is to be divided somewhere in its central portion, this requires intraparenchymal dissection and division within the substance of the liver. If a division of the middle hepatic vein at its origin is required, there are two approaches that can be used. An extrahepatic division can be accomplished by encircling the middle hepatic vein with a clamp in its usually short extrahepatic course. The middle vein can be encircled above the liver but is much more easily encircled once the right hepatic vein has been divided, as there is now excellent exposure of the right side of the middle hepatic vein (Fig. 19.12). The origin of the middle hepatic vein can also be approached by splitting the liver back to it with identification from an intraparenchymal exposure. Regardless of the approach, it is of critical importance to protect the outflow of the left hepatic vein, since compromise of this vein will result in venous ischemia of the remnant left

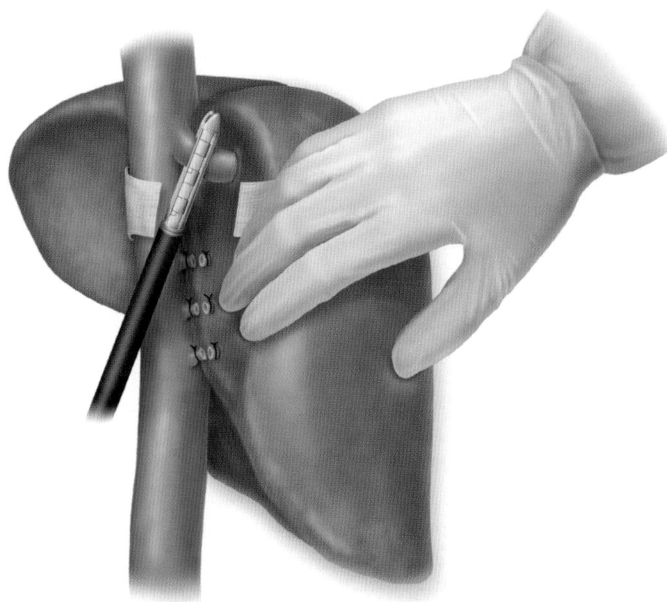

**Figure 19.11** The right hepatic vein has been dissected and encircled. It is then most easily divided with a vascular stapler. Alternatively, the vein can be clamped, divided, and oversewn.



liver, as well as torrential hemorrhage as the liver will be devoid of venous outflow. To ensure that the left hepatic vein is intact, the presumed middle hepatic vein can be clamped with patent left-sided inflow. If there is compromise of the left hepatic vein, venous congestion will be seen grossly. In addition, the outflow can be tested with Doppler ultrasound. In experienced hands, the left hepatic vein can be reconstructed if necessary.

## Parenchymal Transection

A right hepatectomy requires division of the hepatic parenchyma in the main portal scissura in the plane of the middle hepatic vein. If possible, the middle hepatic vein should be preserved to optimize venous drainage of the remnant. In this situation, the transection line is just to the right of the middle hepatic vein. This requires

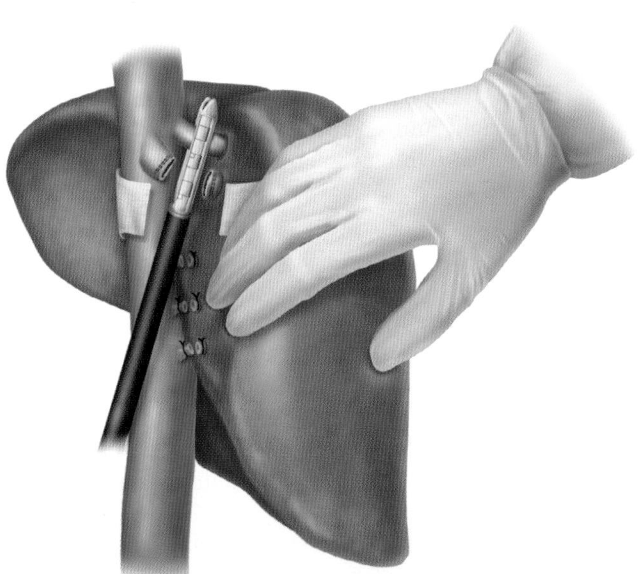

**Figure 19.12** The middle hepatic vein can be approached within the substance of the liver during parenchymal transection or in its extrahepatic location. Once the right hepatic vein has been divided, the middle hepatic vein can usually be encircled and divided with a vascular stapler. Preservation of the left hepatic vein is critical.

dissection of the right-sided branches of the middle hepatic vein, with careful identification and ligation. There is typically a large branch off the middle hepatic vein to segment VIII that must be carefully controlled. A right hepatectomy can also be performed in this central plane to the left of the middle hepatic vein with preservation of segment IV.

An extended right hepatectomy removes some or all of segment IV, in addition to segments V to VIII, and the plane of transection is typically along the right side of the umbilical fissure, back toward the origin of the middle hepatic vein (depending on how much of segment IV is to be removed) (see Fig. 18.6). This requires dissection at the base of segment IV where the line of transection turns transversely to the right, protecting the left bile duct and left inflow structures. This mandates careful dissection and previous lowering of the hilar plate.

There are numerous instruments and methods used to transect hepatic parenchyma, none necessarily better than the other (see Figs. 18.10 and 18.11). Among the many techniques, some prefer use of instruments such as the Cavitron ultrasonic aspirator (CUSA), others prefer pre-coagulation with radiofrequency ablation devices and still others prefer a simple clamp-crushing technique with a Kelly clamp. The preferred technique is dependent on training, comfort level, instrument availability and local expertise. Regardless of instrumentation, parenchymal transection should be a dissection rather than a frantic effort to control bleeding. Intraparenchymal structures should be anticipated, identified and divided safely with full knowledge of one's location inside the liver. Although the optimal technique for parenchymal transection is debatable, we discourage the use of multiple, blind staple fires or deep coagulation with ablation devices. Our technique is a simple clamp-crushing technique with division of specific vessels using clips, ties, sutures, staplers, or cautery devices. Low CVP anesthesia (see above) minimizes bleeding from hepatic veins. Inflow occlusion (Pringle maneuver) can also be safely used and applied intermittently.

## Special Considerations

- For large tumors of the right liver, classical mobilization as described above may not be possible or safe. Sometimes an anterior approach is necessary. In this technique, the inflow to the right liver is controlled and the parenchymal transection is performed without any mobilization or dissection of the vena cava. The transection is carried out back to the vena cava, and the right hepatic vein (and other retrohepatic venous branches) is encircled and divided. Only then is the liver dissected off of its diaphragmatic and retroperitoneal attachments. This technique has been associated with a survival benefit in patients with large hepatocellular carcinoma of the right liver in a randomized trial.
- The anterior approach can also be facilitated by a "hanging maneuver" in which a large clamp is used to bluntly dissect the plane between the vena cava and the liver inferiorly up to the groove between the right and middle hepatic vein. This clamp is then used to pass a tape underneath the liver which can guide the anterior approach parenchymal transection (Fig. 19.13).

## Adjacent Organs

The most common adjacent involved organs during a right hepatectomy are the diaphragm and the right adrenal gland. If it is suspected that the diaphragm is involved, the surgeon should not hesitate to excise a disc of it with the tumor. The diaphragm is repaired with interrupted non-absorbable sutures. The pneumothorax can be evacuated with a catheter placed through a purse-string stitch into the pleural space and removed under suction. One should also consider placing a chest tube, although we do not think this is mandatory in all cases.

The right adrenal gland can be involved by posterior tumors and should be removed if necessary for tumor clearance. Part of the gland can be transected with a stapler or between sutures, preserving the adrenal vein, or the whole gland can be excised. If the

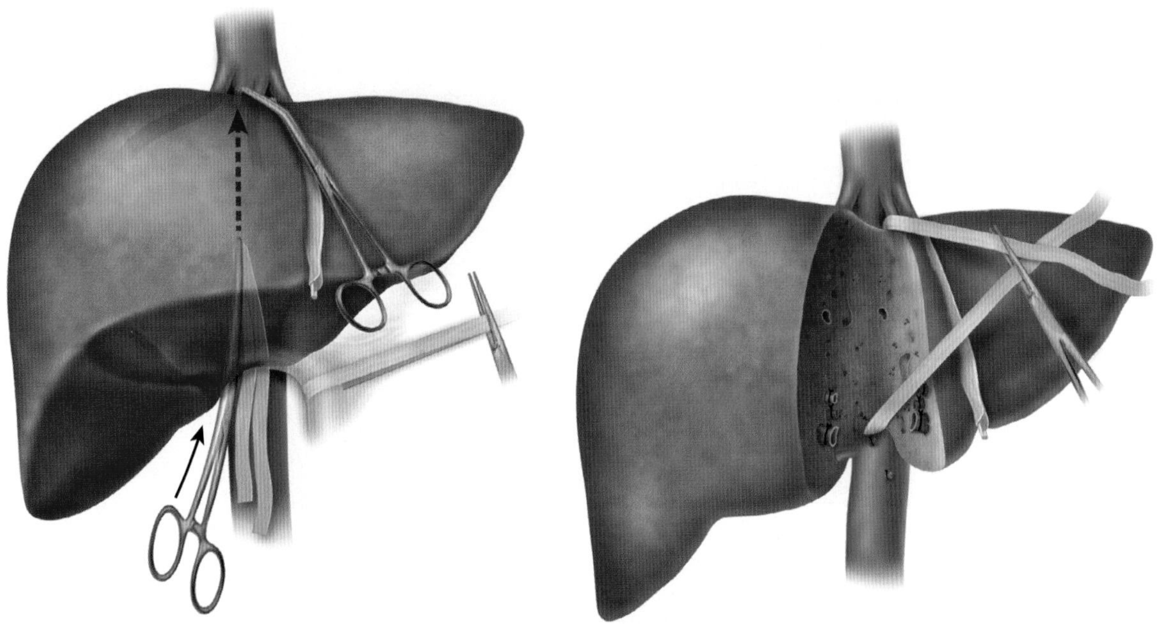

Figure 19.13 The hanging maneuver is illustrated. Briefly, a long clamp is bluntly passed between the liver and vena cava in a plane between the right and the middle hepatic vein. A sling is then passed through this space and used to elevate the central plane of the liver to assist in division of the liver substance.



whole gland is to be excised, the right adrenal vein must be completely dissected and divided as it enters the vena cava.

## Post-resection

- An oozing raw surface is common after resection and requires some degree of hemostasis. Use of the argon beam coagulator is common. Significant bleeding should be sutured. If there is any concern about placing deep sutures and injury to underlying structures, topical hemostatics can be used instead of sutures.
- The falciform ligament is re-attached to prevent extreme rotation of the left liver.
- Perfusion and venous drainage of the remnant liver should be observed grossly and assessed with Doppler ultrasound if necessary.
- Although it is common practice to place drains after a hepatic resection, we do not use drains routinely, since randomized trials have not shown any benefit
- Inspection of the cut surface of the liver and the porta hepatis for bile leaks which should be addressed with fine absorbable suture. If an ongoing bile leak cannot be corrected, a drain should be placed.

# POSTOPERATIVE MANAGEMENT

Fluid resuscitation is generally required in the first 24 to 48 hours but overuse of fluid should be avoided. As in any major operation, early ambulation is critical. Electrolytes, blood counts and prothrombin times should be checked daily; electrolyte replacement is commonly required, particularly potassium and phosphate. In experienced hands, transfusion of packed red blood cells should be uncommon, and we typically use a hemoglobin level of 7 to 8 g/dL as a trigger. The international normalized ratio (INR) should be routinely checked and, although triggers for the transfusion of fresh frozen plasma (FFP) vary, most patients will tolerate having an INR of 1.8 to 2 without problems. We typically transfuse FFP at an INR of 2 or if there are signs of bleeding. Prolonged antibiotics are unnecessary. While venous thromboembolism is uncommon after

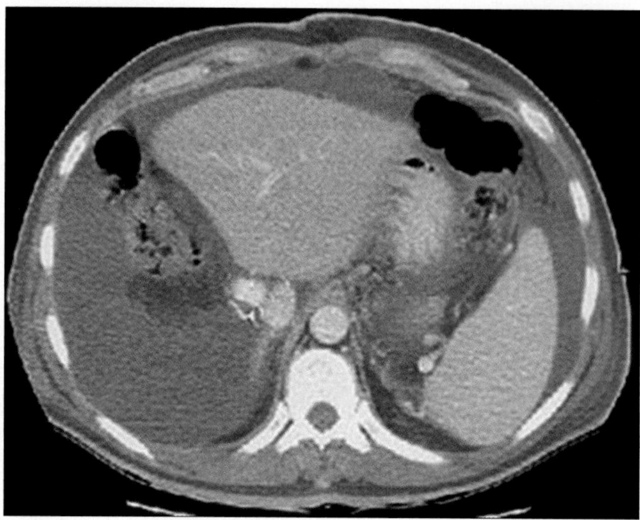

Figure 19.14 A postoperative computed tomography scan illustrates a liver remnant after an extended right hepatectomy with accompanying ascites.

major hepatic resection, one should consider prophylactic doses of subcutaneous heparin once the INR approaches normal.

## COMPLICATIONS

- Significant complications that require special attention include ascites, abscess and/or biloma, biliary stricture and liver dysfunction. Patients are also at risk for generalized cardiopulmonary complications.
- Transient portal hypertension and ascites can occur and can be troublesome if leaking through a wound (Fig. 19.14). This requires aggressive treatment with diuretics and often a course of Spironolactone for a period of time postoperatively. If there is no resolution, radiologic assessment of the portal and the hepatic venous flow is indicated.
- A right hepatectomy can often leave a large dead space that can accumulate fluid or bile. If infected or symptomatic (fever, elevated white blood cells, etc.) percutaneous drainage is indicated. Almost all bile leaks will heal with drainage and do not generally require biliary drainage or operative repair.
- Biliary strictures are rare after resection but should be considered if there is unexplained jaundice postoperatively. Biliary drainage is indicated to prevent liver failure. Ultimately, attempts at balloon dilatation are worth trying but delayed operative repair may be necessary.
- Postoperative liver dysfunction is usually manifested as rising serum bilirubin and INR. Most often, this is transient and is resolving by postoperative day 5. If liver dysfunction persists, imaging is indicated to assess portal and hepatic venous flow as well as biliary dilatation; each of which should be addressed if possible. Rarely, postoperative liver failure occurs with no explanation, and unfortunately is often lethal.

## RESULTS

While morbidity for these operations has generally remained around 40% (half of which is minor), mortality has significantly decreased, with mortality rates generally below 5%.

## Recommended References and Reading


Belghiti J, Guevara OA, Non R, et al. Liver hanging maneuver: a safe approach to right hepatectomy without liver mobilization. *J Am Coll Surg.* 2001;193(1):109–111.

Bruix J, Castells A, Bosch J, et al. Surgical resection of hepatocellular carcinoma in cirrhotic patients: prognostic value of perop-erative portal pressure. *Gastroenterology.* 1996;111(4):1018–1022.

D'Angelica M, Maddineni S, Fong Y, et al. Optimal abdominal incision for partial hepatectomy: increased late complications with Mercedes-type incisions compared to extended right subcostal incisions. *World J Surg.* 2006;30(3):410–418.

Farges O, Belghiti J, Kianmanesh R, et al. Portal vein embolization before right hepatectomy: prospective clinical trial. *Ann Surg.* 2003;237(2):208–217.

Fong Y, Brennan MF, Brown K, et al. Drainage is unnecessary after elective liver resection. *Am J Sur.* 1996;171(1):158–162.

Jarnagin WR, Gonen M, Fong Y, et al. Improvements in perioperative outcome after hepatic resection: Analysis of 1,803 consecutive cases over the past decade. *Ann Surg.* 2002;236(4): 397–407.

Launois B, Jamieson GG. The importance of Glisson's capsule and its sheaths in the intrahepatic approach to resection of the liver. *Surg Gynecol Obstetrics.* 1992;174(1):7–10.

Liu CL, Fan ST, Cheung ST, et al. Anterior approach versus conventional approach right hepatic resection for large hepatocellular5 carcinoma: a prospective randomized controlled study. *Ann Surg.* 2006:244(2):194–203.

Melendez JA, Arslan V, Fischer Me, et al. Perioperative outcomes of major hepatic resections under low central venous pressure anesthesia: blood loss, blood transfusion and the risk of postop-erative renal dysfunction. *J Am Coll Surg.* 1998;187(6):620–625.

Poon RT, Fan ST, Lo CM, et al. Improving perioperative outcome expands the role of hepatectomy in management of benign and malignant hepatobiliary diseases; analysis of 1222 consecutive patients from a prospective database. *Ann Surg.* 2004;240(4):698–708.

# 20 Left and Extended Left Hepatectomy

**J. Peter A. Lodge**

## Introduction

Anatomic left-sided hepatic resections can be described as left lateral sectionectomy (resection of segments 2 and 3), left hemihepatectomy (resection of segments 2, 3, and 4 ± 1) and left hepatic trisectionectomy (or extended left hepatectomy, resection of segments 2, 3, 4, 5, and 8 ± 1) (see Fig. 18.6). En bloc resection of the caudate lobe (segment 1) may be performed in conjunction with left or extended left hepatectomy for various diagnoses (see Chapter 22).

Left lateral sectionectomy is commonly performed laparoscopically today and the laparoscopic technique is described in Chapter 31. This is one of the most minor hepatectomies and a detailed description is not necessary. It is mentioned here only for completeness.

Left hemihepatectomy is more challenging and is most usually performed by an open surgery, although more expert laparoscopic surgeons are beginning to carry it out.

Left hepatic trisectionectomy was first described in detail by Starzl as left trisegmentectomy in 1982. The procedure has recently been renamed because of an international confusion in nomenclature: Terms such as extended left hepatectomy have become ill-defined. It remains a procedure used in few highly specialised units primarily for the treatment of extensive and advanced hepatic or biliary diseases: I reported my own unit's experience with 70 cases of left hepatic trisectionectomy in 2005 and this experience now extends to 100 cases of this difficult operation. Despite the advances in surgical and anesthetic techniques made in recent years, left hepatic trisectionectomy is still thought to be associated with higher rates of morbidity and mortality than other resections. This is mainly attributable to the aggressive nature of the (usually malignant) disease being treated, but may also be related to the extent of liver volume being resected, estimated at approximately 80% by several authors. It should be noted, however, that the volume of the liver remnant after left trisectionectomy (segments 6 and 7) is generally greater than that remaining after right trisectionectomy (segments 2 and 3). Despite this, we have demonstrated that it is possible to extend the procedure to include parts of segments 6 and 7. This procedure has enabled the resection of advanced tumors with curative intent. Despite advances in surgical technique and perioperative management, it remains the most challenging of the major anatomic hepatectomies with higher complication rates than other hepatic, and worldwide experience remains small. The infrequency with which it is performed and the absence of surface landmarks to guide the resection both contribute to the higher morbidity. Although several authors have focused on this complicated hepatectomy, few reports have described the results of large series and long-term follow-up has rarely been considered.

The comments below, therefore, relate primarily to left hemihepatectomy and left hepatic trisectionectomy.

## Patient Selection

### Cardiorespiratory Assessment

Before considering a surgical procedure of this scale, it is essential to be as sure as possible that the patient is fit enough to withstand the operation. It is important to take a detailed history of previous cardiovascular diseases, including myocardial infarction, angina pectoris, and hypertension. Clearly, a history of smoking or peripheral vascular disease should raise the clinical suspicion of coronary artery disease. Respiratory diseases, particularly emphysema and chronic bronchitis, are quite prevalent in the elderly population and clinical examination with chest radiology can be helpful.

Resting and exercise electrocardiography are the standard cardiologic objective assessment tests in our center. Failure to achieve an adequate heart rate for true stress testing can be a problem in the elderly population, most often due to osteoarthritis of the hips and knees. In this situation, a great deal of useful information can be gained from echocardiography, with measurement of end diastolic and systolic volumes to calculate left ventricular ejection fraction, or by radioisotope assessment with dobutamine stress. Failure to complete these investigations or a significant depression of the ST segment on the exercise ECG is a clear indication for coronary artery angiography. This procedure is carried out in 3% of major liver surgery candidates in our experience, ruling out surgery in 1% but providing reassuring information in the rest. Only a few patients in our experience have been suitable for preoperative coronary artery angioplasty, stenting or bypass grafting prior to liver surgery, but these are clearly potential treatment options to consider.

Routine lung function tests including vital capacity and forced expiratory volume form part of our standard assessment as well as chest radiology. Useful information is also gained from the chest CT, which is done primarily to look for lung metastases and diaphragm involvement by the hepatic tumor. The CT appearances of emphysema in particular are characteristic. In our northern UK population, because of the high incidence of emphysema and chronic obstructive airways disease, we occasionally consider blood gas sampling preoperatively.

### Hepatic Reserve Assessment (see Chapter 18)

Preoperative blood tests necessary before proceeding to major resection include full blood count, urea and electrolytes, liver function tests, clotting screen and tumor marker studies. Prothrombin time, bilirubin and albumin give a fairly accurate indication of global hepatic function, but in some cases, a liver biopsy of the residual tumor-free liver will also be necessary if there is a doubt about hepatic reserve, in particular, when considering resection for hepatocellular carcinoma. This is particularly important in the group of patients with a previous history of excess alcohol consumption or if there is serologic evidence of hepatitis B or C. It is also useful when dealing with cholangiocarcinoma, as there may be underlying sclerosing cholangitis.

It is inevitable that a degree of temporary hepatic failure will be induced in some patients undergoing very major resection. More work needs to be done in this interesting area. If the tumor-free segments are affected by biliary obstruction, it is our current practice to attempt biliary decompression by endoscopic or percutaneous techniques a few days in advance of surgery as this may speed up the postoperative recovery and reduce risks for morbidity and mortality in major liver surgery. In most cases of major left hepatectomy, the volume of the right liver remnant, even if only segments 6 and 7, is generally adequate, and preoperative portal vein embolization is usually unnecessary. We have not used portal vein embolization routinely.

### Radiology Assessment

Although MRI is the imaging method of choice for the liver in our center, other groups routinely use CT arterioportography with similar results. Three dimensional CT and MRI imaging technology continue to improve and may be of value in planning the surgical approach. It is our current practice to use CT scanning of chest, abdomen and pelvis to exclude extrahepatic disease for all tumor types, but FDG-PET scanning is also used in selected cases, particularly biliary tract cancers. Screening for primary site recurrence (e.g., colonoscopy) is also clearly important. An isotope bone scan may be useful in patients with advanced disease.

## PREOPERATIVE PREPARATION

Routine blood tests in our unit include full blood count, urea and electrolytes, liver function tests, coagulation screen, C-reactive protein (CRP), blood group and save, and tumor marker studies (primarily carcinoembryonic antigen [CEA], CA19-9, and alpha feto protein) immediately before surgery as a baseline. A low molecular weight heparin may be administered on the night before surgery to reduce the risk of deep vein thrombosis and pulmonary embolism for patients admitted preoperatively and at the end of surgery admitted on the day of surgery. Broad spectrum antibiotics are given at the time of anesthetic induction.



# Anesthesia

It is our routine to place a central venous line and a urinary catheter for careful monitoring. A warm air flow device covers the patient as well as a standard warming blanket underneath. We use an air–oxygen-desfurane-based anesthesia which has been shown to minimise the derangement of postoperative liver function, with infusions of n-acetyl cysteine and antioxidants to confer hepatic protection. We use an accepted methodology for low central venous pressure anesthesia and we use an epidural catheter for central venous pressure manipulation as well as postoperative analgesia, although vasodilators are sometimes necessary in addition. Inotropic/vasoconstrictor support, primarily with norepinephrine or phenylephrine, is often necessary for the elderly patients to support blood pressure during surgery.

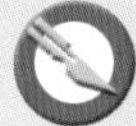

## OPERATIVE TECHNIQUE

### Left Lateral Sectionectomy

A strictly anatomical approach is unnecessary. Left lateral sectionectomy is considered for tumors obliterating much of hepatic segments 2 and 3 or compromising the portal triad structures for these segments. A lesser resection should usually be planned for more peripheral tumors and parenchyma-sparing techniques offer the patient a potential lifeline for re-resection if a further liver tumor occurs in the future. A resection of segment 2 or 3 individually (see Chapter 24 and Figs. 24.5 and 24.6) or wedge excisions for smaller peripheral tumors can be performed. This can often be combined with a right liver resection (Fig. 20.1). The use of ultrasonic dissection (CUSA, Valleylab, Inc., Boulder, CO) or alternative appropriate parenchymal-dissection techniques negates the need for vascular control in most cases.

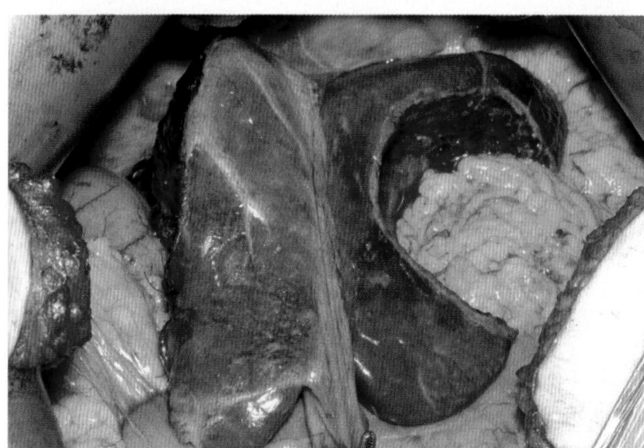

**Figure 20.1** A lesser resection should usually be planned for more peripheral tumors and parenchyma sparing techniques offer the patient a potential lifeline for re-resection if a further liver tumor occurs in the future. This can often be combined with a right liver resection; in this case, right hemihepatectomy.

If vascular control is needed, a simple Pringle maneuver (portal triad clamping) should suffice. The segment 2 and 3 portal triad structures can be divided within the liver parenchyma using clamps and suture ligation or surgical staplers. The left hepatic vein is similarly divided, taking care not to compromise the middle hepatic vein at its common insertion into the inferior vena cava. Thus, this procedure usually lends itself well to laparoscopic approaches.

In some circumstances, a more careful dissection of the left portal pedicle is required, for example in patients with segmental Caroli's disease affecting the segment 2/3 hepatic duct. In these cases, it is preferable to use a Pringle maneuver to allow division of the left hepatic vein at an early stage. It is then possible to lift the left lateral section with some traction to enable a more accurate dissection of the left hepatic duct, or a division closer to segment 4 but without further compromise of the liver parenchyma.

## Left Hemihepatectomy

After operability assessment, portal triad dissection is commenced with ligation and division of the cystic duct and artery, as cholecystectomy is a necessary part of this operation. After mobilization of the left liver (by division of the falciform and left triangular ligaments), the left portal vein and the left hepatic artery are divided separately at the base of the umbilical fissure, and a demarcation between the left and right hemi livers is observed (Fig. 20.2). In cases planned for caudate lobe (segment 1) resection, the left portal vein and the left hepatic artery are divided at their origins to interrupt the blood supply to the caudate lobe. It is our usual practice to use a surgical stapling device for portal vein transection except in cases of tumor encroachment, where division between vascular clamps and suture ligation may be more appropriate to ensure tumor clearance. Our approach is intra-Glissonian and no attempt is made to ligate or divide

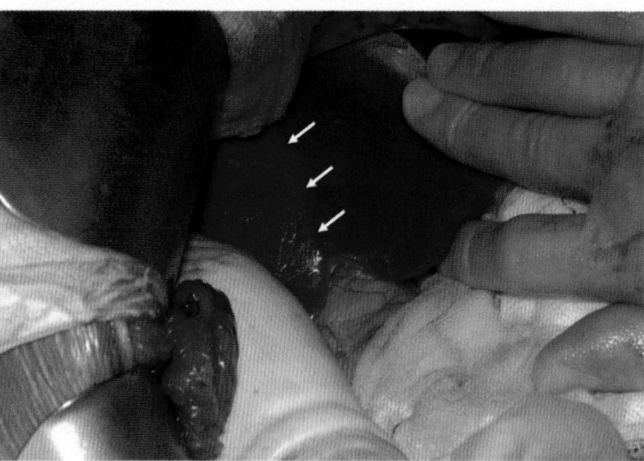

**Figure 20.2** Demarcation between the left and right hemi livers is observed (*arrows*). In this case, the gallbladder has just been removed.

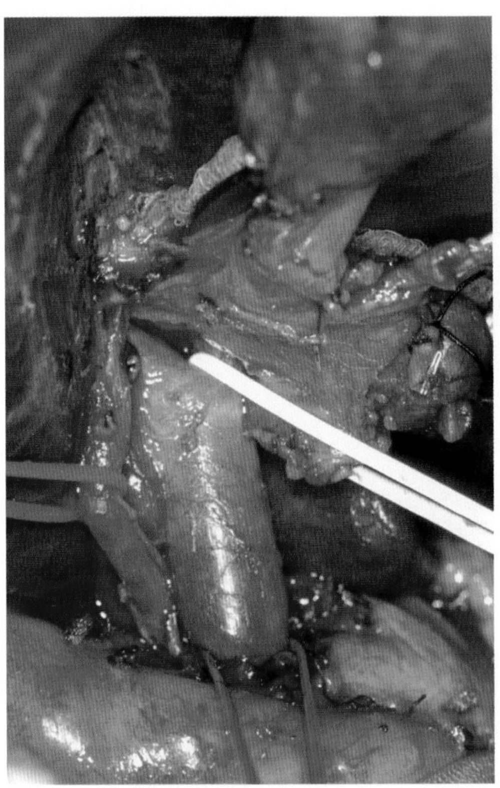

Figure 20.3 In cases of hilar cholangiocarcinoma, regional or extended (regional + paraaortic) lymphadenectomy along with division of the common bile duct within the superior aspect of the head of the pancreas allows biliary excision, lymphadenectomy and neurectomy of the portal triad region. In this case, there is an abberant right hepatic artery from the superior mesenteric artery (*red sling*) and this can be life saving. The left portal vein is about to be divided (*white sling*).



the left hepatic duct at this stage as variant anatomy is common and it is safer to divide the biliary tree later during liver parenchymal transection (see Fig. 17.9). The lesser omentum is divided (ligating any accessory left hepatic arterial branches). In cases of hilar cholangiocarcinoma (see Chapter 26), these aspects are preceded by regional or extended (regional and paraaortic) lymphadenectomy along with division of the common bile duct within the superior aspect of the head of the pancreas to allow biliary excision, lymphadenectomy and neurectomy of the portal triad region (Fig. 20.3). If the caudate lobe is to be excised, it needs to be mobilized from the inferior vena cava, with ligation or suture of its short hepatic veins (Fig. 20.4). No attempt is made to identify or isolate the left hepatic vein at this stage, as this introduces danger to the middle hepatic vein, which almost always has a common insertion into the inferior vena cava with the left hepatic vein.

Liver parenchymal transection is done using the CUSA under low central venous pressure anesthesia (<5 cm $H_2O$), and by lifting the left lateral section ventrally (by traction on the round ligament in most cases) to minimize the venous bleeding by reducing the "central venous pressure" within the liver remnant. An intermittent Pringle maneuver is used when necessary, and rarely have we used total vascular isolation. We have not used

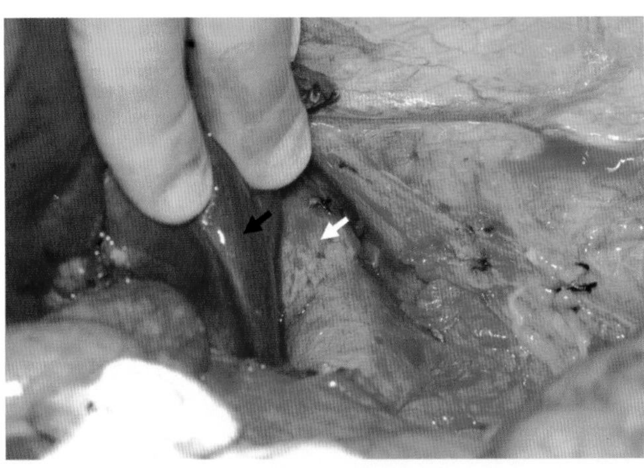

Figure 20.4 If the caudate lobe is to be excised, it needs to be mobilized from the inferior vena cava (*white arrow*), with ligation or suture of its short hepatic veins. In this image, the caudate is retracted upward off the vena cava (*black arrow*).

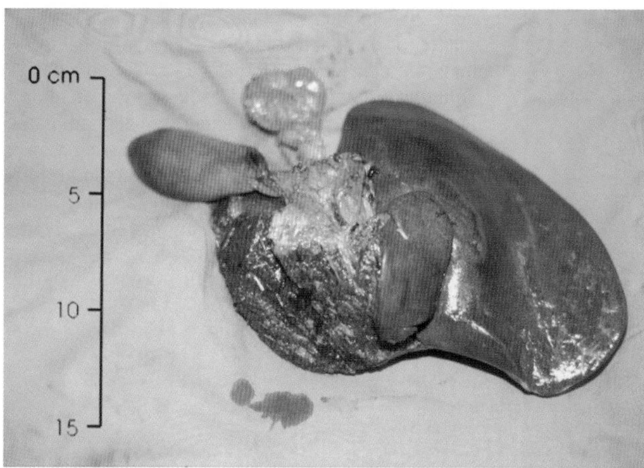


**Figure 20.5** In cases of perihilar cholangiocarcinoma, it is our usual practice to complete all aspects of the parenchymal transection before division of the right hepatic duct or the anterior (segments 5 and 8) and posterior (segments 6 and 7) sectional hepatic ducts, lifting the left liver, dropping the right liver back to divide the ducts as far away from the tumor as possible. Here, the resected specimen is demonstrated.

ischemic preconditioning. Residual vascular and biliary division is done at appropriate stages of the hepatic transaction. Metastases may also be resected from the liver remnant.

In cases of perihilar cholangiocarcinoma, it is our usual practice to complete all aspects of the parenchymal transection before division of the right hepatic duct or the anterior (segments 5 and 8) and posterior (segments 6 and 7) sectional hepatic ducts, lifting the left liver, dropping the right liver back to divide the ducts as far away from the tumor as possible (Fig. 20.5). In cases of other primary liver tumors or metastasis, it is our practice to retain the hepatic duct confluence to avoid biliary injury. In cases with bile duct resection, reconstruction between the right hepatic duct or the sectional hepatic ducts and the jejunum is performed by Roux-en-Y hepaticojejunostomy (Fig. 20.6, Fig. 20.7).

## Left Hepatic Trisectionectomy

Inevitably, operative techniques have developed with increasing experience. Currently, our technique is as follows, and this is largely as described by Blumgart et al. After mobilization of both the right and the left liver, the left portal vein and the left hepatic artery are divided separately at the base of the umbilical fissure (Fig. 20.8). In cases planned for caudate lobe (segment 1) resection, the left portal vein and the left hepatic artery are divided at their origins to interrupt the blood supply to the caudate lobe. The right anterior sectional portal and arterial branches are divided separately by opening the right Glissonian sheath (Fig. 20.9), if possible, or the entire right anterior sectional portal pedicle can be isolated and divided at this stage, staying outside the Glissonian sheath. When the vessels are difficult to identify extrahepatically, they are divided during liver parenchymal transection. The lesser omentum is divided (ligating any accessory left hepatic arterial branches). If the caudate lobe is to be excised, it needs to be mobilized from the inferior vena cava, with ligation or suture of its short hepatic veins (see Chapter 22). This maneuver can usually be accomplished from the left side, but if

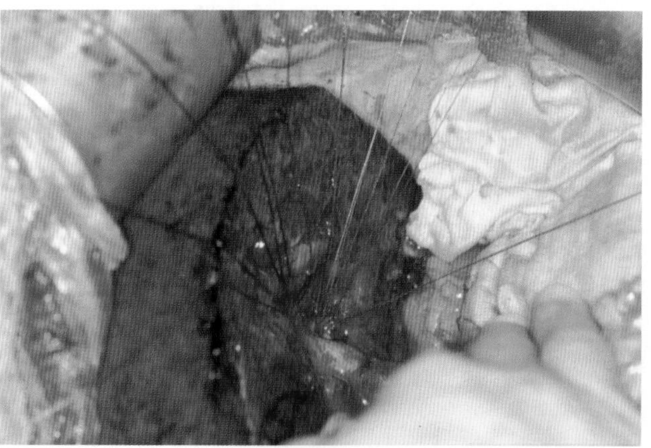

**Figure 20.6** In cases with bile duct resection, reconstruction between the right hepatic duct or the sectional hepatic ducts and the jejunum is performed by Roux-en-Y hepaticojejunostomy. In this case, the portal vein confluence has been resected and there is an anastomosis between the right portal vein and the main portal vein. 4-0 vicryl sutures have been placed for subsequent biliary anastomosis.

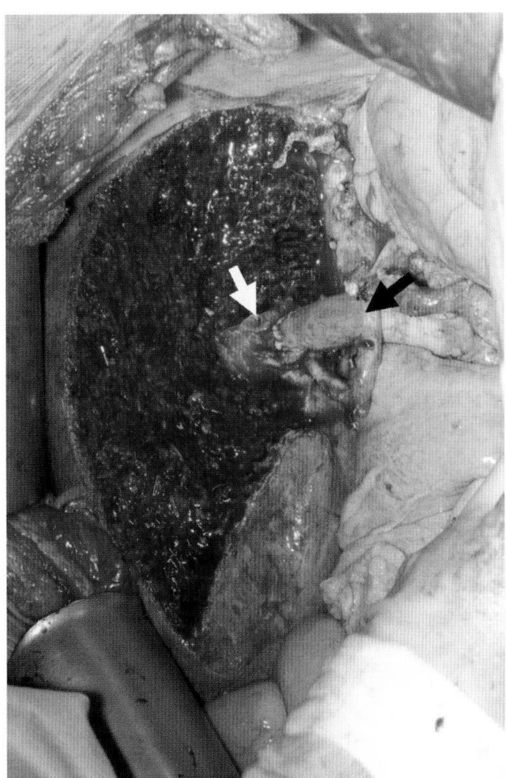

**Figure 20.7** In this further example of left hemi-hepatectomy for hilar cholangiocarcinoma, the portal vein confluence has been resected and there is an anastomosis between the right portal vein and the main portal vein (*black arrow*). The lymphadenectomy has been completed, with resection of nerves and lymphatics from the right hepatic artery and portal vein. The segment 5/8 and 6/7 hepatic duct stumps can be seen anterior to the portal vein anastomosis (*white arrow*).



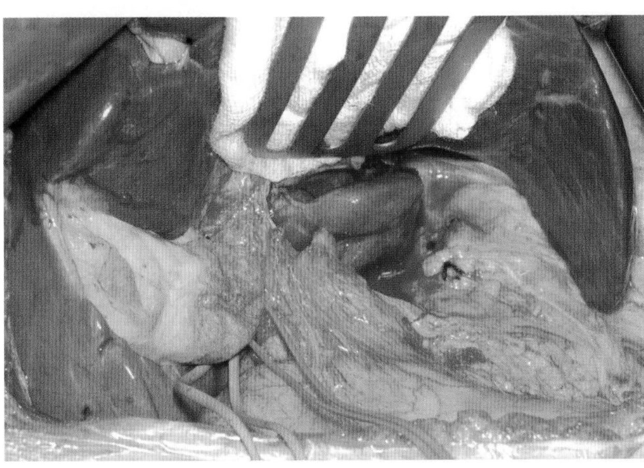

**Figure 20.8** After mobilization of both the right and the left liver, the left portal vein and the left hepatic artery have been divided separately at the base of the umbilical fissure. The slings are isolating and protecting the right posterior sectional hepatic artery and portal vein.

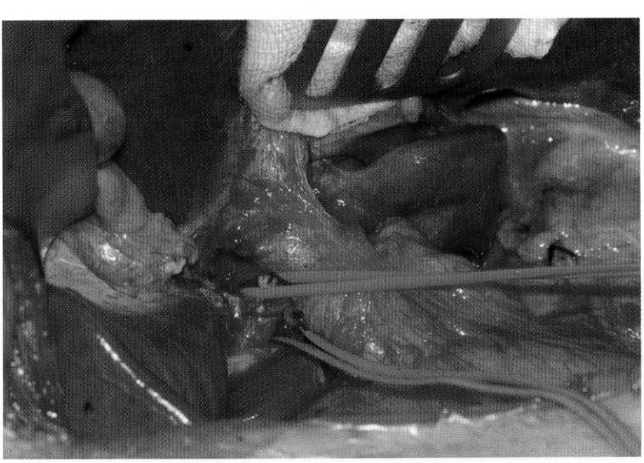

**Figure 20.9** The right anterior sectional portal and arterial branches are divided separately by opening the right Glissonian sheath, if possible as shown here, or the entire right anterior sectional portal pedicle can be isolated and divided at this stage, staying outside the Glissonian sheath. The slings are isolating and protecting the right posterior sectional hepatic artery and portal vein.

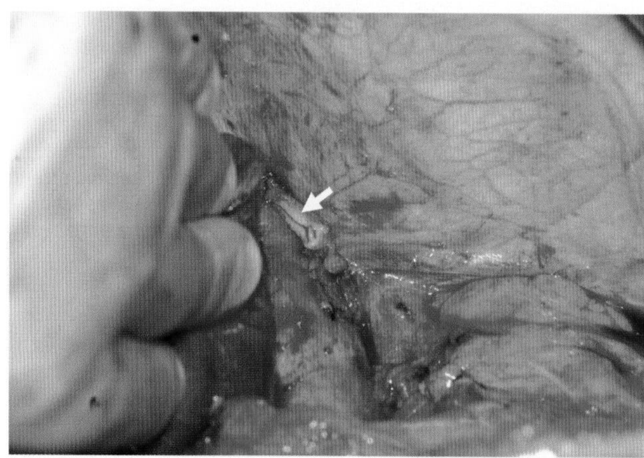

**Figure 20.10** If the right anterior sectional portal vein and the hepatic artery have been divided, then the middle and left hepatic veins should be divided immediately, and our usual practice is to use a surgical stapling device (*white arrow*).

there is significant involvement of the caudate lobe with tumor, then it may be necessary to approach the caudate veins from the right. In this case, it is important to preserve any major inferior or middle right hepatic veins which may be draining segment 6. The hepatocaval confluence is most safely approached from the left side: The middle and left hepatic veins can be isolated and slung together for subsequent division by passing behind these structures anterior to the inferior vena cava to emerge between the middle and right hepatic veins (see Fig. 22.6). If the right anterior sectional portal vein and hepatic artery have been divided, then the middle and left hepatic veins should be divided immediately, and our usual practice is to use a surgical stapling device (Fig. 20.10). However, in the past or in cases of very difficult access, we have used a 3/0 monofilament polypropylene suture after division between vascular clamps. This division creates two distinct advantages: A clear line of demarcation appears at the junction of segments 6 and 7 with 5 and 8 (Fig. 20.11); and the extended left liver to be removed becomes considerably more mobile. If the right anterior sectional portal vein and hepatic artery have not been divided, then division of the left and middle hepatic veins must wait until that point in the parenchymal transection, or the extended left liver will become congested, resulting in more difficult access and increased blood loss. In some cases, it is necessary to divide and reconstruct the major portal and hepatic arterial structures. This is best done after parenchymal transection to gain access for the reconstruction phase. In cases of perihilar cholangiocarcinoma, as extrahepatic bile duct excision is required, the common bile duct is divided in the head of the pancreas. All other points of biliary division are done during parenchymal transection to prevent bile duct injury. Liver parenchymal transection is done in our center using the CUSA (Valleylab, Inc., Boulder, CO) under low central venous pressure anesthesia (<5 cm H2O), and lifting the right posterior section ventrally to minimize the venous bleeding by reducing the "central venous pressure" within the liver remnant (Figs. 20.12–20.16).

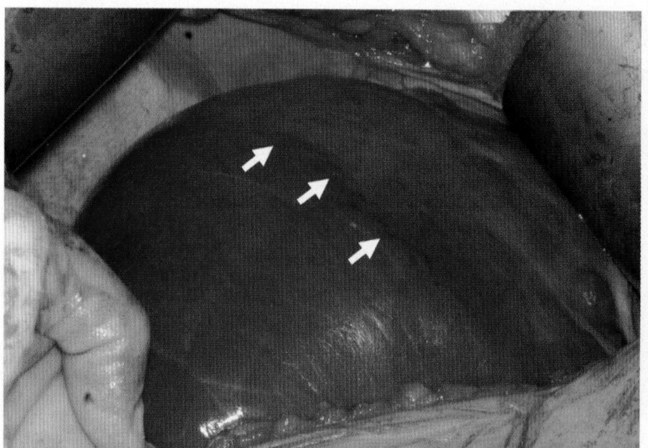

**Figure 20.11** Demarcation appears at the junction of segments 6 and 7 with 5 and 8 (*arrows*).

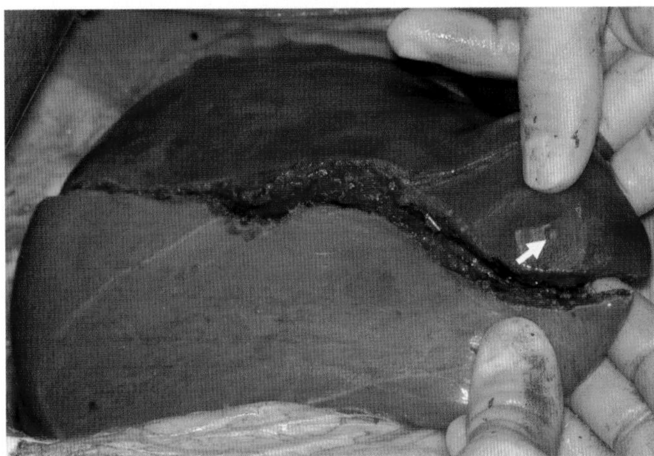

**Figure 20.12** Liver parenchymal transection has begun using the CUSA under low central venous pressure anesthesia. In this case, there is a metastasis in segment 6 and the resection has been extended to include it (*arrow*).

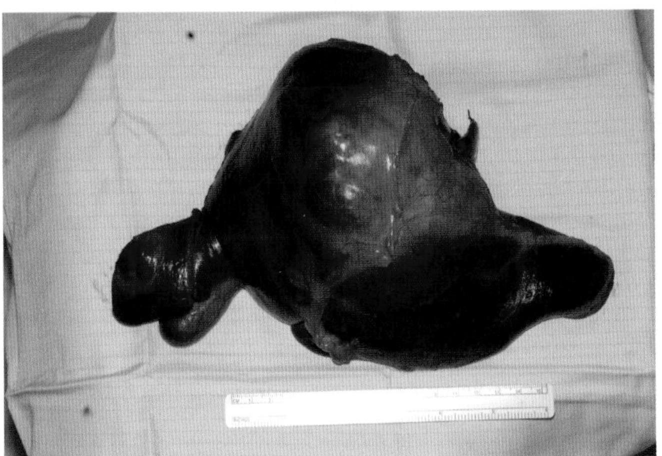

**Figure 20.13** The resected specimen is segments 1, 2, 3, 4, 5, and 8 with the metastasis in segment 6.



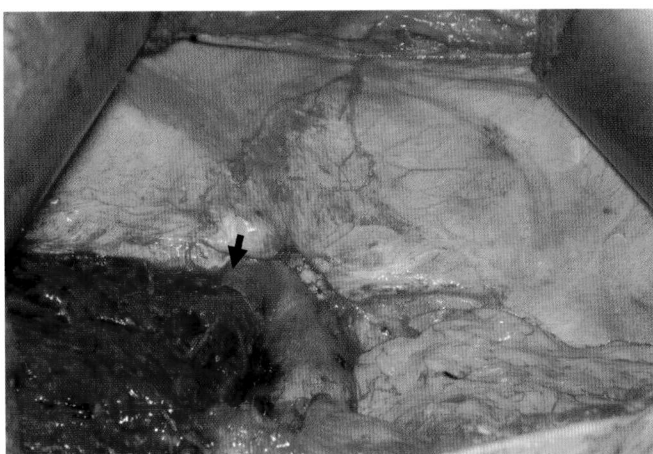

**Figure 20.14** The right hepatic vein can be seen clearly at the resection margin (*arrow*).

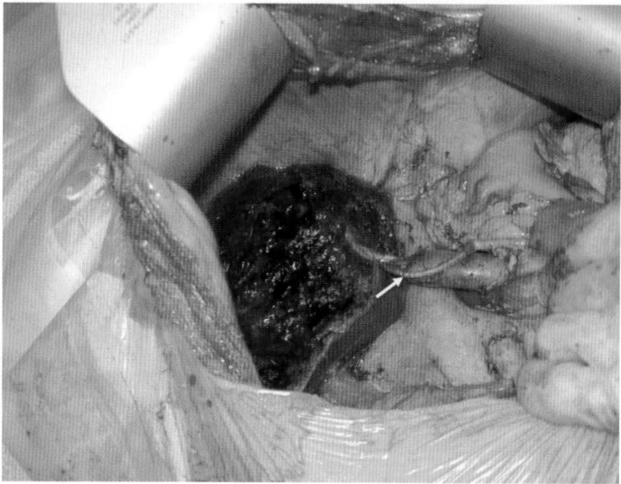

**Figure 20.15** In this example of left hepatic trisectionectomy for hilar cholangiocarcinoma, the portal vein confluence has been resected and there is an anastomosis between the right posterior sectional portal vein and the main portal vein. The lymphadenectomy has been completed. The segment 6/7 hepatic artery can be seen (*arrow*) and the segment 6/7 hepatic duct stump will be anastomosed to a Roux-en-Y.

An intermittent Pringle maneuver is used when the bleeding is considered excessive, and rarely, we have used total vascular isolation (see Chapter 30). Residual vascular and biliary division is done at appropriate stages of the hepatic transection. In cases of perihilar cholangiocarcinoma, it is our usual practice to complete all aspects of the parenchymal transection before division of the segment 6 and 7 hepatic ducts, lifting the extended left liver, dropping the right posterior section back to divide the ducts as far away from the tumor as possible. In cases of metastasis, it is our practice to retain the hepatic duct confluence, dividing the segment 1, 2/3, 4, and 5/8 ducts individually to avoid biliary injury. In cases with bile duct resection, reconstruction between the right posterior sectional bile duct or the segment 6 and 7 bile ducts and the jejunum is performed by Roux-en-Y hepaticojejunostomy.

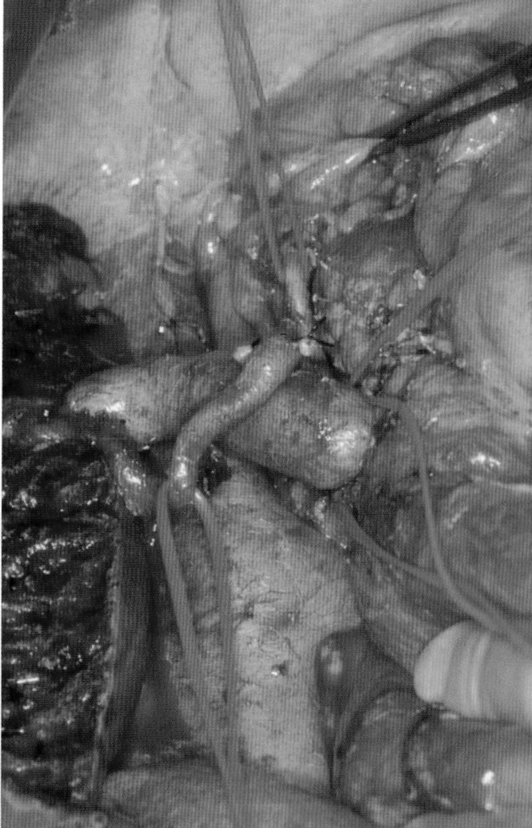

**Figure 20.16** This further example of left hepatic trisectionectomy for hilar cholangiocarcinoma demonstrates the extent of lymphadenectomy.

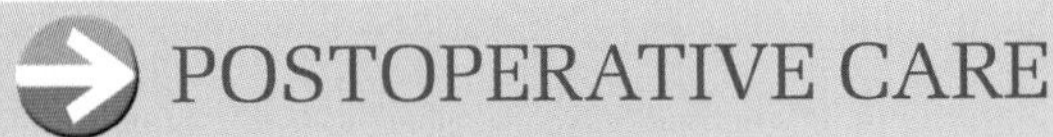

## POSTOPERATIVE CARE

The postoperative care for major liver resection candidates is standardized in most major liver surgery centers. Nursing care should be initially on a high dependency ward or intensive care unit. Rapid mobilization and introduction of enteral nutrition are usually possible. Gastric acid secretion suppression with a proton pump inhibitor is sensible as there is often an associated acute portal hypertension which may be additive to postoperative stress ulceration. The prothrombin time seems to be most predictive of hepatic functional recovery. A daily requirement for fresh frozen plasma (rarely) and 20% human albumin solution (200 ml/day) can be calculated from the blood results. Our group uses n-acetyl cysteine by intravenous infusion for major hepatic resection cases as we have found it to be useful in our fulminant hepatic failure program. In addition, there is usually a requirement for potassium, magnesium, and phosphate supplementation intravenously following very radical resection. The average postoperative stay in our unit is 6 days except in cholangiocarcinoma cases, where recovery is slower (average 14 days). Patients should be expected to feel very tired for 6 to 12 weeks, during liver regeneration, and most will lose weight for 3 to 4 weeks and return to normal weight by 3 months. Quality of life does not appear to be significantly impaired in the long term.

## Recommended References and Readings


Blumgart LH, Baer HU, Czerniak A, et al. Extended left hepatectomy: technical aspects of an evolving procedure. *Br J Surg.* 1993; 80:903–906.

Dasgupta D, Smith AB, Hamilton-Burke W, et al. Quality of life after liver resection for hepatobiliary malignancies. *Br J Surg* 2008;95: 845–854.

Halazun K, Al-Mukhtar A, Aldouri A, et al. Right hepatic trisectionectomy for hepatobiliary diseases: results and an appraisal of its current role. *Ann Surg.* 2007;246:1065–1074.

Lodge JPA. Assessment of hepatic reserve for the indication of hepatic resection: how I do it. *J Heptobiliary Pancreat Surg.* 2005; 12:4–9.

Nishio H, Hidalgo E, Hamady ZZ, et al. Left hepatic trisectionectomy for hepatobiliary malignancy: results and an appraisal of its current role. *Ann Surg.* 2005;242:267–275.

Starzl TE, Iwatsuki S, Shaw BW Jr, et al. Left trisegmentectomy. *Surg Gynecol Obstet.* 1982;155:21–27.

The terminology committee of the IHPBA. The Brisbane 2000 terminology of hepatic anatomy and resections. *HPB.* 2000;2:333–339.

Wong KHV, Hamady ZZ, Malik HZ, et al. Intermittent Pringle manoeuvre is not associated with adverse long-term prognosis after resection for colorectal metastases. *Br J Surg.* 2008:95:985–989.

# 21 Central Hepatectomy

**Jonathan B. Koea**

## Introduction

Central hepatectomy is the only anatomical liver resection that utilizes hepatic venous anatomy rather than the anatomy of hepatic inflow structures as the basis for segmental resection. The procedure removes hepatic parenchyma drained by the middle hepatic vein (Couinaud segments IV, V, and VIII) while preserving inflow to segments II, III, VI, and VII (see Figure 18.6). Resection of the caudate lobe (segment I) can be undertaken in conjunction with the procedure if indicated (see Chapter 22). It is not commonly performed and central resections constitute between 4% and 6% of segmental resections reported from high volume hepatobiliary units. Central hepatectomy is technically more challenging than an extended right hepatectomy, but the additional parenchyma that is preserved translates into a lower risk of postoperative hepatic failure.

The procedure was first described in 1972 by McBride and Wallace. Pack and Miller described middle hepatic lobectomy for cancer in 1961, although this only removed parenchyma between the main interlobar fissure (Cantlie's line) and the umbilical fissure and consequently represents resection of segment IV only. Central hepatectomy has been variously named middle lobectomy, central bisegmentectomy, mesohepatectomy (*meso:* Greek, translates to middle or central), lobectomie médiane totale, hépatectomie or lobectomie médiale, or mixed right intermediate hepatectomy. The Brisbane nomenclature does not assign a single term for the procedure since it comprises a combination of a left medial sectionectomy (segment IV resection) and a right anterior sectionectomy (segments V and VIII resection) although a central bisectionectomy is probably the correct nomenclature. Currently the terms central hepatectomy or mesohepatectomy are used most commonly.

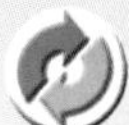

## INDICATIONS

Central hepatectomy is indicated for the resection of tumors located in segments IV, V, and VIII. The tumor must be separate from the left and right hepatic veins such that it can be dissected free of these structures and removed with an adequate surgical margin. Consequently, central hepatectomy can be utilized in the management of the following tumors, if suitably located.

- Symptomatic benign liver tumors (adenoma, focal nodular hyperplasia, hemangioma) and asymptomatic adenoma ≥5 cm in diameter

- Primary malignant tumors of the liver (hepatocellular carcinoma, intrahepatic cholangiocarcinoma)
- Gallbladder carcinoma
- Hilar cholangiocarcinoma
- Metastatic tumors, most commonly colorectal cancer, neuroendocrine carcinoma, melanoma, genitourinary tumors. Generally these patients will have only liver metastatic disease

## CONTRAINDICATIONS

Central hepatectomy cannot be applied to tumors that have spread beyond segments IV, V, and VIII. In particular, tumors that involve either the right or left hepatic veins or the right or left inflow pedicles will require a more extensive resection than central hepatectomy in order to obtain adequate surgical margins.

Central hepatectomy is also contraindicated in the following patients.

- Patients with comorbidities that render them unfit for general anesthesia.
- Patients with normal hepatic parenchyma in whom a central hepatectomy will leave less than 20% hepatic volume since these patients are at significant risk of postoperative liver failure.
- Patients with cirrhosis in whom a central hepatectomy will leave less than 40% of hepatic volume as these patients will be at significant risk of postoperative liver failure.

# Anatomical Considerations

The safe performance of central hepatectomy requires that segments IV, V, and VIII can be isolated and removed while maintaining the vascular inflow and venous and biliary drainage to the remaining five hepatic segments. Several anatomical variations must be recognized preoperatively as they may make safe performance of the procedure impossible or technically difficult.

- The inflow to segment IV is generally constant and is from two discrete branches that arise from the right side of the left main pedicle within the umbilical fissure. Rarely, the main left portal vein arises from the right anterior sectoral pedicle and traverses segment IV supplying it as well as segments II and III (Fig. 21.1). The presence of this variation makes the procedure impossible to perform since the blood supply to segments II and III cannot be preserved, when segment IV is resected.

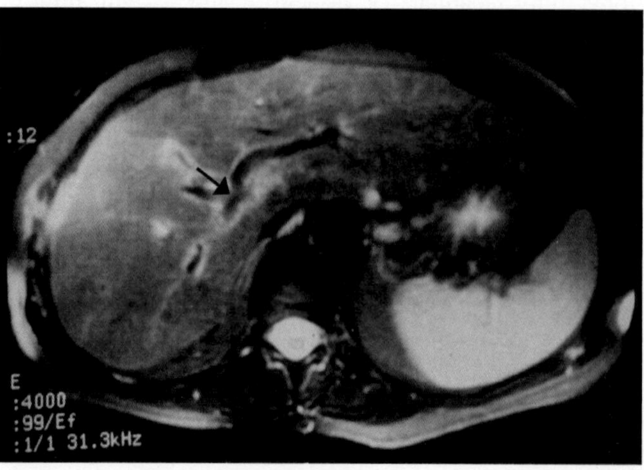


**Figure 21.1** Magnetic resonance scan showing the left hepatic inflow arising from the right inflow pedicle within segment IV (*arrow*).

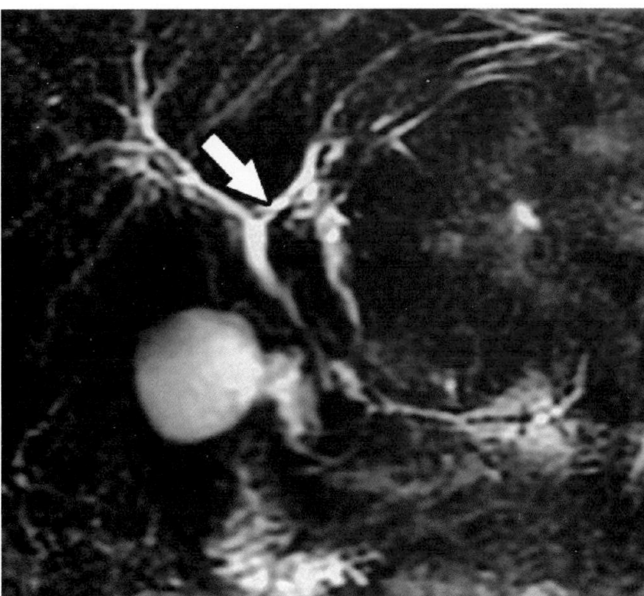

Figure 21.2 Coronal magnetic resonance cholangiogram showing the right posterior sectoral duct joining the proximal left main hepatic duct (*arrow*).

- The right posterior sectoral bile duct drains into the left bile duct in 1% of patients (Fig. 21.2) (see Fig. 17.9). The presence of this variant makes the procedure technically difficult but the posterior sectoral duct generally joins the left main duct close to the hilus and can be isolated and protected, or reconstructed using a Roux-en-Y hepaticojejunostomy.
- The right anterior sectoral duct draining segments V and VIII can arise from the left main pedicle (Fig. 21.3). This does not prevent the procedure from being performed but means that the anterior sectoral branch must be clearly defined and controlled without compromising the main left pedicle.
- The presence of a long common venous trunk formed by the union of the left and middle hepatic veins (Fig. 21.4). This does not prevent the performance of central hepatectomy but emphasizes that the middle hepatic vein must be carefully controlled and isolated without compromising the left hepatic vein.

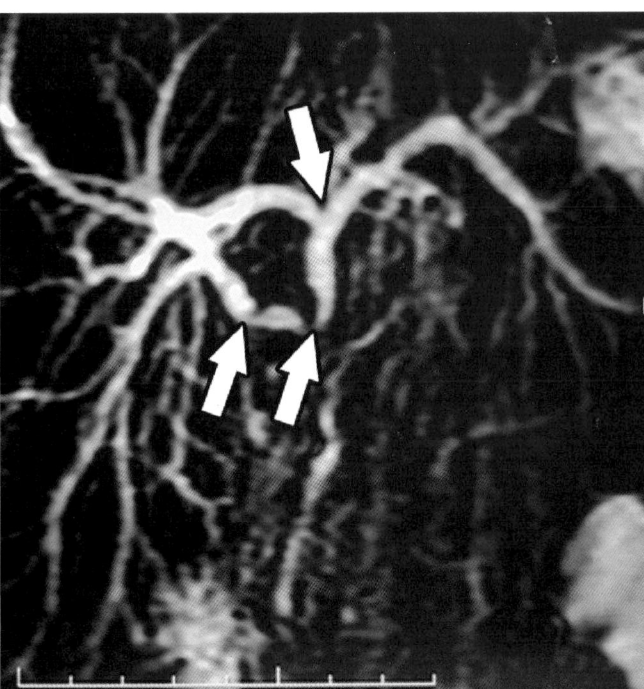

Figure 21.3 Coronal magnetic resonance cholangiogram showing the right anterior sectoral duct draining into the left main duct (*arrow*). The right posterior sectoral duct joins the common hepatic duct inferiorly (*double arrow*).

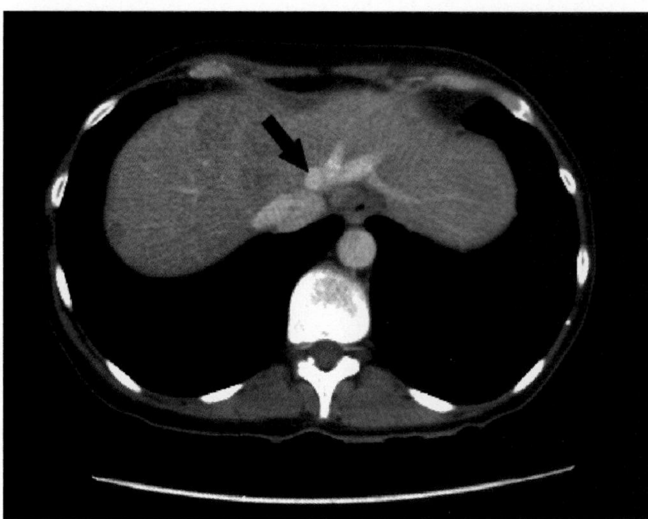

Figure 21.4 CT scan showing the union of left and middle hepatic veins (*arrow*) into a long common venous trunk draining into the vena cava.

## PREOPERATIVE PLANNING

Before surgery a comprehensive assessment of the patient must be carried out. This evaluation should define the patient's overall state of fitness for general anesthesia, the presence of any comorbidities, the functional status of the liver and establish the diagnosis, clinical stage and precise location of the tumor (see Chapter 18).

### Patient Assessment

A thorough history and physical examination should be performed with specific emphasis on defining any underlying cardiovascular, pulmonary, renal, or neurologic disease. If signs of major organ dysfunction or comorbidity are present then these should be investigated appropriately and referred to the relevant specialty for detailed assessment. Measurement of relevant tumor markers such as α-fetoprotein, carcinoembryonic antigen (CEA) and CA19-9 should also be undertaken at this stage.

### Hepatic Function

A physical examination should be conducted looking for stigmata of chronic liver diseases (palmar erythema, flap, gynecomastia, spider nevi, ascites, and edema) and liver function should be formally assessed with measurement of platelet count, prothrombin time or INR, albumin, total protein, bilirubin, alkaline phosphatase, aspartate transaminase, and gamma glutamyl transferase. Cross-sectional imaging should be reviewed for signs of portal hypertension (portal vein dilation, varices, splenomegaly, and ascites) and cirrhosis (ascites, small irregular liver outline). Functional hepatic assessment with indocyanine green retention can also be performed.

### Radiologic Imaging

Most patients who present with hepatic tumors undergo cross-sectional imaging with various modalities. In general, patients are often assessed initially with transabdominal ultrasound and then undergo imaging with computed tomography (CT scan) and/or magnetic resonance imaging (MRI) scans. Staging with computed tomography/positron emission scans (CT/PET) is now also accepted as standard of care for many tumor types, in those centers where it is available. A thorough review of all imaging modalities in a multidisciplinary meeting will generally clarify potential diagnoses based on tumor imaging characteristics and the precise anatomical location. Further review of imaging will assist with staging, the presence of any important anatomical variations, and the expected size and volume of the liver remnant following resection. In addition, discussion in a multidisciplinary context will allow consideration to be given to treatment related issues such as the potential role of neoadjuvant chemotherapy, radiotherapy or the intraoperative placement of catheters for postoperative regional chemotherapy.

# SURGICAL TECHNIQUE

## Anesthesia and Postoperative Analgesia

Patients are managed with general anesthesia and usually require placement of a central venous line, peripheral venous lines, an arterial line, and a urinary catheter. Postoperative analgesia is provided by thoracic epidural analgesia or a single dose of intrathecal morphine depending on the assessment of the anesthetist. All patients are managed intraoperatively with sequential calf compression devices. Subcutaneous administration of unfractionated heparin is begun in the postoperative period when the INR is less than 1.5 and is continued until discharge.



## Positioning

Patients are positioned supine with both arms at right angles from the body taking due care to protect against traction injuries with adequate padding. The urinary catheter and electrocardiogram leads should be kept clear of the sides of the operating table to permit attachment of a subcostal retraction system. The abdomen should be prepped and draped between the nipples and suprapubic area. Upper and lower body warming systems should be applied. If a staging laparoscopy is planned it can be performed at this stage.

## Technique

### Exposure

The abdomen is opened through a right subcostal incision some two finger breadths below the costal margin with a midline extension to the xiphisternum. This provides excellent exposure for central liver tumors. The ligamentum teres should be divided and secured with a ligature (Fig. 21.5). This ligature should be left long as it is a useful mechanism for securing the left side of the liver and opening the parenchyma between segments II/III and IV. The falciform ligament should be divided back to the level of the vena cava. The left (Fig. 21.6) and right coronary ligaments (Fig. 21.7) should be taken down (see Figs. 18.7 and 18.8).

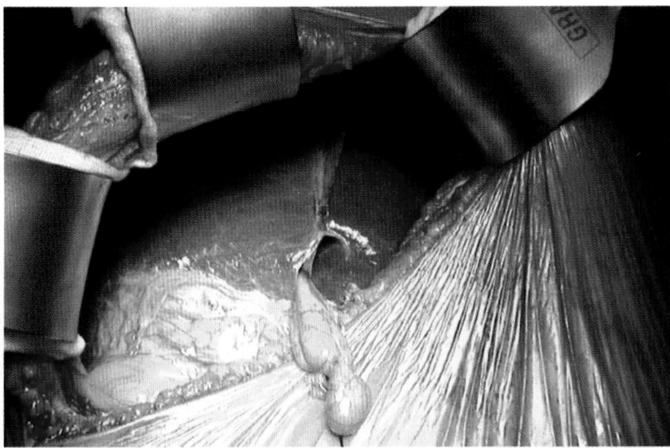

**Figure 21.5** The abdomen has been opened and the liver exposed via a right subcostal incision. A subcostal retractor has been deployed and the ligamentum teres has been secured with a silk tie.

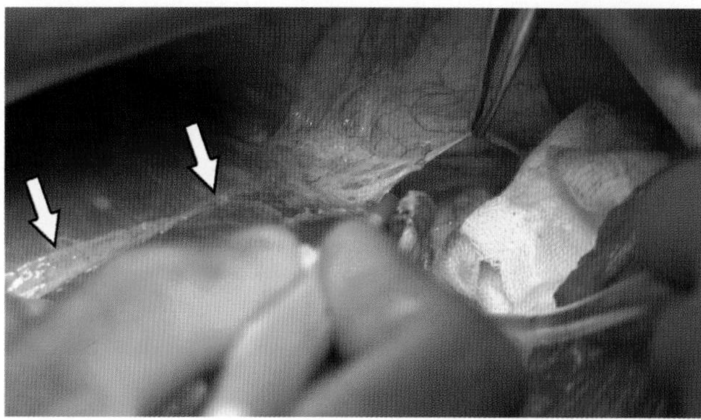

Figure 21.6 Using diathermy the left coronary ligament is divided separating segment II from the diaphragm. The falciform ligament has been divided to the level of the vena cava (*arrows*).

### Initial Assessment and Intraoperative Ultrasound

Intraoperative assessment should first focus on detection of metastatic spread to peritoneum, regional lymph nodes, or the remainder of the liver in operations for malignant disease where these findings may preclude resection (see Fig. 18.9). An assessment should also be made of liver quality noting signs of steatosis or cirrhosis. If portal hypertension is suspected, portal pressures can be measured directly, although this is usually recognized before operation and is best performed in the radiology suite.

An intraoperative ultrasound should be performed. This should verify the position of the tumor within segments IV, V, and VIII and the presence of standard inflow and hepatic venous anatomy. In addition, in operations for malignant disease, a thorough assessment of hepatic parenchyma should be made to locate any intrahepatic metastatic lesions that have not been detected with preoperative imaging investigations.

### Control of Segment IV Inflow

The inflow to segment IV is approached in the umbilical fissure. The anatomy of the fissure is constant (Fig. 21.8). When viewed from the caudal perspective, the left hepatic artery, left bile duct and left portal vein run within the umbilical fissure contained within Glisson's sheath. Branches to the caudate lobe (segment I), segment II and segment III arise sequentially from the left side of the sheath. Branches to segment IVA and IVB arise from the right side of the sheath. Each segmental pedicle contains the respective branch of the hepatic artery, portal vein and bile duct contained within a connective tissue sheath.

The segment IV pedicles can be isolated by gentle dissection within the right side of the umbilical fissure. Segment IVB is approached first using a right angle forceps to develop the plane between Glisson's capsule and parenchyma until the pedicle is encircled (Fig. 21.9). Occasionally a small amount of parenchyma needs to be divided within the line of the falciform ligament to expose the anterior aspect of the IVB pedicle to assist with safe mobilization. If necessary this can be undertaken with intermittent mass

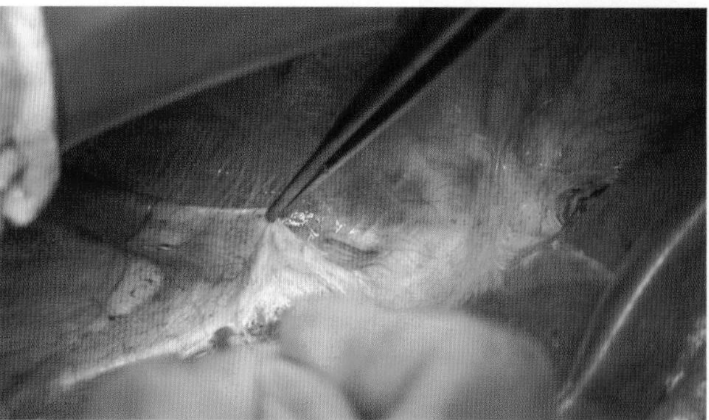

Figure 21.7 The right coronary ligament is divided separating the right lobe of the liver from the diaphragm and exposing the bare area.

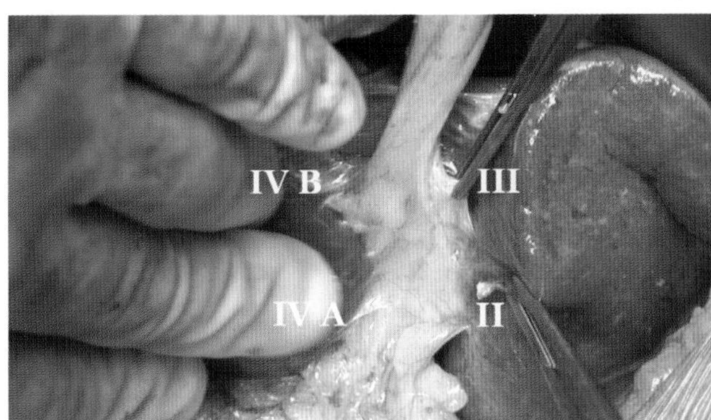


Figure 21.8 The umbilical fissure viewed from a caudal perspective. The liver has been retracted superiorly demonstrating the location of the inflow pedicles to segments IVB, IVA, II, and III. The small bridge of hepatic tissue (the pons hepatitis) that often covers the umbilical fissure has been divided and is secured with forceps.

inflow control (Pringle maneuver). Once the pedicle has been encircled a vascular tape can be passed around it and the pedicle then divided with a linear stapler or between clamps and suture ligated with a 4-0 non-absorbable suture (see Figs. 24.7 and 27.9).

Further dissection within the right side of the fissure will expose the segment IVA pedicle which can be controlled in the same manner and this should be followed by a significant color change in segment IV (Fig. 21.10). Significant branches to segment IV can arise from the posterior aspect of the left pedicle and should be sought if parts of segment IV appear to be vascularized. However, great care must be taken not to damage or occlude the pedicles to segments I, II, and III which arise in the left side of the fissure.



### Control of Segments V and VIII Inflow

Segments V and VIII are usually supplied by the anterior sectoral branch of the right portal inflow pedicle. The anterior sectoral branch then divides into a branch supplying segment V and a branch supplying segment VIII. This inflow to segments V and VIII can be approached in three ways. Most commonly hilar dissection is undertaken dividing the hilar plate and encircling the main right pedicle. Cholecystectomy is performed removing the gallbladder from the liver either anterograde or retrograde and controlling the cystic artery with a ligature and dividing and controlling the cystic duct with an absorbable suture (Fig. 21.11). Caudal retraction on this pedicle and gentle dissection of the parenchyma from Glisson's capsule will sometimes permit the bifurcation of the right main pedicle into anterior (supplying segments V and VIII) and posterior branches (supplying segments VI and VII) to be directly visualized (Fig. 21.12). The anterior pedicle can then be controlled with a vascular tape and a trial occlusion performed. Division can then be undertaken with either a linear cutting stapler or between clamps followed by suture ligation.

This technique can be difficult in patients with anteriorly placed tumors obstructing access to the hilus or in patients with a right pedicle that divides deeply within

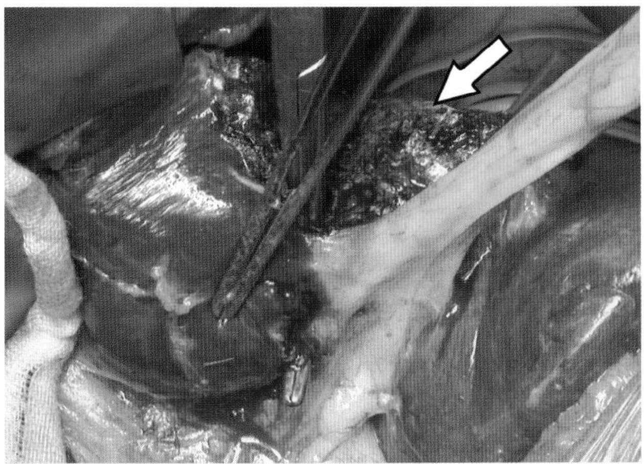

Figure 21.9 The inflow pedicle to segment IVB has been encircled with a right angle forceps prior to division with a linear cutting stapler. The parenchyma lying anterior to the inflow pedicle has been divided (*arrow*) to facilitate its exposure. Once the segment IVB pedicle has been divided the pedicle to segment IVA can be exposed and divided in a similar manner.

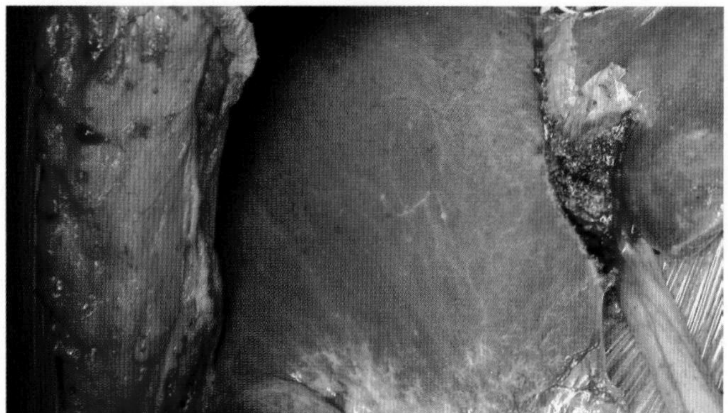

**Figure 21.10** The pedicles to segments IVB and IVA have been divided devascularising segment IV. Inspection of the anterior surface of the liver demonstrates an obvious color change outlining the boundaries of segment IV.

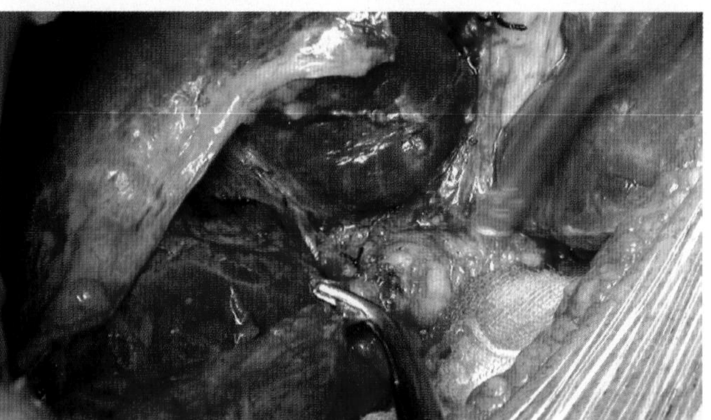

**Figure 21.11** Cholecystectomy has been performed and the cystic artery secured with a silk tie. The cystic duct is controlled with a right-angled forceps prior to suture ligature.

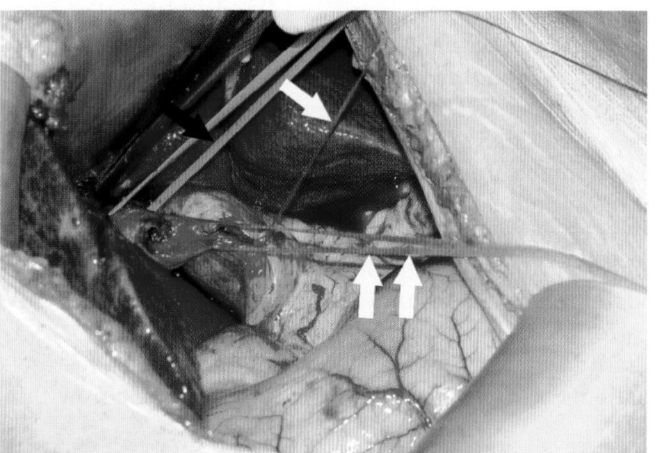

**Figure 21.12** With gentle traction on the hepaticoduodenal ligament the right inflow pedicle has been controlled with an umbilical tape (*double white arrow*). The anterior sectoral pedicle to segments V and VIII has then been mobilized and controlled with an orange vessel loop (*black arrow*). A ligature has been placed around the cystic duct and left long to assist with exposure (*single white arrow*).

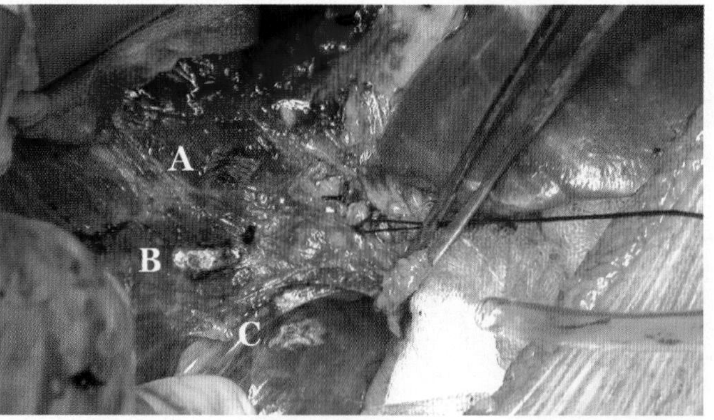


**Figure 21.13** The gallbladder has been removed and small diathermy marks made in the caudate process (*C*), segment V lateral to the gallbladder fossa (*B*), and segment IV medial to the gallbladder fossa (*A*).

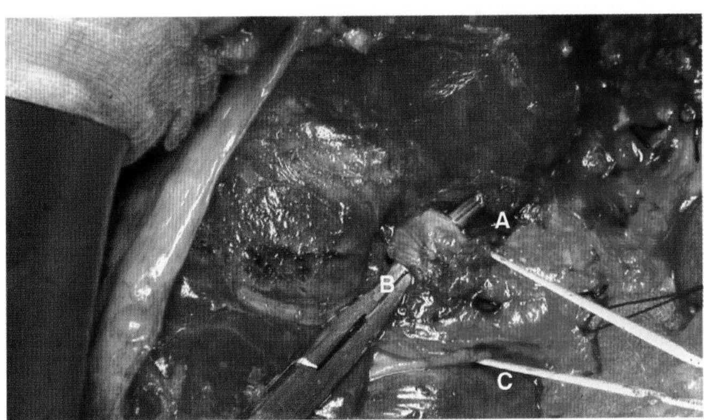


**Figure 21.14** A blue vessel loop has been passed around the main right inflow pedicle via hepatotomies made at points (**A**) and (**C**). The anterior sectoral pedicle to segments V and VIII has been encircled with a right angled forceps passed through a small hepatotomy at point (**B**) and exiting the liver at point (**A**). If necessary, the posterior sectoral pedicle could be controlled in the same way passing a forceps from a hepatotomy at point (**B**) to point (**C**).

the hepatic parenchyma. In these cases two other techniques are available to the surgeon. The line of division between the anterior (segments V and VIII) and posterior sectors (segments VI and VII) of the right hemiliver is marked by the course of the right hepatic vein. Using an intraoperative ultrasound, the course of the right hepatic vein can be mapped from its most anterior and caudal extent to its entry into the vena cava. Under mass inflow control the parenchyma can be carefully divided just medial to the course of the vein. Great care must be taken to ligate all medial branches of the right hepatic vein. The parenchymal division can be deepened and extended until the anterior sectoral pedicle is exposed intraparenchymally. A trial ligation can be performed and then the vessel can be divided with either a linear cutting stapler or following suture ligation. Alternatively, the posterior intrahepatic approach can be used. The anterior inflow pedicle can be controlled by passing a pair of right angled forceps into a small hepatotomy in the base of segment IV medial to the gallbladder bed and anterior to the hilum, angling posterior to the gallbladder and exiting via a small hepatotomy lateral to the gallbladder within segment V (Fig. 21.13). A vascular tape can then be passed through the tract encompassing the anterior pedicle and a trial occlusion performed. This technique is straightforward but relies on the presence of a normal hepatic inflow anatomy which can be assessed on preoperative imaging and the use of an intraoperative ultrasound. Common issues with this technique are damaging the anterior sectoral sheath or branches of the middle hepatic vein within the hepatic substance and subsequent bleeding. Passage of a right angle forceps through the hepatic parenchyma requires a gentle touch and the instrument should slide through without resistance (Fig. 21.14) (see also Fig. 24.4). When resistance is encountered, it is typically the result of a significant structure (either a branch of the middle hepatic vein or the posterior aspect of the Glissonian sheath) and the end of the forceps should be negotiated around the obstruction. Paradoxically this often means pursuing a deeper arc within the hepatic substance. Once the control of the anterior sectoral branch has been verified this can be ligated or divided with a linear cutting stapler.

### Control of the Middle Hepatic Vein (see Chapter 19)

The middle hepatic vein can also be approached in three ways. Pack and Miller describe exposure of the middle vein via the suprahepatic approach by placing caudal traction on the liver following division of the falciform ligament and the tissues lying anterior to the suprahepatic vena cava. Division of these tissues exposes the suprahepatic vena cava and caudal traction on the liver allows visualization of the origins of the left, middle, and right hepatic veins. If the origin of the middle vein can be clearly visualized, then it can be encircled and ligated prior to parenchymal division. However, in practice, this technique is dangerous and technically difficult. In most patients the middle vein joins the left hepatic vein intraparenchymally and both veins join the inferior vena cava as a common trunk. Isolation of the middle vein via a suprahepatic approach under these circumstances risks ligation of both the middle and the left vein. In addition, a common indication for central hepatectomy is a large centrally placed tumor and, in these cases, gaining adequate visualization and access to the suprahepatic vena cava can be limited.

Ogura et al. describe ligation and control of the middle vein by taking an intraparenchymal approach. Parenchymal transection is undertaken in the line of the falciform ligament following control of the inflow structures to segment IV within the umbilical fissure. Parenchymal transection is continued craniad until the anterior surface of the vena cava and the origin of the middle vein is exposed and divided. This approach is technically straight forward but requires precise parenchymal dissection in order to avoid significant hemorrhage. In addition, this approach can compromise the surgical margin when used to remove large tumors that lie close to the middle hepatic vein origin.

The most straight forward approach is to visualize and control the middle hepatic vein using a retrohepatic approach prior to parenchymal division and following inflow control. This approach was first fully described by Lortat-Jacob in 1952. Using this technique the liver is mobilized by dividing the falciform ligament as well as the right and left coronary ligaments, opening the bare area and exposing the vena cava. A full caval mobilization is performed taking all the venous branches draining into the vena cava from the caudate lobe and caudate process. Small branches can be divided following the application of titanium clips while larger branches can be controlled with 2-0 silk ties or 4-0 suture ligatures. The retrohepatic caval ligament (Makuuchi ligament) should be encircled and divided (see Fig. 19.6). This often contains a small arterial vessel and should be divided between clamps and suture ligated or formally divided with a linear cutting stapler. Division of this ligament exposes the lateral side of the right hepatic vein. This vein can then be controlled by creating a tunnel under direct vision by carefully separating the areolar tissue that lies between the right and middle vein and then passing a vessel loop around the right hepatic vein (Fig. 21.15).

The caudate lobe should be fully mobilized off the vena cava if it is being resected en bloc with segments IV, V, and VIII. If the caudate lobe is to be preserved then it should be mobilized taking all small venous branches but preserving the large branch that lies superiomedially (see Fig. 22.9). The left hepatic vein can then be accessed by retracting segments II and III anteriorly, opening the lesser omentum and dividing the ligamentum venosum (the obliterated remnant of the ductus venosus) between 2-0 silk ties (Fig. 21.16) (see also Fig. 22.6). This exposes the left side of the left hepatic vein and the inferior edge can be directly seen. A tunnel can be created around the left hepatic vein using a right angle forceps between the inferior edge of the left hepatic vein and parenchyma, gently encircling the vein (Fig. 21.17). Superiorly the sulcus between the middle and left hepatic veins can be visualized and the end of the right angle forceps can be exteriorized at this point. The left hepatic vein can then be controlled with a vessel loop (Fig. 21.18). In cases where the left vein joins the middle vein forming a common trunk, a small hepatotomy may need to be made anterior to the sulcus between the common trunk and the right hepatic vein.

This vessel loop can then be transferred to the middle vein by passing the inferior end to a forceps placed in the tunnel between the right and middle hepatic veins. The middle vein can be ligated and divided prior to parenchymal division. In complex resections such as central hepatectomy, it is good practice to have vascular tapes around the remaining veins, in this case the right and left veins, to permit control during parenchymal division if it is required (Fig. 21.19).

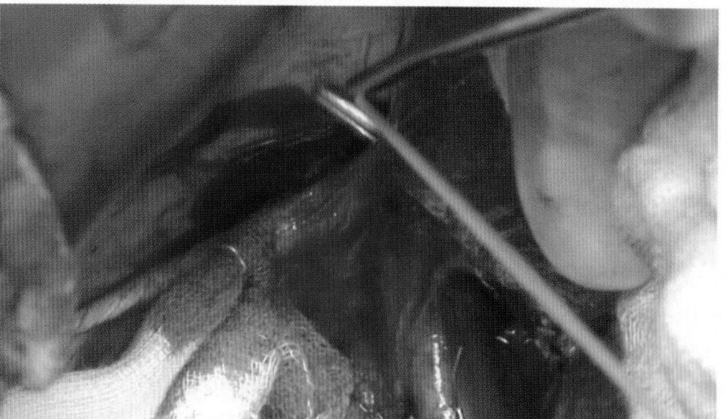

**Figure 21.15** The right lobe of the liver has been fully mobilized off the diaphragm and the vena caval ligament (Makuuchi ligament) divided. A tunnel has been created medial to the right hepatic vein and a right-angled forceps is placed in this tunnel before securing the vein with a blue vessel loop.

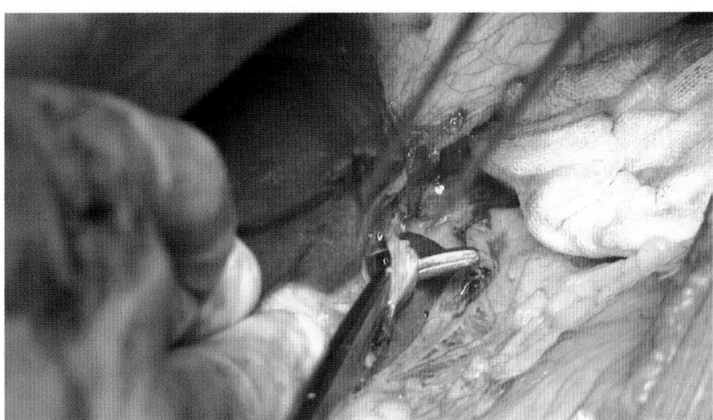

Figure 21.16 Segments II and III have been retracted anteriorly. The ligamentum venosum has been mobilized with a right-angled forceps prior to ligation and division.

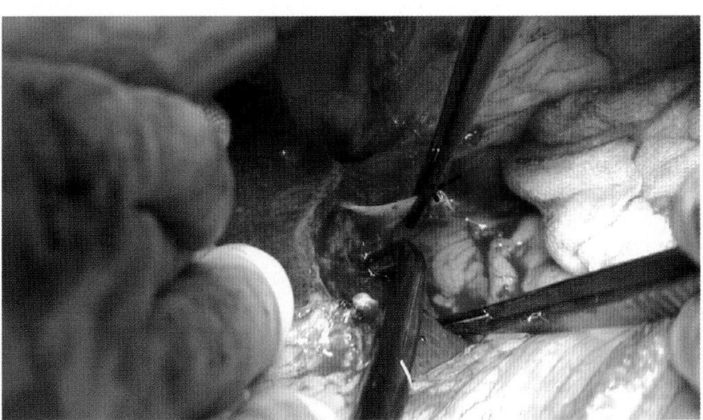

Figure 21.17 Segments II and III have been retracted anteriorly and the superior end of the divided ligamentum venosum is retracted toward the midline. Division of the ligamentum venosum exposes the left hepatic vein and a right-angled forceps can be used to create a tunnel around its inferior edge by gently separating the vein from surrounding parenchyma.

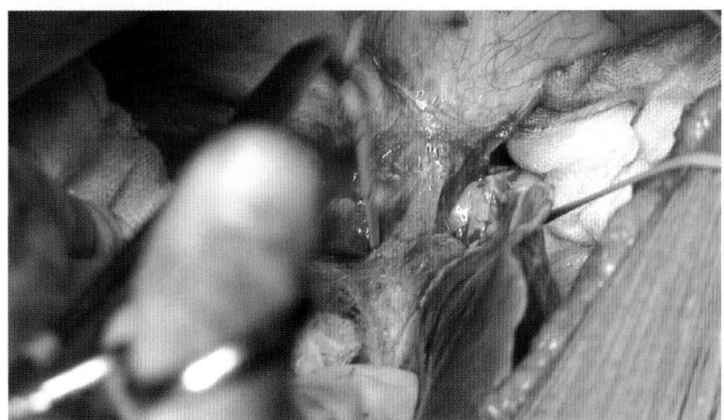

Figure 21.18 A right-angled forceps has been used to complete a tunnel around the left hepatic vein by gently opening the fissure between the left and middle hepatic vein. The left hepatic vein has been controlled with a blue vessel loop.

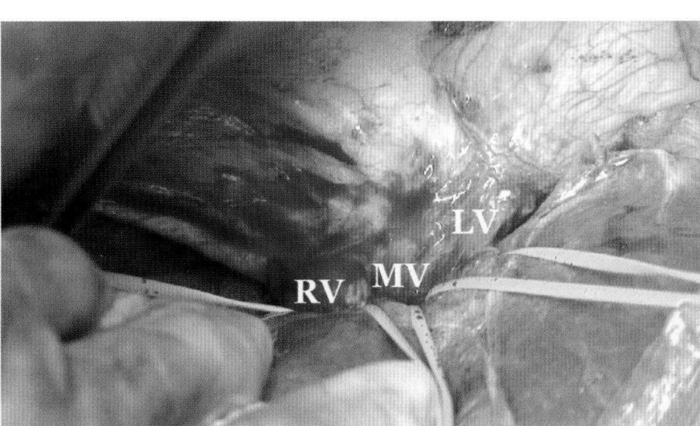


Figure 21.19 The middle hepatic vein (MV) has been secured with a blue vessel loop. The right hepatic vein (RV) and left hepatic vein (LV) has also been secured.

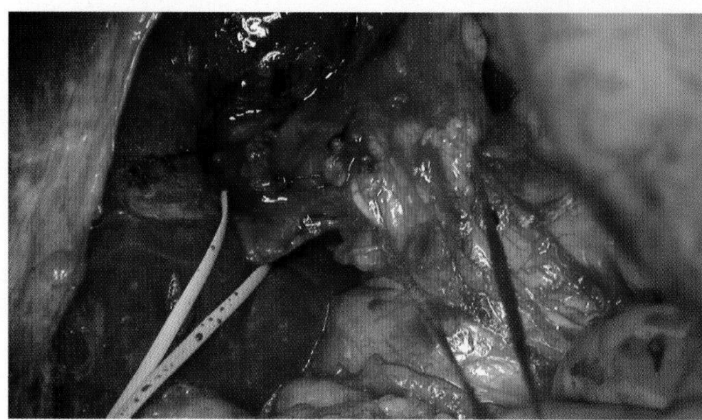

Figure 21.20 An umbilical tape has been passed around the hepatic inflow in the hepaticoduodenal ligament to provide mass inflow control (Pringle maneuver). The right inflow pedicle has also been controlled with a blue vessel loop.

**Parenchymal Division**

The majority of parenchymal division will take place following control of both hepatic inflow and the middle hepatic vein. In the circumstance where the decision is made to locate the anterior sectoral pedicle intrahepatically, the inflow to segment IV can be divided and the middle hepatic vein controlled. Parenchymal division can then be carried out just medial to the course of the right hepatic vein. Mass inflow control can be used to keep the operative field dry by placing a vascular tape around the hepaticoduodenal ligament and securing it with a plastic snugger (Fig. 21.20). Mass inflow control, if required, can be used in 5 minute periods with 2 to 3 minutes recovery. As soon as the anterior sectoral pedicle is secured the middle hepatic vein can be divided and mass inflow control released.

In cases where the inflow to segments IV, V, and VIII and the middle hepatic vein have been divided mass inflow control is not routinely needed as it is generally possible to divide parenchyma, in these circumstances, with minimal blood loss and the presence of vascularised and devascularised areas in the liver is a useful guide to resection.

The hepatic parenchyma can be divided using a number of techniques. The crushing technique using a Kelly clamp (Kelly-clysis), an ultrasonic dissector, a waterjet dissector, and a harmonic scalpel have all been utilized. The harmonic scalpel is simple to set up and effective at dividing different types of parenchyma. With the scalpel set to settings of three and five the instrument will divide parenchyma but spare vessels larger than 2 to 3 mm in diameter and these can be controlled with clips or 3-0 ties. The plane of parenchymal division for central hepatectomy extends from the anterior aspect of the umbilical fissure to the vena cava to divide segment IV from segments II and III (Fig. 21.21). This line of division follows the course of the falciform ligament. On the lateral side parenchymal division begins at a point lateral to the gallbladder fossa and extends posterior to the vena cava following the right hepatic vein (Fig. 21.22). Posteriorly the parenchyma must be lifted off the hepatic hilus incorporating the ligated pedicle supplying segments V and VIII and the line of division will

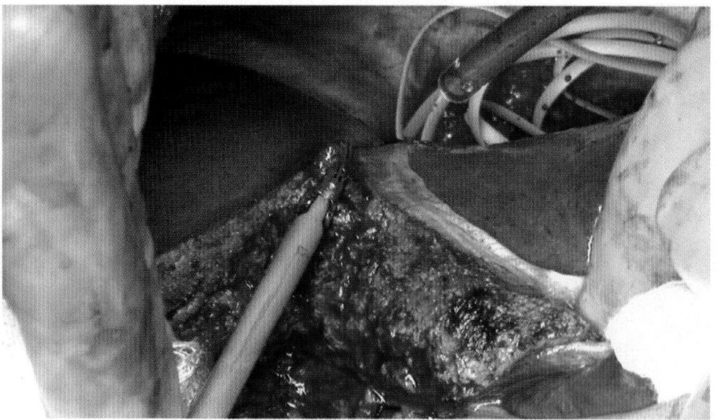

Figure 21.21 The left-sided parenchymal division using the harmonic scalpel. The line of parenchymal division is along the line of the divided falciform ligament, which is visible along the liver surface.

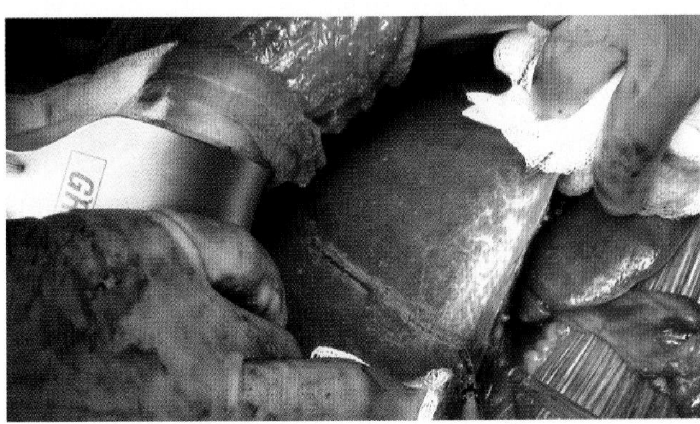

Figure 21.22 The plane of the right-sided parenchymal division has been marked with diathermy separating segments V and VIII from segments VI and VII based on vascular demarcation following division of the segment V/VIII inflow pedicle.



pursue a horizontal course parallel to the hepatic hilus connecting the right and left-sided dissections (Fig. 21.23).

Within the left-sided parenchymal division there are a few significant structures and generally the separation of segment IV from segments II and III is straightforward. Posteriorly the left and middle hepatic veins lie in close proximity and care must be taken to protect the left hepatic vein. Occasionally (5% of cases) the large vein draining segment IV will drain directly into the junction of the middle and left hepatic veins and this must be controlled without compromising the left vein. On the right side the right hepatic vein gives two to three large branches to segments V and VIII and these must be carefully divided without compromising the main venous trunk. In 3% of cases a vein will drain directly from segment VIII into the vena cava.

### Concomitant Caudate Lobectomy (see Chapter 22)

Concomitant caudate lobectomy has been described in conjunction with central hepatectomy. In this case, the caudate lobe is fully mobilized off the vena cava and bought laterally so that it lies fully on the right side of the cava. The small inflow pedicle to the caudate, arising from on the left side, is divided under direct vision after opening the lesser omentum. The left-sided parenchymal dissection then extends from the anterior surface of the liver to the vena cava posteriorly. The right-sided parenchymal division also extends to the vena cava. The caudate lobe can then be removed *en bloc* with segments IV, V, and VIII.

### Concomitant En Bloc Resections of Bile Duct and Portal Vein

Ogura et al. have described concomitant resection of portal vein and the central bile ducts for gallbladder carcinoma (see Chapter 27). In this technique the inflow to the right and left hemilivers is dissected extrahepatically by opening the Glissonian sheath. The involved segments of portal vein are resected between clamps and reconstructed either with primary anastomosis or a small venous interposition graft. The central bile ducts are resected with the specimen and a Roux-en-Y hepaticojejunostomy fashioned incorporating direct

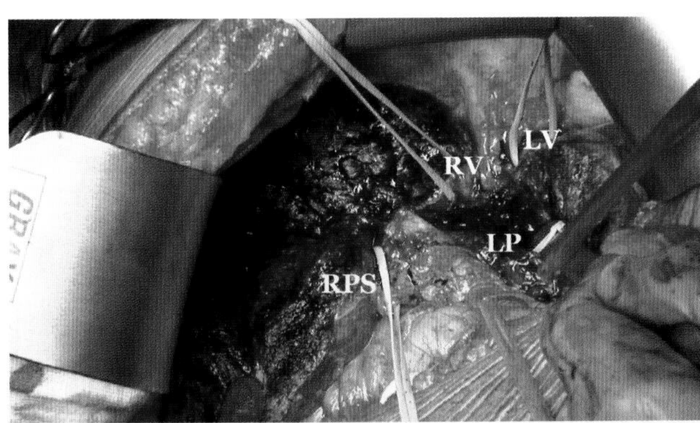


Figure 21.23 The operative field at the completion of the resection demonstrating the remaining left (LV) and right (RV) hepatic veins, the right posterior sectoral pedicle (RPS) to segments VI and VII and the left inflow (LP) supplying segments II and III.

anastomosis to the right posterior duct and the main left duct at the base of the umbilical fissure. Other investigators have described en bloc resection of abdominal wall and diaphragm.

#### Surgical Drainage

Following completion of the resection the operative site is monitored for bleeding while the central venous pressure is increased to physiologic levels (8 to 10 mm water) with intravenous fluid loading. Bleeding points are carefully oversewn with 4-0 prolene. A damp surgical pack is held against the parenchyma surface and carefully inspected for any indication of bile leak. Any open bile ducts at the parenchymal edge are oversewn with 4-0 non-absorbable sutures.

Surgical drains can be left at this point, although many hepatobiliary units do not drain after routine hepatectomies. When used the drains should be soft in consistency, placed within the parenchymal defect and drain to bile bags. Suction drainage is not used.

#### Abdominal Closure

With hemostasis verified, the ligamentous attachments of the liver should be reconstituted to prevent torsion of the remnants. The left coronary ligament is reconstituted with interrupted 3-0 prolene and the edge of the right lobe is loosely secured to the adjacent diaphragm. The abdomen is closed in layers using 0 PDS to the midline aponeurosis posterior rectus sheath and internal oblique. A further suture is placed in the anterior rectus sheath and external oblique layers. An absorbable subcuticular suture is used to close the skin and a dressing is applied.

## POSTOPERATIVE MANAGEMENT

Following liver resection all patients should be closely monitored, generally in an intensive care or high dependency setting. The role of monitoring is to diagnose complications early and institute appropriate treatment. Patients must be closely observed for signs of respiratory depression, particularly those treated with intrathecal morphine, signs of postoperative bleeding, and signs of early hepatic insufficiency. At least once daily, measurement of full blood count, prothrombin time or INR, serum urea and electrolytes, creatinine, albumin, total protein, bilirubin, alkaline phosphatase, aspartate transaminase, and gamma glutamyl transferase should be undertaken.

For the patient pursuing an uncomplicated postoperative course, solid food is instituted as tolerated as soon as they are awake and mobilization to a chair and around the hospital ward is commenced on day 1 postoperation. In general, intravenous fluids are discontinued once oral intake is established. Epidural analgesia is stopped on postoperative day 2 or 3 depending on patient progress. Patients are discharged once stable, comfortable on simple oral analgesia, tolerating a normal diet and independent in personal cares.

### Anticoagulation

All patients are managed intraoperatively with TED stockings and dynamic calf compression. Anticoagulation with twice daily subcutaneous unfractionated heparin is commenced in the postoperative period once the INR is less than 1.5. In patients with epidural catheters, once epidural analgesia has been discontinued, the evening dose of subcutaneous heparin is withheld and the catheter is removed the following morning. Anticoagulation and TED stockings are continued until patient discharge.

### Follow-up and Imaging

Patients are followed up within 1 week of hospital discharge to check on their progress. Further follow-up is defined by the underlying pathology; patients with benign diagnoses can be followed up for several months before discharge while patients with malignancy enter a formal program of lifelong clinical review. All patients are reimaged 6 weeks following surgery to obtain a new baseline picture of the liver. Patients with malignant diagnoses will continue to be reimaged at regular intervals.

## COMPLICATIONS (SEE CHAPTER 18)

### Specific

#### Postoperative Hemorrhage

Postoperative hemorrhage following hepatic resection is rare. The common sites are from the caudate veins, parenchymal vessels or due to failure of ligatures used to control portal vein or hepatic artery branches. Patients present with postoperative hypotension, a falling hemoglobin and abdominal distension. If drains have been placed there may be increased drainage of heavily blood stained fluid. The management is an immediate return to theatre, mobilization of the liver and direct suture ligation of the bleeding point.

In general, postoperative hemorrhage can be prevented by careful dissection and control of all vascular structures. Portal vein and hepatic artery branches should be controlled with sutures rather than ties or divided with linear staplers. The parenchyma should be carefully inspected after specimen removal for bleeding points and these controlled with sutures. In patients managed with low central venous pressure anesthesia intravenous fluid loading should take place at the end of parenchymal division to raise the central venous pressure to physiologic levels. This will permit localization of any small open veins.



#### Hepatic Insufficiency and Liver Failure

Hepatic insufficiency and liver failure are now the most common causes of death following elective hepatectomy. The risk factors for postoperative liver failure are the presence of cirrhosis, a remnant volume of less than 20% of total liver volume, compromise to the blood supply, venous or biliary drainage of the remnant, prolonged inflow occlusion, and shock. Diagnosis is made by a rising plasma bilirubin and lactate with reduced hepatic synthetic function causing a falling albumin, rising INR and edema. Treatment is directed at managing any reversible causes, maintenance of normal physiology and prevention of sepsis. Patients usually require support with intravenous albumin, fresh frozen plasma and nutritional support, usually via an enteral route. Prophylactic antibiotics should be commenced and laxatives should be administered regularly to prevent the development of encephalopathy.

#### Bile Leak/Biloma/Biliary Fistula

Postoperative biliary leaks with the formation of bilomas and occasionally biliary fistulae are reported in approximately 5% of hepatectomies. Most commonly the bile leak develops from a small intraparenchymal bile duct at the edge of the surgical field. Generally these are ducts that have initially sealed during parenchymal division but reopen in the postoperative period causing an accumulation of bile within the surgical field. Diagnosis is made by a rising plasma bilirubin level, usually between postoperative days 3 and 7, and confirmed with CT scan showing a fluid collection at the operative site. Patients may have signs of sepsis with local tenderness, fever and raised inflammatory markers. Treatment is with percutaneous drainage. ERCP is also useful as it will demonstrate if the leak originates from a major bile duct and transampullary stent placement will reduce intrabiliary pressure and assist in resolution of the leak. Rarely operative intervention is required for those patients with bile peritonitis, an injury to a major duct that requires reconstruction, or in the management of a cutaneous biliary fistula.

#### Torsion of the Remnant

Torsion of the hepatic remnant is rare but catastrophic since infarction occurs and the patient then becomes anhepatic. Acute transplantation is the only possible treatment. Following central hepatectomy segments II and III and VI and VII are freely mobile. In addition, the left and right hepatic veins have been skeletonized and lack support of the surrounding parenchyma making them vulnerable to torsion and partial obstruction. Torsion can be prevented by reconstituting the left and right coronary ligaments at the end of the procedure with non-absorbable sutures.

#### Portal Vein Thrombosis

Portal vein thrombosis is a rare postoperative complication. Thrombosis usually occurs against a background of reduced flow, either due to narrowing postsurgery or in low flow states associated with shock and sepsis. Patients present with signs of liver failure and the sudden development of ascites. Diagnosis is made with duplex ultrasound and/or CT scan. If diagnosis is made within 24 hours of thrombosis, surgical thrombectomy is associated with improved long-term patency particularly if any underlying obstructive cause is addressed. After the thrombosis has been established for 24 hours, surgical thrombectomy is not indicated and treatment is with anticoagulation.

### General

#### Respiratory

Pleural effusion and atelectasis are seen in most patients following a liver resection—particularly those who have undergone right-sided resections. Generally these are self limiting and asymptomatic and can be managed with early mobilization and chest physiotherapy. Occasionally large sympathetic effusions require drainage when they become symptomatic. Pneumonia may also develop in patients who are slow to mobilize or who have a background of chronic lung disease. Treatment is with appropriate antibiotic therapy, respiratory support and physiotherapy.

#### Cardiac

Cardiac complications are common following abdominal surgery in elderly patients. They may present with signs of myocardial ischemia (chest pain, hypotension, dyspnoea) or with arrhythmia and signs of organ failure such as deteriorating renal function. Ischemia should be initially investigated using an ECG and checking circulating troponin levels. Cardiac ischemia is also a common cause of cardiac arrthymia but atrial tachyarrthymias (atrial flutter and atrial fibrillation) can be observed in patients developing a hypermetabolic septic state or in fluid overload as well as in electrolyte disorders.

#### Gastrointestinal

Gastrointestinal complications are rare following hepatectomy. Ileus is unusual since the bowel does not lie near the operative field and hepatectomy can usually be undertaken without exteriorizing or exposing the small bowel to the environment. Similarly bowel obstruction is also unusual and generally related to adhesions from previous surgery or a secondary procedure. Peptic ulceration is a recognized complication in critically ill patients. Prophylactic administration of proton pump inhibitors should be part of the routine care of all patients undergoing hepatectomy. Hematemesis or an unexplained fall in hemoglobin should be investigated with an upper gastrointestinal endoscopy.

#### Cerebral

The most common cause of postoperative delirium in patients undergoing hepatectomy is hepatic encephalopathy which is always associated with a flap and deteriorating liver function tests. Treatment is with regular laxatives and by optimizing hepatic function.

Cerebovascular accident is also rare but should be suspected in any patient who develops focal neurologic signs. Investigation with a CT or MRI of the brain will confirm whether ischemic or hemorrhagic changes are present. Duplex ultrasound of the carotid arteries may also be required.

### Deep Vein Thrombosis

Thromboembolic complications are rare in patients undergoing elective hepatectomy. The rise in INR observed after hepatic resection, the use of TED stockings, intraoperative calf compression and early mobilization have all contributed to reducing the incidence of deep venous thrombosis and pulmonary embolus. Prophylactic subcutaneous heparin can also be commenced in the postoperative phase once the patient's INR has decreased below 1.5. Patients experiencing thromboembolic complications have usually pursued a complex postoperative course due to sepsis or some other complication and have developed a hypercoagulable state, often in the context of greatly reduced mobilization. Diagnosis of deep venous thrombosis and pulmonary embolus is by duplex ultrasound and CT scan respectively and patients are managed with systemic anticoagulation.

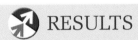

## RESULTS

In comparison to many other liver resections, central hepatectomy is only rarely performed. This reflects the low numbers of suitably placed and staged tumors as well as the relative technical challenge of the procedure. Most investigators report operative times between 5 and 7 hours with blood losses ranging between 700 cc and 5,000 cc. No investigator has reported positive surgical margins following central hepatectomy. Significant complications have been reported in between 20% and 37% of cases with postoperative bile leak, pleural effusion and pneumonia being the most common. Mortality rates of less than 1% are routine. Wu et al. have compared patients undergoing central hepatectomy with those undergoing extended hepatectomy (either extended right or left hepatectomy) for hepatocellular carcinoma. Central hepatectomy was associated with a longer mean operating time (7.9 hours vs. 5.8 hours) but similar intraoperative blood loss, transfusion requirement and hospital stay. Postoperative complication rates were reduced in the central hepatectomy group although this did not reach statistical significance and survival was comparable between the two groups.

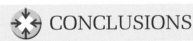

## CONCLUSIONS

Central hepatectomy is a unique procedure where the limits of resection are defined by the position of the right and left hepatic veins rather than the hepatic inflow. It should be considered in all patients who present with tumors located in segments IV, V, and VIII. Central hepatectomy can be technically more difficult than extended hepatectomies (right or left) but preserves parenchyma and therefore carries a lower risk of hepatic failure. Successful completion of the procedure requires accurate preoperative imaging to precisely define the position of the tumor and any anatomical variants present, intraoperative assessment with ultrasound, palpation, and careful trial dissection. For centrally placed tumors, central hepatectomy offers an excellent alternative to extended hepatectomy whereby clear surgical margins can be obtained with the conservation of significant parenchymal volume.

## Recommended References and Readings


Aldameh A, McCall JL, Koea JB. Is routine placement of surgical drains necessary after hepatectomy? Results from a single institution. *J Gastrointest Surg.* 2005;9:667–671.

Billingsley KG, Jarnagin WR, Fong Y, et al. Segment-orientated hepatic resection in the management of malignant neoplasms of the liver. *J Am Coll Surg.* 1998;187:471–481.

Bourgeon R, Guntz M. Noveau traite de technique chirurgicale, tome XII, fascicule premier. Foie, voies biliaires intra-hepatiques. Voies Ba, Paris: Masson & Cie; 1975.

Couinaud C. Controlled hepatectomies and exposure of the intrahepatic bile ducts. Anatomical and technical study. Paris, France: Dépôt légal 3e trimestre 1981.


Part II: Liver

Foster JH, Berman MM. Solid liver tumors. Major Problems in Clinical Surgery XXII. Philadelphia, London, Toronto: WB Saunders; 1977:298–299.

Hasegawa H, Makuuchi M, Yamazaki S, et al. Central bisegmentectomy of the liver: Experience in 16 patients. *World J Surg.* 1989; 13:786–790.

Koea JB, Young Y, Gunn K. Fast track liver resection: The effect of a comprehensive care package and analgesia with single dose intrathecal morphine with gabapentin or continuous epidural analgesia. HPB 2009, Article ID 271986. http://www.hindawi.com/journals/hpb/2009/271986.html Accessed March 9 2010.

Launois B, Jamieson GG. The posterior intrahepatic approach for hepatectomy or removal of segments of the liver. *Surg Gynecol Obstet.* 1992;174:155–158.

Lortat-Jacob JL, Robert HG, Henry C. Un cas d'hépatectomie droite reglee. *Memoires de l'Academie de Chirurgie.* 1952;78:244–251.

McBride CM, Wallace S. Cancer of the right lobe of the liver. A variety of operative procedures. *Arch Surg.* 1972;105:289–296.

Ogura Y, Matsuda S, Sakurai H, et al. Central bisegmentectomy of the liver plus caudate lobectomy for carcinoma of the gallbladder. *Dig Surg.* 1998;15:218–223.

Pack GT, Miller TR. Middle hepatic lobectomy for cancer. *Cancer.* 1961;14:1295–1300.

Terminology Committee of the International Hepato-Pancreato-Biliary Association. IHPBA Brisbane 2000 terminology of liver anatomy and resections. *HPB.* 2000;2:333–339.

Tung TT. *Les Résections Majeures et Mineures du Foie.* Paris: Masson & Cie; 1979.

Wu C-C, Ho W-L, Chen J-T, et al. Mesohepatectomy for centrally located hepatocellular carcinoma: an appraisal of a rare procedure. *J Am Coll Surg.* 1999;188:508–515.

# 22 Hepatic Caudate Resection

**Michael G. House**

## Introduction

The caudate lobe (segment I) lies posterior to the hilum and anterior to the inferior vena cava (IVC) (Fig. 22.1; see also Fig. 18.6) and is composed of three parts: the caudate lobe proper or Spiegel lobe extends to the left of the vena cava and under the lesser omentum, which separates it from segments II and III; the paracaval portion of the caudate lies anterior to the IVC and extends cephalad to the roots of the major hepatic veins; the caudate process is located between the main right glissonian pedicle and the IVC and fuses with segment VI of the right lobe.

The caudate lobe is surrounded by major vascular structures, which can make resection technically challenging. The posterior and superior borders are formed by the retrohepatic IVC and the confluence of the left and middle hepatic veins, respectively, while the left portal vein and hepatic hilum serve as the anterior border. The ligamentum venosum, the obliterated ductus venosus, courses along the medial aspect of the caudate from the umbilical portion of the left portal vein to the inferior border of the left hepatic vein. The rightward extent of the caudate is typically small and is indistinctly delimited by the posterior surface of segment IV and the medial surfaces of segments VI and VII. The middle hepatic vein is adjacent to the right side of the caudate, and may be the source of significant hemorrhage if injured during resection. The posterior edge of the caudate on the left has a fibrous component (the hepatocaval ligament or dorsal ligament) that attaches to the crus of the diaphragm and extends posteriorly behind the vena cava to join segment VII on the right side of the IVC. In a large proportion of patients, this fibrous tissue is replaced by hepatic parenchyma (Fig. 22.1).

Both the left and right portal pedicles contribute to the blood supply and biliary drainage of the caudate. Portal venous blood is supplied by two to three branches from the left portal vein and the main right or right posterior sectoral portal vein. From a practical standpoint, the left branch is much more constant and supplies a greater proportion of the lobe than the right branch(es). During left or extended left hepatectomy, it is important to identify and spare this left-sided branch if the caudate is to be preserved. The caudate is the only hepatic segment whose entire hepatic venous drainage

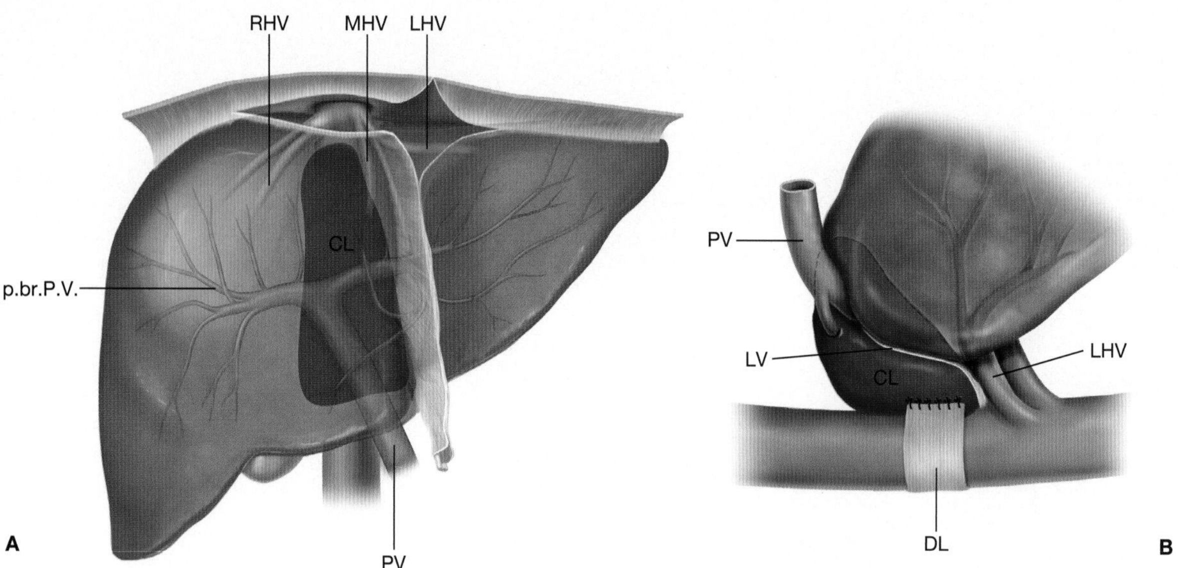


Figure 22.1 Two views of the caudate lobe (*shaded*), from above (**A**) and from the left, with the left lateral segment retracted upward and to the patient's right (**B**). The extent of the caudate, from the hilus to the insertion of the hepatic veins is clearly shown. A plane from the origin of the right posterior sectoral portal vein (*p.br.P.V.*) to the confluence of the right hepatic vein (*RHV*) and inferior vena cava approximates the right border of the caudate (**right**). The ligamentous attachment, hepatocaval ligament or dorsal ligament (*DL*), extending from the caudate to the IVC and segment VII is shown (**A**). CL, caudate lobe; PV, main portal vein; MHV, middle hepatic vein; LHV, left hepatic vein; LV, ligamentum venosum.

is directly into the IVC, through a variable number of short venous branches that completely bypasses the major hepatic veins (Fig. 22.2).

Many anatomical features of the caudate are thus unique relative to the other hepatic segments. Consideration of its embryogenesis provides a clearer understanding of the caudate lobe anatomy in the adult (Fig. 22.3). During the second trimester of fetal life, the persistent left umbilical vein enters the liver via the umbilical fissure and empties into the left portal vein. The ductus venosus is suspended within the dorsal mesentery of the liver and shunts placental blood from the left portal vein directly into the vena cava. As the liver enlarges and rotates counterclockwise, a small portion extends behind the ductus venosus mesentery anterior to the IVC. The extrahepatic portion of the ductus venosus and its mesentery progressively shorten, and the caudate lobe arrives at its final position between the IVC and the left portal triad. The ductus venosus obliterates shortly after birth and persists as the ligamentum venosum.

Safe resection of the caudate lobe requires resolute preoperative cross-sectional imaging to determine the anatomic relationships between any target lesion(s) and the major inflow and outflow vessels within the liver and the IVC. The natural confinement of the caudate between the vena cava posteriorly and the left portal vein and middle

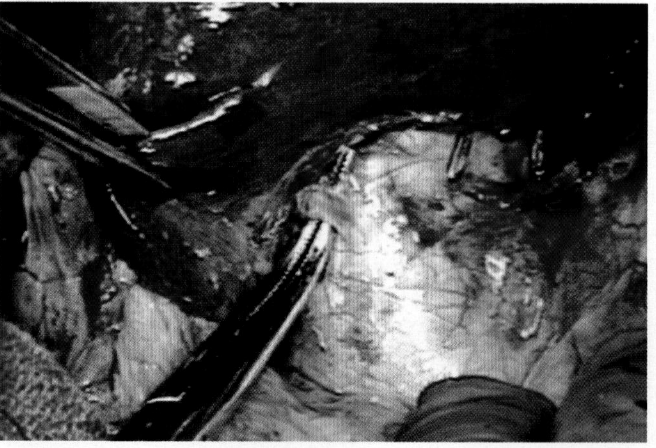

Figure 22.2 Intraoperative photo showing mobilization of the caudate lobe off the IVC. The Spiegel lobe portion of the caudate is retracted upward and to the patient's right. One of several small caudate veins draining directly into the IVC has been isolated and is being prepared for ligation and division. (Reprinted with permission: Figure 8–9, Techniques of Hepatic Resection. In: Blumgart LH, Fong Y, Jarnagin WR, eds. *Hepatobiliary Cancer,* Hamilton, Ontario: BC Decker; 2001: p. 165)

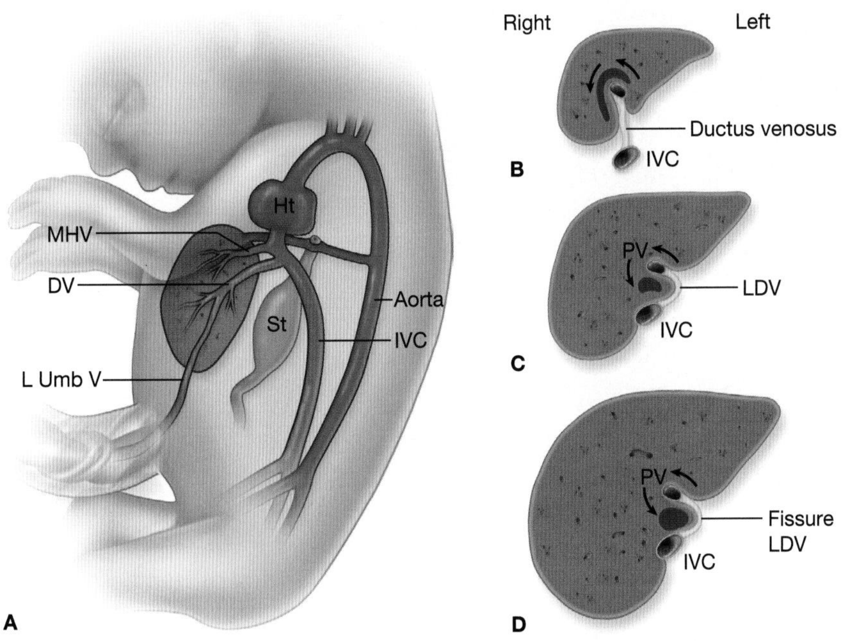


Figure 22.3 Schematic representation of the ductus venosus and the fetal circulation (**A**). The left umbilical vein (*L Umb V*) carries placental blood to the left portal vein, which is shunted directly into the inferior vena cava (*IVC*) by the ductus venosus (*DV*). MHV, middle hepatic vein; Ht, heart. The figure at right (**B**) depicts the counterclockwise rotation of the liver as it enlarges, and the resulting insertion of the caudate lobe between the ductus venosus and IVC (**C,D**). PV, left portal vein; LDV, ligament of the ductus venosus.



and left hepatic veins anteriorly and superiorly contributes to the technical difficulty of caudate resection. Isolated caudate hepatectomy, using an open technique for a large hepatic adenoma, was first described by Lerut et al. in 1990. Even though operative parenchymal transection techniques and pre- and intraoperative imaging have improved over the past two decades, the underlying principles guiding careful hepatectomy originate with mastery of the extra- and intrahepatic anatomy. Laparoscopic caudate hepatectomy has recently been reported, but the technical considerations necessary for a safe open resection should not be compromised. This chapter focuses on the technical aspects of performing a caudate resection, either in isolation as a monosegmentectomy or in combination with a partial hepatectomy, the latter being the most common.

## INDICATIONS

When indicated, benign and malignant tumors within the caudate should be considered for operative resection. Depending on location, tumors isolated to segment I are often amenable to monosegmentectomy without the need for contiguous major hepatectomy. Large solitary, benign tumors within the caudate (e.g., hepatic adenoma, vascular malformation, cysts, etc.) can present with upper abdominal pain or symptoms of gastric impingement. Compression of the IVC can occur, but complete occlusion is uncommon, especially with benign tumors. Primary and secondary (i.e., metastatic) cancers of the liver can present within the caudate either as uni- or multifocal disease. Liver directed therapies aimed at tumor downsizing, for example, hepatic artery embolization, are applicable for palliative situations. Extrahepatic tumors arising from the stomach, duodenum, or retroperitoneal organs can invade the caudate directly and might be amenable to en bloc resection. Perihilar and intrahepatic bile duct cancers that involve the left hepatic ducts require caudate resection, typically in continuity with a major hepatectomy, for optimal tumor clearance.

Contraindications for isolated caudate resection include tumors extending into adjacent hepatic segments (i.e., II, III, IV, VI, and VII), main or left portal vein invasion, direct invasion of the middle hepatic vein, left hepatic vein, or vena cava. Under these circumstances, caudate resection should be performed in continuity with other segmentectomies

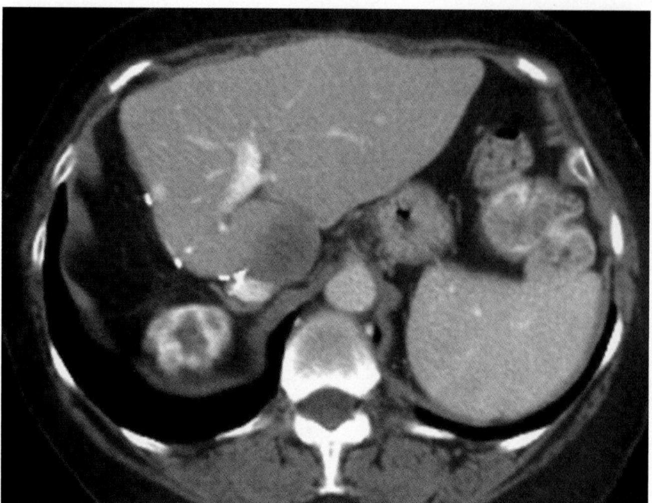

**Figure 22.4** CT scan showing isolated colon cancer metastasis to the hepatic caudate. Patient had undergone a prior right hepatectomy for metastatic colon cancer 2 years ago.

or hemihepatectomy. Hepatic vein occlusion in the setting of Budd–Chiari syndrome along with advanced hepatic cirrhosis and portal hypertension are contraindications for caudate resection (see Chapter 18).

##  PREOPERATIVE PLANNING

A careful clinical history and physical examination should determine the presence of hepatic cirrhosis and portal hypertension. Standard serum liver function tests are routine. Serum tumor marker levels can be tested to aid diagnosis or future surveillance.

Computed tomography (CT) and magnetic resonance imaging (MRI) delineate the boundaries of solid and cystic tumors within the caudate (Fig. 22.4) and can determine direct invasion of adjacent hepatic segments, major vascular structures (e.g., retrohepatic vena cava and main portal vein), and adjacent organs (e.g., stomach and duodenum). Radiographic staging of malignant tumors with cross-sectional imaging, with or without a functional component (i.e., positron emission tomography), will help to determine the presence of multifocal disease within the liver, regional lymphadenopathy (e.g., periportal, celiac, aortocaval), and distant extrahepatic metastases. Ultrasound with duplex can assess patency and direct tumor invasion of major inflow and outflow blood vessels of the liver. Endoscopic or magnetic resonance cholangiography can determine the extent of extra- and intrahepatic ductal involvement associated with perihilar and intrahepatic bile duct cancers.

##  OPERATIVE TECHNIQUE

The lesser omentum (gastrohepatic ligament) is divided to expose and inspect the caudate. Careful palpation and liver ultrasonography should be used to exclude occult tumors not detected on preoperative imaging and to delineate the boundaries of the tumor and relationships to the liver inflow and outflow vessels, especially the middle hepatic vein. The left triangular ligament is divided across the falciform tent, and the left hepatic vein is exposed. Division of the ligamentum venosum between ties allows the left hepatic vein to be dissected along with the common trunk shared with the middle hepatic vein (Fig. 22.5) which can be encircled with a loop for safe clamping when necessary later. The caudate is exposed fully by rotating segments II and III over the liver.

Three orderly operative steps provide safety during caudate resection.

1. *Control inflow to the caudate.* The hilar plate is lowered. The caudate branches off the left portal vein and hepatic artery are dissected along the base of the umbilical

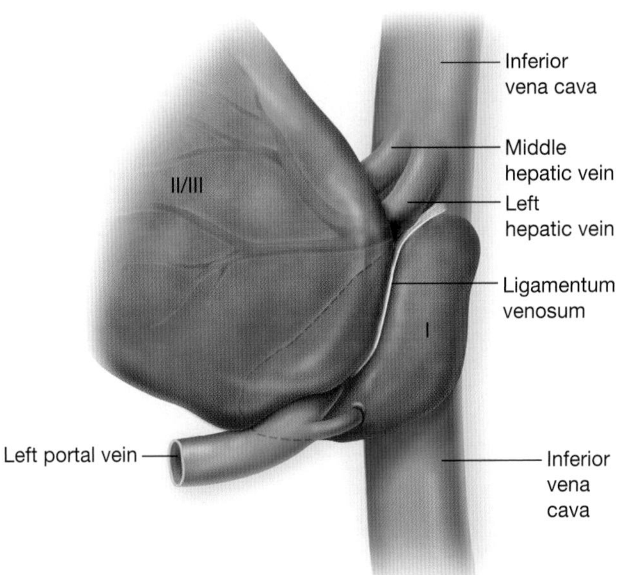


**Figure 22.5** Segments II and II have been rotated over to expose the caudate. The pertinent anatomic landmarks in reference to the caudate are indicated. IVC, inferior vena cava; LV, ligamentum venosum; MHV, middle hepatic vein; LHV, left hepatic vein; LPV, left portal vein.



fissure, ligated, and divided (Fig. 22.6). Perihilar bile duct tumors and larger tumors involving the caudate may require major portal vein resection and reconstruction.

2. *Control outflow of the caudate.* The left hepatocaval ligament is divided, which frees the spigelian caudate for elevation away from the IVC (Fig. 22.7A). This dissection is probably best performed sharply (Fig. 22.8), which along with maintenance of low CVP, will help avoid inadvertant injury to the IVC. Dissection of the retrocaudate hepatic veins is conducted with careful individual ligation (Figs. 22.7B and 22.9). Occasionally, and especially with bulkier tumors, the retrocaudate veins can be approached more easily from the right of the vena cava after mobilization of the right hemiliver (Figs. 22.9 and 22.10). A right-sided approach to the retrocaudate hepatic veins should be used when the caudate is resected in continuity with a right or extended right hepatectomy. Direct invasion of the retrohepatic vena cava requires partial cavectomy with reconstruction when patency can be preserved.

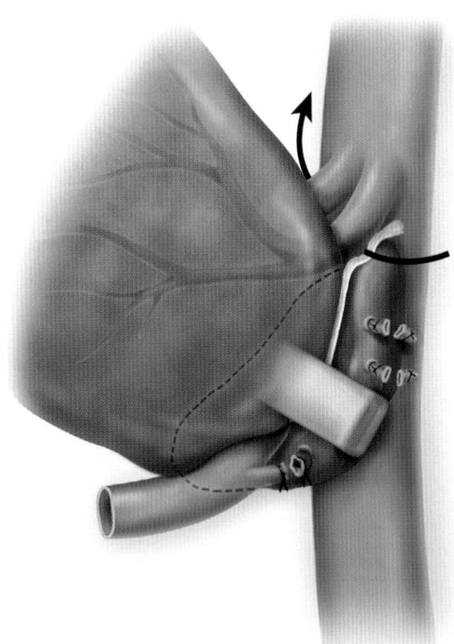

**Figure 22.6** The caudate vein off the left portal vein is ligated and divided. The caudate branch off the left hepatic artery is divided similarly (not shown). The spigelian caudate has been rotated away from the IVC, and retrocaudate hepatic veins are individually dissected, ligated, and divided. After the ligamentum venosum has been divided, the left and middle hepatic veins can be controlled with a loop.

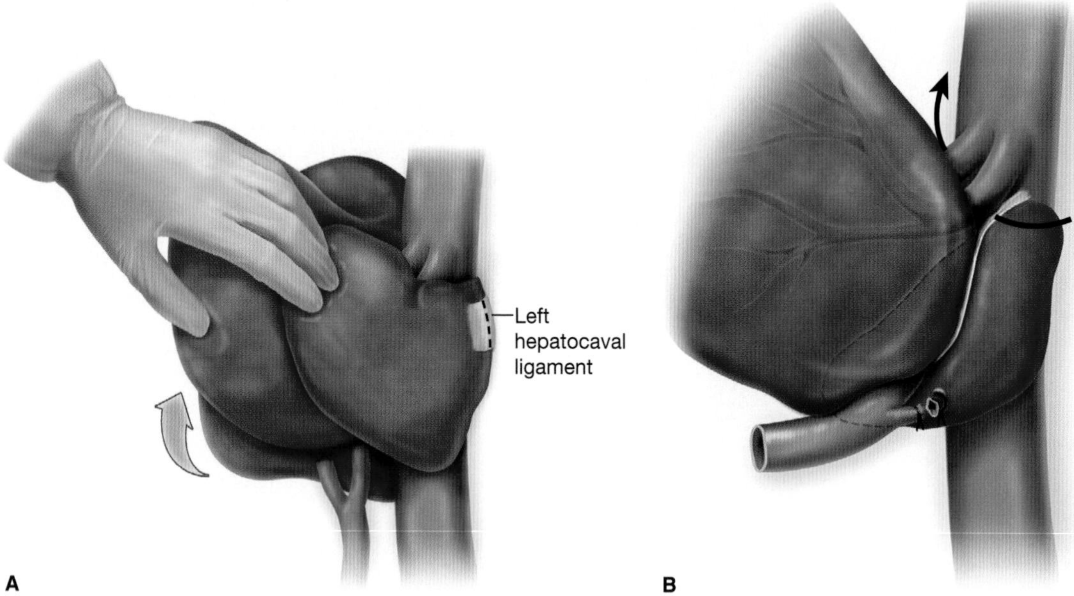


Figure 22.7 A division of the left hepatocaval ligament, also called the caudate-caval ligament (CCL), allows the spigelian caudate to be rotated and elevated off the IVC.

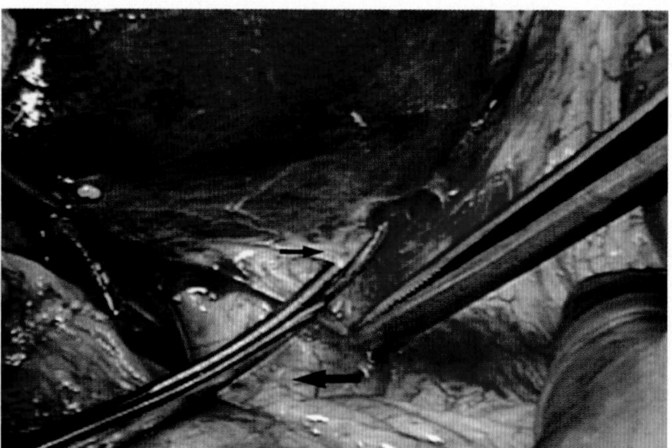

Figure 22.8 Intraoperative photo showing sharp division of the hepatocaval or dorsal ligament (*small arrow*). The Spiegel lobe portion of the caudate is retracted upward and toward the patient's right, away from the IVC (*large arrow*).

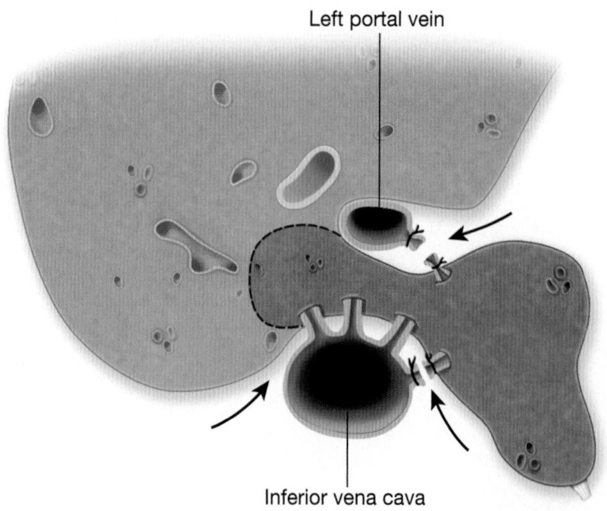


Figure 22.9 After division of the caudate inflow from the left portal vein (LPV), the retrocaudate hepatic veins can be dissected using an approach from either the left or right sides of the inferior vena cava (IVC).

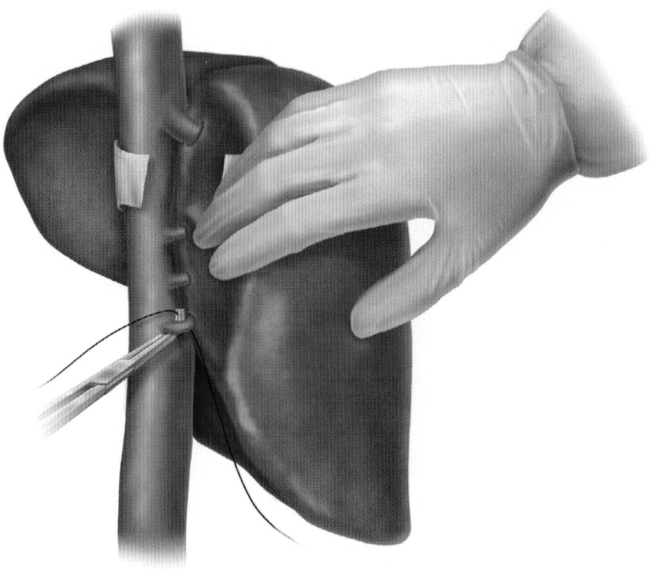

Figure 22.10 The retrohepatic caudate veins are approached from the right side of the vena cava after full mobilization of the right hemiliver.



3. *Division of liver parenchyma shared with the caudate.* Isolated caudate resection requires dissection and transection of the parenchyma between the caudate and segment IV anteriorly and segments VI and VII laterally (Fig. 22.11). Ligation of caudate bile ducts shared with the left hepatic ducts should be conducted carefully. If necessary, exposure of the paracaval caudate can be approached anteriorly with a split liver technique (Fig. 22.11).

## POSTOPERATIVE MANAGEMENT

Routine use of surgical drains is not advocated unless a bilio-enteric anastomosis has been performed (e.g., perihilar bile duct tumor resection) (see Chapter 18). Intravenous circulating volume should be repleted aggressively, and liver function should be monitored closely in the early postoperative period. Upward trends in transaminase levels should raise suspicion for ongoing hepatocellular injury resulting from outflow impedance or more commonly inflow obstruction (i.e., portal vein thrombosis). Duplex ultrasonography can assess blood flow alterations in the remnant liver. Although unlikely after isolated caudate resection, hepatic insufficiency and associated coagulopathy are

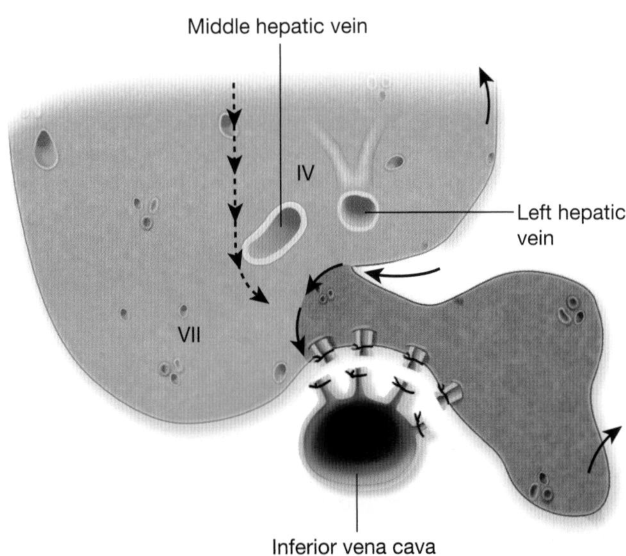


Figure 22.11 The caudate parenchyma is dissected between segments VI, VII, and the base of segment IV. The left (*LHV*) and middle hepatic vein (*MHV*) are encountered in close proximity to the superior tip of the caudate. A split liver technique uses an anterior hepatotomy plane (*dashed arrow*) along the right aspect the MHV to gain exposure to the paracaval caudate.

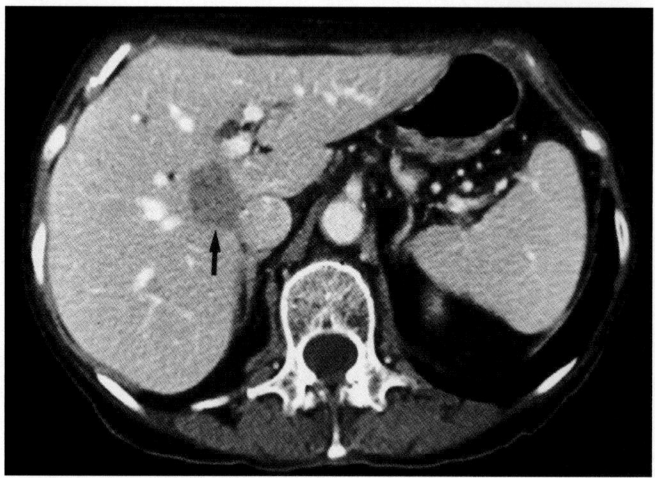

Figure 22.12 Axial contrast-enhanced CT scan image showing a metastatic tumor (*arrow*) involving the caudate process extending to the paracaval portion. Isolated caudate lobectomy is not feasible in this situation, as a positive medial margin is likely. Complete resection will require a major hepatectomy en bloc with the caudate.

common after caudate resection performed in continuity with a right and especially extended right hepatectomy.

## 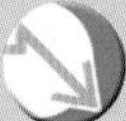 POSTOPERATIVE COMPLICATIONS

- Infectious (surgical site, deep organ space)
- Bleeding (IVC)
- Partial liver necrosis and abscess
- Bile leak (biloma)
- Portal vein thrombosis
- Hepatic vein thrombosis
- Cardiac (infarction, dysrhythmia)
- Organ failure (renal, pulmonary)

##  RESULTS

Because of anatomic constraints, wide margin clearance is usually not achieved after monosegmentectomy for tumors located within the hepatic caudate, especially the paracaval area (Fig. 22.12). As a result of the central liver location of most caudate-involving tumors, the majority of caudate resections will be performed in continuity with a hemihepatectomy. Major vascular resections and reconstructions of the IVC and portal vein are more likely in patients who undergo caudate resection compared to other hepatectomies. In a large series of caudate resections, performed as a monosegmentectomy or in continuity with a major hepatectomy, postoperative complications were recorded in 55% of patients and were likely to be infectious in etiology. Because of the association of caudate resection with larger tumor size and extensive hepatectomy with major vascular resection, postoperative mortality has been reported in 6% of patients.

## 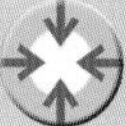 CONCLUSIONS

- Caudate resection can be performed as a monosegmentectomy or in continuity with a partial hepatectomy
- Caudate resection for larger tumors may require major vascular resection and reconstruction of the IVC and/or portal vein
- Tumor involvement of the left hepatic duct and/or left portal vein requires caudate resection for optimal margin clearance

- The anatomic relationship of the caudate and the middle hepatic vein should be recognized at all times
- Ligation of the inflow to the caudate should precede dissection of the retrocaudate hepatic veins

## Recommended References and Readings

Hawkins WG, DeMatteo RP, Cohen MS, et al. Caudate hepatectomy for cancer: a single institution experience with 150 patients. *J Am Coll Surg.* 2005;200:345–352.

Kokkalera U, Ghellai A, Vandermeer TJ. Laparoscopic hepatic caudate lobectomy. *J Laparoendosc Adv Surg Tech A.* 2007;17(1):36–38.

Lerut J, Gruwez JA, Blumgart LH. Resection of the caudate lobe of the liver. *Surg Gynecol Obstet.* 1990;171:160–162.

Yamamoto J, Kosuge T, Shimada K, et al. Anterior transhepatic approach for isolated resection of the caudate lobe of the liver. *World J Surg.* 1999;23:97–101.

# 23 Right Anterior and Posterior Sectionectomy (Bisegmentectomy)

**M.B. Majella Doyle, Adeel S. Khan, and William C. Chapman**

## Introduction

The liver is comprised of eight anatomic segments that are defined by the distribution of the hepatic and portal venous system (Fig. 23.1). These segments can be grouped into four sections or sectors: The right anterior section (segments V and VIII), right posterior section (segments VI and VII), left medial section (segment IV), and left lateral section (segments II and III). Each segment is a functionally independent unit with its own vascular inflow, outflow, and biliary drainage. Consequently, it is possible to remove individual segments (and sectors) without disrupting the blood flow or biliary drainage of the remaining liver (see Chapter 24). Anatomic segment or sector based resections are not only just oncologically superior to non-anatomic resections but also allow for maximal conservation of normal liver parenchyma. In this chapter we will discuss our technique of right anterior and posterior sectorectomy.

##  INDICATIONS/CONTRAINDICATIONS

### Indications

The most common indication is resection of benign or malignant hepatic lesions that meet the criteria for resection (see Chapter 18) and involve all or part of segments V and VIII (anterior sector) or VI and VII (posterior sector). Less common indications include benign biliary strictures of the anterior or posterior sectoral bile duct or retroperitoneal tumors that involve the posterior sector secondarily.

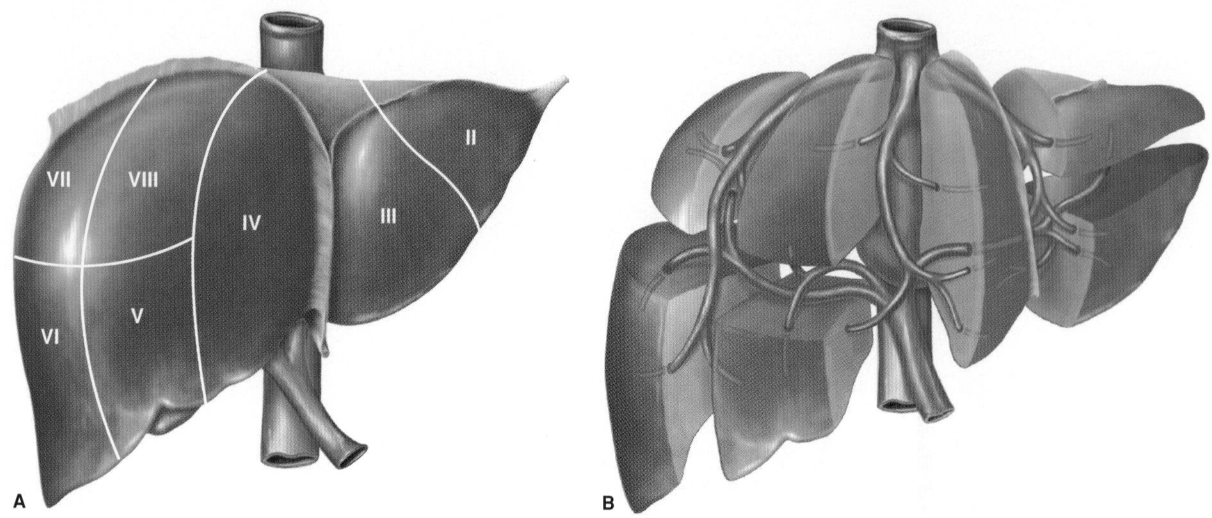


**Figure 23.1** Diagrammatic representation of the segmental anatomy of the liver as defined by Couinaud. Segment I (Caudate lobe) is not seen. Each segment of the liver has its own vascular inflow (portal vein and hepatic artery), outflow (hepatic veins) and biliary drainage. This allows successful removal of individual segments (and sectors) without disrupting the blood supply to the remaining liver. LHV, left hepatic vein; MHV, middle hepatic vein; PV, portal vein; RHV, right hepatic vein.

## Contraindications

Absolute contraindications include presence of wide spread metastatic disease, advanced cirrhosis (Childs Pugh class C) or inability of the patient to tolerate general anesthesia.

# PREOPERATIVE PLANNING

Preoperative investigation includes liver and renal function tests, complete blood count, and coagulation profile. All patients should have cross-sectional imaging either with a contrast-enhanced abdominal computed tomography (CT) scan or magnetic resonance imaging (MRI). The lesion under question must be localized to either right anterior or posterior sector and must be resectable (Figs. 23.2, 23.3). Invasion or thrombus of the portal vein outside the area of resection must be ruled out. An attempt should be made to assess the function of the remaining liver and evaluate for extent of cirrhosis, steatosis, or chemotherapy induced hepatic damage. Volumetric analyses may be necessary in these patients especially when additional hepatic resections are required. Older

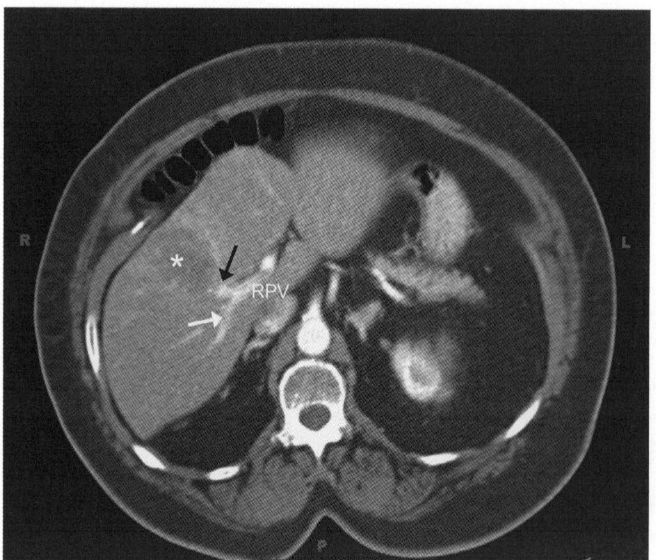


**Figure 23.2** Computed tomography (CT) image of a patient with metastatic colon cancer to the right anterior sector. The classic hypo-attentuating lesion (*asterix*) can be seen in segment V. Note the relationship of the tumor with anterior (*black arrow*) and posterior (*white arrow*) sectoral branches of the right portal vein (RPV).

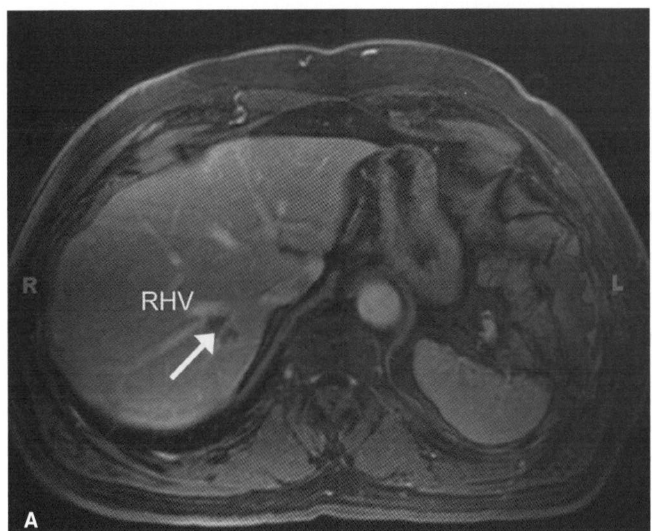

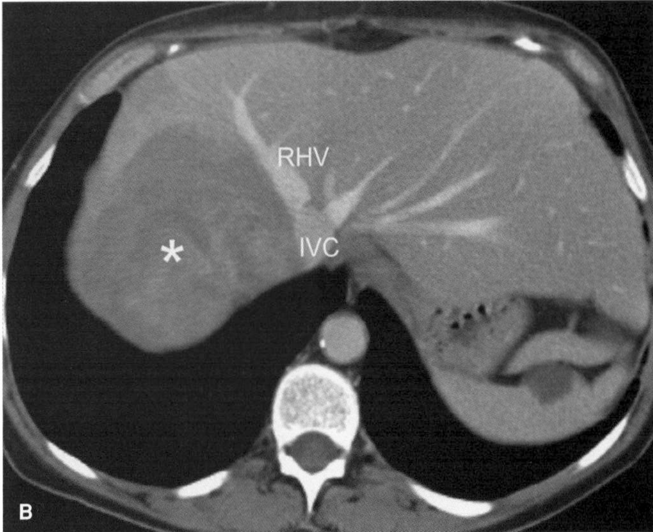


Figure 23.3 **A:** Computed tomography (CT) image of the patient with colorectal metastasis to the posterior sector of the liver. Small hypo-attenuating lesion (*white arrow*) can be seen in segment VII. Note the relationship with right hepatic vein (RHV). **B:** CT image of patient with sarcoma involving segment VII (*asterix*) seen posterior to the RHV. Note abutment of the tumor against the inferior vena cava (IVC).



patients and all patients with significant medical comorbidities must undergo thorough cardiopulmonary assessment and clearance before proceeding with surgery. At Washington University in St. Louis, an image-guided planning system to reconstruct the cross-sectional images as 3D images where the hepatic and portal veins are displayed along with the tumor and a resection plane can be drawn and manipulated to achieve the desired resection margin (Fig. 23.4). The future liver remnant (FLR) volume is also calculated in an automated fashion (see Chapter 18).

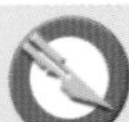

# SURGICAL TECHNIQUE

## Anatomy

The liver can be divided into right and left hemi-livers by the middle hepatic vein, which runs in the mid-hepatic plane designated as "Cantile's Line," which runs from the gallbladder fossa to the suprahepatic vena cava. The right liver is further divided

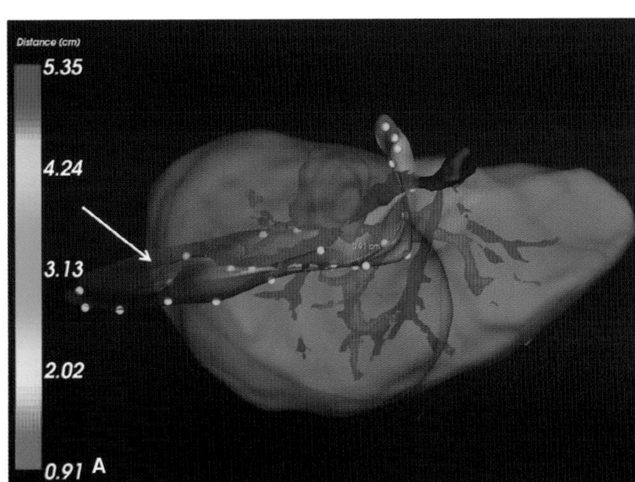

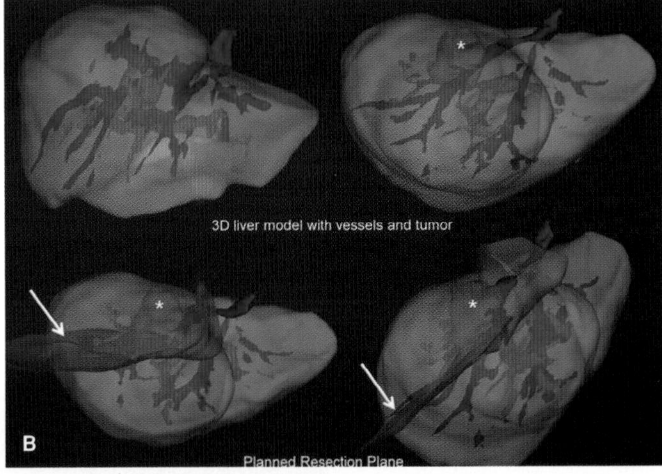


Figure 23.4 3D reconstruction image showing resection plane (*white arrow*) with heat map to calculate planned resection margin. Tumor location is marked with asterix.

into an anterior sector and a posterior sector by the right portal scissura containing the right hepatic vein (RHV). The anterior sector is made up of two segments—segment V caudally and segment VIII cranially. Similarly, the posterior sector comprised of segment VI caudally and segment VII cranially (see Fig. 18.6). All of these landmarks can be identified on intraoperative ultrasound, which should be an essential component of any major liver resection procedure. It is imperative that all hepatobiliary surgeons be very comfortable with this imaging modality (see Fig. 18.9).

## Positioning

The patient is positioned supine with arms in or out. All bony prominences are suitably padded.

## Technique

### Right Anterior Sectionectomy (Bisegmentectomy—Segments V and VIII)

1. Skin incision: The choice of incision depends on surgeon's experience and comfort. Some of the commonly used incisions include unilateral or bilateral subcostal incision with midline extension, midline incision, or by a thoracotomy extension from right subcostal incision. We favor the right subcostal with midline extension (see Fig. 18.7) (see also Figs. 19.3 and 21.5) or bilateral subcostal with midline extension ("Mercedes Benz" incision).
2. Careful inspection of abdominal cavity to rule out extra hepatic disease.
3. Take down falciform ligament over anterior surface of the liver.
4. Perform intraoperative ultrasound (IOUS) of the liver to delineate vascular anatomy and relationship of the tumor with the hepatic veins and portal pedicles (Fig. 23.5). The RHV is identified at its point of entry into the vena cava and moving the probe caudally along the liver allows it to be followed into the hepatic parenchyma. The RHV separates the anterior sector from the posterior sector and therefore is an important landmark. It is important to check for a common variant where the anterior sector is drained by a large branch draining directly into the middle hepatic vein.

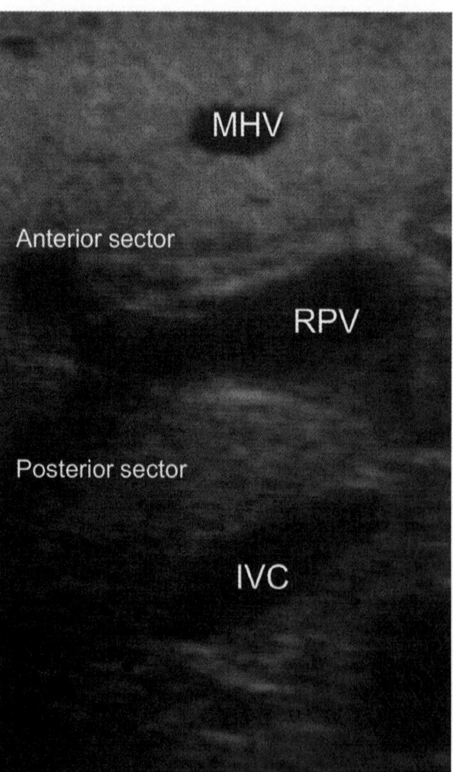


**Figure 23.5** IOUS of the liver demonstrating relevant anatomy for right anterior and posterior sectoral resection. RPV can be seen bifurcating into anterior sectoral and posterior sectoral branches. MHV, Middle hepatic vein; IVC, inferior vena cava; RPV, right portal vein.

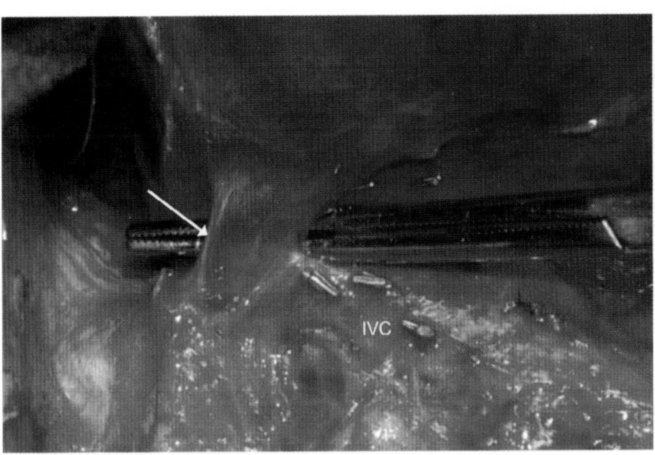


Figure 23.6 Circumferential dissection of RHV (*white arrow*). Lateral view; IVC, inferior vena cava; RHV, right hepatic vein.



The main portal vein is next identified at the base of segment IV and followed till the bifurcation into the right and left portal pedicles is visualized. By scanning toward the right liver, the main right portal triad can be seen dividing into anterior and posterior sectoral branches. The anterior sectoral branch supplies superior branches to segment VIII and inferior branches to segment V.

5. Completely mobilize the right liver and obtain circumferential control of the extra hepatic portion of the RHV (outflow) (Fig. 23.6) (see also Figs. 19.6 and 19.11).
6. Perform cholecystectomy with ligation of cystic duct.
7. Carefully lower the hilar plate and identify the right main portal pedicle (see Figs. 21.14 and 24.4).
8. Dissect along the right main portal pedicle until it is seen bifurcating into the right anterior and posterior sectoral pedicles (Figs. 23.7, 23.8). IOUS can be used to get a rough estimate of the bifurcation point. Alternately, if the bifurcation point is too distal, minor hepatotomies can be made to allow access to origin of the anterior sectoral pedicle.
9. Test clamp the anterior sectoral pedicle (inflow) to visually confirm demarcation of segments V and VIII (Figs. 23.9, 23.10).
10. Divide the anterior pedicle as far distally as possible to avoid injury to the posterior pedicle. The right posterior bile duct is especially prone to injury where it hooks around the right posterior sectoral portal vein.

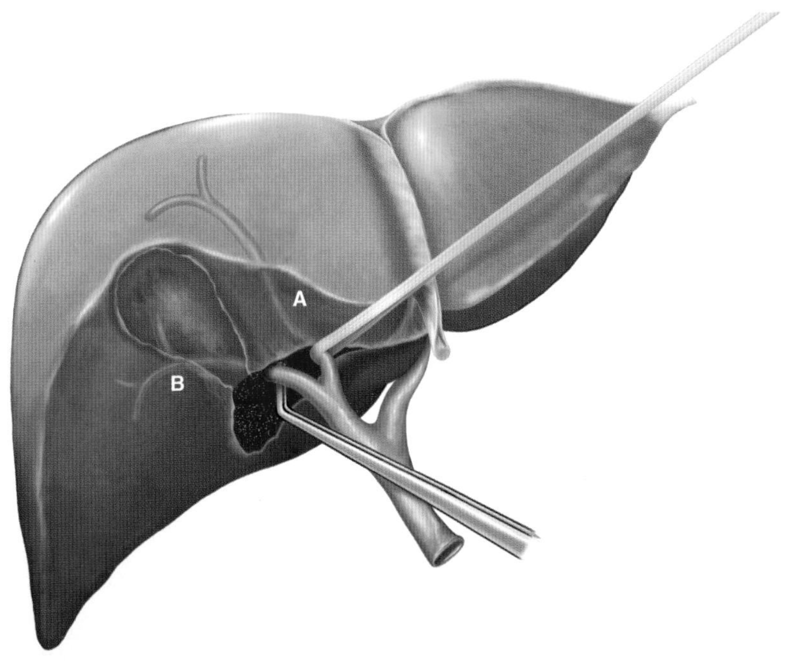


Figure 23.7 Isolation of right anterior **(A)** and posterior **(B)** sectional (sectoral) pedicles. The right main portal vein branches into the right anterior sectional and the right posterior sectional pedicles. The fissure of Ganz (Fig. 23.8) is a useful landmark to locate the right posterior sectional pedicle.

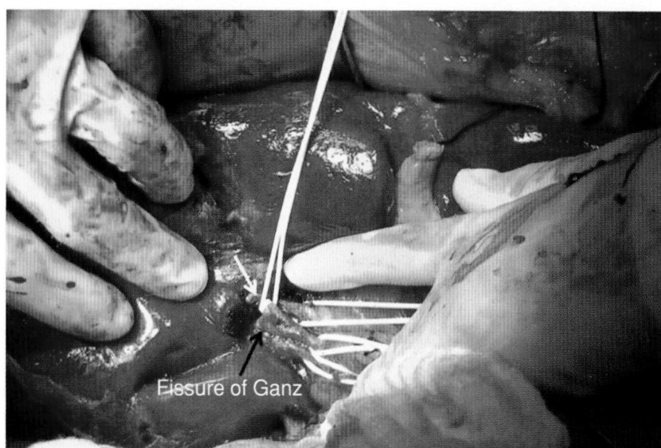


Figure 23.8 Dissection and control of the right anterior portal pedicle. Note the RPV dividing into right anterior sectoral branch (*white arrow*) and right posterior sectoral branch (*black arrow*). RPV, right portal vein.

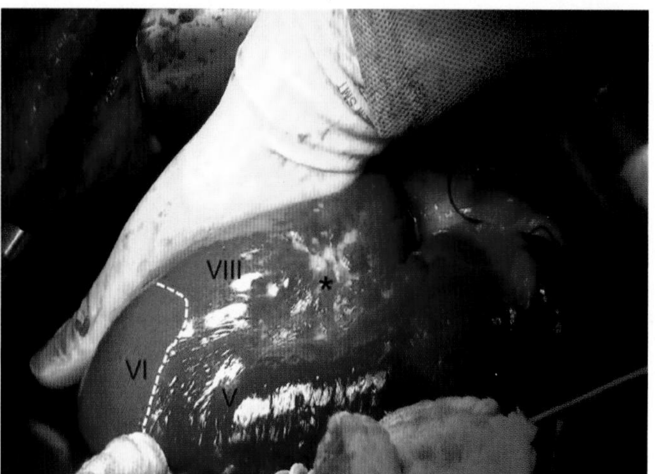


Figure 23.9 Anterolateral view of the liver after clamping of right anterior sectoral pedicle. The line of demarcation (*white dotted line*) can be seen separating the right anterior sector (segments V and VIII) and posterior sector (segments VI and VII). The tumor can be seen where it comes close to the anterior surface of the liver (*asterix*).

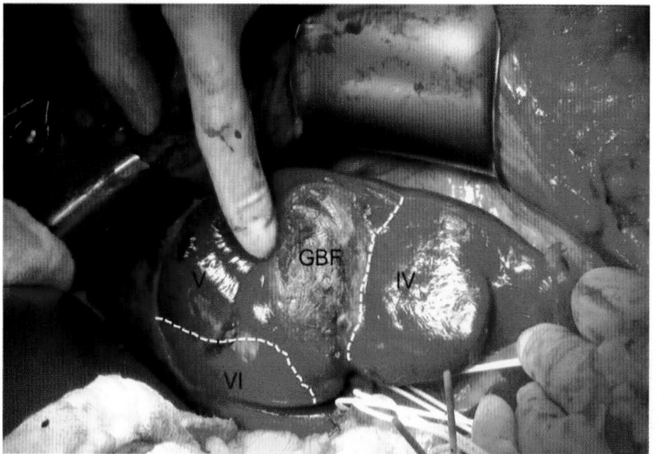


Figure 23.10 Posteriolateral view of the liver after clamping of right anterior pedicle. Note the lines of demarcation (*white dotted line*) separating segment V of the anterior sector from segments VI (part of posterior sector) and segment IV. GBF, gallbladder fossa.

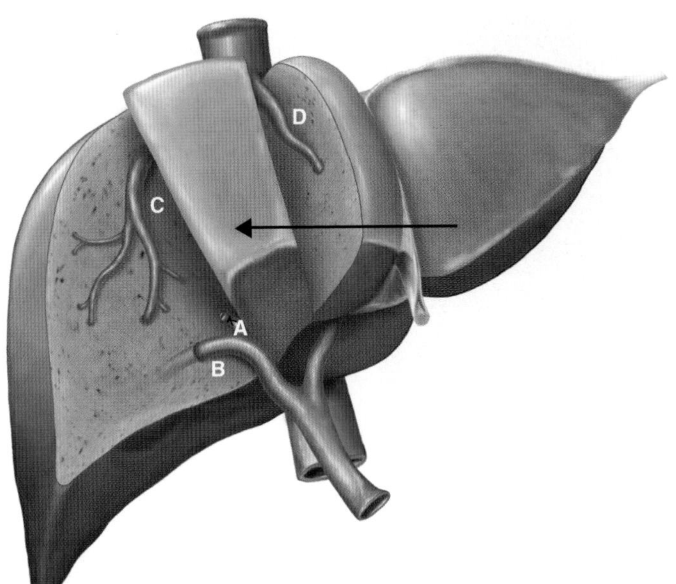


**Figure 23.11** The right anterior section is defined by clamping and ligation of the right anterior pedicle **(A)**. The pedicle to the right posterior section **(B)** is preserved. The anterior section (*black arrow*) is then removed by parenchymal transection along the mid-hepatic plane (Cantlie's line) and the plane of the RHV **(C)** until they meet posteriorly. The RHV **(C)** is usually preserved while the middle hepatic vein **(D)** may need to be divided. RHV, right hepatic vein.



11. Begin parenchymal transection along the sagittal plane at the line of demarcation of anterior sector with segment IV till RHV is visualized. Then follow the plane anterior to the RHV laterally until the hepatectomy is completed. In some cases, the middle hepatic vein may be sacrificed, if necessary for tumor clearance, with the expectation that the umbilical vein will provide adequate venous drainage of segments IVA and IVB (Fig. 23.11).
12. Check vascularity of the posterior sectoral pedicle.
13. Inspect the transected liver surface for hemostasis and leakage of bile.
14. Leave an external drain connected to bulb suction in selected cases.

**Right Posterior Sectionectomy (Bisegmentectomy—Segments VI and VII)**

1. Make the skin incision as for right anterior sectionectomy.
2. Careful inspection of abdominal cavity to rule out extra hepatic disease.
3. Take down falciform ligament over the anterior surface of the liver.
4. Perform IOUS of the liver to delineate vascular anatomy and relationship of tumor with the hepatic veins and portal pedicles. The RHV is identified as it drains into the vena cava and is followed proximally to the hepatic parenchyma. In 20% of the population, segment VI drains directly into the vena cava via a large right inferior hepatic vein (Fig. 23.12). This can be seen by IOUS posterior to the main right portal vein (RPV) as it enters the right anterolateral portion of the retrohepatic vena cava. The main portal vein can be identified at the base of segment IV and followed till the bifurcation into the right and left portal pedicles is identified. The right portal pedicle can then be traced laterally until it is seen dividing into the right anterior and posterior sectoral pedicles. Evaluation of the posterior portions of segments VI and VII may require scanning from the inferior or lateral liver surface.
5. Completely mobilize the right liver (Fig. 23.13) and obtain circumferential control of the extra hepatic portion of the RHV (Fig. 23.14). Obtain control of accessory right inferior hepatic vein if present (Fig. 23.12) (see also Figs. 19.5 and 19.6).
6. Proceed with cholecystectomy and ligation of cystic duct.
7. Carefully lower the hilar plate and identify the right portal pedicle (see Figs. 21.14 and 24.4).
8. Dissect along the right portal pedicle until the point of bifurcation to right anterior and posterior pedicles. Circumferential control of posterior pedicle is obtained (Fig. 23.15). Some times the right posterior pedicle can be visualized and controlled at the base of the fissure of Ganz which is a helpful surface landmark present in

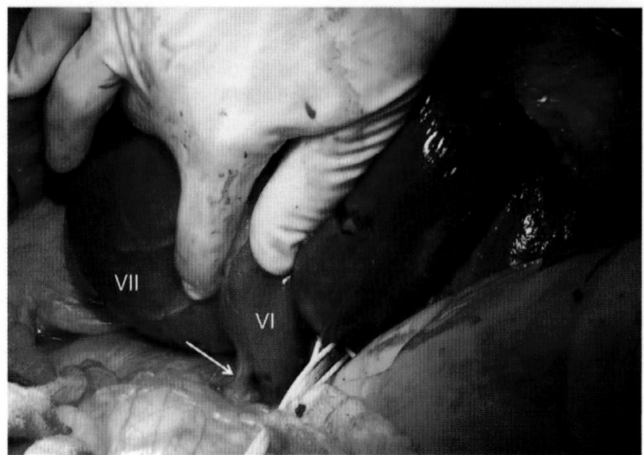


Figure 23.12 Lateral view of the mobilized right liver showing a large right inferior hepatic vein (*white arrow*) draining segment VI directly into the IVC. This anomaly is seen in 20% of the population and can be identified on intraoperative ultrasound prior to mobilization of the liver. This vein is routinely divided during a right posterior sectionectomy but it is essential to recognize and preserve it during a right anterior sectionectomy that includes resection of the right hepatic vein, as it may provide the only venous drainage for the posterior sector.

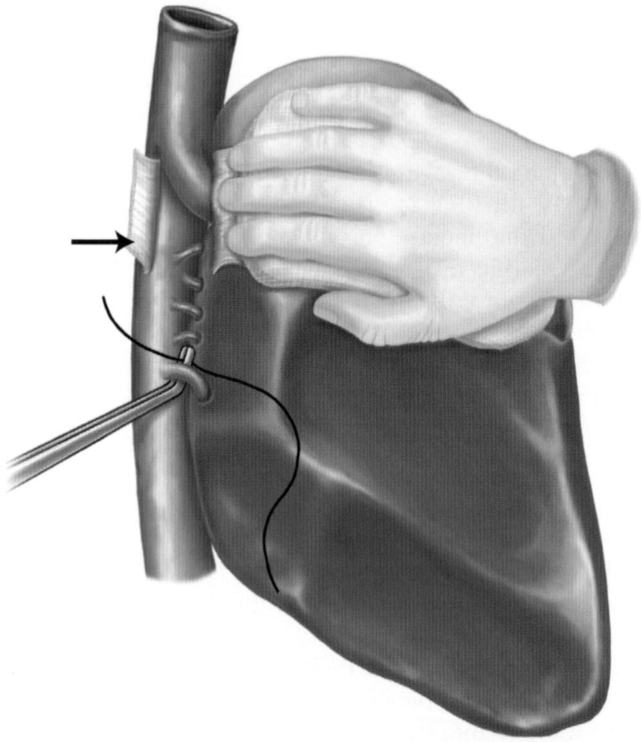

Figure 23.13 Mobilization of the right liver with division of short hepatic veins. The caval ligament (*black arrow*) is divided to facilitate exposure of the RHV. RHV right hepatic vein.

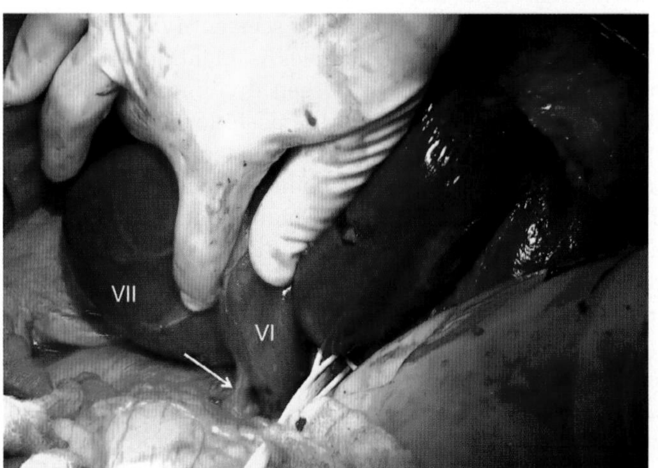


Figure 23.14 Dissection of RHV (*white arrow*) after mobilization of the right liver. Anterior view. IVC, inferior vena cava (suprahepatic portion).

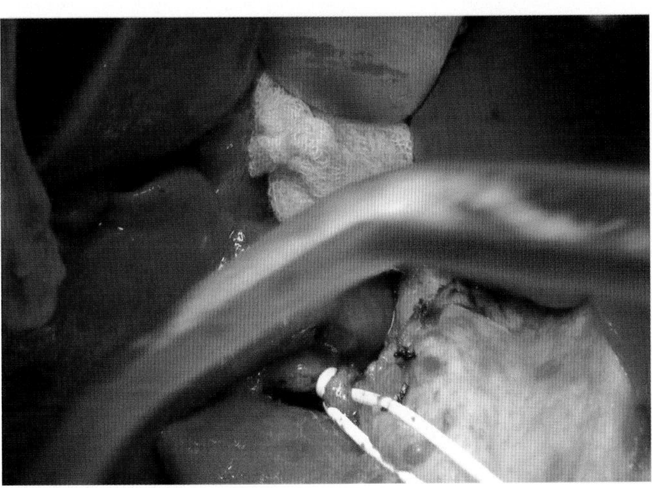

Figure 23.15 Control of right posterior pedicle with vessel loop.



70% of patients (Fig. 23.7). Alternately separate hepatotomies can be made for pedicle control. The location of these hepatotomies can be guided by IOUS.

9. Test clamp right posterior pedicle to visually confirm demarcation of segments VI and VII (Fig. 23.16).
10. Divide the right posterior sectoral pedicle. Our preference is to use the GIA stapler with a vascular load.
11. Divide the accessory right inferior hepatic vein if present.
12. Proceed with parenchymal transection along the demarcation plane. Remember the transection plane is in a lateral-to-medial direction (Fig. 23.17). The RHV may be preserved or sacrificed depending on the relationship with the tumor (Fig. 23.18).
13. Inspect the transected liver surface for hemostasis and leakage of bile (Fig. 23.19).
14. Leave an external drain connected to bulb suction.
15. Examine the specimen on the back table (Fig. 23.20).

## Intraoperative Considerations

Excessive intraoperative blood loss during hepatectomy is a major determinant of adverse perioperative outcome. Therefore every attempt must be made to keep blood loss at a minimum. Vascular inflow and outflow control and low central venous pressure anesthesia (CVP <5) are essential. CVP can be kept low by judicious use of intravenous fluids and blood products. Ideal monitoring is with intraoperative echocardiography when available.

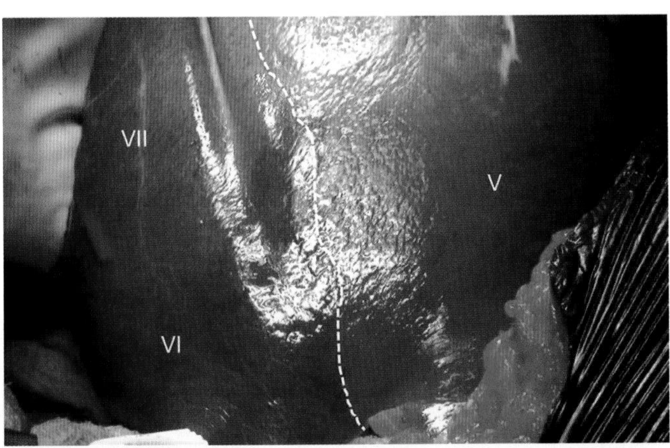


Figure 23.16 Visual confirmation of demarcation (*white dotted line*) of right posterior sector (segments VI and VII) after test clamping of right posterior pedicle. Right liver is rotated anteriorly for demonstration purposes.

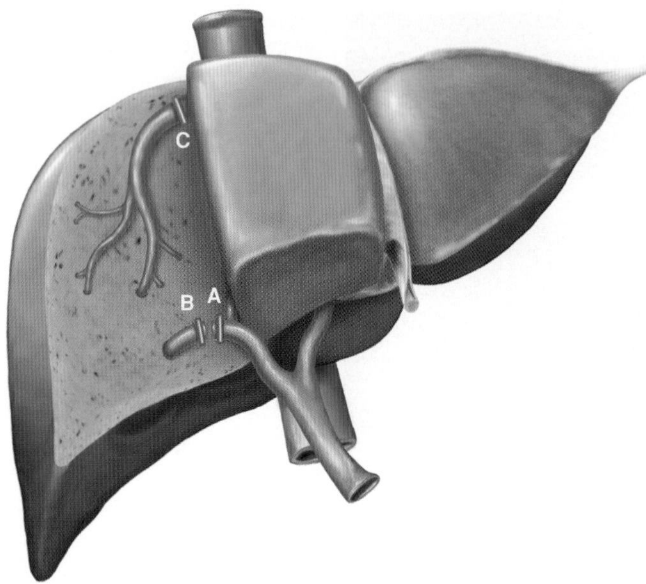


Figure 23.17 Right posterior sectionectomy. The right posterior pedicle **(B)** is divided after test clamping and demonstration of line of demarcation. The anterior sectoral pedicle **(A)** is preserved (anterior sector is not shown). The decision to divide the right hepatic vein **(C)** is made on individual basis. The plane of parenchymal transection runs from medial to lateral along the plane of the RHV. RHV, right hepatic vein.

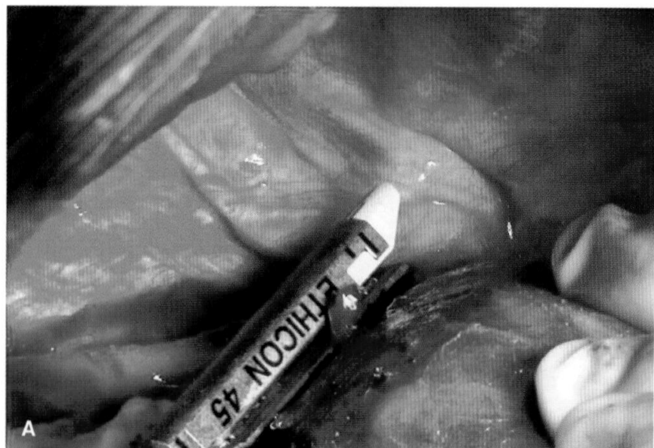


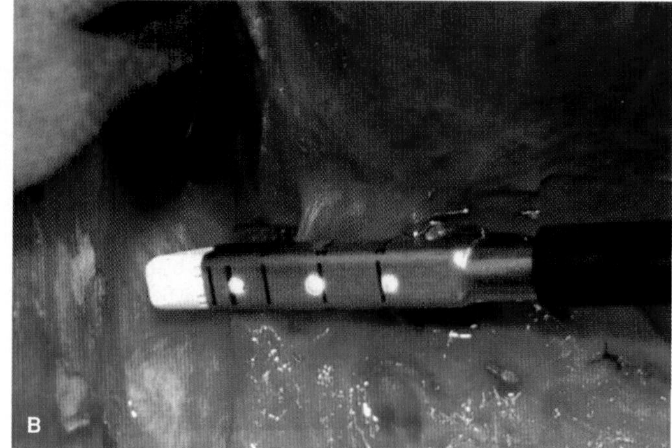


Figure 23.18 Division of the RHV with Endo GIA stapler. Anterior **(A)** and lateral **(B)** views. RHV, right hepatic vein.

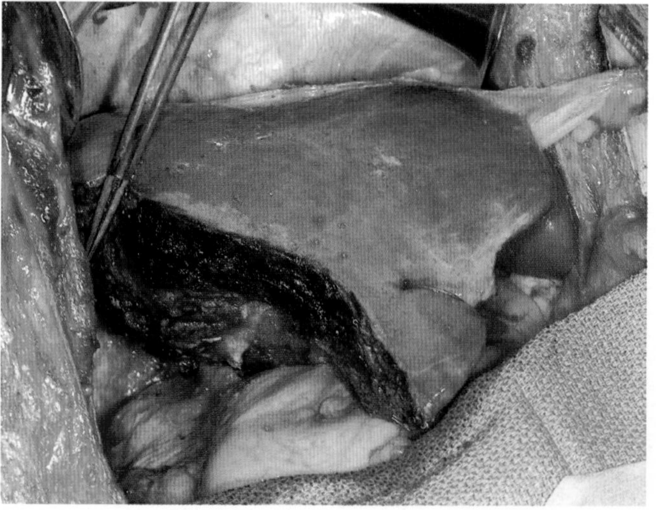

Figure 23.19 Transected liver surface.

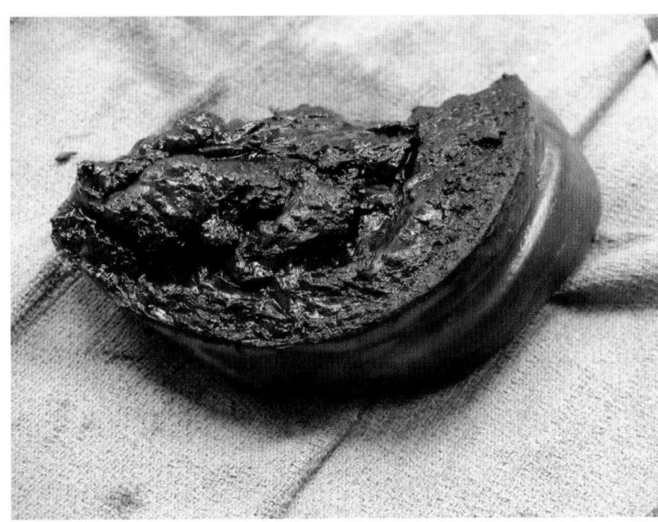

**Figure 23.20** Liver specimen for examination.



### Postoperative Management

Initial postoperative monitoring is carried out in an intensive care or step down unit. Vitals are measured periodically and drain output carefully monitored. Tachycardia and hypotension may indicate postoperative bleeding. The synthetic function of the liver is also closely monitored, especially in cirrhotics, for any sign of hepatic insufficiency. Serum electrolytes are checked and repleted as required. Bile staining of drain fluid for the first few days after surgery is not unusual and usually represents leakage from small ducts at the site of parenchymal transection but must be investigated if the volume is high or if it persists beyond the first few days. Intravenous narcotics must be judiciously used, as their metabolism may be impaired. We strongly encourage early ambulation and frequent incentive spirometry in the postoperative period.

## COMPLICATIONS

With advancement in anesthesia, techniques of parenchymal transection and postoperative care, the overall mortality and morbidity after segment-oriented resection has considerably decreased. Most high volume cancer centers have a perioperative mortality and morbidity of 1% to 4% and 25% to 40%, respectively.

Pulmonary complications such as atelectasis, pneumonia, and respiratory failure are the most common sources of morbidity in the postoperative period. Surgery specific complications include postoperative bleeding, hepatic insufficiency, bile leaks, intraabdominal fluid collections, abscess, and wound infection. Most of these complications can be managed non-operatively. The burden of these complications can be lowered by meticulous intraoperative techniques, adherence to basic principles of hepatic surgery (e.g., inflow and outflow control and hemostasis) and very close monitoring in the postoperative period. Predictably, morbidity and mortality is higher in patients with hepatocellular carcinoma (HCC) and underlying cirrhosis (see Chapter 18).

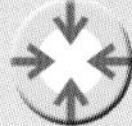

## CONCLUSION

This standardized technique of right bisegmentectomy (anterior or posterior sectorectomy) is a safe and effective alternative to right hepatectomy in selected patients. It avoids unnecessary sacrifice of functioning hepatic parenchyma with all the oncologic and "hemostatic" benefits of an anatomic resection. This technique may increase resectability rate in patients with bilateral disease and provide more options of repeat resections in patients with recurrent disease.

## Recommended References and Readings

Billingsley KG, Jarnagin WR, Fong Y, et al. Segment-oriented hepatic resection in the management of malignant neoplasms of the liver. *J Am Coll Surg.* 1998;187:471–481.

Blumgart LH, et al. *Surgery of the Liver, Biliary Tract and Pancreas.* Philadelphia: Saunders; 2004:1440–1451, 1484–1524.

Chouillard E, Cherqui D, Tayar C, et al. Anatomical bi- and trisegmentectomies as alternatives to extensive liver resections. *Ann Surg.* 2003;238:29–34.

DeMatteo RM, Palese C, Jarnagin WR, et al. Anatomic segmental hepatic resection is superior to wedge resection as an oncologic operation for colorectal liver metastases. *J Gastrointest surg.* 2000;4:178–184.

Hasegawa K, Kokudo N, Imamura H, et al. Prognostic impact of anatomic resection for hepatocellular carcinoma. *Ann Surg.* 2005; 242:252–259.

Jarnagin WR, Gonen M, Fong Y, et al. Improvement in perioperative outcome after hepatic resection: analysis of 1,803 consecutive cases over the past decade. *Ann Surg.* 2002;236:397–406.

Lau WY, Leung KL, Lee TW, et al. Ultrasonography during liver resection for hepatocellular carcinoma. *Br J Surg.* 1993;80:493–494.

Liau KH, Blumgart LH, DeMatteo RP. Segmented oriented approach to liver resection. *Surg Clin North Am.* 2004;84:543–561.

Machado MC, Herman P, Meirelles Jr RF, et al. Bisegmentectomy V-VIII as alternative to right hepatectomy: an intrahepatic approach. *J Surg Oncol.* 2005;90:43–45.

Makuuchi M, Hashikura Y, Kawasaki S, et al. Persona experience of right anterior sectionectomy (segments V and VIII) for hepatic malignancies. *Surgery.* 1993;114:52–58.

Strasberg SM. Nomenclature of hepatic anatomy and resections: a review of the Brisbane 2000 system. *J Hepatobiliary Pancreat Surg.* 2005;12:351–355.

Terminology Committee of the IHPBA. Terminology of liver anatomy and resections. *HPB Surg.* 2000;2:333–339.

Torzili G, Procopio F, Cimino M, et al. Anatomic segmental and subsegmental resection of the liver for hepatocellular carcinoma. A new approach by means of ultrasound-guided vessel compression. *Ann Surg.* 2010;251(2):229–235.

# 24 Hepatic Segmental Resections

**William R. Jarnagin, Charbel Sandroussi, and Paul D. Greig**

## Introduction

Better understanding of hepatic anatomy has been pivotal in the evolution of safe liver surgery (see Chapter 18 and Figs. 17.6, 18.6 and 23.1). Compared to lobar and extended lobar resections, segmental liver resections, where appropriate, allow preservation of liver parenchyma without compromising oncologic results. The ability to resect one or two segments rather than the entire lobe allows parenchymal preservation, which is critical in patients with diseased parenchyma and in those with extensive disease and/or a high likelihood of requiring future liver directed therapy. The latter are particularly relevant in patients with metastatic disease. Segmental vascular inflow control may facilitate the resection by precisely mapping the transection plane, although this is not always possible. In addition, such anatomically based resections involving the removal of a hepatic segment confined by tumor-bearing portal tributaries may, in fact, be more sound from an oncologic standpoint.

## Anatomy and Terminology

The segmental anatomy of the liver originated from the original descriptions of Couinaud in 1952. Couinaud's work showed that the liver consists of eight independent segments, each with its own vascular inflow, hepatic venous outflow, and biliary drainage and each amenable to resection. These segments form the foundation of current hepatic nomenclature (Fig. 24.1A and B; see also Fig. 18.6). The Brisbane Terminology eliminates confusing terminology of lobes and sectors used in past descriptions of liver anatomy. The terms hemi-liver (first order division), section (second order division), and segments (third order division) are not interchangeable and provides common terminology for better communication among surgeons, radiologists, and other physicians.

The first order division separates the right (segments 5 to 8) and left (segments 1 to 4) **hemi-livers** (or liver) along the principal resection plane or Cantlie's line, delineated by the middle hepatic vein (MHV), coursing along a line from the gallbladder fossa to the IVC. The second order division separates the right and left hemi-livers into liver

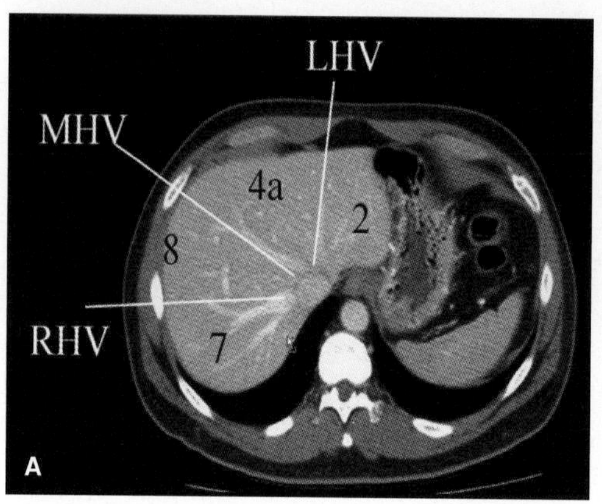


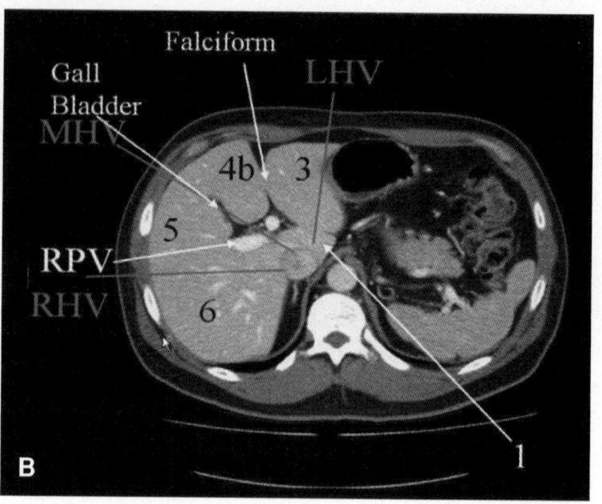


**Figure 24.1** **A:** Axial CT scan image through the upper liver demonstrating the anatomic boundaries of segments 1, 2, 4a, 8, and 7. **B:** Axial CT scan image through the lower liver demonstrating the anatomic boundaries of segments 1, 3, 4b, 5, and 6. RHV, right hepatic vein; MHV, middle hepatic vein; LHV, left hepatic vein. From: W.R. Jarnagin (ed.), *Blumgart's Surgery of the Liver, Biliary Tract and Pancreas, 5th Edition,* Elsevier, 2012.

**sections** based on the portal distribution (i.e., the primary divisions of the right and left portal pedicles) and the hepatic venous drainage. The right liver is divided into right anterior (segments 5 and 8), and right posterior (segments 6 and 7) sections, separated by the right hepatic vein (RHV). The left liver is divided into left lateral (segments 2 and 3) and left medial (segments 4a and 4b) sections by the umbilical vein, which runs along a line delineated by the falciform ligament. Together, segments 2 and 3 are commonly, but erroneously, referred to as the left lateral segment.

The third order division separates segments into segments (numbers 1 to 8) and is defined by hepatic arterial supply and biliary drainage (see Figs. 17.6 and 18.6).

# Selection of Patients

Anatomically based resections should be the gold standard in most cases, excluding fenestration of liver cysts (see Chapter 28), wedge excisions of superficial lesions, and enucleation of certain lesions such as metastatic neuroendocrine tumors (see Chapter 25). A clear understanding of the patient's segmental liver anatomy is essential to a safe, controlled resection. Segmental resections are not limited by indication nor by the presence of hepatic parenchymal disease.

Achieving a balance between parenchymal sparing resections and adequate tumor clearance is clearly an important consideration for all resections but is critical in patients with diseased livers. In patients with hepatocellular carcinoma (HCC), where cirrhosis is frequently present, segmental liver resection forms a bridge between the major hepatectomy and non-anatomic resection to preserve the maximum liver volume to prevent postoperative liver failure. Since HCC have a propensity for intraportal extension and dissemination, segmental resections, by removing the parenchyma supplied by the principal segmental portal vein branch, are likely to be more effective than non-anatomic resections from an oncologic standpoint. Segmental liver resection is also preferred in patients with multifocal colorectal metastasis treated extensively with preoperative chemotherapy, which frequently results in hepatic dysfunction and impaired regeneration due to steatosis (see Fig. 18.1).

# PREOPERATIVE PLANNING

The planning of a segmental-based resection must take into account anatomic variations and their relationship to the plane of transection (Fig. 24.2) (see Figs. 17.9, 19.2, and 21.1 to 21.4). Resection has been facilitated by the precision digital imaging provided by computerized tomography, magnetic resonance imaging (MRI), and ultrasound (US), allowing interpretation of intrahepatic vascular and biliary anatomy (see Chapter 18) and the ability to manipulate and scroll through reconstructions in the axial, coronal, or sagittal planes using software such as picture archiving and communication system

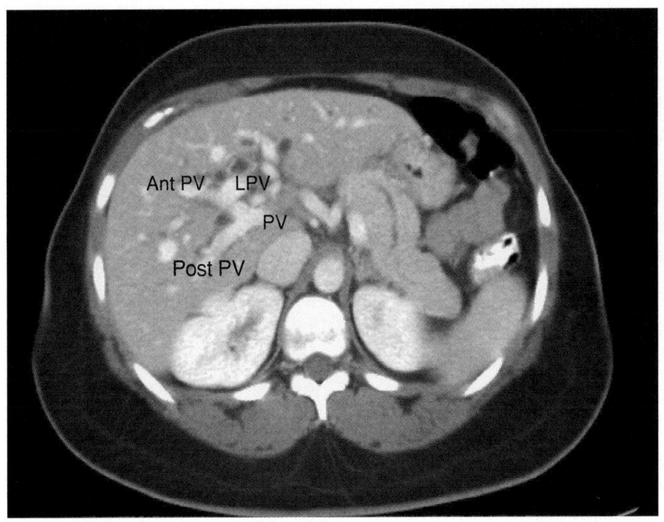


Figure 24.2 Axial CT image showing variant portal venous anatomy, with the left portal vein (LPV) arising as a branch of the right anterior sectoral branch (Ant PV) and the posterior sectoral branch (Post PV) branching separately from the main portal vein (MPV).



(PACS). With the appropriate protocol for arterial and venous enhancement, the third and fourth level vascular structures can be accurately defined. More sophisticated software is available that may facilitate the preoperative planning. These easily manipulated, three-dimensional reconstructions that create a virtual reproduction of the liver can be used to determine the proposed plane of transection, taking into account the minimum resection margin, and residual volume of liver (Fig. 24.3).

# General Operative Principles

## Preoperative Assessment and Anesthesia

The preoperative assessment and preparation of the patient for a liver resection are described in Chapter 18. Comorbidities should be identified and optimized. Careful assessment of liver function, particularly in those with intrinsic liver disease is important. Preoperative biliary decompression and/or portal vein embolization are infrequently required for patients undergoing segmental compared to more extensive resections (see Chapters 18, 19, 20, and 26). Particular attention should be paid to the reduction of the central venous pressure during transection in order to reduce blood loss, and measures to prevent hypothermia, infections, and venous thromboembolism are required.

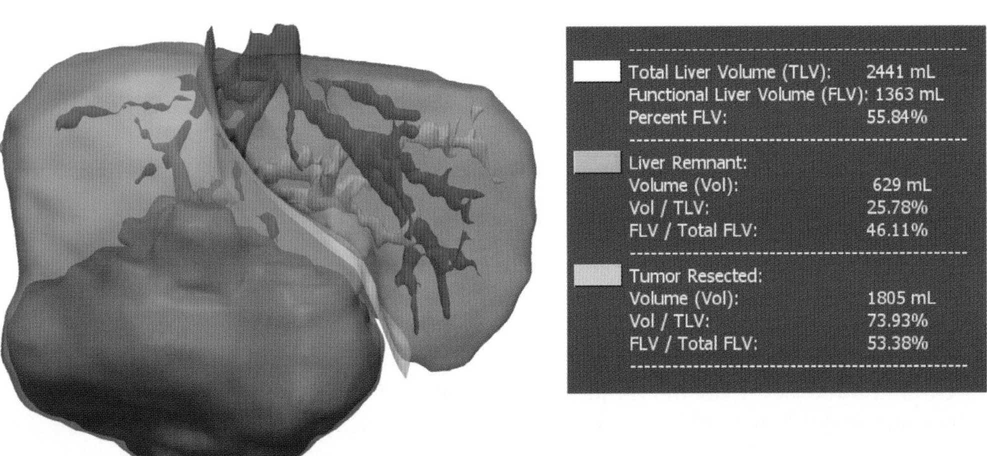

Total Liver Volume (TLV): 2441 mL
Functional Liver Volume (FLV): 1363 mL
Percent FLV: 55.84%
Liver Remnant:
Volume (Vol): 629 mL
Vol / TLV: 25.78%
FLV / Total FLV: 46.11%
Tumor Resected:
Volume (Vol): 1805 mL
Vol / TLV: 73.93%
FLV / Total FLV: 53.38%


Figure 24.3 Three-dimensional model generated from a preoperative CT scan using Scout™ software system (Pathfinder Therapeutics, Inc, Nashville, TN). The planned resection plane is shown. The total liver volume, the functional liver volume (total volume—tumor volume), and future liver remnant volumes are shown.

### Exposure and Mobilization

Segmental resections may be performed laparoscopically (see Chapter 31) or at laparotomy. For open resections, exposure can be achieved through a variety of incisions (see Figs. 18.7, 19.3 and 21.5), including right subcostal with midline extension (hockey-stick) or its modification (J-shaped), or a bilateral subcostal incision with (Mercedes incision) or without (chevron) midline extension. A long midline incision may be used for selected liver resections, particularly if combined with a left or sigmoid colon or rectal resection; thoracoabdominal is seldom required. Following laparotomy and general inspection, the liver is mobilized by transection of the obliterated umbilical vein and division of the falciform ligament as it triangulates onto the IVC to identify the origins of the hepatic veins (see Fig. 19.4). Mobilization of the right and left livers requires division of the triangular ligaments in order to free the liver fully from the hemidiaphragms. During the division of the lesser omentum (gastro-hepatic ligament), attention should be given to the presence of an accessory or replaced left hepatic artery arising from the left gastric artery (see Chapter 20). Full mobilization of the right liver requires division of the coronary ligaments; if resection of one of the posterior right segments is planned (6 and/or 7), then the right adrenal gland must be separated and allowed to retract into the retroperitoneum and dissection of the retrohepatic IVC must be performed, as one would for more extensive procedures (see Chapters 19 and 23, Figs. 19.5, 19.6, and 23.12).

### Intraoperative Assessment

The intraoperative assessment of the liver requires correlation of the findings of inspection and palpation of the mobilized liver with those of the preoperative imaging (see Chapter 18). Intraoperative ultrasound is used to localize the lesion, confirm the preoperative imaging findings, and further stage the proposed remnant liver (see Fig. 18.9). Operative US of the liver may be valuable to identify venous tumor thrombus and to assess the proposed plane of transection and its three-dimensional relationship with major hepatic veins and portal triads. Anatomically based segmentectomy and subsegmentectomy by intraoperative ultrasound (IOUS)-guided finger compression has been described. With this technique, IOUS-guided finger compression of the vascular pedicle feeding the segment results in demarcation of the parenchyma, allowing a complete resection.

### Transection Techniques

Over the years, the method of transecting the liver parenchyma has received much attention, and several devices have evolved for facilitating this portion of the operation (see Chapter 18). In truth, for resections that are anatomically based and performed using proper intraoperative management (i.e., low central venous pressure) and meticulous technique, the method of parenchymal transection is a secondary issue. The Cavitron ultrasonic aspirator (CUSA, Valleylab, Boulder, CO), which reduced blood loss compared with the clamp crushing technique in one study is now widely used for liver transection, even in cirrhotic livers. Clamp crushing, the conventional method of liver transection is used in some centers, and when properly done, allows precise delineation of intrahepatic vascular and biliary structures. The hydro-jet dissector (ERBE, Teubingen, Germany) is also widely used. The goal of all of these approaches is to selectively clear away the liver parenchymal tissue to expose the vascular and biliary structures for ligation. There is no evidence supporting one particular technique, and hence the technique chosen for transection is often dependent on local expertise.

Techniques that rely on destructive control of the parenchyma before division include linear cutting staplers, in-line radiofrequency ablation (Habib, Angiodynamics Queensbury NY) and bipolar cautery (Gyrus-Gyrus ACMI Southborough MA, Ligasure-Covidien Boulder CO). In-line radiofrequency ablation allows some surgeons to perform minor and major hepatectomies with low blood loss and low blood transfusion requirements. However, this device has raised serious concerns regarding preservation of venous drainage of the remnant liver and the risk of tissue necrosis and postoperative

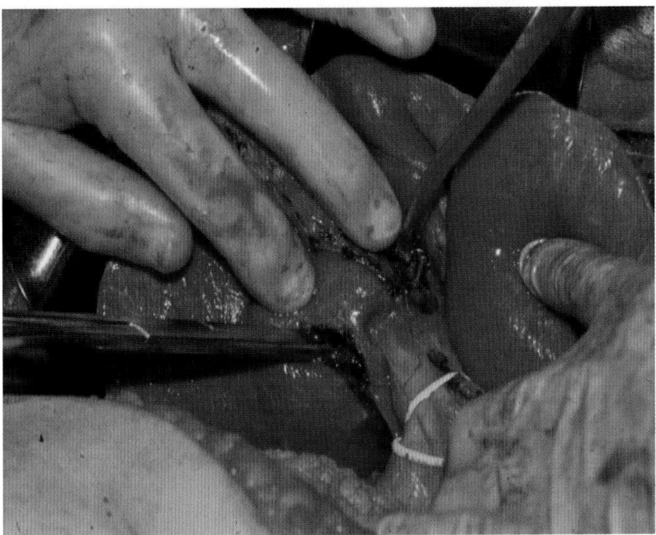

**Figure 24.4** A clamp has been passed around the right portal pedicle after making two small hepatotomies in the gallbladder fossa and posteriorly along the caudate process. Further dissection will help identify the segmental pedicles, which can be confirmed with initial clamping, and then divided with a vascular stapler.



bile leakage. The role of this technology probably is limited to small peripheral resections because of the substantial risk of bile duct injury when this instrument is used near the liver hilum and its inability to control bleeding from large venous branches. The Aquamantys [Salient Surgical Technologies (Formerly TissueLink Medical), Dover, NH] is another device that uses radiofrequency energy to divide the liver parenchyma, although in a more controlled fashion, combined with saline and configured as a bipolar tip for coagulating small pedicle and venous structures.

Pretransection vascular control is used by many surgeons, with potential oncologic and hemostasis implications. Early occlusion of the hepatic venous outflow of the resected segment(s) may reduce the risk of venous tumor emboli. Occlusion of the hepatic artery and portal vein to the segment(s) being resected facilitate the procedure by defining the line of division between ischemic segments to be removed and the viable remnant liver, thereby potentially reducing blood loss. Occlusion of the inflow to sectors of the right hemi-liver (6/7 and 5/8) or to the segments of the left lobe (2, 3, 4a, and 4b) can be performed either by dissection and division of the artery and vein outside the liver, leaving the transection of the hepatic duct and remaining hilar plate for later in the procedure, or by the Glissonian technique in which the sectoral or segmental pedicle is encircled (using either an anterior or posterior intrahepatic approach) and then exposed by incising the reflection of Glisson's capsule and clearing away overlying parenchymal tissue. The portal triad to the segment or segments of interest can then be divided en masse, either by suture or a linear stapler (Fig. 24.4) (see also Fig. 21.14).

# Procedures

Mono- and bi-segmental resections

### Segment 1 Resection

Segment 1 is difficult to access, lying between the IVC and the left portal vein; it receives inflow predominantly from the left PV and HA (see Chapter 22). The biliary drainage of segment 1 is variable, and the segment 1 bile duct runs in the hilar plate and enters the posterior aspect of either left or right hepatic duct. Posteriorly, segment 1 rests on the IVC and most of its outflow is directly into the IVC via a series of small veins. Tumors arising in the caudate lobe are closely related to the posterior aspect of the left hepatic vein (LHV) and the middle hepatic vein (MHV).

The anatomy and technical aspects of resection of the caudate lobe are addressed in detail in Chapter 22.

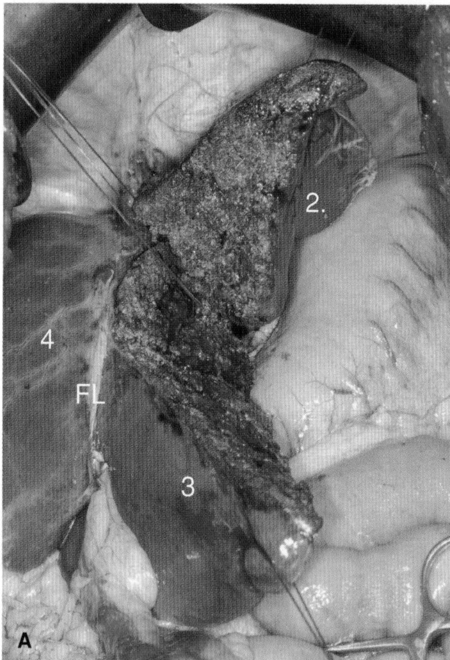


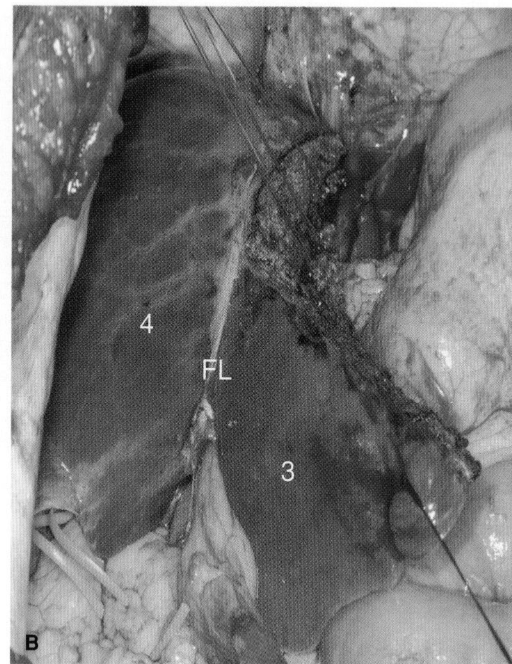


Figure 24.5 Isolated resection of segment 2. **A:** Suture ligatures have been placed around the segment 2 pedicle and the LHV, which are divided along the left border of the falciform ligament (FL), separating segments 4 from 2 and 3. **B:** The resection is completed. A healthy appearing segment 3 is shown.

## Segment 2 or 3 Resection

Isolated resection of segments 2 or 3 are possible, although given their frequent small size, they are often resected in combination as a left lateral sectionectomy. However, as more aggressive resections are pursued, particularly in patients with hepatic colorectal metastases, with bilobar lesions in chemotherapy-damaged livers, parenchymal sparing approaches are critical. When either of these segmentectomies is planned, the plane of resection is by either side of the LHV (left and posterior for segment 2 resection, and right and anterior for segment 3). The LHV can be sacrificed during isolated resection of segments 2 or 3, if necessary, provided the fissural or segment 4 vein is preserved; this branch , also referred to as the umbilical vein in Couinaud's original description, runs in the liver parenchyma in a line delineated by the falciform ligament and is capable of draining the residual liver in the left lateral section. The inflow is approached on the left side of the falciform ligament, by incising the peritoneal reflection onto the liver and identifying the segment 2 (Fig. 24.5) or 3 portal pedicle (Fig. 24.6). Once the inflow is divided, the line of parenchymal transection becomes prominent between the ischemic segment to be resected and the normally perfused residual segment.

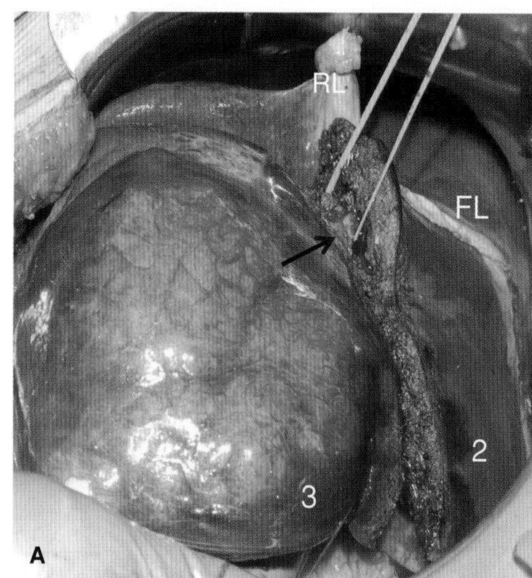


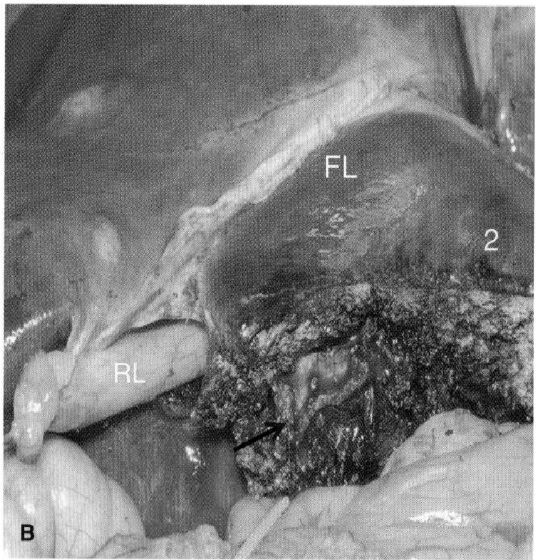


Figure 24.6 Isolated resection of segment 3 as part of a debulking procedure for metastatic neuroendocrine carcinoma. **A:** Dissection within the umbilical fissure, just to the left of the falciform ligament (FL) and round ligament (RL) allows identification of the segment 3 pedicle, which has been encircled. The parenchyma along the border of segments 2 and 3 has been divided (*arrow*). **B:** The completed resection, showing the stapled stump of the segment 3 pedicle.

## Combined Resection of Segments 2 and 3 (Left Lateral Sectionectomy)

The left lateral section is mobilized by division of the falciform ligament and the left triangular ligament (see Chapter 20). The extrahepatic portion of the LHV can be lengthened by dividing the fibrous tissue to the left of the IVC down to the level of the fissure for the ligamentum venosum. The ligamentum venosum is then ligated and divided as it enters the posterior aspect of the LHV allowing encircling of this vein if the point of entry into the MHV is extrahepatic. Dissection of the LHV outside the liver is generally recommended when tumor is in close proximity to its confluence with the IVC; otherwise, the isolation of the LHV is delayed until completion of the parenchymal transection. The inflow to segments 2 and 3 is usually isolated during transection of the parenchyma to the left of the falciform ligament, leaving the portal vein intact to supply segments 4a and 4b. Occasionally, pedicles to segment 2 and 3 can be identified and encircled outside the liver in the left side of the umbilical fissure; in some patients, these pedicles arise from a common trunk. The plane of parenchymal transection follows the falciform ligament. As the liver is divided, the portal structures to segment 2 and 3 will become apparent and can be electively ligated and divided. Once this is done and the parenchyma surrounding the LHV has been dissected, the vein can also be ligated and divided. The transection is completed by dividing the parenchyma anterior to the caudate lobe, in the fissure for the ligamentum venosum.



## Segment 4 Resection

Segment 4, like the left lateral section, is frequently small in size and is not commonly resected in isolation, but rather as part of a larger procedure, such as central hepatectomy (see below and also Chapter 21) or segmentectomy 4b/5 for gallbladder carcinoma (see below and also Chapter 27). Segment 4a is very rarely resected alone, unlike segment 4b, given its peripheral location and easy access; although a segment 4a/8 resection for a high central tumor may be preferred over a central hepatectomy. Segment 4 is bordered posteriorly by the IVC, by the falciform ligament and umbilical vein on the left, and by the MHV on the right. Inferiorly, the left portal pedicle runs along the base of segment 4, just below the hilar plate (see Figs. 17.5A and 17.6). Inflow and biliary drainage are provided by branches of the main left portal pedicle within the umbilical fissure, directly opposite the pedicle branches to the left lateral section. Venous drainage of segment 4 is predominantly through the MHV, with a contribution from the umbilical vein.

After mobilization of the left liver and division of the falciform (see Chapter 20), the confluence of the LHV and the MHV with the IVC is identified (the left-middle groove identifies the apex of segment 4a), and the inflow pedicles are now approached. By incising the peritoneal reflection on the right side of the umbilical fissure, the segment 4a and 4b pedicles can be identified, encircled, and divided (see Fig. 27.9). Alternatively, these pedicles may be identified within the substance of the liver, just to the right of the falciform, and divided in the course of parenchymal transection (Fig. 24.7) (see also Figs. 19.10 and 21.8–21.10). The parenchymal demarcation should be seen along the principal resection plane or Cantlie's line on the right and the divided falciform ligament on the left, and transection of the parenchyma should proceed along these lines. As the resection proceeds toward the base of segment 4, care must be taken to avoid injury to the left portal pedicle, and particularly the left hepatic duct, which lies just below the hilar plate, anterior and cephalad to the left portal vein. As the transection continues superiorly to the level of the suprahepatic IVC, care should be taken to avoid injury to the major hepatic venous branches. The LHV and MHV commonly join within or just outside of the liver to form a common trunk, which then inserts into the IVC. The dissection of the right side is along Cantlie's line, to the left of the MHV. Several tributaries to the MHV (the 4a and 4b veins) will need to be identified and ligated. If necessary, the MHV may be sacrificed during resection of segment 4, with the bulk of the venous drainage then provided by the LHV (segments 2 and 3) and the RHV (segments 5 and 8). Once the medial border of the hilar dissection has been reached the parenchymal transection is then done in a transverse plane to complete the separation of segment 4.

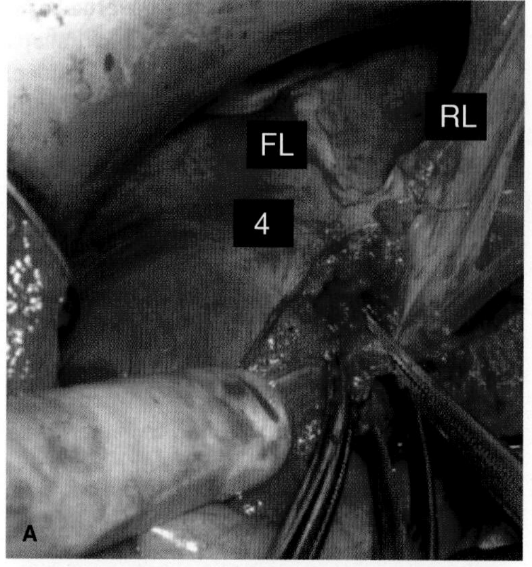


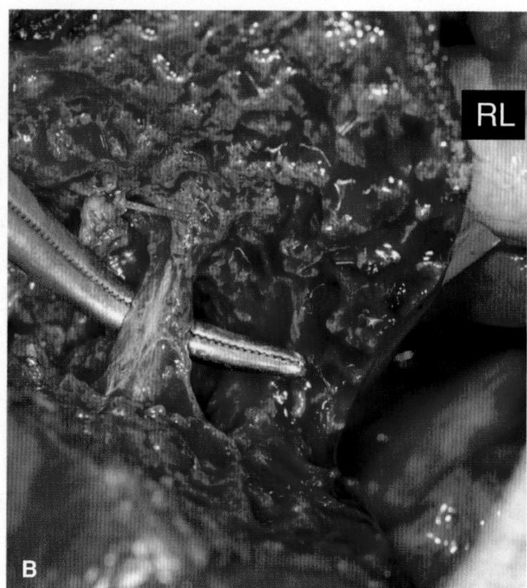


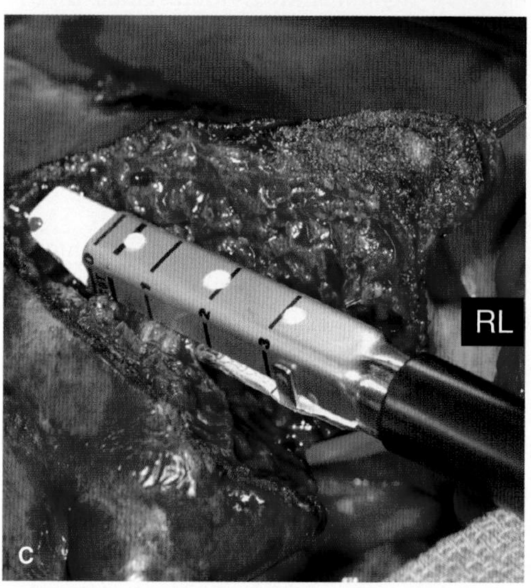


Figure 24.7 Resection of segment 4. **A:** Initial parenchymal transection along the right side of the falciform ligament (FL) and round ligament (RL) allows identification of the pedicles to segment 4B (and ultimately 4A more cephalad, **panel B**). **C:** The pedicles may be divided with a vascular stapler.

## Segment 5 or 8 Resection

These segments comprise the right anterior sector or section. The bifurcation of the right portal pedicle into anterior and posterior pedicles is intrahepatic, and primary ligation prior to parenchymal transection can be difficult, especially for segment 8. Therefore some parenchymal transection along Cantlie's line toward the pedicle is generally performed to expose the pedicles. The segment 5 pedicle emerges anteriorly and runs anteroinferiorly, while the segment 8 pedicle emerges posteriorly and runs superiorly. The axial plane of transection for an isolated segment 5 or segment 8 resection runs through the liver at the level of the bifurcation of the portal vein, with segment 5 below and segment 8 above this line. The medial and lateral limits of the resection are the MHV and the RHV, respectively.

## Segment 5 Resection

Isolated segment 5 resection begins with division of the liver on the undersurface up the centre of the gallbladder fossa and anteriorly along Cantlie's line half-way up toward the IVC. Continued parenchymal transection in this plane will ultimately lead to the major right portal pedicles. With careful dissection, the anterior pedicle, and its component branches to segment 5 and 8, are identified (see Fig. 27.13, which illustrates isolation of the segment 5 pedicle during resection of gallbladder cancer). In some

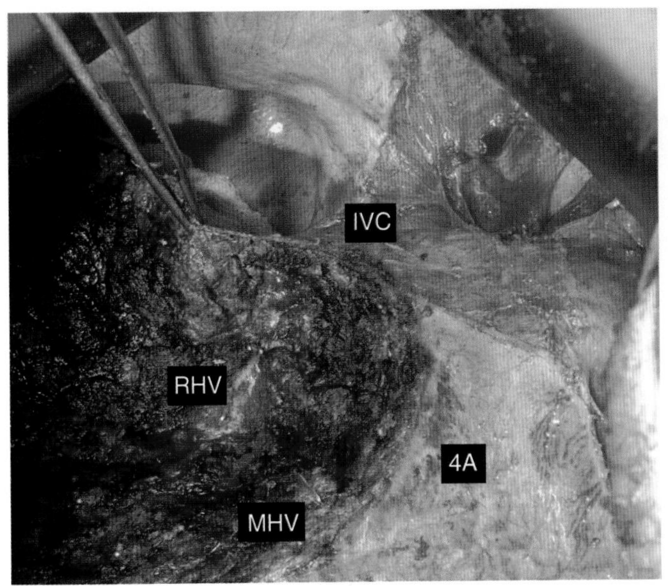


**Figure 24.8** Resection of segment 8, bounded by the RHV and the MHV.



patients, the pedicle to segment 7 arises from the anterior sector; recognition of this anatomical variation is important in order to avoid compromising the integrity of this segment. The parenchyma between the MHV on the left and RHV on the right is then divided, up to the take of the segment 8 pedicle superiorly.

## Segment 8 Resection

Isolated resection of segment 8 is challenging as there are few external landmarks delimiting its boundaries, which consist of the IVC posteriorly, Cantlie's line or the MHV medially and the RHV laterally (Fig. 24.8). The segment 8 pedicle corresponds to the ascending division of the right anterior sectorial pedicle and is most commonly identified after initial division of liver parenchyma between segments 4 and 5 in the sagittal plane, along the level of the portal bifurcation. The horizontal transection should proceed in a coronal plane anterior to the RHV to its intersection with the sagittal plane that includes Cantlie's line and the MHV down to the anterior surface of the IVC. Mobilization of the right liver, as one would do for a major right hepatectomy, is necessary to free the posterior aspect of segment 8 (see Chapter 19 and Figs. 19.5 and 19.6; see Chapter 23 and Figs. 23.12 and 23.13). Care must be taken during the parenchymal division to adhere to the correct transection plane posteriorly. This allows resection of all the liver in segment 8 while avoiding injury to the RHV.

## Combined Resection of Segments 5 and 8

The combined resection of segments 5 and 8 constitutes an anterior sectionectomy, a procedure that can be performed in place of a right hepatectomy, when appropriate, provided the integrity of the procedure is not compromised from an oncologic standpoint. This procedure, and its counterpart posterior sectionectomy (resection of segments 6 and 7), are covered in detail in Chapter 23.

## Segments 6 or 7 Resection

Segments 6 and 7 comprise the posterior section. The right posterior sectorial pedicle can be identified in the *incisura dextra of Ganz,* which corresponds to the horizontal fissure lateral to the gallbladder fossa. The pedicle to segment 6/7 can be isolated after initial division of the liver parenchyma in this area. Alternatively, the posterior sectoral branches of the hepatic artery and portal vein may be isolated with dissection within the proximal porta hepatis, but this approach is not always possible (see Figs. 23.7 and 23.17). The pedicle for an isolated resection of segment 6 or 7 is therefore usually

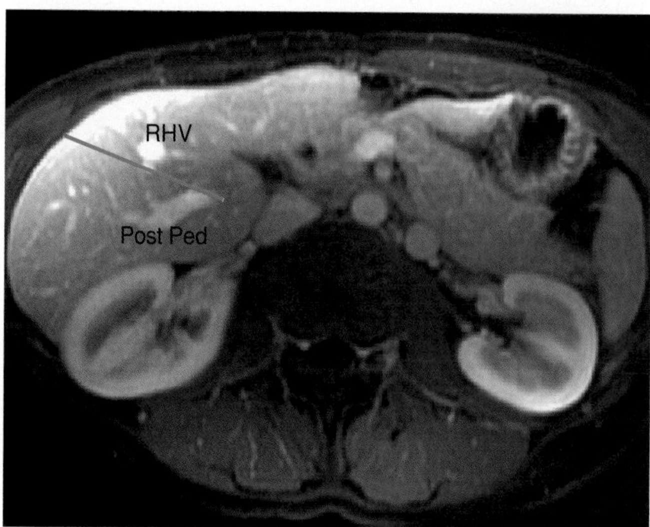


Figure 24.9 Relationship of the RHV and the posterior sectoral pedicle (Post Ped). Note the line of parenchymal transection in the sagittal plane, indicated in red and is posterior to the RHV and anterior to the posterior pedicle at its origin with the main right pedicle.

approached and controlled from within the liver, during parenchymal transection. It is important to bear in mind that the sagittal transection plane between the anterior and posterior sectors is oblique, approximately half way between the horizontal and vertical planes (Fig. 24.9). A resection of segment 6 or 7 requires complete mobilization of the right lobe of the liver with division of the retrohepatic veins draining into the IVC (Fig. 24.10). A combined resection of segments 6 and 7, or posterior sectionectomy, can be performed with preservation or sacrifice of the RHV.

## Segment 6 Resection

Isolated segment 6 resection is among the more straightforward of the isolated segmental resections, similar to resection of segment 3, given its very peripheral location. The resection begins with an oblique transection line along the *incisura dextra of Ganz* on the under surface of the liver and anteriorly approximately half-way toward the IVC, posterior to the plane of the RHV. The axial transection plane is at the level of the portal vein bifurcation. The posterior pedicle will be encountered medially, at the intersection of the transection planes. Care must be taken at this point to fully expose the pedicle branches and avoid injury to the segment 7 inflow.

## Segment 7 Resection

Isolated segment 7 can be performed with initial transection of the parenchyma in the axial plane, just above the bifurcation of the portal vein, which corresponds to the

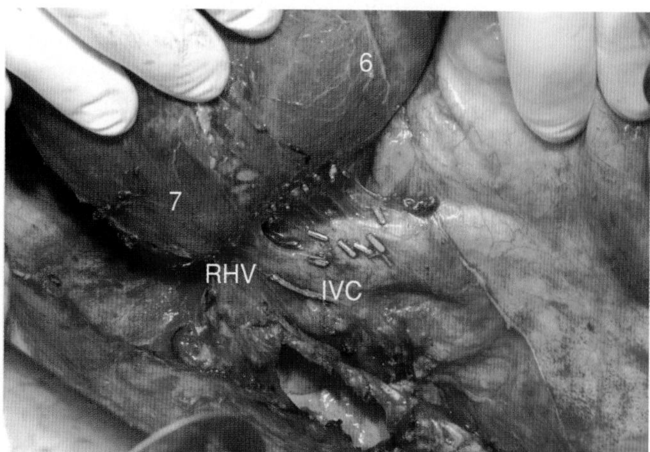


Figure 24.10 Mobilization of the right liver is required for resections of the posterior pedicles (6 and 7). Here, the right liver has been mobilized off the diaphragm and out of the retroperitoneum. The inferior vena caval (IVC) has been completed and the RHV exposed and can be clamped or divided if necessary.

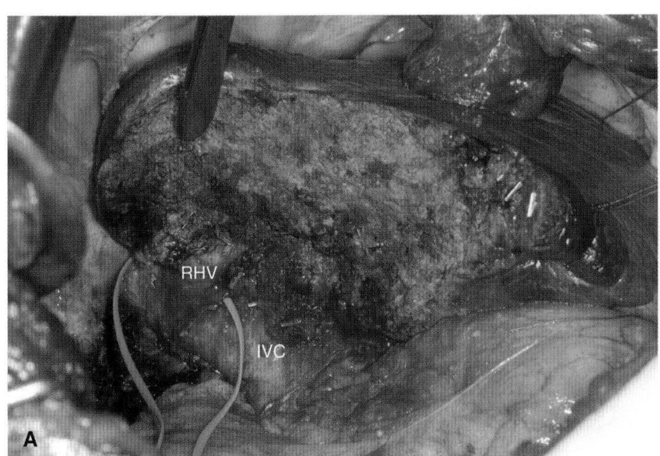


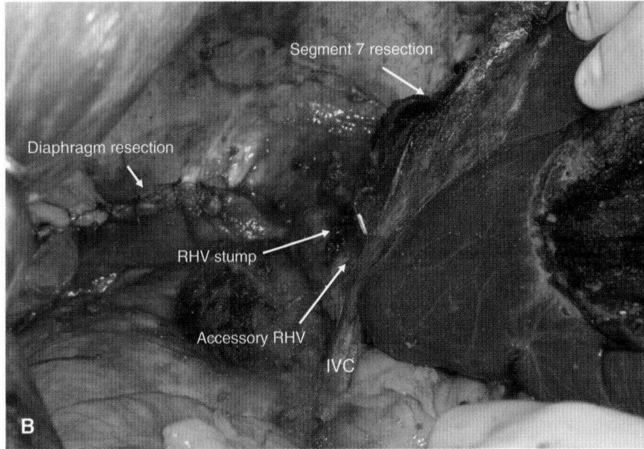


Figure 24.11 Segment 7 resection. **A:** Preservation of the RHV. **B:** Sacrificing the RHV in the presence of a large accessory hepatic vein. (Photo courtesy of Dr. Michael D'Angelica.)



horizontal resection line for a segment 6 resection. The resection continues medially to the lateral margin of the RHV; it is during this portion of the transection that the pedicle branches to segment 7 are encountered. The horizontal transection line runs obliquely through the liver lateral and posterior to the RHV (Fig. 24.11A). Resection of segment 7 can be done to include the RHV, provided there is a reasonable sized accessory hepatic vein draining segment 6 directly into the IVC (Fig. 24.11B).

## Combined Resection of Segments 6 and 7

Resection of segments 6 and 7 together constitutes a right posterior sectionectomy, a procedure that can be performed as an alternative to a right hepatectomy when the anterior sector can be spared without compromising is the completeness of the resection, especially in patients with diseased parenchyma. Posterior sectionectomy is described in detail in Chapter 23.

## Combined Resection of Segments 5 and 6

Resection of these two segments is very commonly performed. The vertical plane of transection is along Cantlie's line between segments 4b and 5, to the right of the MHV from the edge of the liver to half-up toward the IVC, with the axial transection plane being at the level of the portal vein confluence, as it would be for an isolated segment 5 resection. The portal pedicles to segment 5 and 6 are usually divided during the parenchymal transection (Fig. 24.12). This resection requires mobilization of the right lobe from the retroperitoneum and diaphragm with division of the accessory hepatic veins in the anterior surface of the IVC. It is convenient to start the transection in the middle of the gallbladder fossa along Cantlie's line up to the level of the right portal pedicle. The axial transection plane is then developed from the top of the vertical plane, with the pedicle branches identified and divided in the course of parenchymal transection. Branches of the RHV will be encountered and require division in the course of this resection. Once again, care must be taken to accurately identify the pertinent pedicles for division and avoid injury to adjacent structures.

## Resection of Segments 4b and 5

Segmentectomy 4b and 5 is commonly performed for gallbladder cancer and combines the elements of resecting each segment individually, as described above. This procedure may include en bloc resection of the extrahepatic biliary tree and porta hepatis lymphatic tissue and is discussed in more detail in Chapter 27.

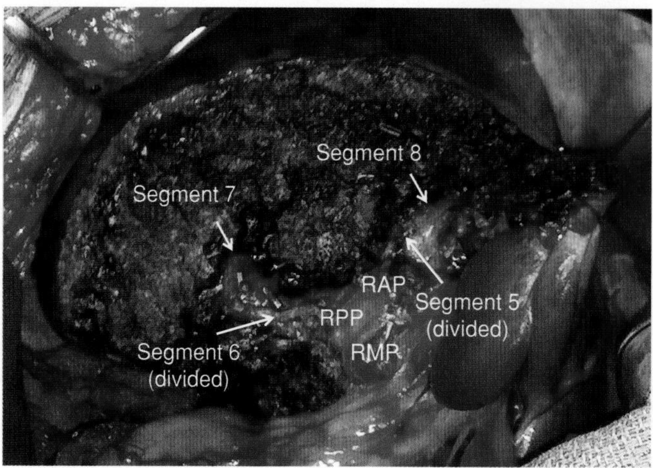


**Figure 24.12** Combined resection of segments 5 and 6. The pedicles to segment 5 and 6 have been divided with a vascular stapler, as shown, while the pedicles to segments 7 and 8 have been preserved. The main right portal pedicle (RMP), right anterior pedicle (RAP) and right posterior pedicle (RPP) are indicated.

## Resection of Segments 4, 5, and 8 (Central or Mesohepatectomy)

This resection is indicated primarily for large central tumors where an extended right or left hepatectomy risks leaving behind a liver remnant of insufficient volume. The technical aspects of central hepatectomy are described in detail in Chapter 21.

## Recommended References and Readings


Abulkhir A, Limongelli P, Healey AJ, et al. Preoperative portal vein embolization for major liver resection: a meta-analysis. *Ann Surg.* 2008;247:49–57.

Agrawal S, Belghiti J. Oncologic resection for malignant tumors of the liver. *Ann Surg.* 2011;253:656–665.

Ayav A, Jiao LR, Habib NA. Bloodless liver resection using radiofrequency energy. *Dig Surg.* 2007;24:314–317.

Ayav A, Jiao L, Dickinson R, et al. Liver resection with a new multiprobe bipolar radiofrequency device. *Arch Surg.* 2008;143:396–401.

Baer HU, Maddern GJ, Blumgart LH. New water-jet dissector: initial experience in hepatic surgery. *Br J Surg.* 1991;78:502–503.

Belghiti J, Ogata S. Preoperative optimization of the liver for resection in patients with hilar cholangiocarcinoma. *HPB (Oxford).* 2005;7:252–253.

Billingsley KG, Jarnagin WR, Fong Y, et al. Segment-oriented hepatic resection in the management of malignant neoplasms of the liver. *J Am Coll Surg.* 1998;187:471–481.

Bismuth H, Castaing D, Garden OJ. Segmental surgery of the liver. *Surg Annu.* 1988;20:291–310.

Bismuth H, Houssin D, Castaing D. Major and minor segmentectomies "reglees" in liver surgery. *World J Surg.* 1982;6(1):10–24.

Clavien PA, Selzner M, Rüdiger HA, et al. A prospective randomized study in 100 consecutive patients undergoing major liver resection with versus without ischemic preconditioning. *Ann Surg.* 2003;238:843–850.

Couinaud C. Segmental and lobar left hepatectomies. *J Chir (Paris).* 1952a;68:821–839.

Couinaud C. Segmental and lobar left hepatectomies; studies on anatomical conditions. *J Chir (Paris).* 1952b;68:697–715.

Couinaud C. Contribution of anatomical research to liver surgery. *Fr Med.* 1956;19:5–12.

Couinaud C. *Surgical Anatomy of the Liver Revisited.* Paris: C. Couinaud; 1989.

Curro G, Habib N, Jiao L, et al. Radiofrequency-assisted liver resection in patients with hepatocellular carcinoma and cirrhosis: preliminary results. *Transplant Proc.* 2008;40:3523–3525.

Fan ST, Lai EC, Lo CM, et al. Hepatectomy with an ultrasonic dissector for hepatocellular carcinoma. *Br J Surg.* 1996;83:117–120.

Figueras J, Lopez-Ben S, Lladó L, et al. Hilar dissection versus the "glissonean" approach and stapling of the pedicle for major hepatectomies: a prospective, randomized trial. *Ann Surg.* 2003; 238:111–119.

Hasegawa K, Kokudo N, Imamura H, et al. Prognostic impact of anatomic resection for hepatocellular carcinoma. *Ann Surg.* 2005;242:252–259.

Imamura H, Seyama Y, Kokudo N, et al. One thousand fifty-six hepatectomies without mortality in 8 years. *Arch Surg.* 2003; 138:1198–1206.

Jarnagin WR, Gonen M, Fong Y, et al. Improvement in perioperative outcome after hepatic resection: analysis of 1,803 consecutive cases over the past decade. *Ann Surg.* 2002;236:397–406.

Kim J, Ahmad SA, Lowy AM, et al. Increased biliary fistulas after liver resection with the harmonic scalpel. *Am Surg.* 2003;69:815–819.

Kooby DA, Fong Y, Suriawinata A, et al. Impact of steatosis on perioperative outcome following hepatic resection. *J Gastrointest Surg.* 2003;7(8):1034–1044.

Launois B, Jamieson GG. The importance of Glisson's capsule and its sheaths in the intrahepatic approach to resection of the liver. *Surg Gynecol Obstet.* 1992;174:7–10.

Liau KH, Blumgart LH, DeMatteo RP. Segment-oriented approach to liver resection. *Surg Clin North Am.* 2004;84:543–561.

Lin TY. A simplified technique for hepatic resection: the crush method. *Ann Surg.* 1974;180:285–290.

Little JM, Hollands MJ. Impact of the CUSA and operative ultrasound on hepatic resection. *HPB Surg.* 1991;3:271–277.

Lupo L, Gallerani A, Panzera P, et al. Randomized clinical trial of radiofrequency-assisted versus clamp-crushing liver resection. *Br J Surg.* 2007;94:287–291.

Machado MA, Herman P, Machado MC. A standardized technique for right segmental liver resections. *Arch Surg.* 2003;138:918–920.

Makuuchi M, Takayama T, Kosuge T, et al. The value of ultrasonography for hepatic surgery. *Hepatogastroenterology.* 1991;38: 64–70.

Polk W, Fong Y, Karpeh M, et al. A technique for the use of cryosurgery to assist hepatic resection. *J Am Coll Surg.* 1995;180(2):171–176.

Scheele J, Stang R, Altendorf-Hofmann A, et al. Resection of colorectal liver metastases. *World J Surg.* 1995;19:59–71.

Takayama T, Makuuchi M, Kubota K, et al. Randomized comparison of ultrasonic vs clamp transection of the liver. *Arch Surg.* 2001; 136:922–928.

The Brisbane 2000. Terminology of liver anatomy and resections. *HPB (Oxford).* 2002;4:99–100.

Torzilli G, Procopio F, Cimino M, et al. Anatomical segmental and subsegmental resection of the liver for hepatocellular carcinoma: a new approach by means of ultrasound-guided vessel compression. *Ann Surg.* 2010;251:229–235.

Wakai T, Shirai Y, Sakata J, et al. Anatomic resection independently improves long-term survival in patients with T1-T2 hepatocellular carcinoma. *Ann Surg Oncol.* 2007;14:1356–1365.

# 25 Enucleation of Hepatic Lesions

**Florencia G. Que and Mark D. Sawyer**

## Introduction

Enucleation is a useful parenchymal-sparring technique for the treatment of many hepatic lesions. While mostly suited to benign lesions such as adenomas and symptomatic hemangiomas, enucleation may be useful in situations where debulking of malignant disease is indicated clinically, such as ovarian and neuroendocrine metastases. The operative techniques are generally straightforward, and lesions near the hepatic surface may lend themselves well to laparoscopic techniques. Enucleation may be used in combination with resection and/or radiofrequency or microwave ablation. As the tumors amenable to enucleation are by their nature not invasive, anatomic structures are usually displaced rather than invaded making it possible to remove large masses (see Fig. 25.1); and in the case of neuroendocrine metastases, large total numbers of tumors may be present with a relatively small impact on hepatic anatomy and functional hepatic mass.

## Selection of Candidates

The lesions usually amenable to enucleation are hemangiomas, cystadenomas (provided that the presence of malignant change can be reliably excluded, see Chapter 28), hepatic adenomas and focal nodular hyperplasia, simple and hydatid cysts, and neuroendocrine metastases. Patient selection should also take into consideration whether or not an anatomic resection (see Chapter 18) or nonresectional technique, such as ablation, may provide equivalent results with lower morbidity than enucleation.

A distinct advantage of enucleation is that it may be employed when anatomic lesions abut major vascular and ductal structures, such as in the case of a centrally located hemangioma. While radiofrequency ablation may be used near major vascular structures, it generally should not be used within a centimeter of major ductal structures due to the elevated risk of bile duct injury.

Metastatic neuroendocrine lesions are often good candidates for treatment by enucleation whether as the solitary technique employed or in conjunction with anatomical resection or ablative techniques. As the goal in such cases is often debulking rather than

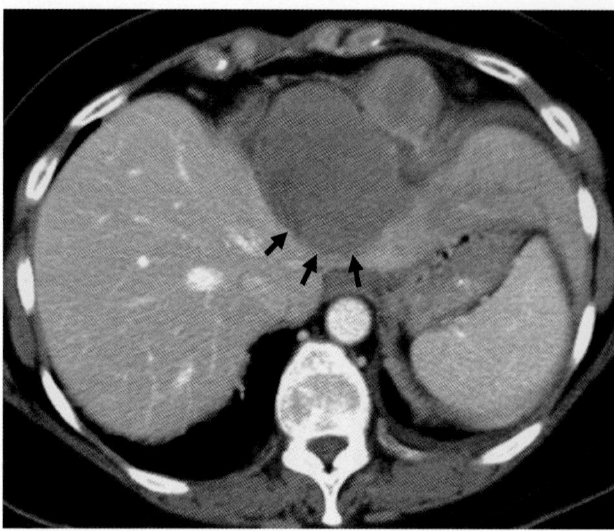

**Figure 25.1** Large metastatic ovarian tumor to the left liver. Notice that the tumor is compressing the liver rather than invading the parenchyma (*arrows*).

a curative resection, a flexible, varied, and multifaceted approach will often yield the best results.

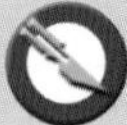

## OPERATIVE TECHNIQUES

### General

Operative technique in enucleation has four main elements: division of overlying hepatic parenchyma (approach), separation of the lesion from the surrounding rim of compressed hepatic tissue, division of the small vessels that feed and drain the lesions, and hemostasis.

Optimal approach generally entails division of the hepatic parenchyma overlying the lesion at its most superficial point, although, in the case of more deeply seated lesions, a pathway along the interlobar or intersegmental planes will entail less perturbation of surrounding hepatic anatomic structure and less attendant risk of bleeding or biliary leak (see Fig. 25.2). The hepatotomy should be of sufficient length to allow adequate exposure to circumferentially to separate the lesion from the surrounding hepatic tissue, and safely ligate and divide bridging vessels.

The technique of separating the lesion from the surrounding hepatic parenchyma is similar regardless of the underlying lesion, and a number of techniques may be used depending upon surgeon preference (see Chapter 18). In the hands of a surgeon comfortable with a particular technique, Cavitron ultrasonic surgical aspirator (CUSA), finger fracture, electrocautery, and water jet dissection all accomplish the purpose of separating the lesion from the surrounding hepatic parenchyma with similar results; the particular technique utilized is more the function of the surgeon's familiarity with it rather than any purported technologic superiority.

Ligation of the bridging vessels should be as meticulous as with any other hepatic resection. While vessel clips may be utilized on the lesional side, the author prefers to minimize or avoid the use of clips on the hepatic side, as they may cause artifactual interference at future radiologic imaging and may be dislodged during the resection as the lesion is retracted from one direction to another. Other alternatives are coagulative/division devices such as the Ligasure™ (Covidien, Boulder, CO) and harmonic scalpel, which coagulate and divide vessels up to 7 mm. While the underlying physics of the two devices are disparate—the harmonic scalpel simultaneously coagulates and divides tissue with harmonic vibrations at 20,000 Hz, and the Ligasure™ is essentially a bipolar cautery device which coagulates, then divides—the vessel size they are capable of dividing safely and effectively (and therefore the end result) is essentially the same.

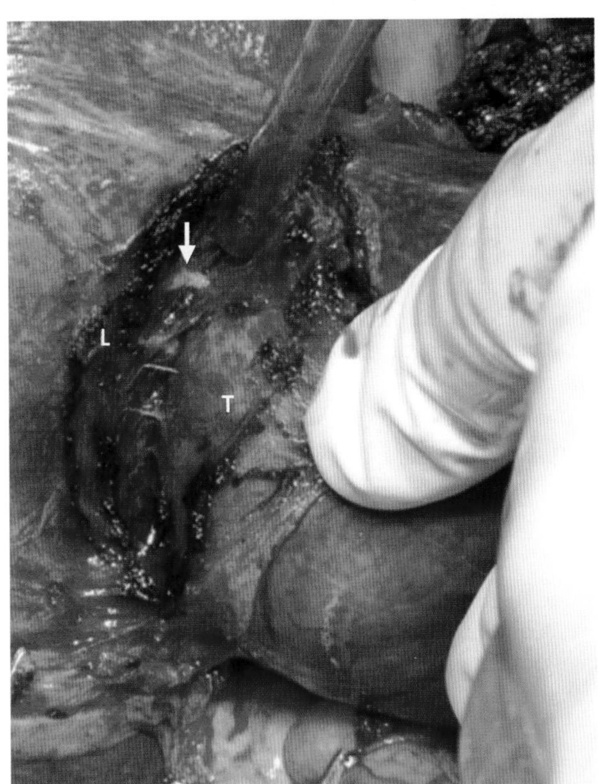


**Figure 25.2** Enucleation of a metastatic endocrine tumor. The overlying liver parenchyma has been incised. Dissection within the interface between the tumor (*T*) and compressed liver parenchyma (*L*) reveals a number of feeding vessels (*arrow*) that must be controlled.



Hemostasis is best achieved as an ongoing endeavor during the separation phase and as a final measure after the completion of the resection. Inflow occlusion may not be necessary in the most superficial lesions, but will substantially decrease blood loss for enucleation of most lesions in proportion to their size, depth, and multiplicity. Electrocautery, argon beam coagulation, and saline-coupled radiofrequency coagulation are all useful techniques to obtain hemostasis. A number of surface coagulative agents—Surgicel® (Ethicon, San Angelo, TX), Gelfoam® (Pharmacia, Kalamazoo, MI), fibrin glue, thrombin spray, etc.—may also be utilized as adjunctive measures to ensure complete hemostasis during the resection and after the lesion is removed.

## Exposure

As in any other hepatic surgery, exposure and mobilization is an important key to success (see Chapter 18). Division of the ligamentum teres and the falciform ligament is almost always useful, save for the most anterior–inferior lesions. Lesions in the posterior right lobe are aided by exposure of the bare area of the liver by division of the right coronary and triangular ligaments, especially the right lateral peritoneohepatic reflection (see Chapters 19 and 23). This allows the liver to be rotated medially on its vertical axis to gain access to the posterior right lobe. Access to the caudate lobe is aided by division of the gastrohepatic ligament. Self-retaining retractors are useful in maintaining steady and unwavering exposure, especially in difficult areas.

## Laparoscopic Techniques

Laparoscopic technique in enucleation utilizes the same basic principles as open enucleation (see Chapter 31). Currently it is most useful for fairly superficial and anterior lesions, although as in almost every area in laparoscopic surgery, the boundaries are being extended. The most important considerations in laparoscopic enucleation are those fundamental to any laparoscopic procedure: an adequate number of properly placed ports, meticulous technique, and thorough hemostasis as the resection proceeds. Differences from open surgical technique are threefold. Firstly, while in the open technique dissection may proceed in one vector as long as is comfortable, laparoscopic resection often utilizes a "corkscrew" technique, progressing circumferentially around the lesion, deeper with each successive pass around the periphery. Secondly, ligature is not the most convenient means of vessel control and division during laparoscopic enucleation. While the use of clips is more convenient and readily available, a perhaps more favorable method is the use of coagulative/division devices such as the harmonic scalpel or Ligasure™ to avoid the issues with clips delineated above. Laparoscopically, the author prefers to avoid the use of surgical clips, if possible, for the reasons described above. The third consideration is whether or not the anatomic location of the lesions lends itself to the laparoscopic technique. More superficial, and therefore technically less challenging lesions, may be better candidates for a laparoscopic approach.

## Lesion-specific Considerations

### Hemangioma

Symptomatic hemangiomas are well suited to enucleation, and recurrence after enucleation is rare. The usual indication for surgery is abdominal pain, and resection results in symptom relief in most of the patients. Hemangiomas usually have a major feeding vessel; identifying this preoperatively is helpful during the subsequent resection (Fig. 25.3A, and B).

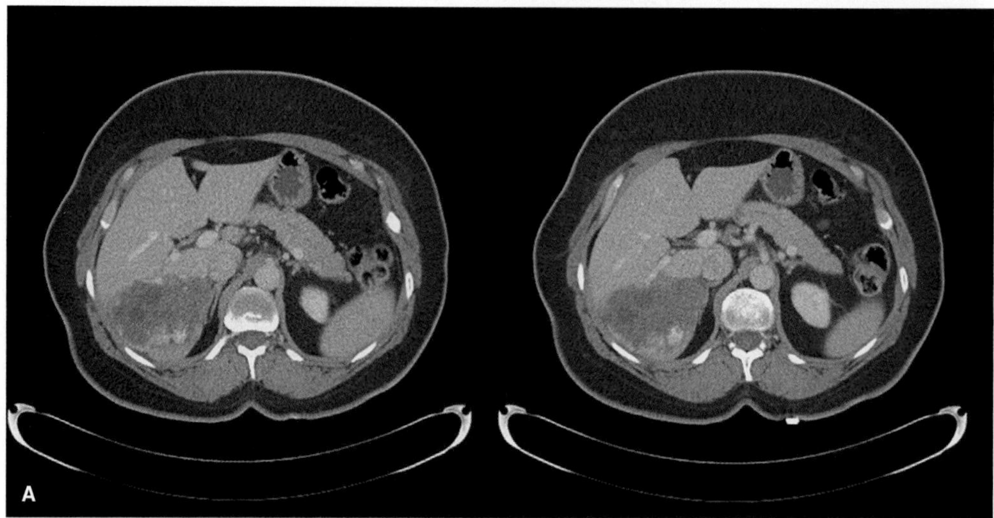

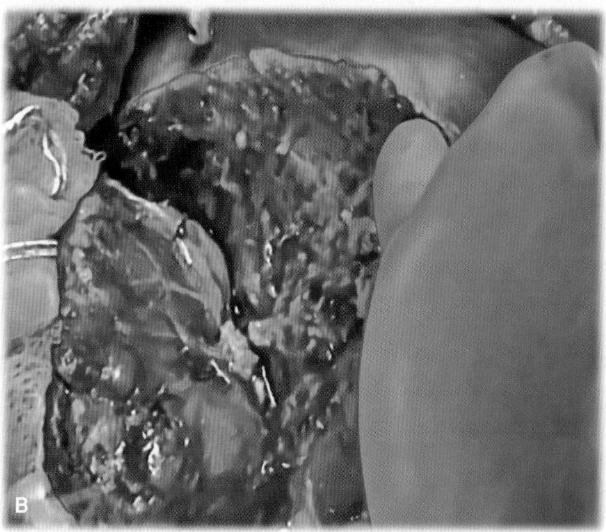

**Figure 25.3 A:** Posteriorly located hemangioma. **B:** Intraoperative photo of the enucleation plane and the feeding central vessel (*arrow*).

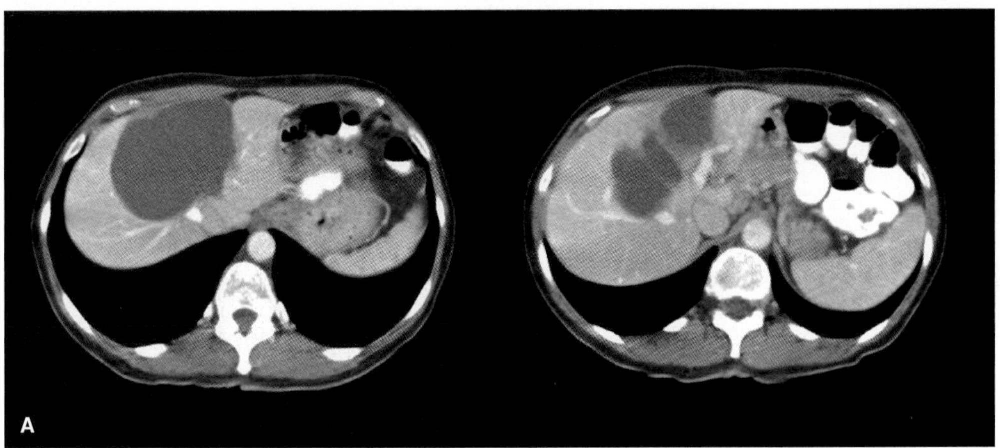


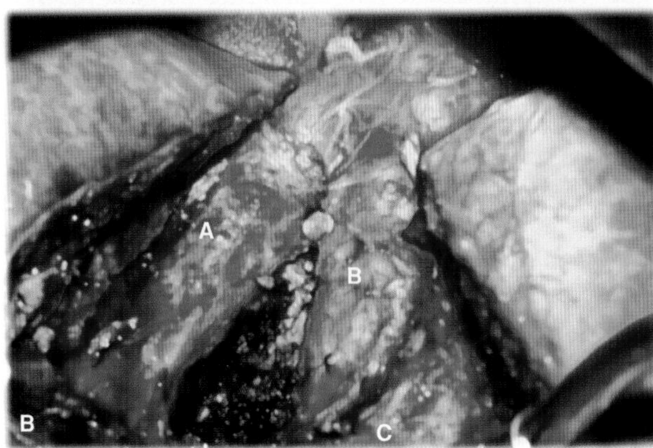


Figure 25.4 **A:** Centrally located mucinous cystadenoma abutting three hepatic veins, vena cava, and the porta hepatis. **B:** Photo of tumor bed after enucleation of mucinous cystadenoma. *A* is the right hepatic vein. *B* is the middle hepatic vein. *C* is the left portal vein.



As might be expected, peripherally located lesions are more easily resected than centrally located lesions, with lower blood loss and complication rates.

## Cystadenoma

Biliary cystadenomas should be resected, as up to 15% may have malignant degeneration of a portion of their walls. Recurrence after partial resection may be as high as 50%, so complete removal is important. Thomas et al. were able to resect one-third of their patients with enucleation. However, careful consideration must be given before enucleation is used; if the preoperative evaluation raises any concerns for the possibility of malignancy, then anatomic resection is the preferred treatment (see Chapter 28). Figure 25.4A and B shows the CT images and an intraoperative view, respectively, of a patient with a centrally located mucinous cystadenoma.

## Hepatic Adenoma and Focal Nodular Hyperplasia

Because of the risk of malignant change and hemorrhage, large hepatic adenomas are generally resected; however, as with cystadenomas, enucleation is satisfactory if the likelihood of malignant degeneration appears to be low. Resection of focal nodular hyperplasia is rarely performed but may be indicated if the patient is symptomatic or the diagnosis is uncertain.

## Parasitic and Non-parasitic Cysts (see Chapter 18)

In non-parasitic cysts (exclusive of cystadenomas), fenestration is usually adequate treatment; enucleation is usually only performed if the diagnosis is uncertain. Surgical intervention in echinococcal cysts is usually reserved for those refractory to percutaneous treatment ("PAIR"—puncture, aspiration, injection, and reaspiration) because of complications such as secondary bacterial infection, communication with the biliary tree, or obstruction. As such, anatomic resection may be less troublesome than attempting an enucleation under these circumstances. Whatever technique is used, chemotherapy with benzimidazole-class anti-parasitic chemotherapy is an integral part of treatment.

## Hepatic Neuroendocrine Tumor Metastases

The chief goal in the treatment of neuroendocrine hepatic metastases is the removal of as much tumor burden as possible while preserving hepatic parenchyma (see Fig. 25.5). Due to the prolonged natural history, patients can live for years with disease, and debulking, while almost never curative, may increase both survival and quality of life. Enucleation of neuroendocrine metastases is a preferred technique for several reasons. Firstly, a large tumor burden can be removed while preserving functional hepatic parenchyma in cases where a standard 1 cm margin would devastate the remaining hepatic reserve. Secondly, the recurrence rate in the enucleation bed is low. Thirdly, management

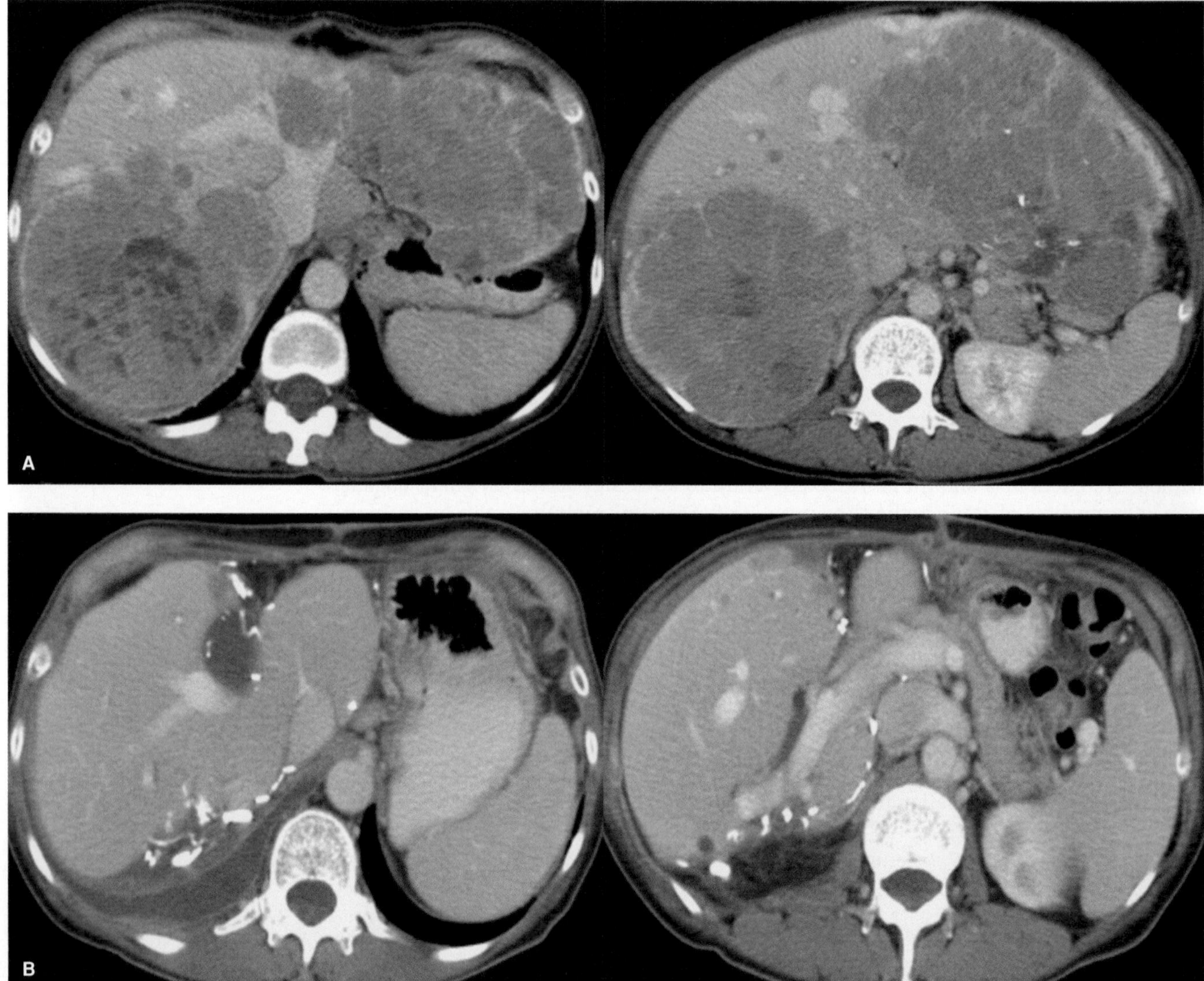


**Figure 25.5** Metastatic neuroendocrine disease to the liver. **A:** Preoperative CT scan showing a large burden of disease in the right and left sides; there are two dominant lesions and several smaller tumors. **B:** Postoperative view after a debulking procedure. Note that the dominant lesions have been enucleated, sparing a large amount of functional parenchyma; the smaller residual disease was treated, in this case, with hepatic artery embolization after recovery from surgery.

of recurrences with percutaneous ablative techniques is usually feasible and straightforward; and lastly, enucleation allows preservation of major portal venous and biliary structures allowing patients to undergo repeat resection, if indicated and appropriate. Deeply seated lesions less than 3 cm in diameter may be primarily treated with radiofrequency ablation, although, enucleation is thought to have a lower rate of recurrence. In the case of a large tumor burden predominant in one lobe, a formal lobar resection with enucleation and/or radiofrequency ablation of disease the contralateral lobe may give the best results. The strategy for maximal debulking of disease includes enucleation of superficial lesions and radiofrequency ablation for lesions that are deep or centrally located. Intraoperative ultrasound is used extensively in such cases to accurately locate, remove, and ablate as much of the tumor burden as possible.

# Summary

Enucleation is a valuable technique in the hepatobiliary surgeon's armamentarium. A variety of lesions lend themselves well to the technique, either alone or in combination with other methodologies. For lesions amenable to enucleation, morbidity and mortality are usually lower than anatomic resective techniques, given the preservation of hepatic parenchyma. Careful patient selection, proper exposure, and meticulous technique are the keys to success.



## Recommended References and Readings


Carson JG, Huerta S, Butler JA. Hepatobiliary cystadenoma: a case report and a review of the literature. *Curr Surg.* 2006;63(4):285–289.

Choi BY, Nguyen MH. The diagnosis and management of benign hepatic tumors. *J Clin Gastroenterol.* 2005;39(5):401–412.

Dixon E, Sutherland F, Burak K, et al. Cystadenoma of the liver without mesenchymal stroma in a female following hormonal therapy for acne. *HPB (Oxford).* 2001;3(2):183–186.

Hamaloglu E, Altun H, Ozdemir A, et al. Giant liver hemangioma: therapy by enucleation or liver resection. *World J Surg.* 2005; 29(7):890–893.

Herman P, Pugliese V, Machado M, et al. Hepatic adenoma and focal nodular hyperplasia: differential diagnosis and treatment. *World J Surg.* 2000;24(3):372–376.

Langer JC, Rose DB, Keystone JS, et al. Diagnosis and management of hydatid disease of the liver. A 15-year North American experience. *Ann Surg.* 1984;199(4):412–417.

Makdissi FF, Surjan RC, Machado MA. Laparoscopic enucleation of liver tumors. Corkscrew technique revisited. *J Surg Oncol.* 2009; 99(3):166–168.

Ozden I, Emre A, Alper A, et al. Long-term results of surgery for liver hemangiomas. *Arch Surg.* 2000;135(8):978–981.

Sanchez H, Gagner M, Rossi ML, et al. Surgical management of nonparasitic cystic liver disease. *Am J Surg.* 1991;161(1):113–118; discussion 118–119.

Sarmiento JM, Heywood G, Rubin J, et al. Surgical treatment of neuroendocrine metastases to the liver: a plea for resection to increase survival. *J Am Coll Surg.* 2003;197(1):29–37.

Smego RA Jr, Sebanego P. Treatment options for hepatic cystic echinococcosis. *Int J Infect Dis.* 2005;9(2):69–76.

Thomas KT, Welch D, Trueblood A, et al. Effective treatment of biliary cystadenoma. *Ann Surg.* 2005;241(5):769–773; discussion 773–775.

Xiao-Hui F, Chun Hung LE, Xiao-Ping Y, et al. Enucleation of liver hemangiomas: is there a difference in surgical outcomes for centrally or peripherally located lesions? *Am J Surg.* 2009;198(2):184–187.

Yoon SS, Charny CK, Fong Y, et al. Diagnosis, management, and outcomes of 115 patients with hepatic hemangioma. *J Am Coll Surg.* 2003;197(3):392–402.

# 26 Resection for Hilar Cholangiocarcinoma

**Yugi Nimura**

##  INDICATIONS/CONTRAINDICATIONS

The indication for resection of hilar cholangiocarcinoma should be determined according to the local extension of the disease and surgical risk to the patient; the presence of distant metastases represents a clear contraindication. As local excision of the proximal bile duct can hardly contribute to radical resection of the tumor with free margins, combined liver and bile duct resection has been the standard surgical procedure for most patients with hilar cholangiocarcinoma during the last decade, and the extent of liver resection depends on the extent of the tumor along the intrahepatic sectional and/or segmental bile ducts.

Although local invasion of the portal bifurcation, main portal vein and/or hepatic arteries had been considered as a sign of unresectable cancer, recent progress in vascular surgical techniques have enabled combined portal vein and hepatic artery resection and reconstruction for locally advanced hilar cholangiocarcinoma (see Chapter 30). Hyperbilirubinemia, cholangitis, and major hepatectomy are considered as risk factors in surgical resection of biliary cancer patients. Functional capacity of the future remnant liver is estimated by CT volumetry and liver function tests, including the indocyanine green clearance (see Chapter 18).

Distant organ metastasis and peritoneal dissemination generally contraindicate resection. However, some value of aggressive paraaortic node dissection for possible lymph node metastasis has been suggested but must be carefully estimated by prospective studies.

##  PREOPERATIVE PLANNING

As most patients with hilar cholangiocarcinoma have obstructive jaundice at the time of diagnosis, ultrasonography followed by multidetector row-CT (MDCT) should be performed for staging of the lesion before biliary drainage. As an expected surgical procedure and future remnant liver can be designed by MDCT, unilateral biliary drainage of the future remnant liver should be carried out with endoscopic nasobiliary drainage (ENBD) or percutaneous transhepatic biliary drainage (PTBD). These external

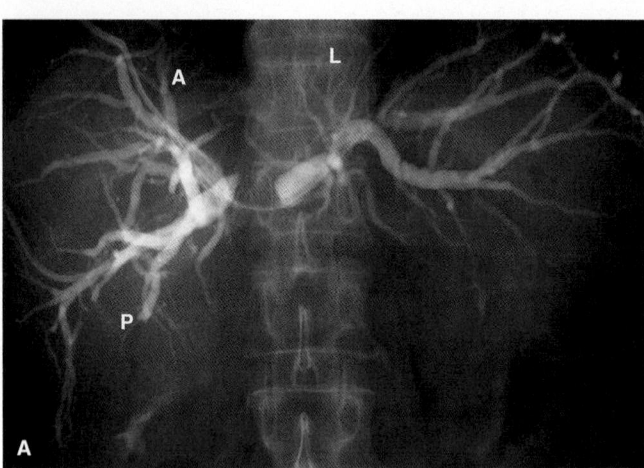


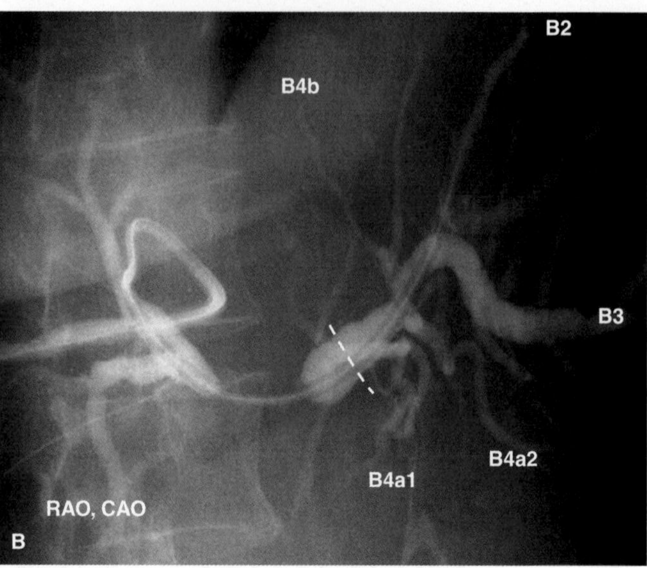


**Figure 26.1** Selective cholangiography through PTBD catheters. **A:** PTBD cholangiography through the right anterior (A) and posterior (P) sectional ducts. The tip of the PTBD catheter A is introduced into the LHD (L) across the hilar lesion. **B:** Selective cholangiography through the catheter A in a right anterior oblique (RAO) and caudo-anterior oblique (CAO) position clearly demonstrates the proximal extension of the tumor and define the site of resection of the LHD (*dotted line*). B2, left lateral superior duct; B3, left lateral inferior duct; B4, left medial duct.

drainage procedures have another advantage in taking selective cholangiography to make precise diagnoses of progress of cancer along the intrahepatic segmental ducts (Fig. 26.1). Percutaneous transhepatic or peroral cholangioscopy is sometimes useful to define the extension of superficially spreading cholangiocarcinoma. From these findings, resection and reconstruction of the intrahepatic sectional, segmental, and/or subsegmental ducts can be planned prior to surgery. If segmental cholangitis develops prior to surgery, urgent PTBD should be performed to drain the contralateral side of the intrahepatic duct or isolated intrahepatic segmental or subsegmental ducts.

In cases of major hepatectomy, particularly right hepatectomy, and right or left trisectionectomy, portal vein embolization (PVE) should be considered to increase the volume and functional capacity of the future remnant liver (see Chapter 18). It is important to note, however, that many patients have atrophy of the ipsilateral lobe, which results in significant hypertrophy of the future liver remnant, thereby obviating the need for PVE. Volumetric assessment is an important preoperative maneuver.

Bile replacement during external biliary drainage should be performed to restore the intestinal barrier function and prevent bacterial translocation. Also synbiotic agents should be administered pre- and postoperatively to prevent perioperative infectious complications.

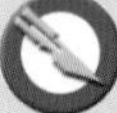

## SURGICAL TECHNIQUE

As biliary branches for the caudate lobe are involved in most of the cases of hilar cholangiocarcinoma, which separate the right and left hepatic duct, the caudate lobe resection (see Chapter 22) is usually performed to establish an R0 resection, and the smallest necessary hepatic segmentectomy or sectionectomy with caudate lobectomy was designed to minimize the volume of the impaired cholestatic liver resection during 1980s. After developing preoperative PVE, hemihepatectomy, or trisectionectomy has been performed to increase the resectability of advanced carcinoma and safety of major hepatectomy (Figs. 26.2, 26.3). Advances in vascular surgical techniques in hepatobiliary surgery have allowed combined liver and portal vein and/or hepatic artery resection and reconstruction with acceptable morbidity and mortality rates for locally advanced tumors.

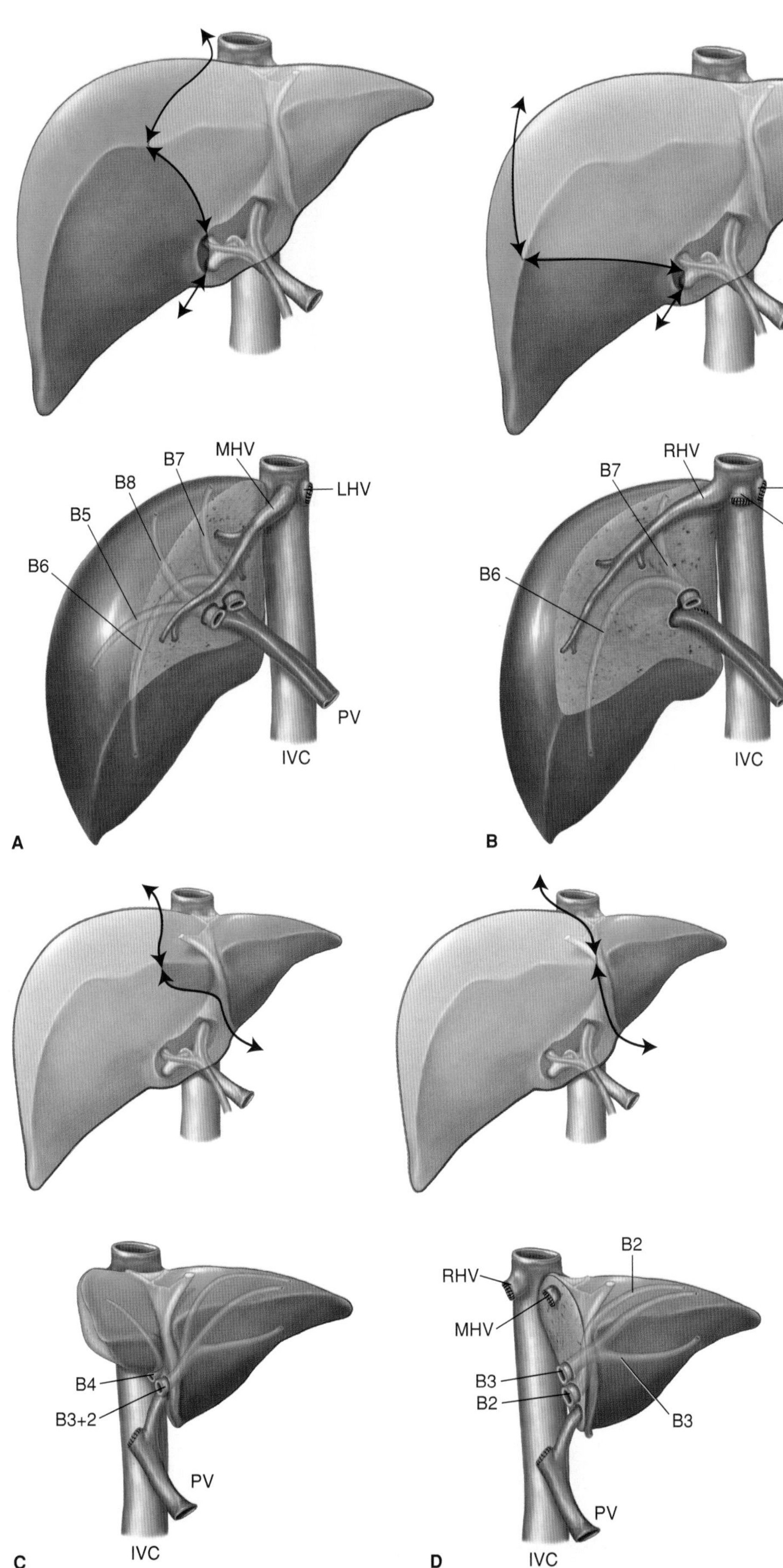


**Figure 26.2** Type of hepatectomy. Type of hepatectomy according to the extent of tumor along the separated sectional and segmental ducts. **A**, left hepatectomy; **B**, left trisectionectomy; **C**, right hepatectomy; **D**, right trisectionectomy; **E**, left medial sectionectomy; **F**, Central bisectionectomy; **G**, Extended central bisectionectomy. IVC, inferior vena cava; RHV, right hepatic vein; MHV, middle hepatic vein; LHV, left hepatic vein; PV, portal vein; B2, left lateral superior segmental duct; B3, left lateral inferior segmental duct; B4, left medial segmental duct; B5, right anterior inferior segmental duct; B6, right posterior inferior segmental duct; B7, right posterior superior segmental duct; B8, right anterior superior segmental duct. (*continued*)

Figure 26.2 (*Continued*)

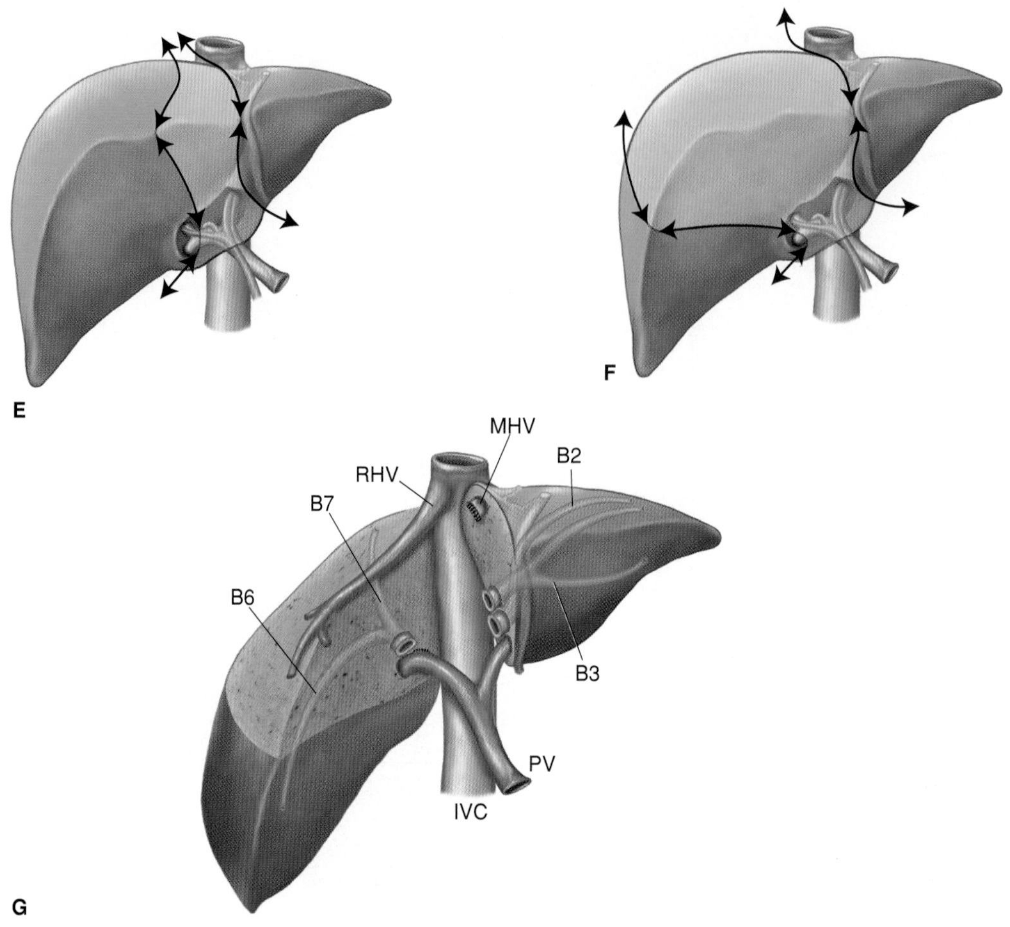


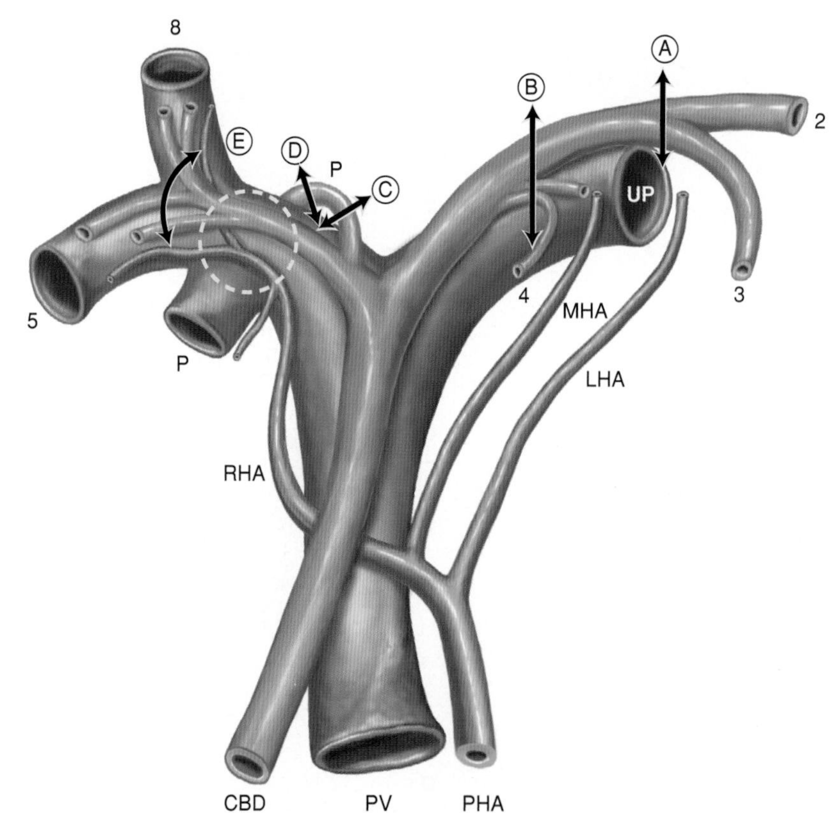


Figure 26.3 Proximal resection line of intrahepatic segmental and subsegmental ducts according to type of hepatectomy. A, right trisectionectomy; B, right hepatectomy; C, E, left hepatectomy; D, left trisectionectomy; numerals indicate the number of Couinaud's segment. UP, umbilical portion; P, posterior sectional branch; LHA, left hepatic artery; MHA, middle hepatic artery; RHA, right hepatic artery; PHA, proper hepatic artery; PV, portal vein; CBD. common bile duct.

1. Skin incision
The peritoneal cavity is entered through a right or bilateral subcostal incision with an upper midline extension to widely expose the upper abdominal cavity including the whole liver using bilateral costal retractors (see Figs. 18.7, 19.3 and 21.5).
2. Intraoperative ultrasonography
Intraoperative ultrasonography (IOUS) is performed to assess the vascular anatomy of the liver, the extent of cancer along the intrahepatic biliary branches, to define the expected resection line of the ducts and to detect unexpected portal vein thrombosis extending beyond the portal bifurcation in case of preoperative PVE (see Chapter 18).
3. Regional connective tissue and lymph node dissection is carried out to expose and isolate the common hepatic artery (CHA), proper hepatic artery (PHA), right and/or left hepatic artery (RHA, LHA), portal vein (PV), right portal vein (RPV) and left portal vein (LPV). The common bile duct (CBD) is exposed and divided above or in the pancreatic head with a free margin. Next, dissection of the hilar lymphatic tissue is pursued up to the hepatic hilus and the RHA or LHA is ligated and divided at its origin, and the caudate lobe branches of the portal vein are ligated and divided before dividing the RPV or LPV, resulting in a demarcation along the Cantlie line.
4. Mobilization of the right and left liver and the caudate lobe.
The right and/or left liver are mobilized in the usual manner, detaching the coronary and triangular ligaments (see Chapter 21, Figs. 21.6 and 21.7). In case of right-sided hepatectomy (see Chapter 19), the posterior liver is further mobilized to be detached from the inferior vena cava (IVC) by ligating and dividing all short hepatic veins (SHV) ((see Figs. 19.5, 19.6, 23.12 and 23.13)). Finally, the right hepatic vein (RHV) is clamped, divided and sutured in a traditional manner or divided with an endosurgical stapler (see Figs. 19.11, 19.12 and 23.18).
In case of the left-sided hepatectomy (see Chapter 20), the caudate lobe is mobilized from the left to the right to be detached from the IVC and all SHVs are ligated and divided, and the distal end of the Arantius canal is ligated and divided close to the left hepatic vein (LHV) or the IVC. Then the posterior surface of the caudate lobe is completely detached from the IVC (see see Chapter 22 and Figs. 22.8 and 22.9).
The LHV may be dissected and exposed outside the liver. The left and middle hepatic veins typically form a common trunk before entering the IVC. It is therefore difficult to isolate the LHV separately; it is technically much easier to encircle the common trunk. Alternatively, the LHV and/or middle (MHV) and LHVs may be divided intrahepatically during parenchymal transection.
5. Liver transection and bile duct resection
   (a) Hemihepatectomy
   The liver capsule is coagulated along the demarcation on the Cantlie line and the liver is transected in a surgeon's favorite manner—ultrasonic surgical scalpel or traditional fracture method.
      (1) Right hepatectomy (see Chapter 19)
      Liver dissection is pursued along the MHV and the caudate lobe is turned and pulled toward the right (see Figs. 20.4, 22.8 and 22.9). Finally, the left hepatic duct (LHD) is isolated on the right edge of the umbilical portion (UP) of the LPV and divided with a histologically free margin (Fig. 26.4).
      (2) Left hepatectomy (see also Chapter 20)
      Liver dissection is pursued cranially along the MHV to the confluence of the MHV and LHV. After confirming the anatomical variation of the MHV and LHV, the latter is divided with an endovascular stapler or the traditional manner between vascular clamps. Liver dissection continues posteriorly behind the MHV and right hepatic duct (RHD) is exposed behind the MHV. The posterior wall of the RHD is detached from the anterior wall of the RPV. Also the anterior branch of the right hepatic artery, which runs between the RHD and RPV, is carefully detached and isolated. After complete isolation of the RHD, a stay suture is placed on the RHD, which is divided and the inferior (B5) and superior (B8) branches should be identified internally and

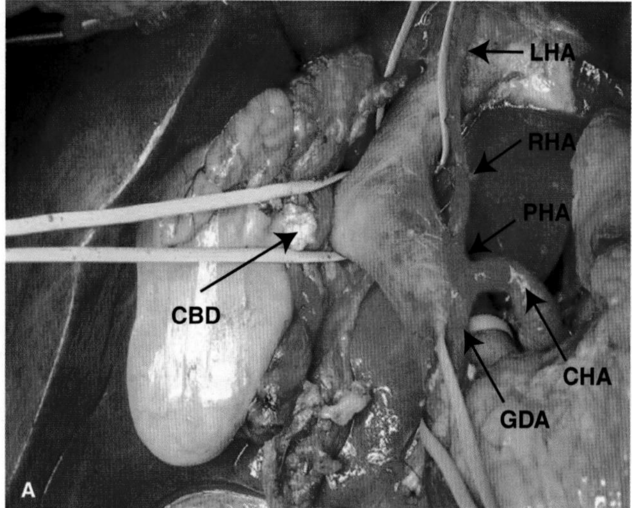


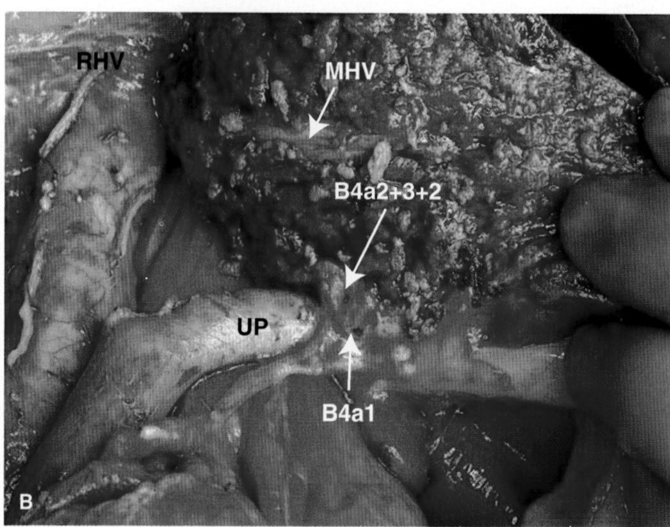


Figure 26.4 Right hepatectomy with caudate lobectomy. **A:** Skeletonization of the hepatic arteries and portal vein. LHA, left hepatic artery; RHA, stump of right hepatic artery; PHA, proper hepatic artery; CHA, common hepatic artery; GDA, gastroduodenal artery; CBD, stump of common bile duct. **B:** After en bloc resection. Resected margins of the segmental and subsegmental duct lines side by side along the umbilical portion (UP) of the left portion vein. RHV, stump of RHV; MHV, middle hepatic vein; B4a1, ventral branch of the segment 4; B4a2+3+2, main left hepatic duct.

externally (Fig. 26.5). Finally, liver transection progresses dorsally between the caudate lobe and the segment 7 along the right edge of the IVC to remove the left liver and the caudate lobe, en bloc.

(b) Trisectionectomy

Trisectionectomy removes a large volume of hepatic parenchyma, particularly on the right side; therefore, in the absence of notable hypertrophy of the future liver remnant (FLR), with atrophy of the contralateral liver, preoperative PVE should be considered. Liver volumetrics should be performed, and a decision made based on this assessment. In general, preoperative PVE is probably not necessary with an FLR volume greater than 25% in a healthy liver or greater than 40% in an abnormal liver (i.e., jaundiced) (see Chapter 18).

(1) Right trisectionectomy (see Chapter 19)

The RHA, the RPV and the caudate lobe branches of the portal vein (P1) are ligated and divided, and the right liver is mobilized and the SHVs and the RHV are ligated, divided, and sutured in the same manner as a right hemihepatectomy.

Next, the feeding vessels for the segment 4 are divided (see Figs. 19.10, 21.8–21.10, 24.7 and 27.9): Middle hepatic artery (MHA) or arterial branches (A4) from the LHA and medial branches (P4) from the umbilical portion (UP) of the LPV, are ligated and divided at the Rex's recesses and the liver is divided along a demarcation on the umbilical fissure. Liver parenchymal transection is advanced cranially and the MHV is ligated and divided near the confluence of the LHV. Then the LHD is isolated and divided just to the right of the UP, and the right trisection of the liver, the caudate lobe and the extrahepatic duct are removed en bloc.

At the resected margin of the LHD, a single duct, representing the confluence of the left lateral sectional duct (B2+3) or each lateral segmental duct, superior (B2) and inferior (B3), are identified according to the anatomical variation of the biliary anatomy (Fig. 26.6).

(2) Left trisectionectomy (see Chapter 20)

The LHA is ligated and divided, and the RHA is dissected more distally and the anterior (RAHA) and posterior (RPHA) branches are skeletonized in the Rouviere's sulcus and the RAHA is ligated and divided. Next, the P1s are ligated and divided and the LPV, anterior (RAPV) and posterior (RPPV)

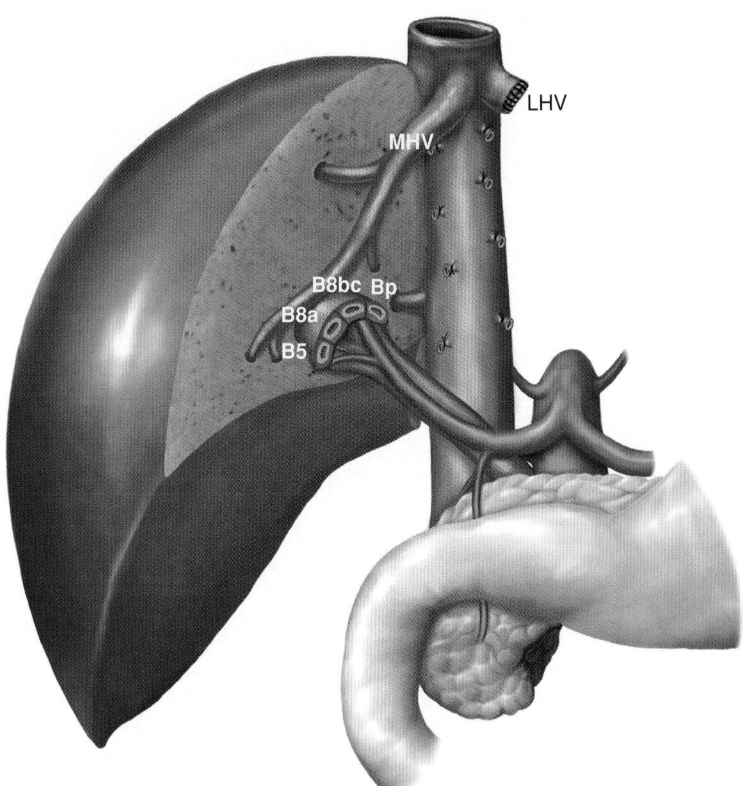


Figure 26.5 Left hepatectomy with caudate lobectomy.
A: Scheme of left hepatectomy with caudate lobectomy. The anterior segmental and subsegmental ducts (B) are divided separately behind the middle hepatic vein (MHV) and the posterior sectional duct (Bp) is located cranially to the RPV. B8a, ventral branch of segment 8; B8bc, lateral and dorsal branch of segment 8 B5, anterior inferior segmental duct.
B: Intraoperative finding. The right anterior segmental and subsegmental ducts are divided behind the middle hepatic vein (MHV). The posterior sectional duct (Bp) is close to the RPV.
C: A variation of the right posterior sectional and segmental ducts. The anterior segmental ducts (B5, B8) are separately divided. The right posterior sectional duct (P) is identified caudally to the RPV and the paracaval branch of the segment 7 (B7d) is found parallel to the IVC.



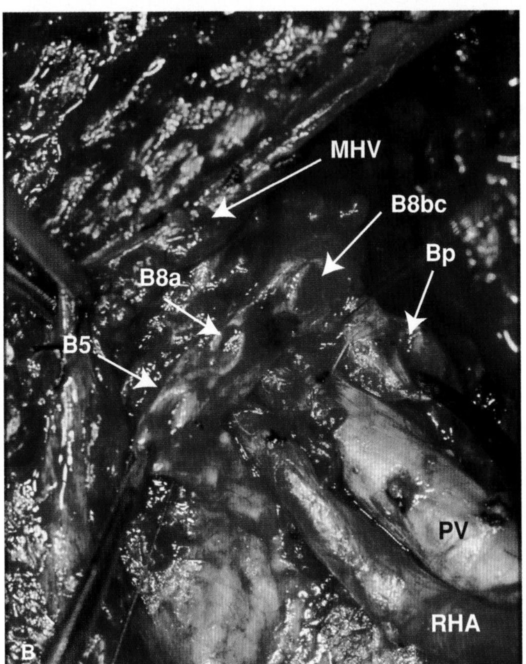


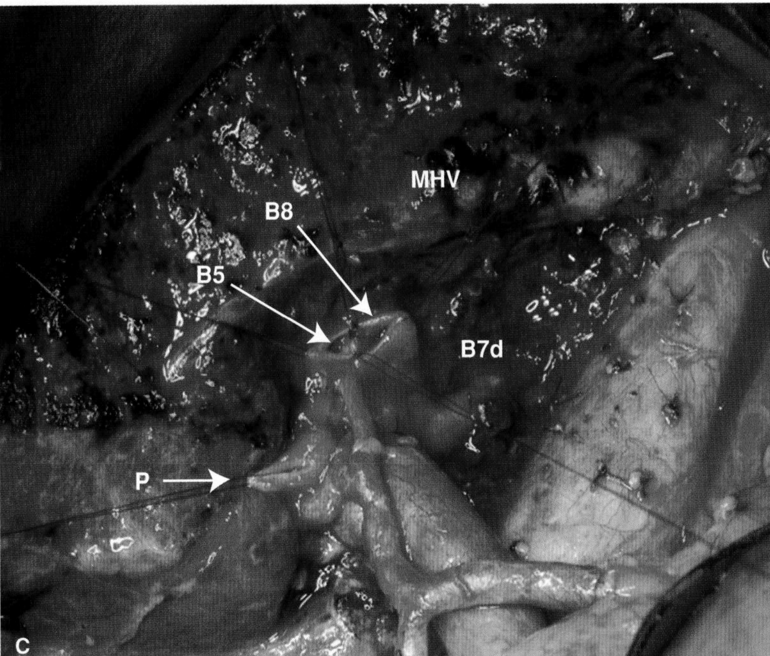


branches of the portal vein are taped, and the LPV and RAPV are ligated and divided. Then a clear demarcation appears on the right portal fissure and a border between the caudate process and S7.

Mobilization of the liver is performed in the same manner of the left hemihepatectomy, and the common trunk of the LHV and MHV are divided and sutured (see Chapter 20). Liver transection is carried out along the demarcation and the RHV is exposed on the raw surface of the liver. Dorsal

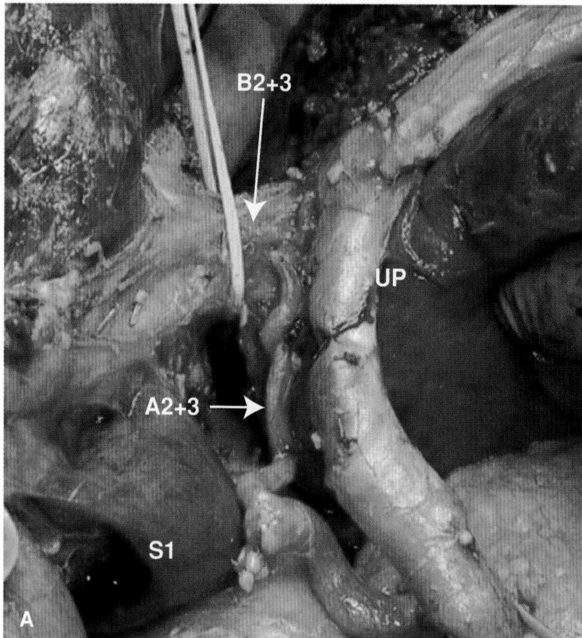


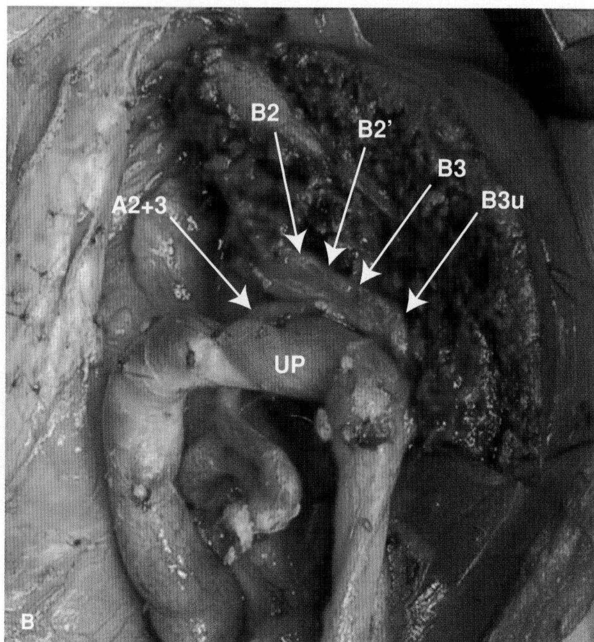


Figure 26.6 Anatomical right hepatic trisectionectomy. **A:** Exposure of the left lateral sectional duct (B2+3) after mobilization of the umbilical portion of the LPV (UP). The hepatic artery for the left lateral section (A2+3) is exposed between the portal vein and the B2+3. S1, caudate lobe; UP, umbilical portion of the LPV. **B:** Left lateral segmental and subsegmental ducts line side by side behind the umbilical portion of the LPV (UP). B2, duct of segment 2; B3, duct of segment 3; B3u, an upper branch of B3.

liver dissection is pursued between the caudate process and the S7 along the right edge of the IVC. Finally, the right posterior sectional duct is isolated cranially to the RPPV and divided at the expected portion, and the left trisection of the liver, caudate lobe and the extrahepatic duct are removed en bloc. At the resected margin of the right posterior sectional duct, a single duct (Bp) is identified at the distal portion of the confluence of the inferior (B6) and superior (B7) branches, or each segmental duct, B6 and B7, is divided separately according to the progress of the tumor (Fig. 26.7).

(c) Central bisectionectomy

Central hepatic bisectionectomy is indicated for the special case of hilar cholangiocarcinoma predominantly involving the left medial (B4) and the right anterior biliary branches (Ba).

Many of the same techniques used for the trisectionectomies are required; however, mobilization of the liver should be performed from the right, but mobilization of the left liver should be minimized to prevent unexpected postoperative

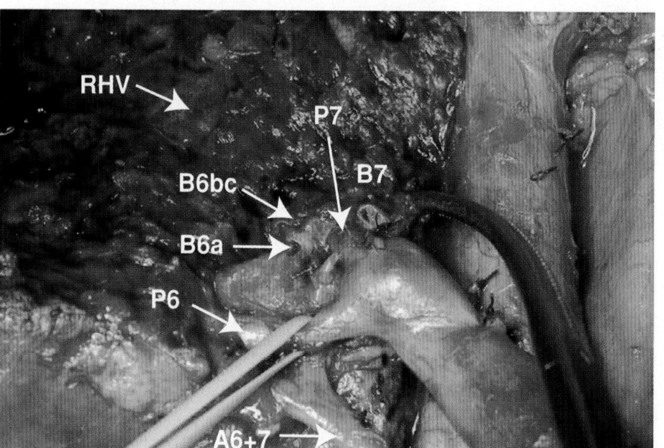


Figure 26.7 Left hepatic trisectionectomy with caudate lobectomy. The right posterior segmental (B6, B7) and subsegmental ducts are separately divided above each segmental portal branch (P6, P7). B6a, ventral branch; B6bc, dorsal and lateral branch; A6+7, right posterior hepatic artery; RHV, right hepatic vein.

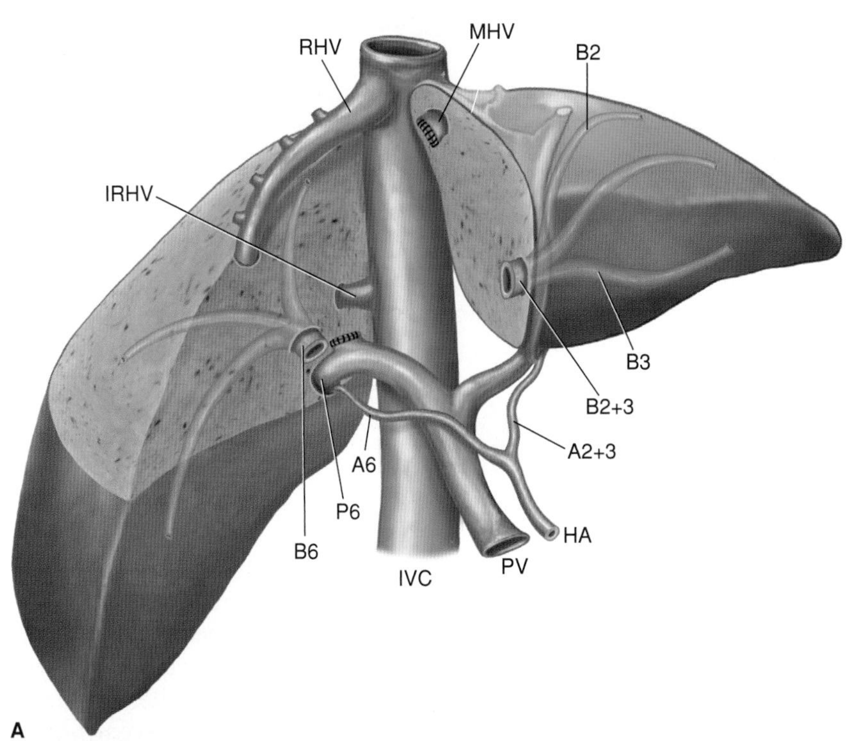


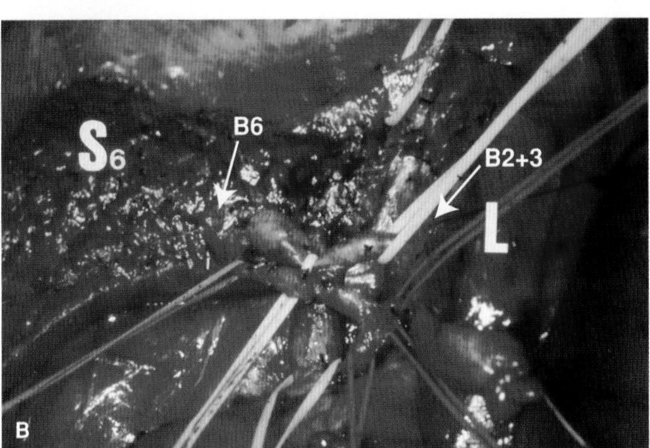


Figure 26.8 Extended central hepatic bisectionectomy. **A:** S1, S4, S5, S7, and S8 are removed en bloc, and the left lateral sectional (B2+3) and right posterior inferior segmental (B6) duct are separately resected. MHV, stump of middle hepatic vein; RHV, right hepatic vein; IRHV, inferior right hepatic vein. **B:** Intraoperative finding—L, lateral section; B2+3, left lateral sectional duct B6, right posterior inferior segmental duct; S6, right posterior inferior segment.



kinking of the LHV. The MHA and/or A4, RAHA, P1, and the RAPV are ligated and divided. Next, the Rex's recessus are opened to ligate and divide the medial branches (P4) of the portal vein from the UP. At this point, clear demarcation appears on the umbilical and right portal fissures.

Liver transaction is stated along the demarcation on the umbilical fissure and the MHV is ligated and divided. The LHD is divided at the expected portion on the right of the UP. Next, the liver is dissected along the demarcation on the right portal fissure to expose the RHV on the raw surface of the liver, and dorsal liver dissection is in progress between the caudate process and the S7. Finally, the Bp is isolated cranially to the RPPV and divided at the expected portion. The central liver, caudate lobe, and extrahepatic bile duct are removed en bloc (Fig. 26.8).

6. Hepaticojejunostomy
Resected margins of the intrahepatic segmental and subsegmental ducts are examined by frozen section, and in the case of multiple small ducts, hepaticoplasty is performed with 5-0 PDS sutures to minimize the number of anastomosis. A Roux-en-Y jejunal limb is pulled up through a retrocolic and retrogastric route and hepaticojejunostomy is started from an anatomically difficult side. In right-sided hepatectomy, resected margins of the left hepatic ducts line side by side perpendicularly on the cranial side of the UP, the caudal (or posterior) side anastomosis should firstly be performed with

a continuous suture of 4-0 or 5-0 PDS and the cranial (or anterior) wall anastomosis later.

In left hepatectomy, caudal (posterior) wall anastomosis should firstly be carried out from the posterior sectional duct to the anterior sectional or segmental ducts and cranial (anterior) wall anastomosis later.

7. Drainage

If the anastomosis(es) are to be stented, a 6-French biliary drainage tube is inserted in each anastomosis from the proximal end of the jejunal limb; however, stents are rarely required and cannot improve the outcome of a poorly conceived or executed anastomosis. Peritoneal drainage tubes are placed routinely in the subphrenic space, behind the hepaticojejunostomy and along the raw surface of the liver.

## POSTOPERATIVE MANAGEMENT

In addition to the routine cardiopulmonary monitoring, special attention should be paid to serum liver function tests, portal blood flow estimated by color Doppler ultrasonography and contents in the peritoneal drainage tubes. The color and volume of externally drained bile can be an index of liver regeneration. Careful management of closed suction drains is important not only to prevent drainage site infections but also for early diagnosis of postoperative complications. In patients with large volume biliary output, early postoperative external nutritional supplementation with bile replacement and synbiotic treatment through a jejunal feeding tube is useful to prevent postoperative infectious complications.

## COMPLICATIONS

Hemorrhage, bile leakage from raw surface of the liver and/or hepaticojejunostomy, wound infection and intraabdominal abscess are among the most common postoperative complications after hepatobiliary resection and reconstruction for hilar cholangiocarcinoma. Infectious complications must be most carefully managed, otherwise they may evolve into liver failure followed by sepsis and multiple organ failure.

Bile leakage from raw surface of the liver and that from the hepaticojejunostomy are distinguished by careful observation of the contents with or without intestinal fluid which should be managed with closed suction drains.

Causative sites of postoperative hemorrhage are raw surfaces of the liver or the ligated and divided hepatic artery. The former usually occurs in the early postoperative period and the latter in the early or late postoperative period after developing intraabdominal infectious complications. In case of massive bleeding from a branch of the hepatic artery, dynamic CT or urgent hepatic arteriography demonstrates pseudoaneurysm which could be treated with selective transcatheter arterial embolization (TAE). However, patients may not be sufficiently stable for this approach, and the only option is emergent reexploration. Also, TAE may result in postprocedure anastomotic insufficiency of the hepaticojejunostomy and/or severe damage of the remnant liver.

Volvulus of the stomach followed by delayed gastric emptying is a rare complication that can develop after left-sided hepatectomy due to adhesion of the stomach to the liver stump; however, this complication can be treated conservatively and prevented by fixation of the gastric omentum to the left upper abdominal wall.

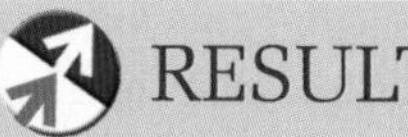

## RESULTS

From 1979, aggressive surgical procedures have been employed for hilar cholangiocarcinoma in the Department of Surgery, Nagoya University Hospital and several types of hepatectomies were performed for 513 (96%) of the 532 resected patients and proximal

TABLE 26.1 Type of Resection

| Type of Resection | Total | | Number of Patients +PD | +PV | +HA |
|---|---|---|---|---|---|
| Right trisectionectomy + S1 | 36 | 96% | 2 | 24 | |
| Right hepatectomy + S1 | 164 | | 40 | 59 | 1 |
| Left trisectionectomy + S1 | 96 | | 8 | 47 | 37 |
| Left hepatectomy + S1 | 180 | | 5 | 55 | 30 |
| Central hepatectomy + S1 | 15 | | 1 | 3 | |
| Other hepatectomies | 22 | | 5 | 1 | |
| Bile duct resection | 19 | | 5 | L | |
| *Total* | *532* | | *66 (12%)* | *190 (36%)* | *68 (13%)* |

PD, Pancreatoduodenectomy; PV, Portal vein resection and reconstruction; HA, Hepatic artery resection and reconstruction; SI, Caudate lobectomy

bile duct resection without hepatectomy for the remaining 19 patients. Combined portal vein resection and reconstruction was applied for 190 patients (36%); of them, hepatic artery resection and reconstruction for 68 patients (13%) and pancreatoduodenectomy for 66 patients (12%) with distal cancer extension. Of the 513 patients, 200 underwent right-sided hepatectomy, 276 left-sided hepatectomy and the remaining 37 central or other resectional procedures (Table 26.1).

Postoperatively several kinds of complications were encountered, and liver failure developed in 16% to 30% of the resected patients during 1980s and 1990s. However, this terrible postoperative complication decreased from 6.0% to 4.0% in the last decade. Postoperative mortality rate was high, 8% to 17% during 1980s and 1990s, but also decreased from 3.0% to 1.1% in the last decade according to the continuous efforts to develop multidisciplinary perioperative managements of high risk patients (Table 26.2).

As we have resected difficult patients with advanced hilar cholangiocarcinoma, 85 patients (16%) with distant metastasis (M1) were included in the 532 resected patients, and R0 resection was possible in 44 patients (8%) of them with paraaortic node dissection.

In 447 M0 patients (84%), R0, R1 and R2 resections were performed in 341 (64%), 92 (17%) and 14 (3%) of the 532 patients. Postoperative 3-, 5- and 10-year survival rates for M0R0, M0R1, and M1R0 to M1R2 patients were 57.3%, 43.6%, 30.2%; 36.8%, 21.1%, 0%; 10%, 0%, 0%, respectively (Fig. 26.9). In the 341 M0R0 patients, histologic regional lymph node metastasis was positive (N1) in 121 patients (35%) and negative in the remaining 220 patients (65%). Postoperative 3-, 5-, and 10-year survival rates for M0R0N0 patients and those for M0R0N1 were 67.4%, 56.0%, 38.6%; 38.2%, 19.9%, and 14.2%, respectively (Fig. 26.10).

TABLE 26.2 Postoperative Liver Failure and Hospital Death

| Period | Number of Patients Resection (Hepatectomy) | Liver Failure | Hospital Death |
|---|---|---|---|
| 1979~1985 | 30 (26) | 6 (20.0%) | 5 (16.7%) |
| 1986~1990 | 43 (41) | 7 (16.2%) | 4 (9.3%) |
| 1991~1995 | 49 (42) | 15 (30.6%) | 4 (8.2%) |
| 1996~2000 | 66 (65) | 13 (19.7%) | 7 (10.6%) |
| 2001~2005 | 167 (164) | 10 (6.0%) | 5 (3.0%) |
| 2006~2009 | 177 (175) | 7 (4.0%) | 2 (1.1%) |
| *Total* | *532 (513)* | *58 (10.9%)* | *27 (5.1%)* |

*1979–2009, Nagoya Univ. Hospital.*

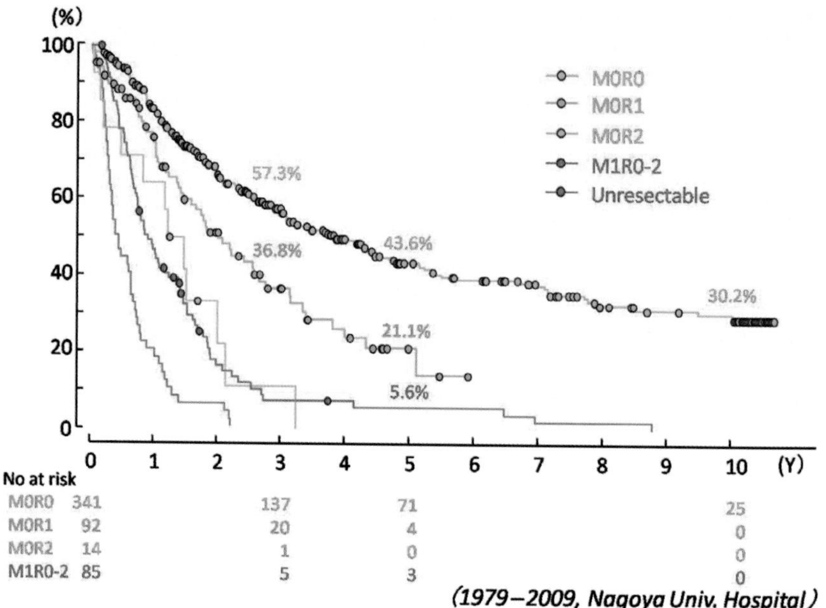


Figure 26.9 Postoperative survival curves for resected 532 patients with hilar cholangiocarcinoma.

## CONCLUSIONS

1. Preoperative staging of hilar cholangiocarcinoma is established by MRC, MDCT, selective cholangiography through PTBD or ENBD catheter with or without cholangioscopic investigation, and resective procedures are preoperatively planned according to the above findings.
2. Advanced surgical techniques have been developed and enable hepatobiliary surgeons to perform extended hepatobiliary resection with vascular resection and reconstruction for locally advanced hilar cholangiocarcinoma.
3. Perioperative management, including biliary drainage, PVE and synbiotic treatment increased the safety of extended hepatobiliary resection and prolonged survival of the resected patient with hilar cholangiocarcinoma.

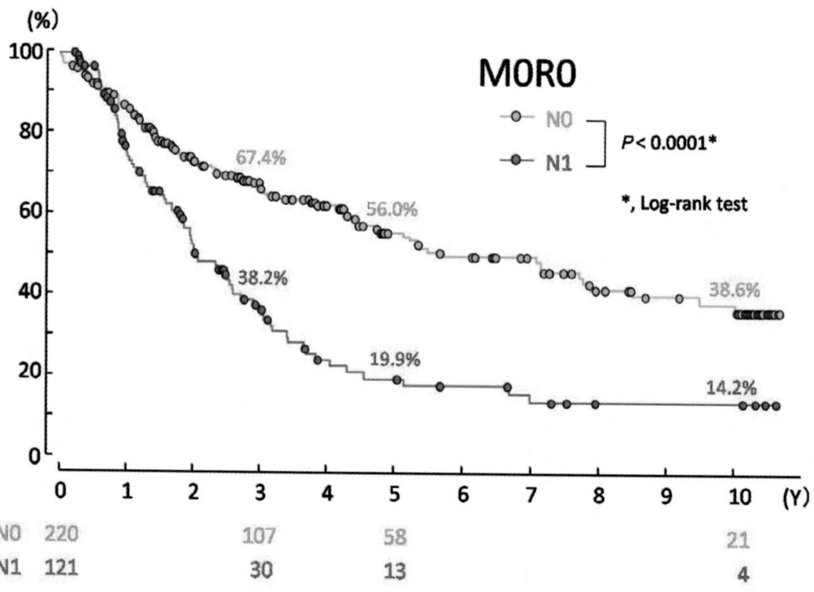


Figure 26.10 Postoperative survival curves for 341 patients without distant metastases according to lymph node metastasis and submitted to complete resection (MOR0).

## Recommended References and Readings


Ebata T, Nagino M, Kamiya J, et al. Hepatectomy with portal vein resection for hilar cholangiocarcinoma: audit of 52 consecutive cases. *Ann Surg.* 2003;238:720–727.

Kamiya S, Nagino M, Kanazawa H, et al. The value of bile replacement during external biliary drainage: an analysis of intestinal permeability, integrity, and microflora. *Ann Surg.* 2004;239: 510–517.

Kanai M, Nimura Y, Kamiya J, et al. Preoperative intrahepatic segmental cholangitis in patients with advanced carcinoma involving the hepatic hilus. *Surgery.* 1996;119:498–504.

Nagino M, Kamiya J, Arai T, et al. "Anatomic" right hepatic trisectionectomy (extended right hepatectomy) with caudate lobectomy for hilar cholangiocarcinoma. *Ann Surg.* 2006;243:28–32.

Nagino M, Kamiya J, Nishio H, et al. Two hundred forty consecutive portal vein embolizations before extended hepatectomy for biliary cancer: surgical outcome and long-term follow-up. *Ann Surg.* 2006; 243:364–372.

Nagino M, Nimura Y, Kamiya J, et al. Changes in hepatic lobe volume in biliary tract cancer patients after right portal vein embolization. *Hepatology.* 1995;21:434–439.

Nagino M, Nimura Y, Kamiya J, et al. Selective percutaneous transhepatic embolization of the portal vein in preparation for extensive liver resection: the ipsilateral approach. *Radiology.* 1996;200:559–563.

Nagino M, Nimura Y, Nishio H, et al. Hepatectomy with simultaneous resection of the portal vein and hepatic artery for advanced perihilar cholangiocarcinoma: an audit of 50 consecutive cases. *Ann Surg.* 2010;252:115–123.

Nimura Y, Hayakawa N, Kamiya J, et al. Hepatic segmentectomy with caudate lobe resection for bile duct carcinoma of the hepatic hilus. *World J Surg.* 1990;14:535–544.

Nimura Y, Hayakawa N, Kamiya J, et al. Combined portal vein and liver resection for carcinoma of the biliary tract. *Br J Surg.* 1991; 78:727–731.

Nimura Y, Kamiya J, Kondo S, et al. Aggressive preoperative management and extended surgery for hilar cholangiocarcinoma: Nagoya experience. *J Hepatobiliary Pancreat Surg.* 2000;7:155–162.

Nimura Y. Staging of biliary carcinoma: cholangiography and cholangioscopy. *Endscopy.* 1993;25:76–80.

Senda Y, Nishio H, Oda K, et al. Value of multidetector row CT in the assessment of longitudinal extension of cholangiocarcinoma: correlation between MDCT and microscopic findings. *World J Surg.* 2009;33:1459–1467.

Sugawara G, Nagino M, Nishio H, et al. Perioperative synbiotic treatment to prevent postoperative infectious complications in biliary cancer surgery: a randomized controlled trial. *Ann Surg.* 2006;244:706–714.

Uesaka K, Nimura Y, Nagino M. Changes in hepatic lobar function after right portal vein embolization. An appraisal by biliary indocyanine green excretion. *Ann Surg.* 1996;223:77–83.

# 27 Gallbladder Cancer

**David Bentrem and Yuman Fong**

## INDICATIONS/CONTRAINDICATIONS

Gallbladder carcinoma (GBC) is the most common biliary epithelial malignancy, with an estimated 9,520 new cases and 3,340 deaths per year. The incidence steadily increases with age, reaching a maximum in the seventh decade of life. GBC predominantly affects women (75% to 85%) and is more commonly found in Native, Alaskan, or Hispanic Americans. There is, in addition, an association between the presence of gallstones and GBC, though this relationship is not well understood. Interestingly, size of gallstones is also a risk factor; patients with stones greater than 3 cm are 10 times more likely to develop GBC compared with patients with subcentimeter-sized gallstones. While cholelithiasis and its associated repeated inflammation may contribute, this relative risk and the influence of environmental toxins (carcinogens in tobacco, diet, etc.) or hormones remain unclear. This disease's insidious nature and typically late presentation place it among the most lethal of invasive neoplasms. Gallbladder cancer spreads early by lymphatic or hematogenous metastasis and by direct invasion into the liver. While surgery may well be curative at early stages, both surgical and nonsurgical treatments remain largely unsuccessful in patients with more advanced disease.

### Indications

- Broadly, surgical therapy is indicated for localized disease that is limited to the gallbladder, liver bed, and regional lymph nodes (Fig. 27.1A, B). Operative strategies differ, however, depending on depth of invasion of the primary lesion and the presence of lymphadenopathy concerning for metastasis.
- Generally, T1a lesions, defined as tumors limited to the gallbladder mucosa without extension to muscular layers of the wall, can be sufficiently treated with cholecystectomy alone without further radical surgical resection. Patients whose disease extends into the muscular layers of the gallbladder and beyond, however, require a more aggressive surgical approach.
- For T1b, T2, or T3 lesions with (or without) associated regional adenopathy, en bloc resection with regional lymphadenopathy is appropriate. Extension of disease proximally to the bile duct may require bile duct excision with reconstruction for biliary drainage. For patients with resected T2 lesions, 30% have been found to have nodal disease and 16% metastatic disease. With resected T3 lesions, 58% were found to

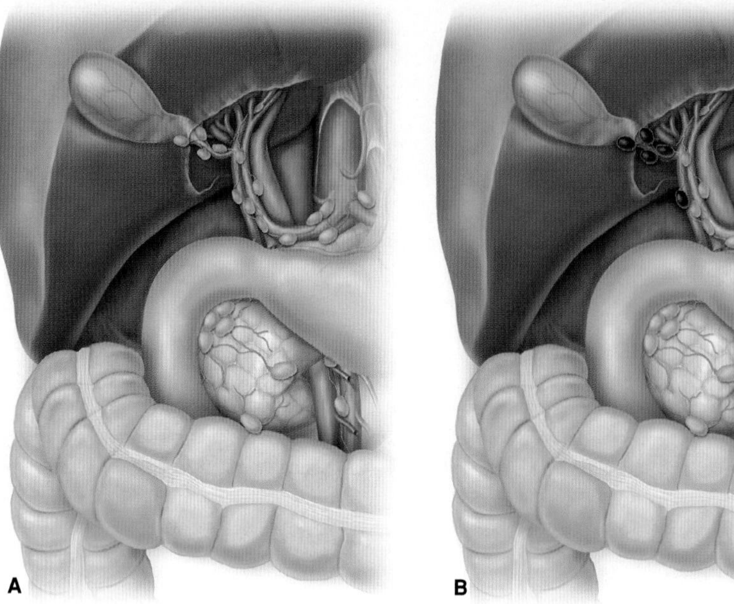


Figure 27.1 **A:** Regional lymph nodes of the gallbladder; **B:** N1 disease is defined as metastasis to regional lymph nodes.

have nodal disease and 42% peritoneal metastases. This leads to a low likelihood of completed resection (27%) for patients with clinically staged T3 tumors.

- Gallbladder wall polyps are not uncommon, and polypoid lesions of the gallbladder are frequently noted on abdominal ultrasonography. The clinical relevance of this finding, however, is not entirely clear. The surgeon's suspicion of growth as well as the evolution of dysplasia and eventual invasive carcinoma serves as the basis for recommending close surveillance, or even resection, for certain polypoid lesions. Concerning features include solitary, large, immobile, or changing lesions. Traditionally, gallbladder polyps greater than 1 cm in size were thought to be at a higher risk for containing GBC foci (Table 27.1).
- Calcifications of the gallbladder (leading to the oft-used term "porcelain gallbladder") have been viewed as a risk factor for developing GBC (Table 27.1). Polk, in 1966, was one of the original proponents of this hypothesis and pointed to two pieces of evidence to substantiate it. More recent literature more specifically defined gallbladder calcifications. A report by Stephen and Berger explicitly classified gallbladder calcifications as intramural ($n$ = 17) or selective mucosal ($n$ = 27). They reported that of gallbladder specimens of the intramural type, no cases of adenocarcinoma were identified, whereas selective mucosal calcifications heralded a 7% malignancy rate.
- With respect to extent of disease related to hepatic parenchyma, critical attention must be given to invasion of the hepatic arteries and ducts. Notably, invasion of the right hepatic artery or duct is not a contraindication to aggressive surgical therapy; while these findings may necessitate a right (or even extended right) hepatectomy, adequate reconstruction can be accomplished.

## Contraindications

- Distant metastases
- Extensive, bilateral liver involvement
- Local extension of disease involving the left hepatic artery, left hepatic duct, or the confluence of the portal vascular or biliary structures is indicative of more extensive disease less likely controlled by surgery (Fig. 27.2A). Similarly, if a tumor progresses distally toward the duodenum and pancreas with (perhaps) invasion of one of those structures, a Whipple procedure may be considered but long-term disease control is doubtful (Fig. 27.2B).

**TABLE 27.1 Series of Gallbladder (GB) Calcifications and Polyps**

| Authors (y) | N | Entity Studied (Calcification or Polyp) | Size, Lesion Characteristics | Association or Incidence of GBC | Conclusion |
|---|---|---|---|---|---|
| Kim et al. (2009) | 9 (of 3,159 inspected) | Calcifications | Pathologically proven porcelain gall bladder | No porcelain GB had GBC; no patients with GBC had calcification | No association between porcelain GB and GBC |
| Ito et al. (2009) | 417 | Polyps | 94% of polyps ≤10 mm, 7% >10 mm | No cases of invasive GBC in 80 surgical specimens | Risk of invasive cancer in GB polyp is extremely low |
| Stephen and Berger (2001) | 150 GBC (of 25,900 inspected) | Calcifications | Selective mucosal $n = 27$, intramural $n = 17$ | 7% of selective mucosal with GBC, none with intramural | Pattern of calcification determines cancer risk |
| Towfigh et al. (2001) | 103 (of 10,741 inspected) | Calcifications ("porcelain" GB) | Partial calcification of wall ($n = 15$) and GBC ($n = 88$) | No porcelain GB had GBC; no patients with GBC had calcification | Porcelain GB/calcifications not associated with GBC |
| Terzi et al. (2000) | 100 | Polyps | 74% benign (20% adenomas, 15% adenomatous hyperplasia) | 26% rate of malignancy | Risk factors for GBC are age >60, size >10 mm, coexistence of gallstones |
| Mainprize et al. (2000) | 38 | Polyps | 11/34 patients with polyps pathologically proven; 7/11 benign cholesterol polyps | All neoplastic disease ($n = 4$) arose in polyps >10 mm | Should perform cholecystectomy for polyps >10 mm |
| Kubota et al. (1995) | 72 | Polyps | 47/72 cholesterol polyps, GBC in 16/72 | 88% of GBC in polyps >18 mm, 56% were sessile | Polyps <18 mm potentially early stage, >18 mm likely advanced |
| Koga et al. (1988) | 32 (of 411 resected specimens) | Polyps | Primarily examined age, size and type (most were cholesterol polyps) | 88% of malignancy in polyps >10 mm, 75% in patients > 60 y | Risk factors for GBC are age >60, size >10 mm |

GBC, gallbladder carcinoma.

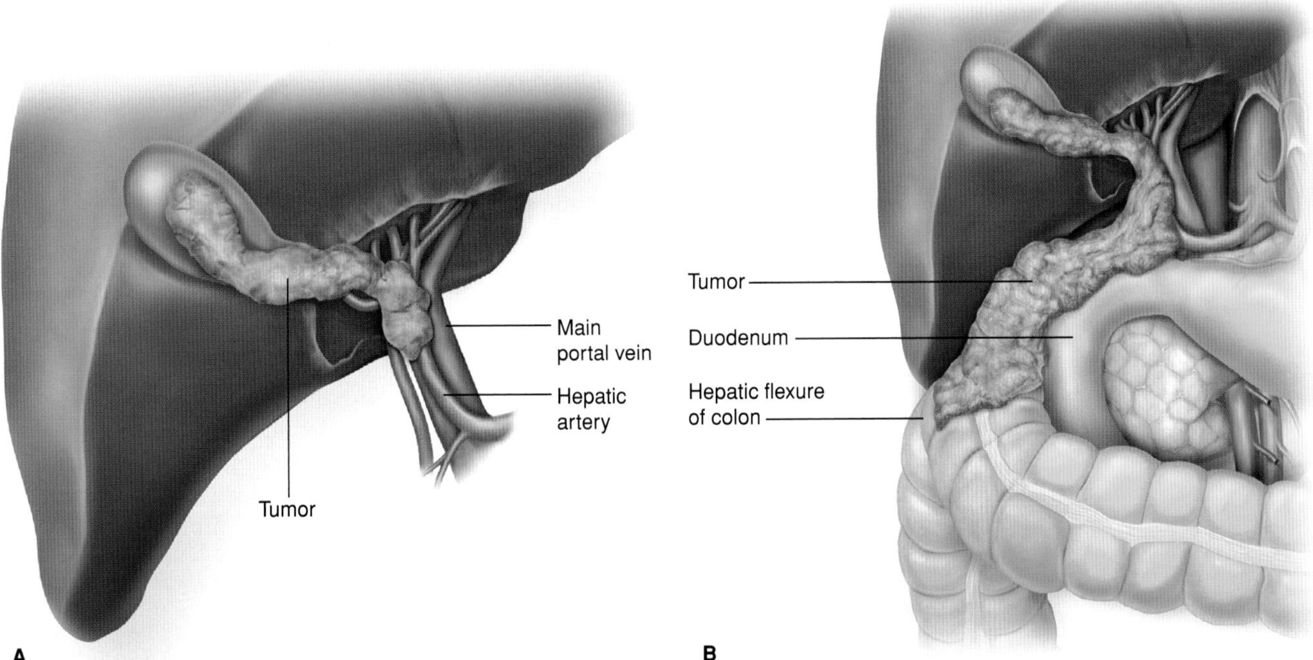


Figure 27.2 **A:** Illustration of a gallbladder cancer extending into the porta hepatis; **B:** Illustration of a gallbladder cancer involving adjacent extrahepatic organs (duodenum, pancreas, colon).

- Lymph node metstases outside the region of the porta hepatis. Nodal spread beyond the hepatoduodenal ligament (celiac, retropancreatic, aortocaval) generally represents metastatic disease.
- Significant comorbidities.

##  PREOPERATIVE PLANNING

### Diagnosis

There is no single clinical physical examination finding, laboratory value, or imaging modality that can unequivocally diagnose early GBC, and rarely are any of these approaches given consideration preoperatively. Symptoms of invasive GBC are notoriously vague and nonspecific. Right upper quadrant pain primarily associated with benign biliary disease may be the first and only presenting symptom. Alternatively, a smaller percentage of GBC patients may present with obstructive jaundice secondary to local disease progression and obstruction of biliary outflow tracts. Other physical signs are limited. The usual clinical scenario is that of incidentally found GBC at the time of cholecystectomy. Approximately 1% of cholecystectomy specimens contain evidence of invasive disease, and this rate is significantly higher in patients greater than 70 years. Mass lesions, focal thickening, or mucosal calcifications on abdominal imaging should raise suspicion of an underlying malignancy.

### Clinical Staging

Cancers of the gallbladder are ultimately pathologically staged according to their depth of penetration and extent of spread. Clinical staging for GBC consists of imaging modalities as well as pathologic specimens when available from prior surgical resections.

For GBC discovered by the pathologist incidentally, subsequent staging depends on pathologic tumor (T) stage. Extent of locoregional disease is directly correlated with the T stage of GBC, with more invasive lesions exhibiting higher rates of lymph node and distant metastases. T stage classification depends on the depth of tumor penetration into the wall of the gallbladder, on the presence of tumor invasion into the liver, hepatic artery, or portal vein, and on adjacent organ involvement. T1a lesions, those that have not breached the muscular layers, require no further staging or treatment. Accurate staging for more advanced, resectable tumors requires that all hilar lymph nodes be removed and analyzed. The hilar nodes include the lymph nodes along the common bile duct (CBD), hepatic artery, portal vein, and cystic duct.

For any tumor that has invaded the muscular layer or beyond, additional postoperative imaging is mandatory for clinical staging. This should include high-resolution 3D imaging of the chest, abdomen, and pelvis, specifically evaluating regional lymphadenopathy or any evidence of distant metastases. In addition, because even sophisticated imaging may understage disease and underestimate the propensity to seed the peritoneal surfaces after the prior operation, staging laparoscopy should be strongly considered. A minority of patients may present not with a tissue diagnosis, but with either (a) an incidentally found mass discovered while imaging the patient for other reasons, or (b) jaundice. Under these circumstances, in addition to the imaging studies described above, one should obtain a complete blood count (CBC), liver function tests, consider adding CA19-9 and carcinoembryonic antigen (CEA) serum markers, and again strongly consider staging laparoscopy, depending on results of the aforementioned tests.

### Imaging

Ultrasonography is the most frequently utilized imaging modality for biliary pathology. Perhaps the only caveat of this approach is the user-dependent nature of both acquiring and analyzing the imaging. For GBC, ultrasound has reported 70% to 90% sensitivity in detecting GBC, but this does not hold true for all stages. A number of sonographic findings are consistent with GBC, though many of them are quite nonspecific; these include gallbladder wall thickening, calcifications, any mass or soft-tissue density interrupting or protruding through the mucosa, and any architectural ambiguity at the gallbladder–liver intersection. Furthermore, ultrasound may be helpful in determining the extent of locoregional disease progression to portal structures including the hepatic artery or portal lymph nodes. Endoscopic ultrasound is an increasingly utilized adjunct in this regard, with the added benefit of a fine needle aspiration tissue biopsy of suspicious regional abnormalities.

Computed tomography (CT) may define advanced (distant) disease and provide specific information about extent of local disease. Most importantly, CT will help delineate T3 and T4 lesions but is not to be relied upon for discrimination of smaller lesions due to the lack of sensitivity in differentiating mucosal and submucosal planes. CT can also be particularly useful for assessing regional lymphadenopathy, predominantly nodes measuring greater than 1 cm. Magnetic resonance is yet one further diagnostic modality that may be utilized if a preoperative diagnosis of GBC is being considered. Magnetic resonance imaging (MRI) may be extremely useful in outlining invasion of carcinoma into surrounding soft tissues. Specifically, MRI can help distinguish the extent of invasion into the surrounding liver parenchyma, presence of tumor around and into adjacent biliary structures that may or may not manifest as biliary narrowing, and obstruction or dilation, and also help define extrahepatic disease. When used as an adjunct to MRI, magnetic resonance cholangiopancreatography (MRCP) may better clarify the extent of biliary pathology and help guide operative management with respect to not only whether resection is appropriate, but also which precise liver segments must be excised.

Fluorodeoxyglucose positron emission tomography (PET) has evolved to become an important test in the management of GBC. It is capable of confirming lymphatic metastases in high risk patients. In a recent series of 126 patients with biliary malignancy, 24% of PET scans influenced therapy. For T3 or T4 GBC, we now consider PET a potentially important staging adjunct in patient selection for radical surgery.



### Neoadjuvant Therapy

There is a paucity of data about the role of neoadjuvant therapy for GBC. In fact, due to low response rates with adjuvant therapy, current standards require aggressive surgical resection for any disease that may be amenable to excision with negative margins. The only sizable series addressing this topic details 23 patients given continuous 5-fluorouracil (5-FU) and 45 Gy of external beam radiation therapy (EBRT) prior to surgical resection. Thus, the authors' conclusions were that neoadjuvant chemoradiation for GBC was not helpful, and in fact may be deleterious. While advances in adjuvant chemotherapy, namely the administration of gemcitabine and cisplatin, have provided guarded optimism, the rarity of this tumor and the general lack of regression in response to chemoradiation mean that, practically, neoadjuvant therapy for GBC should be considered selectively.

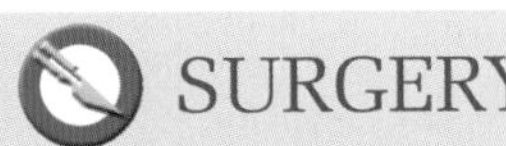

## SURGERY

When performing a cholecystectomy for presumed gallstone disease and intraoperative concern for GBC is raised, the surgeon should convert to an open operation (if begun laparoscopically) and explore the right upper quadrant for evidence of disease; any suspicious findings should prompt pathologic review. If GBC is confirmed and appears confined to the gallbladder, an extended cholecystectomy with en bloc hepatic resection and regional lymphadenectomy is indicated. If the surgeon's comfort with advanced hepatobiliary procedures is in question, then it would be most appropriate to close the incision and transfer the patient to a more experienced surgeon.

The surgical approach to GBC resection has varied historically. The spectrum has ranged from simple cholecystectomy to cholecystectomy with either (a) wedge resection of adjacent liver parenchyma, (b) formal segment IVB–V liver resection, or even (c) complete right/extended right hepatectomy as well as a subhilar lymphadenectomy. When a major hepatectomy is not required by tumor location, determining the optimal extent of the hepatectomy may be difficult, as it has not been well studied. While some investigators have described laparoscopic cholecystectomy (LC) for GBC, there is risk of spillage, tumor dissemination, and port-site recurrence. If there is preoperative suspicion of GBC, the surgeon should plan an open operation. As noted above, simple cholecystectomy is adequate for T1a lesions. For resectable T1b lesions and larger, the standard has become a segment IVB–V liver resection (with, of course, cholecystectomy if the gallbladder has yet to be removed) with regional lymphadenectomy. In addition, this may include resection and reconstruction of the extrahepatic bile ducts.

## Day of Surgery/Positioning

Preoperative medical optimization, with particular emphasis placed on coronary and pulmonary disease, as well as preparation of blood products that may be required, will have been done. At operation, the patient is laid supine on the operating room table with appropriate preinduction measures taken. Communication with the anesthesiologist is critical. Data have shown that low central venous pressure maintained during parenchymal transection can lead to significantly lower blood loss. Likewise, mild Trendelenburg positioning may guard against air embolism during division of the liver. Epidural anesthesia may also be utilized to decrease postoperative narcotic requirements as well as decrease the incidence of postoperative pneumonia. Finally, preoperative preparation should include mobilization of ultrasonography equipment for intraoperative use. A right subcostal (Kocher) incision should provide adequate exposure to the critical structures of the right upper quadrant, with extension in the midline or to a chevron incision if required (see Figs. 18.7, 19.3 and 21.5).

## Subhilar Lymphadenectomy with or without Removal of the Extrahepatic Biliary Tree (see also Chapter 26)

- Once the abdomen is entered, the falciform ligament is divided and the bowel excluded from the operative field. Inspection of the abdomen should be performed to evaluate for metastatic disease.
- A Kocher maneuver will provide access to distant lymph nodes for evaluation, namely celiac, paraaortic, and retropancreatic (Fig. 27.3). Metastases in these nodes represent advanced disease. The portal structures from the duodenum to the hilum of the liver are dissected and inspected.

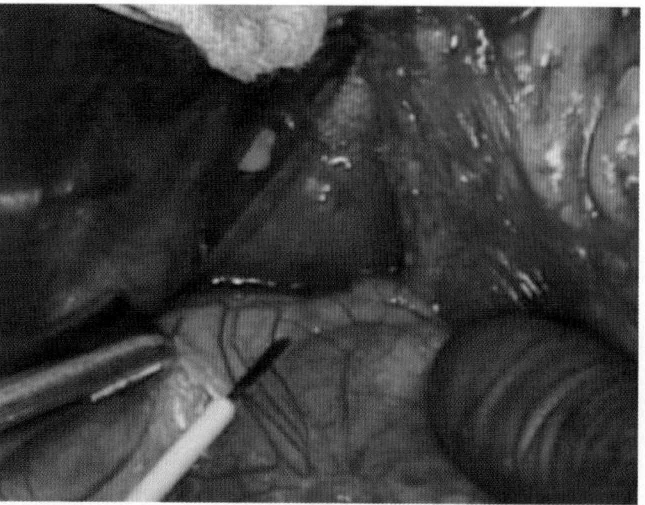

**Figure 27.3** Kocher maneuver.

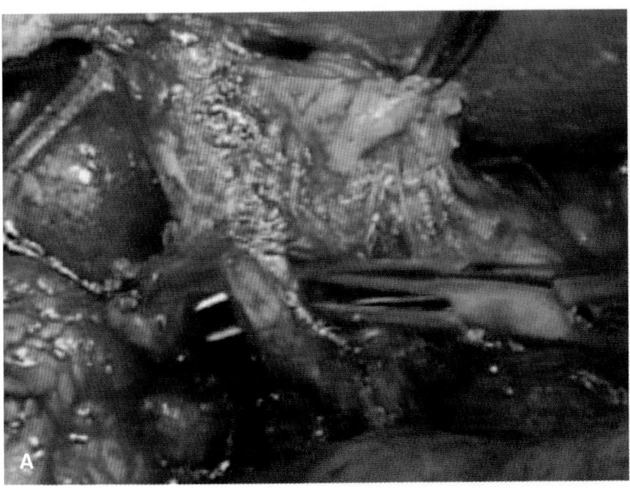


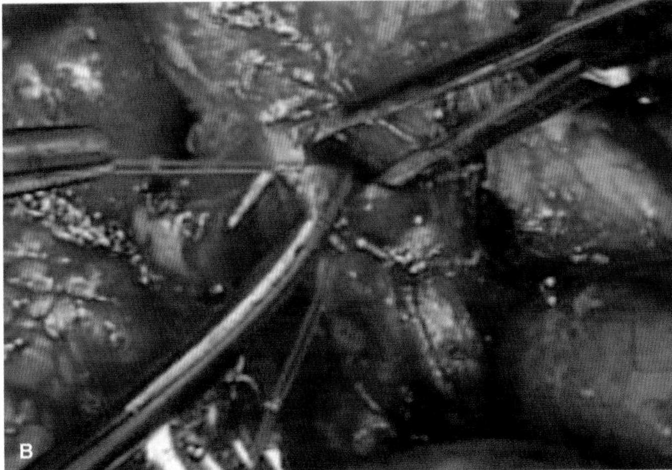


Figure 27.4 CBD is isolated **(A)** and divided **(B)**.



- Right gastric artery is ligated.
- All lymphatic tissue is swept upward and removed. If the CBD is to be removed, it is isolated and divided immediately above the duodenum (Fig. 27.4A, B). Stay sutures remain on the CBD to allow upward traction to expose the anterior surface of the portal vein (Fig. 27.5A, B).
- The subhilar vessels are skeletonized (Fig. 27.6). Arterial or venous involvement in the hepatoduodenal ligament should result in termination of the procedure.
- The hilar plate at the base of segment IV is lowered to identify the left hepatic duct, and the right hepatic artery (Fig. 27.7).

## Segments IVB and V Hepatic Resection

- If tumor is adherent to the right-sided vascular inflow structures, an extended right hepatectomy is mandated for complete resection and is discussed elsewhere (see Chapter 19). Disease in left-sided vascular or biliary structures is less likely controlled by surgery.
- The umbilical fissure is opened and the ligamentum teres is drawn to the patient's left (Fig. 27.8). The inflow vessels to segment IVB are dissected and divided (Fig. 27.9A, B) (see also Figs. 19.10, 21.8–21.10, and 24.7).

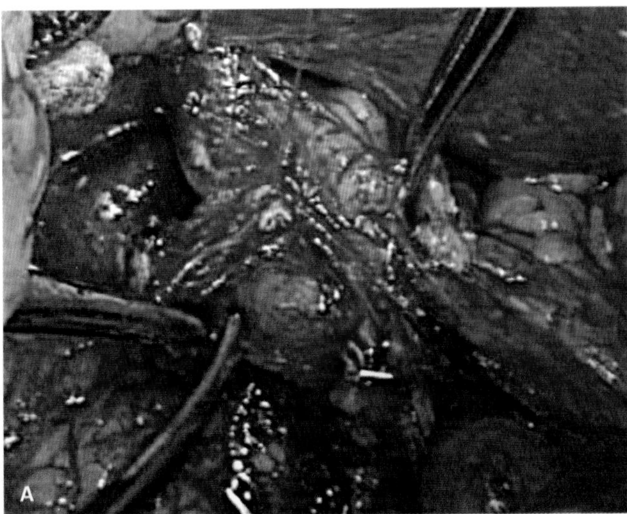


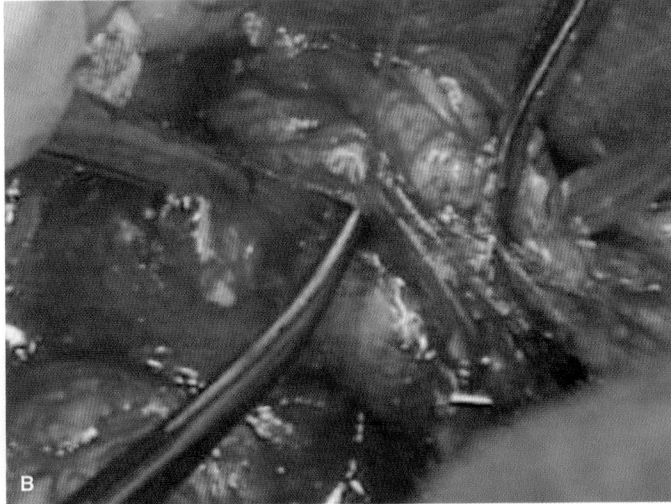


Figure 27.5 All lymphatic tissues are swept upward **(A)** and the anterior surface of the portal vein is exposed **(B)**.

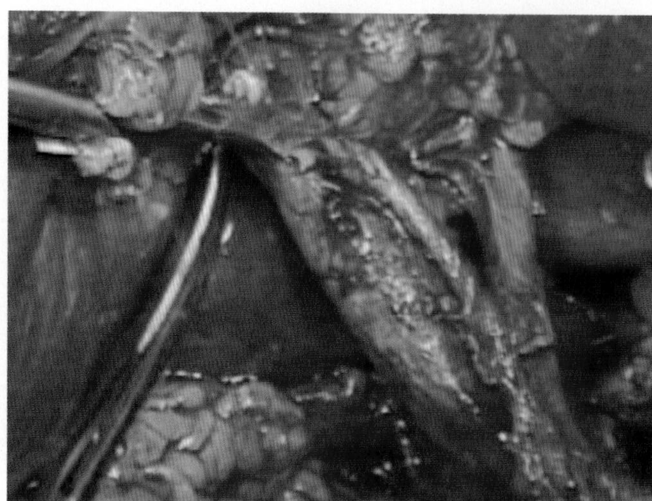

Figure 27.6 Subhilar vessels are skeletonized.

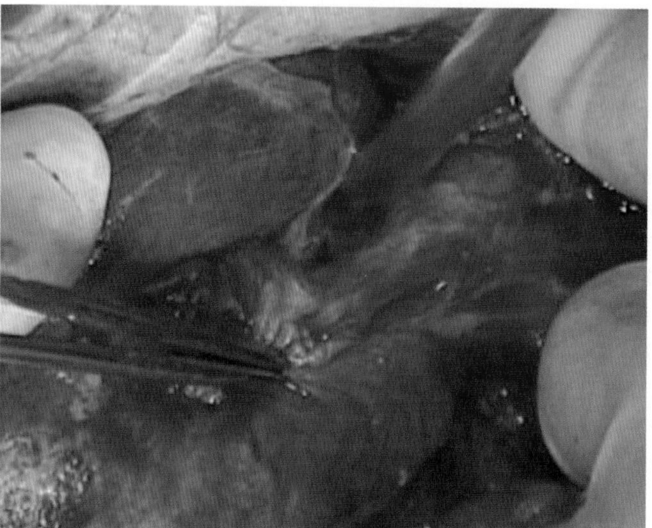

Figure 27.7 Hilar plate at the base of segment IV is lowered to identify the left hepatic duct and right hepatic artery.

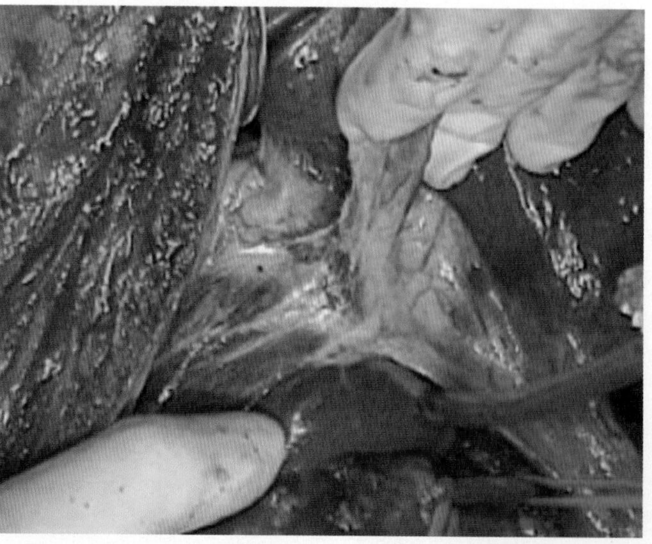

Figure 27.8 Ligamentum teres is drawn to the left.

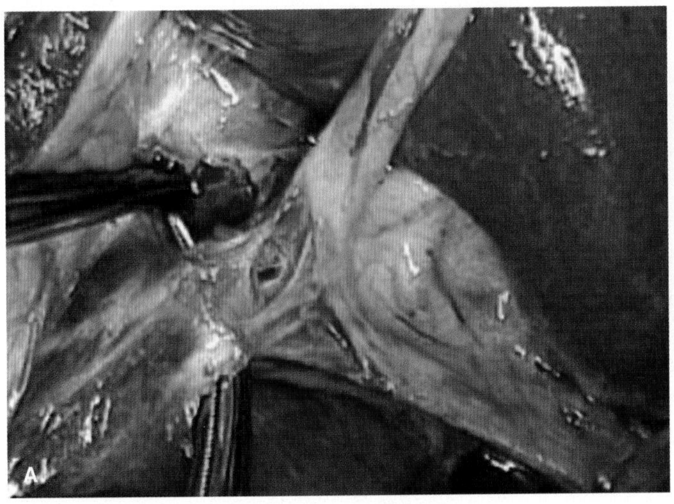


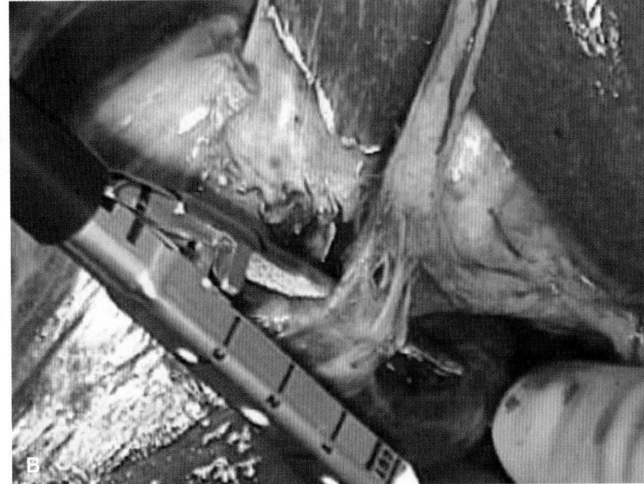


Figure 27.9 Inflow vessels to segment IVB are isolated **(A)** and divided **(B)**.

- Either the CBD or the cystic duct and artery are divided (Fig. 27.10), depending on the need for en bloc bile duct resection.
- The capsule of the liver is scored to mark the line of parenchymal transaction and continued on the inferior surface of the liver to pass anterior to right portal pedicle (if a right lobectomy is not necessary) (Fig. 27.11A).
- Stay sutures are placed and transaction begins medially (Fig. 27.11B). The middle hepatic vein will be encountered and divided (Fig. 27.12). Next, the segment V pedicle will be encountered and divided (Fig. 27.13). The remaining parenchyma between segments V and VI is divided.

Hemostasis is achieved with the argon beam coagulator and a flap of omentum can be placed within the liver bed.

## Hepaticojejunostomy (see also Figs. 17.13–17.15 and Fig 29.8)

- A Roux-en-Y limb is created and brought up in either a retrocolic or anticolic position.
- The left hepatic duct or CBD is prepared for anastomosis (Fig. 27.14). If necessary any caudate ducts can be joined with the left hepatic duct with a vicryl suture (Fig. 27.15). The left duct can also be enlarged with Potts scissors if necessary (Fig. 27.16).
- Anterior sutures can be placed in the bile duct and held on traction. An enterotomy is made in the bowel. Interrupted sutures are placed and serially held. The posterior row is performed first between full thickness of jejunum and bile duct (Fig. 27.17A).

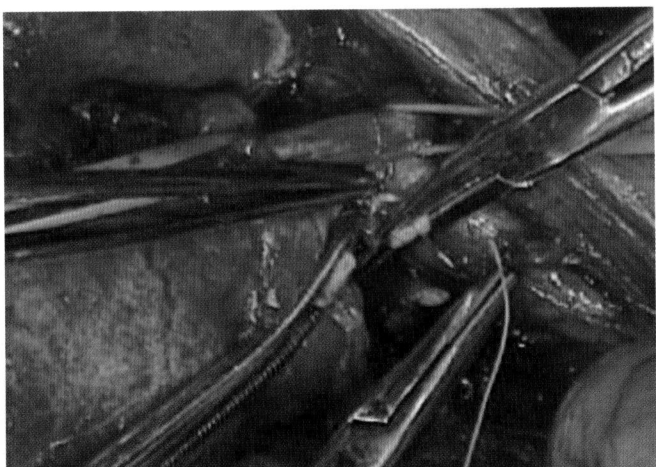

Figure 27.10 Dividing the cystic duct.

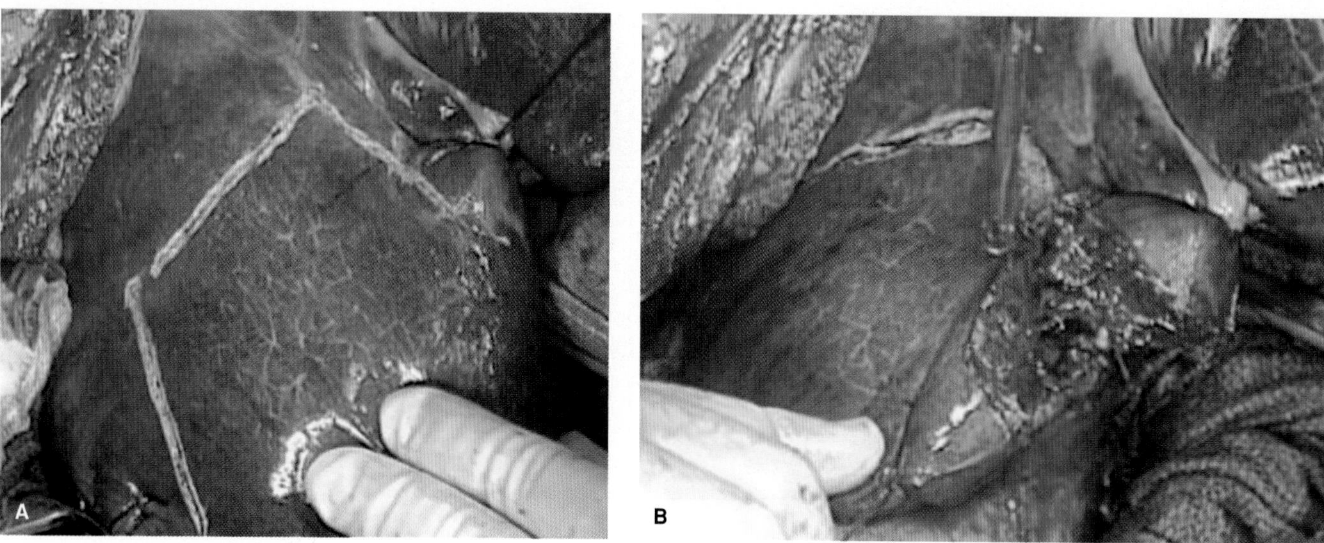

Figure 27.11 Line of transaction for segments IVB and V **(A)**, and parenchymal transection **(B)**.

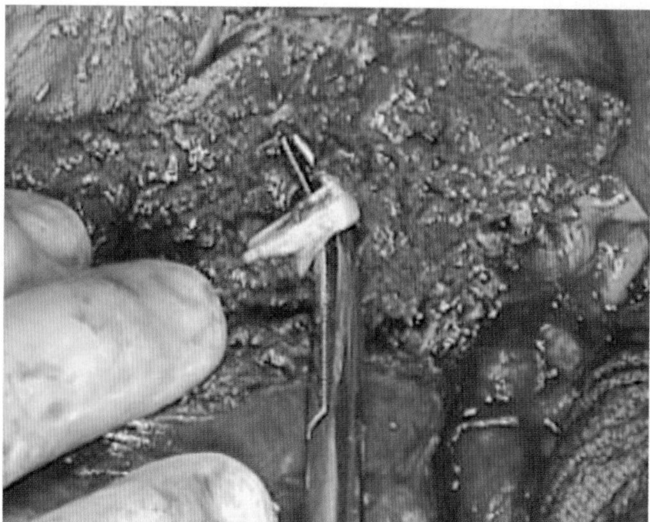

Figure 27.12 Isolating the middle hepatic vein.

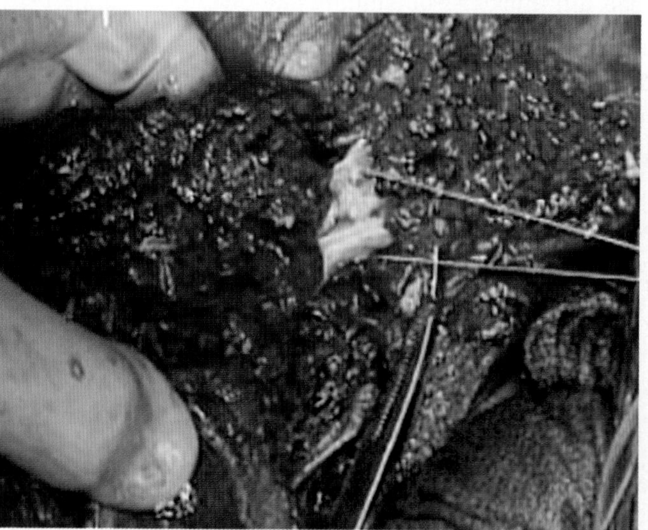

Figure 27.13 Isolation of segment V pedicle.

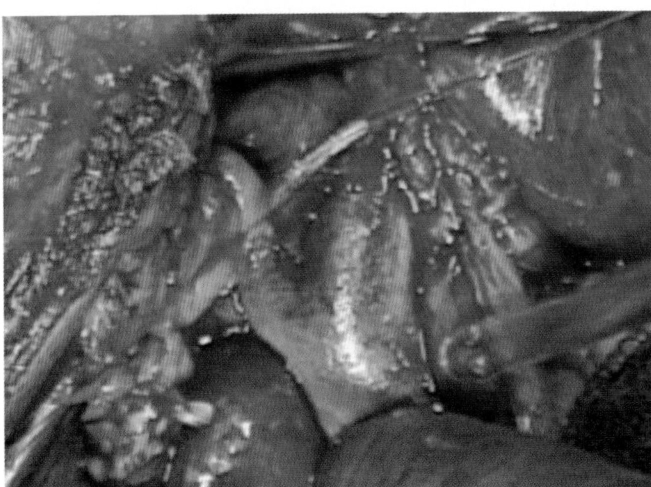

Figure 27.14 Left hepatic duct on stay sutures.

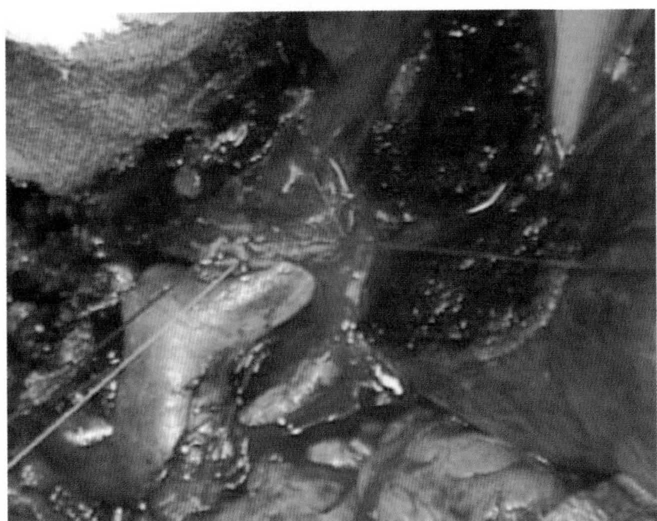

Figure 27.15 Joining the caudate and left hepatic ducts.

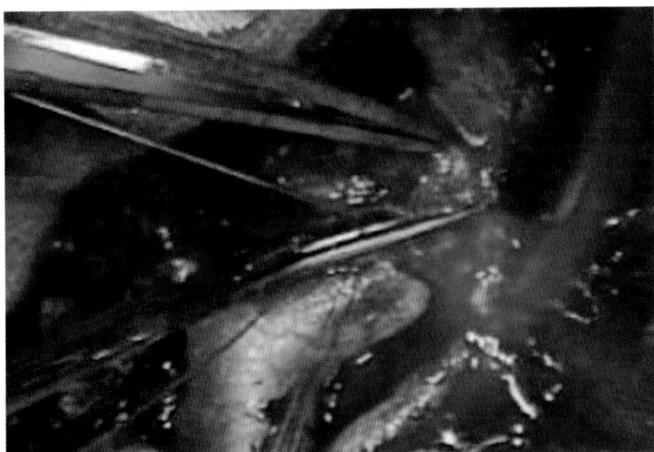

Figure 27.16 Enlarging the left hepatic duct with Pott's scissors.

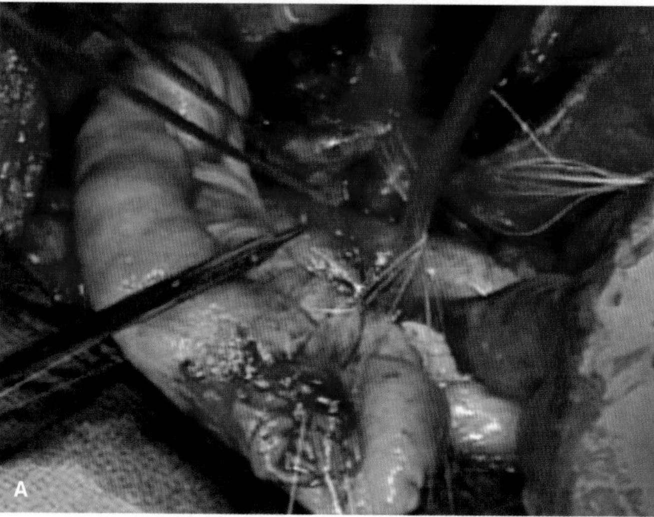


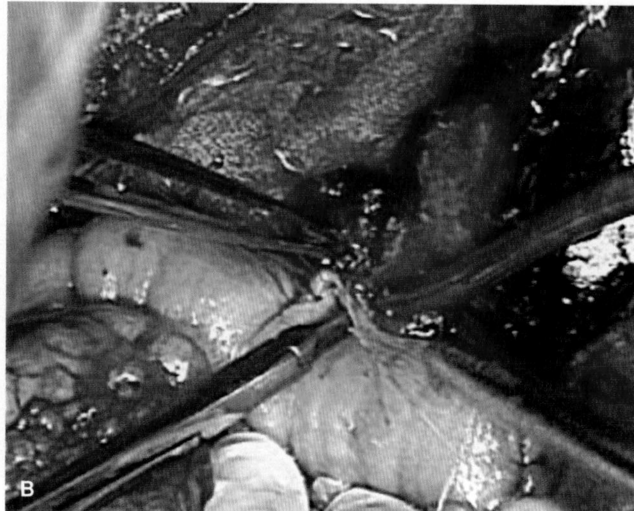


Figure 27.17 Posterior row of hepaticojejunostomy is placed **(A)**, and then the anterior row is completed **(B)**.

- Next the anterior layer is completed with good mucosa-to-mucosa apposition (Fig. 27.17B).
- The ligamentum teres is sutured to the jejunum to limit tension on the anastomosis (Fig. 27.18).

# POSTOPERATIVE MANAGEMENT

Immediately postoperatively, maintaining central venous pressure and close monitoring for symptoms and signs of hemorrhage are important. Hepatic regeneration may require substantial phosphate replacement, and close attention should be paid to this and other electrolyte abnormalities. In the absence of a pronounced ileus, a diet can be introduced and advanced early.

## Follow-up

The majority of recurrences are seen within 2 years of resection. Postoperative follow-up should include biannual 3-dimensional imaging of the chest, abdomen, and pelvis for at least 2 years, though this recommendation is not based on high-quality evidence.

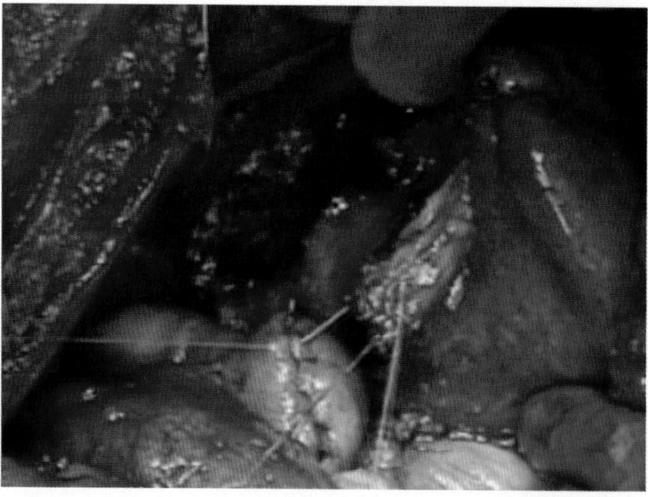

Figure 27.18 Ligamentum teres is secured to the jejunum.

### Adjuvant Therapy

Generally, chemotherapy is indicated for patients with evidence of advanced disease, which is to say, patients with positive margins or known metastases. The question of utilizing chemotherapy for node-positive disease is still unresolved. Traditionally, chemotherapy has been 5-FU based. Special attention should be paid to the increasing use of gemcitabine as an adjunctive therapy. In clinical trials, gemcitabine has been used in variable dosing regimens (800 to 1,000 mg/m$^2$) and with other agents, including pemetrexed, 5-FU/leucovorin, and capecitabine. Median survival in these studies ranged from 6.6 to 16 months. The role of radiation therapy as adjuvant therapy for GBA is even more poorly defined.

## COMPLICATIONS



### Bile Duct Injury/Leak

Perhaps the most feared complication of biliary surgery is unintentional injury of bile ducts that are not involved in resection and, thus, will be critical to biliary drainage from remaining liver segments. Attention should be paid especially when energy devices are used in proximity to essential draining ducts. Simple bile leaks from liver parenchyma will almost always be self-limiting, with adequate internal and/or external decompression (endoscopic stent placement with or without sphincterotomy and percutaneous drainage of the biloma). Furthermore, if a CBD resection has been performed and the reconstruction has, by definition, eliminated the downstream sphincter, this should aid resolution.

### Port-site Disease

Decades of operative experience and the evolution of laparoscopic cholecystectomy have led to the oft-described and universally concerning phenomenon of port-site disease. Evidence for this entity and suggested treatment are born of case series and reports. A Japanese study has published a report of 28 laparoscopic cholecystectomies performed for GBC; three patients developed port-site recurrences. Another large series of 37 patients with undiagnosed GBC who underwent LC demonstrated a 14% port-site recurrence rate. In addition, this and other studies found an increased incidence of disseminated disease when the gallbladder was perforated during LC. With this in mind, the practice of port-site excision at the time of radical resection seems justified, adding minimal morbidity while perhaps eliminating a devastating process.

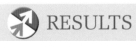

## RESULTS

Survival is closely correlated to stage, with 5-year survival ranging from 60% to 1%, for stage 0–IV disease, respectively, in a retrospective review of 2,500 patients (Fig. 27.19). Patients with less invasive disease will exhibit better long-term disease-free and overall survival, and are more likely to benefit from aggressive surgical therapy. In fact, even patients with carcinoma in regional lymph nodes may enjoy a 45% to 60% 5-year survival with en bloc resection and regional lymphadenectomy. Duffy et al. reported a median survival for all patients in a 10-year study from MSKCC at 10.3 months; substratification revealed median survival of 12.0 and 5.8 months for stages IA–III and IV, respectively. For tumors confined to the gallbladder mucosa, simple cholecystectomy was associated with up to 90% to 100% disease-specific survival. For tumors invading the muscular and serosal layers of the gallbladder, results have varied by extent of disease and extent of resection. The treatment of more extensive tumors invading into the liver and adjacent organs has been more controversial. These tumors tend to be more invasive and require more extensive resections, which previously have not resulted in improved long-term survival with the exception of node-negative tumors.

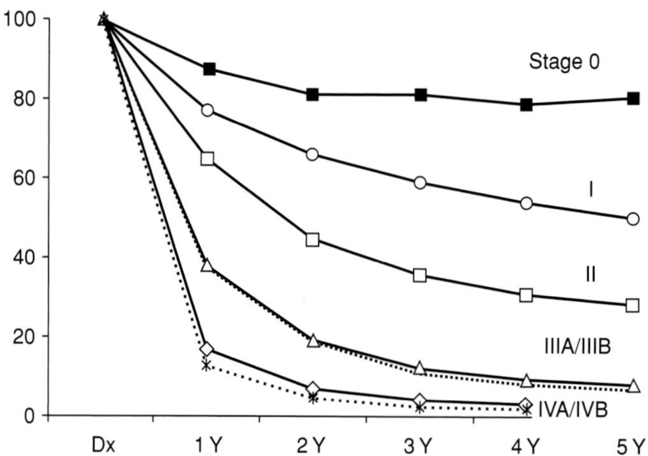


Figure 27.19 Five-year survival based on disease stage.

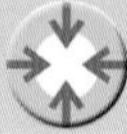

## CONCLUSIONS

GBC remains a dire disease. A fortunate few will be diagnosed at an early stage and cured by aggressive surgical therapy, whereas the majority of patients will be relegated to palliative therapy. Here we have detailed the appropriate workup, indications (and contraindications) for surgery, as well as an accepted operative approach. Resection can (and should) be accomplished with minimal mortality and acceptable morbidity so that a selected cohort of patients can enjoy extended survival. Future improvements in outcome will rely on primarily nonsurgical therapeutics and improved screening/diagnostic mechanisms.

## Recommended References and Readings


Ahmad SA, AE, Spitz FR. Hepatobiliary cancers. In: Feig B, Berger DH, Fuhrman GM, eds. *The MD Anderson Surgical Oncology Handbook*. Philadelphia, PA: Lippincott Williams and Wilkins; 2003:266–302.

Alberts SR, Al-Khatib H, Mahoney MR, et al. Gemcitabine, 5-fluorouracil, and leucovorin in advanced biliary tract and gallbladder carcinoma: a North Central Cancer Treatment Group phase II trial. *Cancer.* 2005;103(1):111–118.

Alberts SR, Sande JR, Foster NR, et al. Pemetrexed and gemcitabine for biliary tract and gallbladder carcinomas: a North Central Cancer Treatment Group (NCCTG) phase I and II Trial, N9943. *J Gastrointest Cancer.* 2007;38(2–4):87–94.

Bach AM, Loring LA, Hann LE, et al. Gallbladder cancer: can ultrasonography evaluate extent of disease? *J Ultrasound Med.* 1998; 17(5):303–309.

Boss P, Lanier AP, Dohan PH, et al. Cancers of the gallbladder and the biliary tract in Alaskan natives: 1970–1979. *J Natl Cancer Inst.* 1982;69(5):1005–1007.

Cho JY, Nam JS, Park MS, et al. A Phase II study of capecitabine combined with gemcitabine in patients with advanced gallbladder carcinoma. *Yonsei Med J.* 2005;46(4):526–531.

Corvera CU, Blumgart LH, Akhurst T, et al. 18F-fluorodeoxyglucose positron emission tomography influences management decisions in patients with biliary cancer. *J Am Coll Surg.* 2008;206(1): 57–65.

D'Angelica M, Dalal KM, DeMatteo RP, et al. Analysis of the extent of resection for adenocarcinoma of the gallbladder. *Ann Surg Oncol.* 2009;16(4):806–816.

de Aretxabala X, Losada H, Mora J, et al. [Neoadjuvant chemoradiotherapy in gallbladder cancer]. *Rev Med Chil.* 2004;132(1):51–57.

Donohue JH, Stewart AK, Menck HR. The National Cancer Data Base report on carcinoma of the gallbladder, 1989–1995. *Cancer.* 1998;83(12):2618–2628.

Duffy A, Capanu M, Abou-Alfa GK, et al. Gallbladder cancer (GBC): 10-year experience at Memorial Sloan-Kettering Cancer Centre (MSKCC). *J Surg Oncol.* 2008;98(7):485–489.

Fong Y, Brennan MF, Turnbull A, et al. Gallbladder cancer discovered during laparoscopic surgery. Potential for iatrogenic tumor dissemination. *Arch Surg.* 1993;128(9):1054–1056.

Fong Y, Heffernan N, Blumgart LH. Gallbladder carcinoma discovered during laparoscopic cholecystectomy: aggressive reresection is beneficial. *Cancer.* 1998;83(3):423–427.

Fong Y, Jarnagin W, Blumgart LH. Gallbladder cancer: comparison of patients presenting initially for definitive operation with those presenting after prior noncurative intervention. *Ann Surg.* 2000;232(4):557–569.

Fong Y, Malhotra S. Gallbladder cancer: recent advances and current guidelines for surgical therapy. *Adv Surg.* 2001;35:1–20.

Fong Y, Wagman L, Gonen M, et al. Evidence-based gallbladder cancer staging: changing cancer staging by analysis of data from the National Cancer Database. *Ann Surg.* 2006;243(6):767–771; discussion 771–774.

Gallbladder Cancer. In: Greene FL, et al, eds. *AJCC Cancer Staging Atlas.* New York, NY: Springer; 2006:134–138.

Hawkins WG, DeMatteo RP, Jarnagin WR, et al. Jaundice predicts advanced disease and early mortality in patients with gallbladder cancer. *Ann Surg Oncol.* 2004;11(3):310–315.

Ito H, Hann LE, D'Angelica M, et al. Polypoid lesions of the gallbladder: diagnosis and followup. *J Am Coll Surg.* 2009;208(4):570–575.

Jemal A, Siegel R, Ward E, et al. Cancer statistics, 2008. *CA Cancer J Clin.* 2008;58(2):71–96.

Kim JH, Kim WH, Yoo BM, et al. Should we perform surgical management in all patients with suspected porcelain gallbladder? *Hepatogastroenterology.* 2009;56(93):943–945.

Koga A, Watanabe K, Fukuyama T, et al. Diagnosis and operative indications for polypoid lesions of the gallbladder. *Arch Surg.* 1988;123(1):26–29.

Krain. Gallbladder and extrahepatic bile duct carcinoma. *Geriatrics.* 1972;27(11):111–117.

Kubota K, Bandai Y, Noie T, et al. How should polypoid lesions of the gallbladder be treated in the era of laparoscopic cholecystectomy? *Surgery.* 1995;117(5):481–487.

Mainprize KS, Gould SW, Gilbert JM. Surgical management of polypoid lesions of the gallbladder. *Br J Surg.* 2000;87(4):414–417.

Melendez JA, Arslan V, Fischer ME, et al. Perioperative outcomes of major hepatic resections under low central venous pressure anesthesia: blood loss, blood transfusion, and the risk of postoperative renal dysfunction. *J Am Coll Surg.* 1998;187(6):620–625.

Nevin JE, Moran TJ, Kay S, et al. Carcinoma of the gallbladder: staging, treatment, and prognosis. *Cancer.* 1976;37(1):141–148.

Onoyama H, Yamamoto M, Tseng A, et al. Extended cholecystectomy for carcinoma of the gallbladder. *World J Surg.* 1995; 19(5):758–763.

Rajagopalan V, Daines WP, Grossbard ML, et al. Gallbladder and biliary tract carcinoma: A comprehensive update, Part 1. *Oncology (Williston Park).* 2004;18(7):889–896.

Shirai Y, Yoshida K, Tsukada K, et al. Radical surgery for gallbladder carcinoma. Long-term results. *Ann Surg.* 1992;216(5):565–568.

Shoup M, Fong Y. Surgical indications and extent of resection in gallbladder cancer. *Surg Oncol Clin N Am.* 2002;11(4):985–994.

Stephen AE, Berger DL. Carcinoma in the porcelain gallbladder: a relationship revisited. *Surgery.* 2001;129(6):699–703.

Terzi C, Sökmen S, Seçkin S, et al. Polypoid lesions of the gallbladder: report of 100 cases with special reference to operative indications. *Surgery.* 2000;127(6):622–627.

Towfigh S, McFadden DW, Cortina GR, et al. Porcelain gallbladder is not associated with gallbladder carcinoma. *Am Surg.* 2001; 67(1):7–10.

Wakai T, Shirai Y, Hatakeyama K. Radical second resection provides survival benefit for patients with T2 gallbladder carcinoma first discovered after laparoscopic cholecystectomy. *World J Surg.* 2002;26(7):867–871.

Wanebo HJ, Vezeridis MP. Treatment of gallbladder cancer. *Cancer Treat Res.* 1994;69:97–109.

Weiland ST, Mahvi DM, Niederhuber JE, et al. Should suspected early gallbladder cancer be treated laparoscopically? *J Gastrointest Surg.* 2002;6(1):50–56; discussion 56–57.

Wibbenmeyer LA, Sharafuddin MJ, Wolverson MK, et al. Sonographic diagnosis of unsuspected gallbladder cancer: imaging findings in comparison with benign gallbladder conditions. *AJR Am J Roentgenol.* 1995;165(5):1169–1174.

Z'Graggen K, Birrer S, Maurer CA, et al. Incidence of port site recurrence after laparoscopic cholecystectomy for preoperatively unsuspected gallbladder carcinoma. *Surgery.* 1998;124(5):831–838.

# 28 Treatment of Liver Cysts

T. Peter Kingham and Ronald P. DeMatteo

## Introduction

Hepatic cysts can be divided into neoplastic and non-neoplastic categories. Non-neoplastic cysts are may be further subdivided into parasitic and non-parasitic cysts, with the latter group comprised of simple hepatic cysts and polycystic liver disease. Benign or simple hepatic cysts are likely a result of congenital malformation of intrahepatic biliary ducts that gradually enlarge over time. Approximately 4% to 7% of the general population has simple hepatic cysts, the majority of which cause no symptoms and rarely affect liver function. Polycystic liver disease is an inherited disorder, commonly associated with polycystic kidney disease, and often causes symptoms that require intervention. Hydatid disease, the most clinically relevant parasitic cystic lesion, is uncommon outside of endemic areas of the world and is the result of infestation with *Ecchinococcus granulosus* or, less commonly, *Ecchinococcus multilocularis.* Biliary cystadenoma or cystadenocarcinoma are the most common neoplastic cystic diseases of the liver but are extremely uncommon. Cystadenomas are benign but premalignant tumors that must be resected completely; it is critical, therefore, to distinguish them from simple cysts. In addition, it is important to recognize that some malignant liver lesions may have a large cystic component but are not typically considered as hepatic cysts (Fig. 28.1).

Treatment of cystic liver lesions varies and is critically dependent on the diagnosis and the presence or absence of symptoms. Imaging plays a central role in diagnosis and establishing the most appropriate therapy. Simple cysts, the most common diagnosis encountered in clinical practice, are generally sharply demarcated from the surrounding liver parenchyma. Simple cysts are comprised of thin, clear fluid, usually clear in color and appear as homogeneous hypodense lesions on CT (Fig. 28.2A). Other imaging modalities, however, particularly US and MRI, provide more useful for evaluating cystic lesion. On US, simple cysts are characteristically thin walled, with a uniform appearance of the intracystic contents and posterior acoustic shadowing (Fig. 28.2B). On MRI, simple cysts are uniformly hyperintense on T2-weighted images (Fig. 28.2C) and show no evidence of perfusion on the post-gadolinium sequences (Fig. 28.2D). The classic imaging appearance of simple cysts may be altered, however, by changes in the cyst contents. Intracystic hemorrhage, in particular, can result in accumulation of proteinaceous debris that results in a complex appearance on imaging (i.e., heterogeneous, thick walled, internal septae Fig. 28.3A, B), that is difficult to distinguish from biliary cystadenoma (Fig. 28.4). Polycystic liver disease and hydatid disease are both associated with multiple cysts. Hydatid disease is characterized by multiple, clustered, thick-walled daughter cysts (Fig. 28.5); the

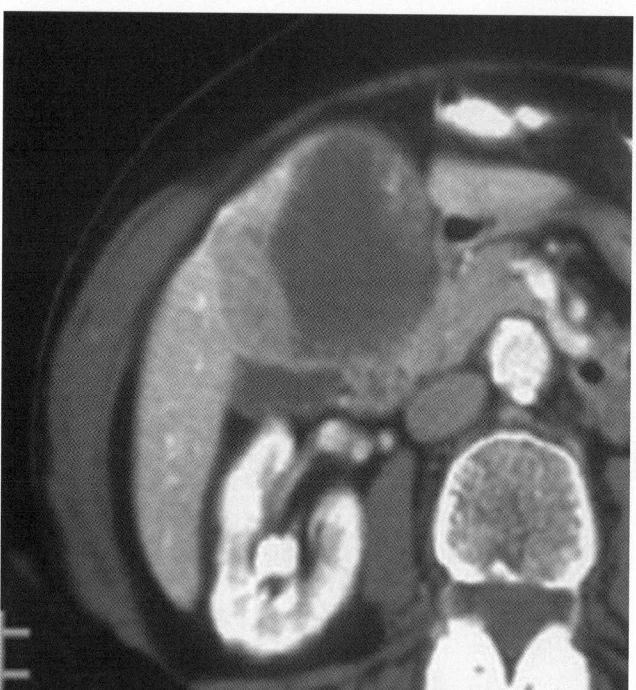

**Figure 28.1** Primary leiomyosarcoma of the liver with a large cystic component. Note the irregular cyst wall.

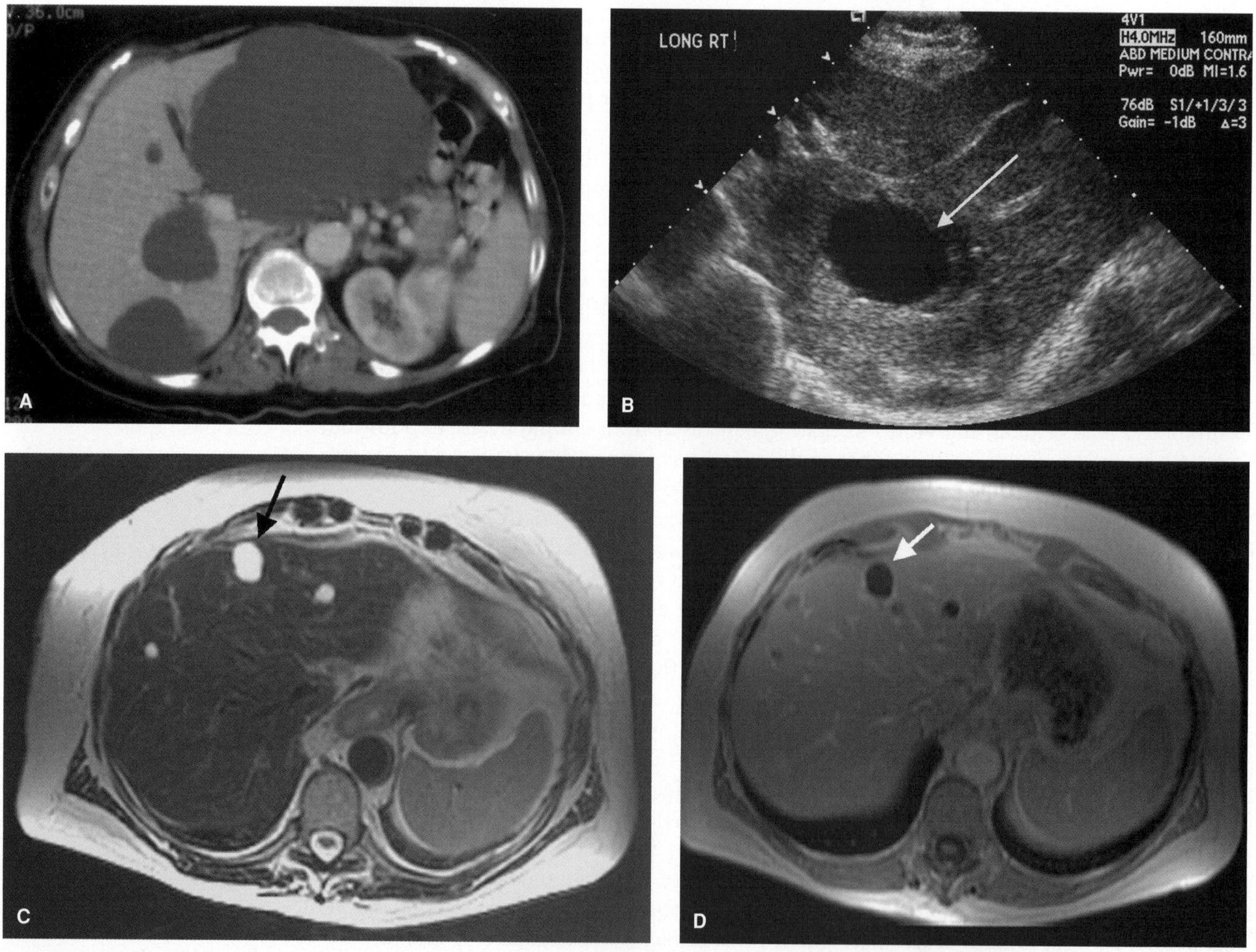

**Figure 28.2** CT scan with hypodense appearance of simple hepatic cyst (**A**). Ultrasound demonstrates a simple thin-walled cyst (**B**). T2-weighted MRI image shows a simple hyperintense cyst (**C**). MRI post-gadolinium sequences demonstrate no evidence of perfusion of the cyst (**D**).

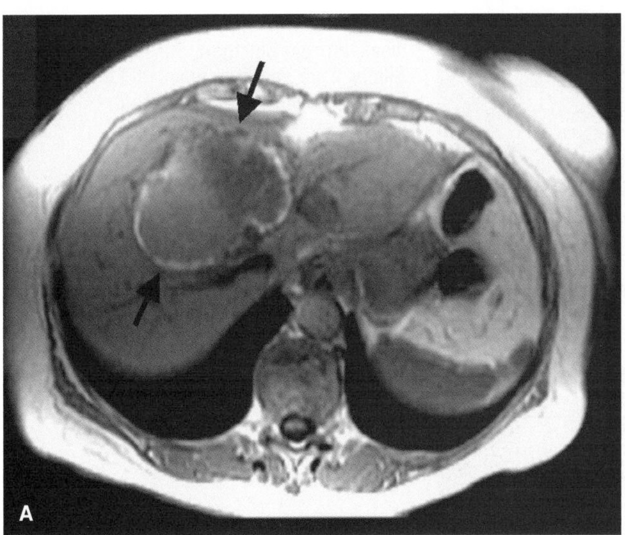


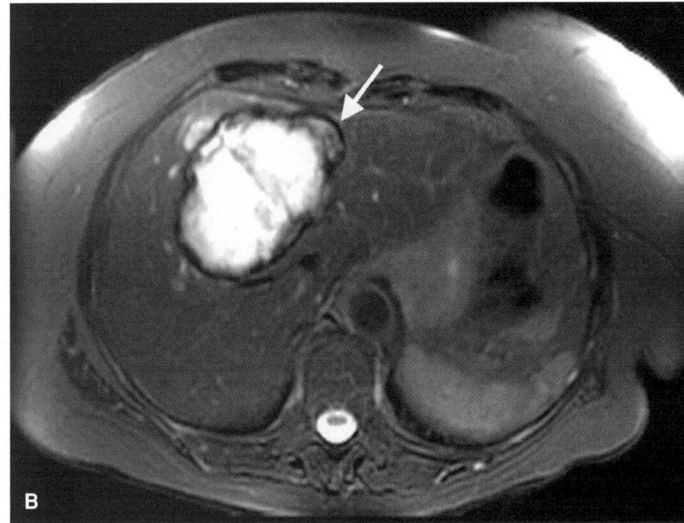


**Figure 28.3** MRI of cyst demonstrates intracystic hemorrhage with thick-walled rim (*arrows,* **A**). MRI of cyst with hemorrhage and a heterogeneous appearance of the cyst (*arrow,* **B**).

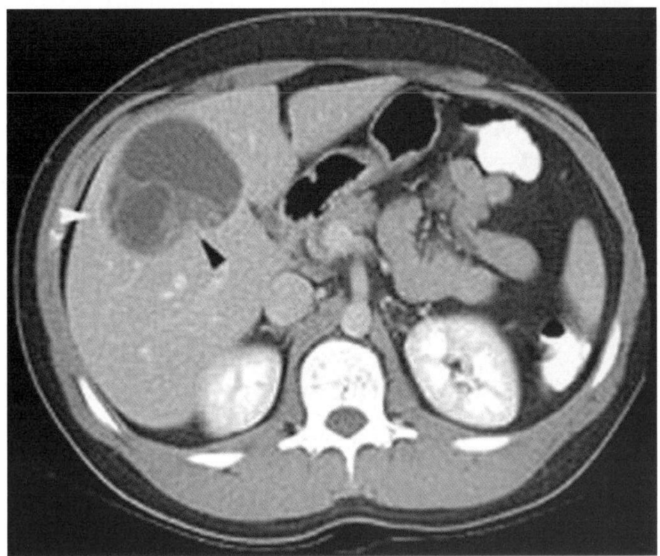

**Figure 28.4** CT scan of biliary cystadenoma with thickened septum.

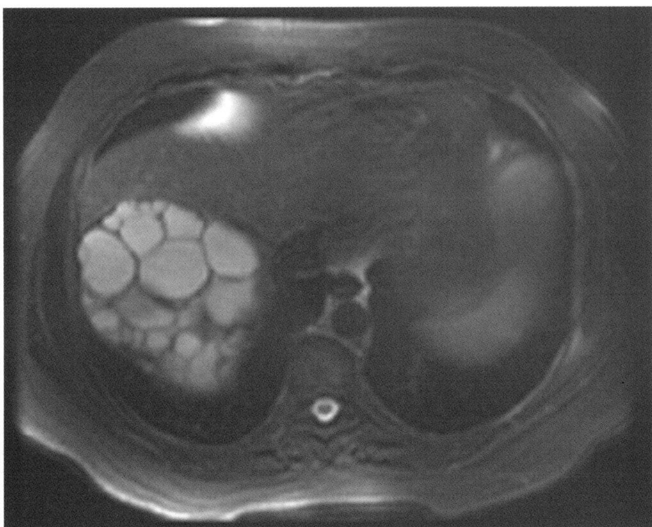

**Figure 28.5** MRI demonstrates hydatid cyst with multiple, clustered, thick-walled daughter cysts.

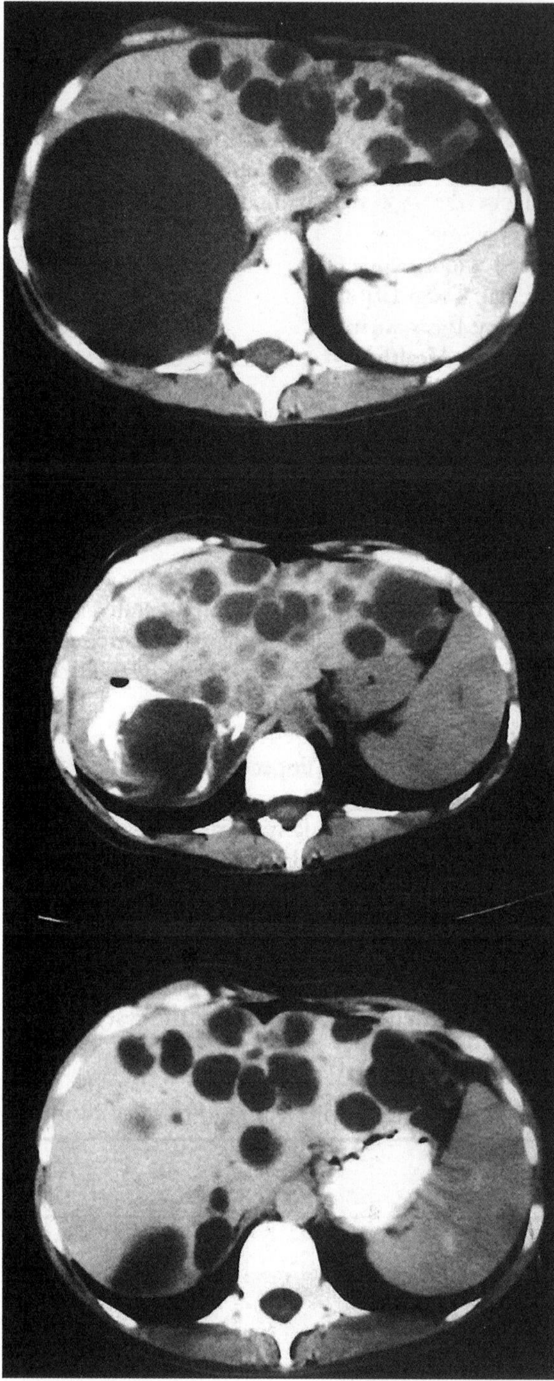

**Figure 28.6** Demonstration of polycystic liver disease (from Blumgart, Surgery of the Liver, Biliary Tract and Pancreas, 4th Edition, Saunders, 2007, with permission).

diagnosis is confirmed with a history of exposure in an endemic area and elevated ecchinococcal titers. Polycystic liver disease, on the other hand, appears as diffuse involvement of the liver with innumerable simple cysts (Fig. 28.6).

Treatment of cystic lesions include:

- Aspiration
- Sclerosis
- Enucleation
- Fenestration
- Resection

When indicated, primarily for symptoms, unroofing or fenestration of simple cysts is the procedure of choice. Unroofing or fenestration of hepatic cysts was first described in 1968. More recently, minimally invasive techniques have been utilized for laparoscopic unroofing. Before one proceeds with cyst fenestration as the definitive procedure, one must exclude other entities. Cystadenoma or cystadenocarcinoma are the most common confounding diagnoses and must be resected rather than opened; hydatid disease rarely causes diagnostic confusion, as discussed above. One option in such cases is laparoscopic or open excisional biopsy of the cyst wall with frozen section histology, which can usually distinguish simple from neoplastic cysts. Percutaneous drainage and sclerosis of simple cysts has been described, but reaccumulation of cyst fluid is common, and this procedure is currently reserved for patients with an infected cyst or patients who cannot tolerate general anesthesia. Extreme care must be taken to prove that there are no cyst-biliary tree connections before introducing a sclerosant.

## INDICATIONS/CONTRAINDICATIONS

Non-parasitic cysts:

Indications for treatment include:

- Infection
- Jaundice
- Cyst rupture and hemorrhage
- Early satiety
- Pain

Contraindications include:

- Asymptomatic cysts
- High concern for neoplastic diagnosis

## PREOPERATIVE PLANNING

There are several important preoperative investigations that assist in diagnosing and surgical planning, both generally and specifically related to cystic lesions (see also Chapter 18):

1. History: Polycystic kidney disease, abdominal pain, early satiety
2. Clinical examination: Jaundice, abdominal tenderness, stigmata of portal hypertension
3. Laboratory evaluations: Bilirubin, alkaline phosphatase, AST, ALT, serology if concern for hydatid disease, tumor markers (CEA, CA 19-9)
4. Radiologic work-up:
   a. US: Evaluates the patency of main hepatic pedicles and veins, the location of the cyst, the degree of biliary dilatation. Ultrasound is perhaps the most useful modality for assessing the cyst wall and cyst contents (Fig. 28.7).
   b. CT scan: Useful to determine the location of the cyst within the liver, the volume of the normal liver, whether a laparoscopic or open approach is appropriate (Fig. 28.8A, B).
   c. MRI: Provides additional information if there is a question on the CT scan as to the etiology of the cyst (Fig. 28.9).

## SURGICAL TECHNIQUE

### Unroofing of a Simple Cyst

Open or laparoscopic approaches can be utilized for unroofing of a simple cyst. Laparoscopic approaches are ideal for the majority of simple hepatic cysts. Open approaches may be required for cysts deep within the liver or in the posterior sector.

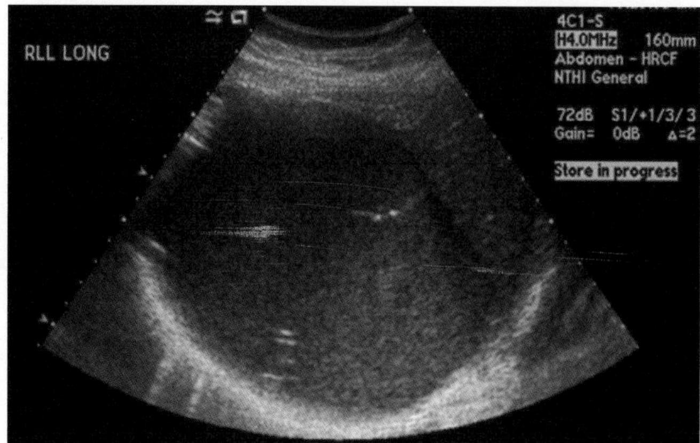


**Figure 28.7** Preoperative ultrasound of a right lobe hepatic cyst (arrow points to cyst). Note the single simple septum and smooth border of the cyst.

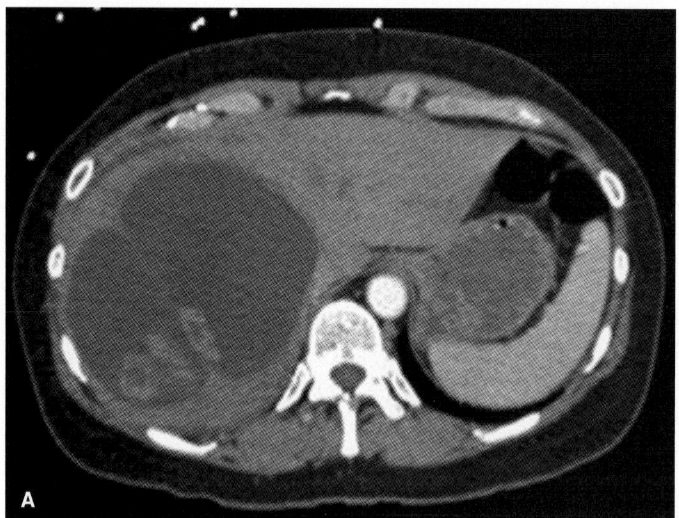


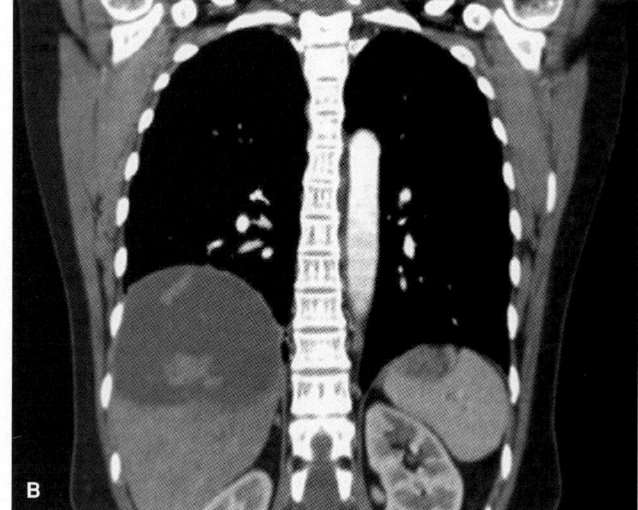


**Figure 28.8** Preoperative CT scan in axial (**A**) and coronal (**B**) sections of a right lobe hepatic cyst with hemorrhagic debris (arrow points to debris).

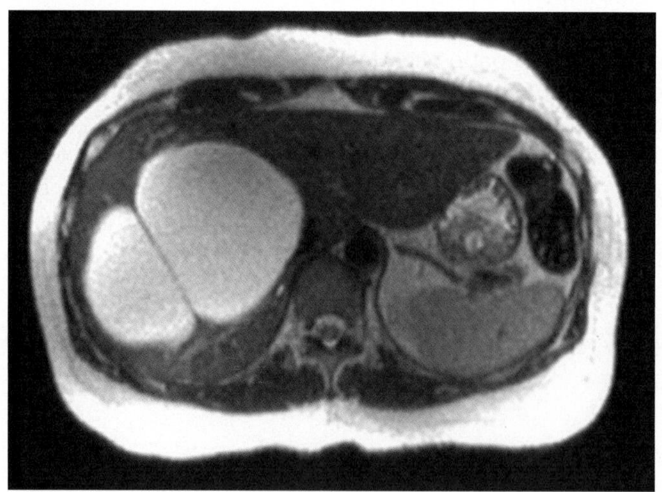

**Figure 28.9** Preoperative MRI of a right lobe hepatic cyst hyperintense on T1 imaging with a single simple septum.

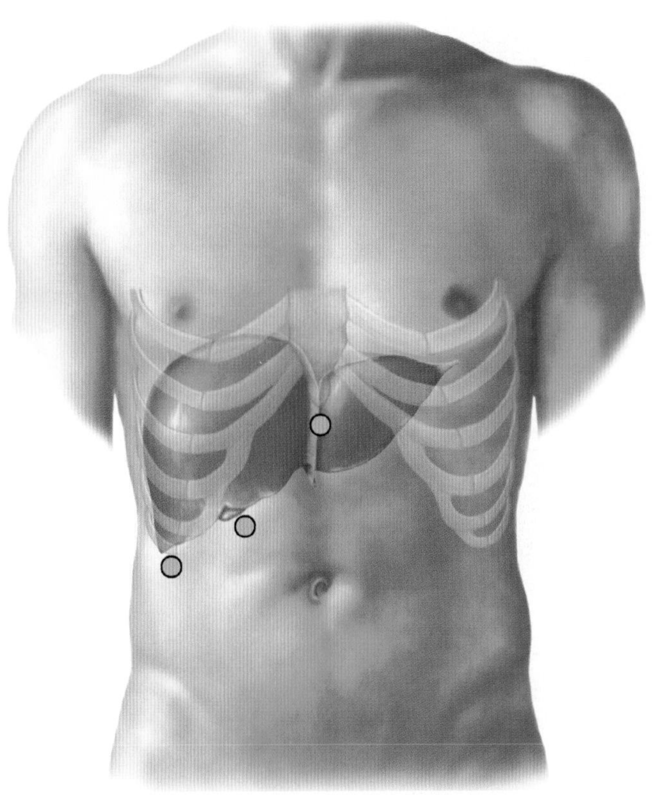

Figure 28.10 Port placement site for deroofing of the right hepatic lobe cyst demonstrated in Figures 28.7–28.9.



## Laparoscopic Unroofing of Hepatic Cysts

### Positioning

Patients are placed supine in the split leg position. A foley catheter and orogastric tube are placed on induction. Three ports are generally adequate to accommodate various combinations of a 30-degree camera, cutting instrument (harmonic scalpel, cautery, or scissors), a retracting forceps for holding the cyst wall, and a suction device. Port placement should be similar to port sites used during laparoscopic liver resections (Fig. 28.10) (see Chapter 31). If the cyst is large and extends to the mid-abdomen, ports can be placed at the level of the umbilicus in order to allow adequate space between the ports and the cyst (Fig. 28.11). Although it is possible to perform some cases with 5 mm ports, a 10 mm port may be required for utilizing 10 mm clips, vascular staplers, and a laparoscopic ultrasound probe.

### Surgical Technique

Hepatic ultrasound should be performed to help delineate the borders of the cyst and liver parenchyma (Fig. 28.12). In order to unroof the cyst, the dome of the cyst wall is elevated with a grasper and a small incision (the appropriate size to introduce a suction device) is made in the cyst wall (Fig. 28.13A–C). Draining the cyst contents makes the cyst wall pliable and thus easier to manipulate. Fluid from simple cysts is usually thin and clear; however, intracystic hemorrhage can result in fluid that is discolored and thicker in consistency. Adhesions from the cyst to the diaphragm and abdominal wall should be left intact until after the cyst has been drained, as once the cyst wall is pliable there will be a visible delineation between cyst wall and liver parenchyma (Fig. 28.14A).

Next, the visible cyst wall is excised with a harmonic scalpel, ligasure or stapling devices; electrocautery may be used but it should be kept in mind that the cyst wall is comprised of hepatic tissue and contains vascular structures that may bleed if not well controlled (Fig. 28.14B). The resection line should be at the interface between the normal liver parenchyma and the cyst wall. This allows for as complete a fenestration as

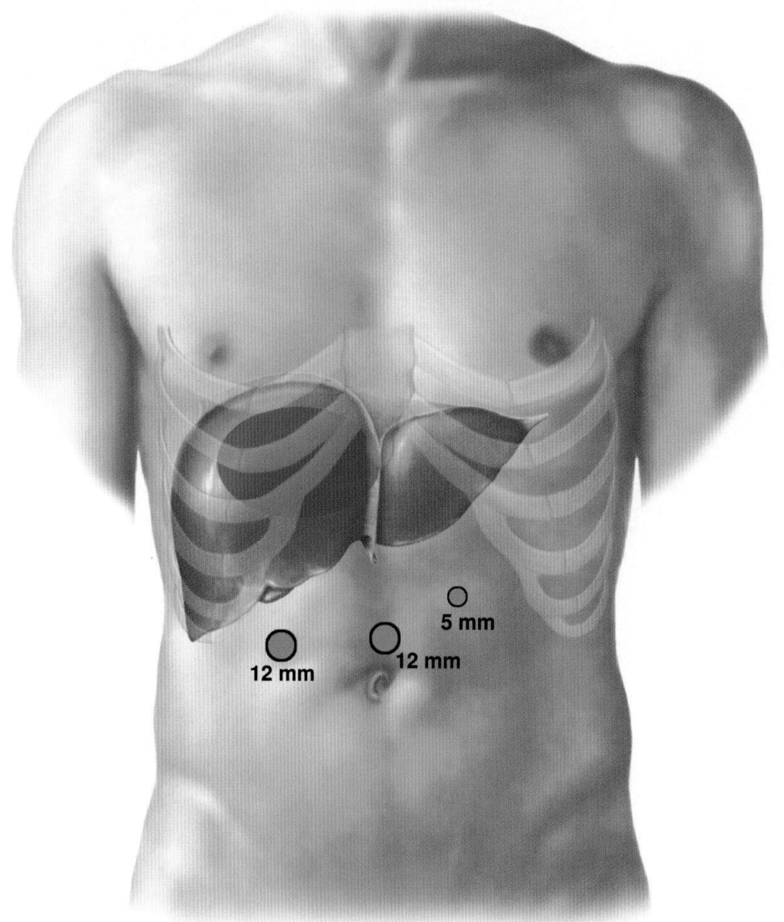


Figure 28.11 Port placement for large cysts of the right lobe and left lobe cysts.

possible and retraction of the intrahepatic cyst wall remnant to prevent the edges of the cyst from reapproximating, resulting in cyst recurrence. If the cyst is complex and has mural nodules, cytology of cyst fluid should be performed, and the cyst wall should be examined with frozen section histology if there is any question regarding the diagnosis, as described above. It is important to assure hemostasis at the remnant cyst wall after unroofing the cyst as this is a hypervascular area.

After the cyst is unroofed, the cyst cavity and residual cyst wall should be inspected. If there are remaining mural nodularities they should be biopsied. If less than 50% of

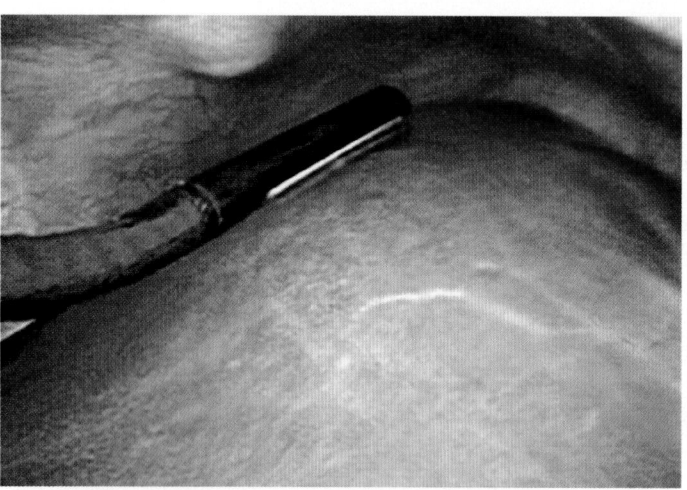

Figure 28.12 Laparoscopic ultrasound of simple cyst in dome of liver to determine borders.

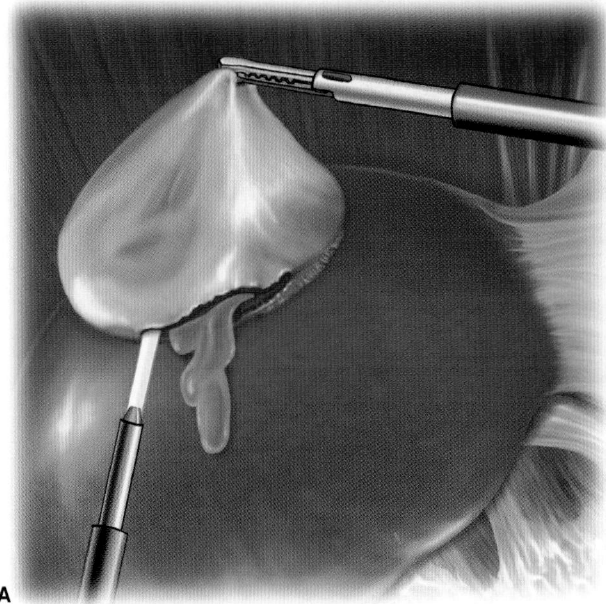

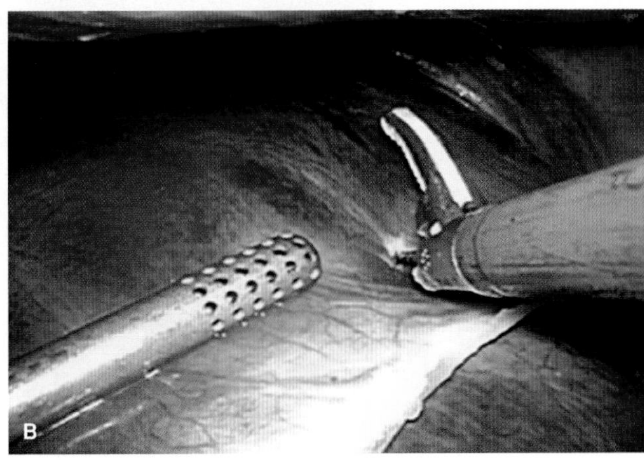

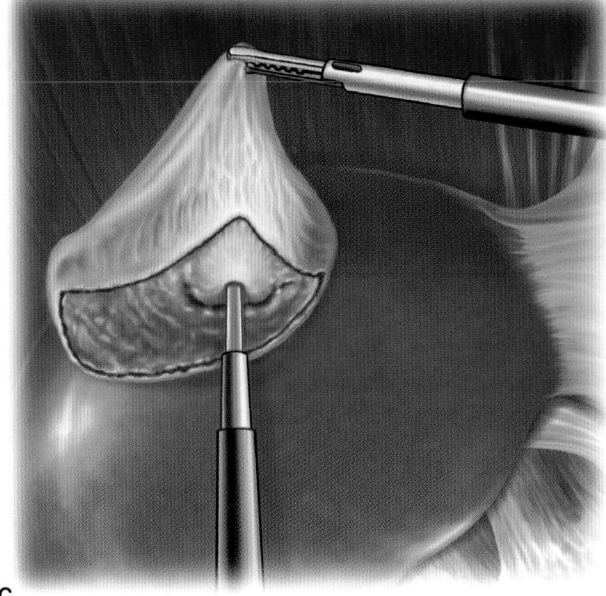

Figure 28.13 Laparoscopic cyst unroofing is initiated by grasping and elevating the cyst wall (**A**) and making a small incision to allow introduction of a suction device into the cyst cavity (**B**). (**C**) After aspirating the fluid, the lining of the wall should be inspected to ensure that it is consistent with a simple cyst. A generous portion of the cyst wall is then excised in order to prevent re-approximation of the edges and re-accumulation of fluid.



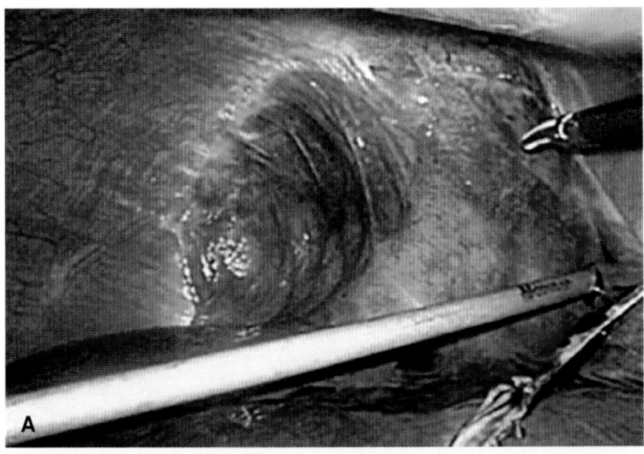

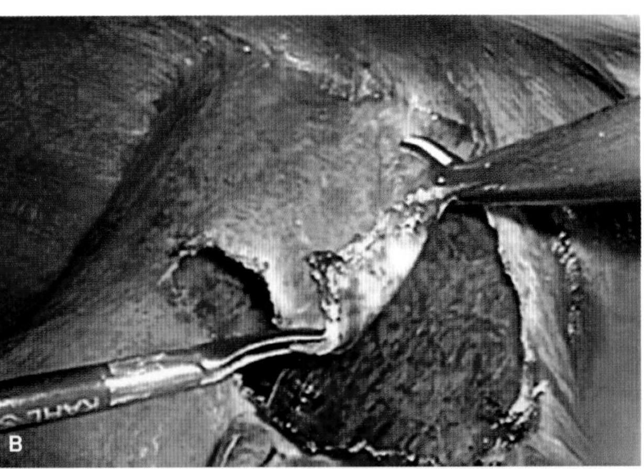

Figure 28.14 After draining the cyst, the border between the cyst, normal liver parenchyma, and diaphragm become obvious (**A**). The cyst wall can be removed with a cautery device (**B**) and the laparoscope can then be inserted into the cyst to inspect the cyst cavity.

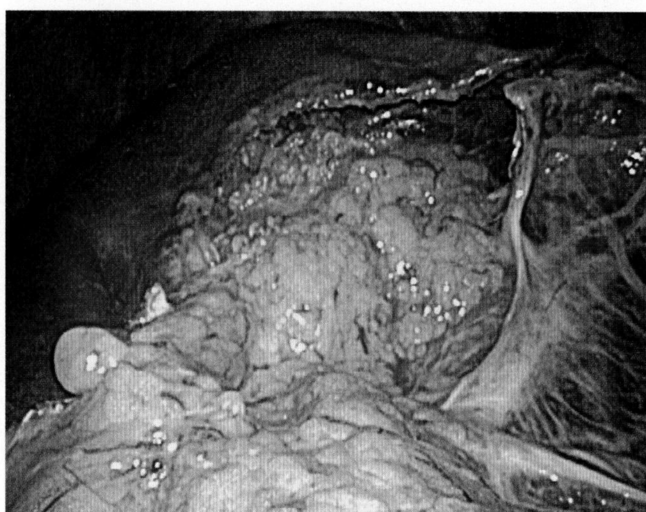

Figure 28.15 The omentum can be placed into the liver cyst cavity to assist in preventing the peritoneum and abdominal wall from trapping fluid in the cyst cavity.

the cyst wall has been removed, the remaining cyst wall can be ablated with cautery or argon beam coagulation. It is not known if this reduces the recurrence rate. Similarly, omentoplasty can be used to fill the cyst cavity but it is unclear if this helps promote resolution of the cyst cavity.

## Open Unroofing of a Simple Cyst

### Pertinent Anatomy

The open approach is sometimes used for cysts located in segments 7 and 8 where it can be difficult to obtain laparoscopic access. Open fenestration follows the same principles as laparoscopic cyst drainage as described above.

### Positioning

The patient is in the supine position. A right subcostal or midline incision is made.

### Technique

1. The triangular ligament and coronary ligament are divided to mobilize the liver toward the midline.
2. At the end of the unroofing there should be no cyst wall external to the liver parenchyma.
3. The cyst is inspected for blood vessels and bile ducts. Any leaking bile ducts should be sutured shut. The omentum can be placed into the cavity if it is available. No drains are utilized (Fig. 28.15).

# POSTOPERATIVE MANAGEMENT

Peri-operative surveillance should be in accordance with the amount of liver resected. Postoperative follow-up should similarly mirror that utilized after common hepatic procedures. Postoperative imaging can be performed 1 to 2 months after cyst drainage to evaluate for cyst recurrence (Fig. 28.16).

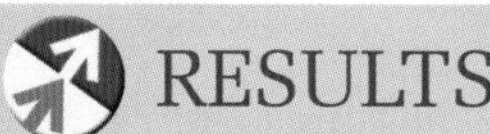

# RESULTS

Historically, image-guided percutaneous aspiration has a recurrence rate of nearly 100%. This rate is lower if sclerosants are injected into the cyst cavity after aspiration

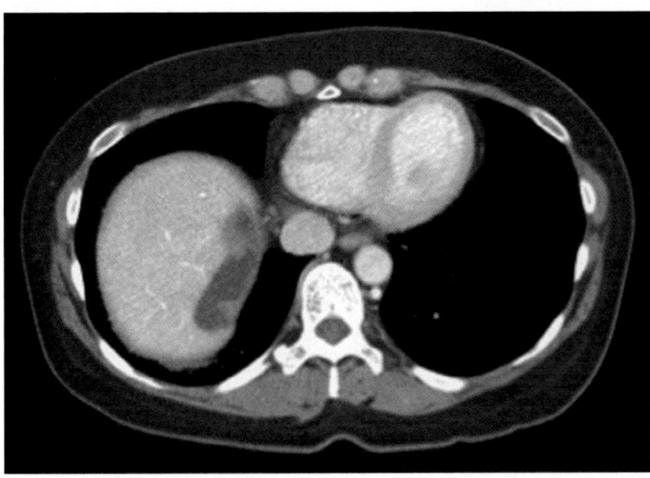

Figure 28.16 CT scan 1-month post laparoscopic cyst drainage of right hepatic cyst seen in Figures 28.1–28.3.



but rates are still as high as 17%. Aspiration can also induce hemorrhage within the cyst (Fig. 28.17).

There are several retrospective series that have evaluated recurrence rates and surgical approaches to liver cysts. One study of 131 patients over a 17-year period who were treated for liver cysts reported that recurrence rates with open deroofing were 8% with simple hepatic cysts and 0% with polycystic liver disease. Recurrence rates with laparoscopic unroofing of simple cysts were 2% and 0% with laparoscopic unroofing in patients with polycystic liver disease. Another retrospective series examined 51 patients who were treated with laparoscopic resection for symptomatic hepatic cysts. With a median follow-up of 13 months all patients had relief of symptoms. Two of the 51 patients required reoperation for cyst recurrence.

## Enucleation of Biliary Cystadenomas (see Chapter 25)

Biliary cystadenomas are complex multilocular cysts that derive from biliary epithelium. Although these tumors are benign, there is a small chance of neoplastic transformation to a cystadenocarcinoma, thus they are treated by surgical enucleation or resection. Resection is usually the most appropriate treatment, since the presence of malignancy cannot be confidently excluded preoperatively.

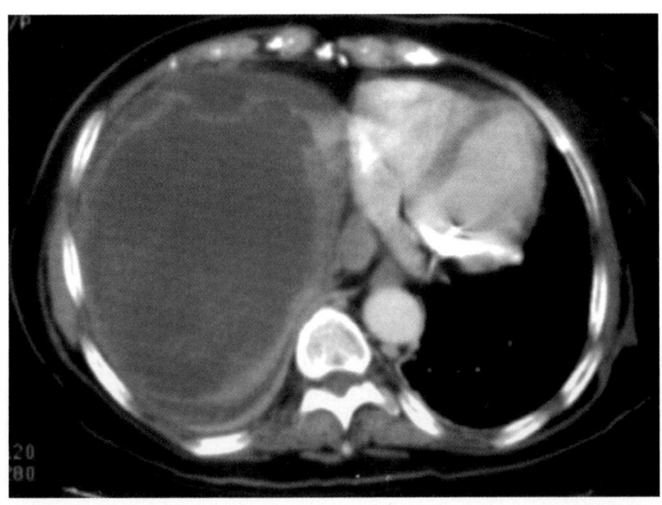

Figure 28.17 Hemorrhage into a simple cyst after percutaneous cyst needle aspiration.

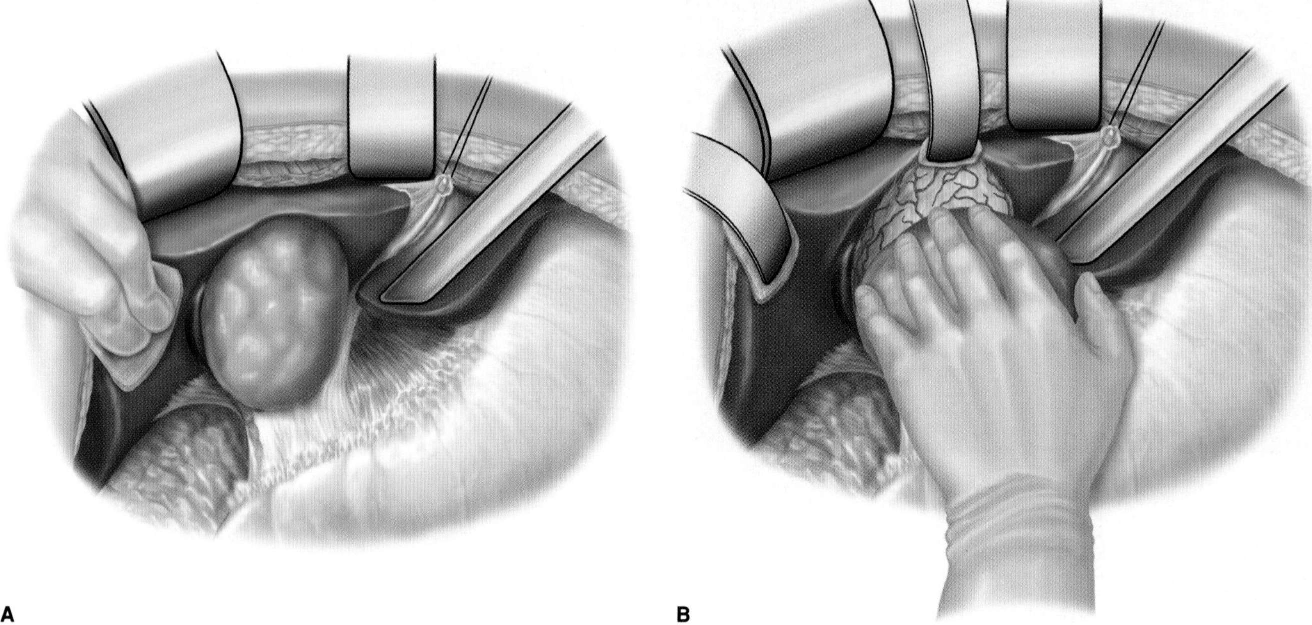


**Figure 28.18** Enucleation of biliary cystadenomas begins with exposure of the cyst (**A**; gallbladder is obscured by large cyst) followed by dissection of the border between normal liver parenchyma and the cyst wall (**B**).

The first step is to mobilize the side of the liver with the cyst. With countertraction applied by the nondominant hand of the surgeon, the border between the normal liver parenchyma and cyst wall is developed (Fig. 28.18A, B). Generally biliary cystadenomas have thick walls that help prevent cyst rupture during their enucleation. While completing the circumferential dissection of the cyst, hepatic veins, arteries and bile ducts should be preserved as often as possible. After enucleation, frozen section histology should be used to rule out cystadenocarcinoma; however, the possibility of misdiagnosis due to sampling error must be recognized.

Major hepatic ducts are potentially at risk for injury during enucleation of large lesions in segment 4B, particularly if they extend to the base of the liver, adjacent to the biliary confluence. If bile ducts are injured during enucleation they should be repaired with 4-0 or 5-0 interrupted sutures. The hepatic ligament should be accessible throughout this procedure in order to utilize a Pringle maneuver to control bleeding.

# Laparoscopic Resection of Cysts

In general, simple hepatic cysts do not require formal hepatic resection, but this approach is appropriate and indicated for other diagnoses, including cystadenoma, cystadenocarcinoma and hydatid disease; resection is also reasonable in the face of diagnostic uncertainty. Cystic lesions in any location may be resected laparoscopically but particularly when located in accessible areas (i.e., left lateral sector or anterior segments [segments 4B, 5, or 6]) (see Chapter 31). Four ports are generally used and their placement depends on the location of the lesion. Parenchymal dissection can be performed with devices such as the CUSA, Tissuelink, Harmonic Scalpel, or surgical staplers. The thin parenchyma around the borders of cystic lesions often allows for use of stapler to seal the superior and inferior edges of the transection line, minimizing blood loss (Fig. 28.19A). If the normal parenchyma is too thick for stapler transection, other devices, such as the Harmonic Scalpel or Ligasure, can be used, with the stapler reserved for the pedicle (Fig. 28.19B).

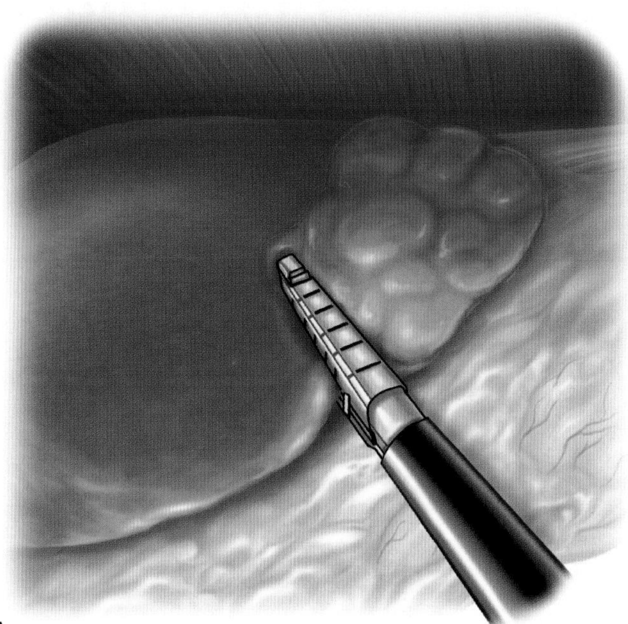


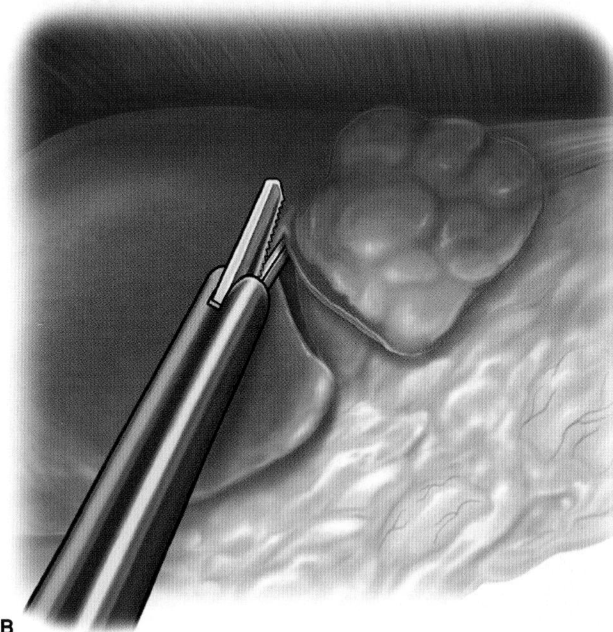


Figure 28.19 Laparoscopic resection of cysts that meet criteria for resection in the left lateral sector can be performed with either stapled parenchymal transection (**A**) or harmonic scalpel dissection (**B**).



After the parenchyma has been transected, the transection line is inspected for hemostasis and biliary leakage. Pneumoperitoneum should be released for at least 5 minutes, followed by reinsufflation and reinspection of the liver bed to ensure no hemorrhage or bile leak developed with normal intraperitoneal pressure.

# Hydatid Liver Disease

Hydatid cysts are the result of a parasitic infection with Echinococcus, as described above. The mordbidity from these cysts is related to the rupture of the cyst causing an anaphylactic reaction or bacterial super-infection of the cyst. Hydatid cysts are treated with two objectives in mind:

1. Remove the parasite surgically
2. Avoid spilling the parasitic cyst contents intraoperatively to avoid spreading it throughout the peritoneum.

Optimal treatment of hydatid disease is "en-bloc" removal of the cyst with maximal sparing of normal liver parenchyma. There is debate as to whether this can be accomplished with a formal liver resection or pericystectomy. In many cases, hepatic resection is the most appropriate approach.

## Preoperative Evaluation

Patients should be treated with albendazol 10 to 14 mg/kg/day orally in two doses beginning 2 to 4 weeks before surgery and continuing for a similar time period after surgery.

Indications for resection include:

1. Resectable hydatid cyst

Contraindications for resection include:

1. Contraindication to general liver resection
2. Major vascular invasion within the liver that precludes liver resection

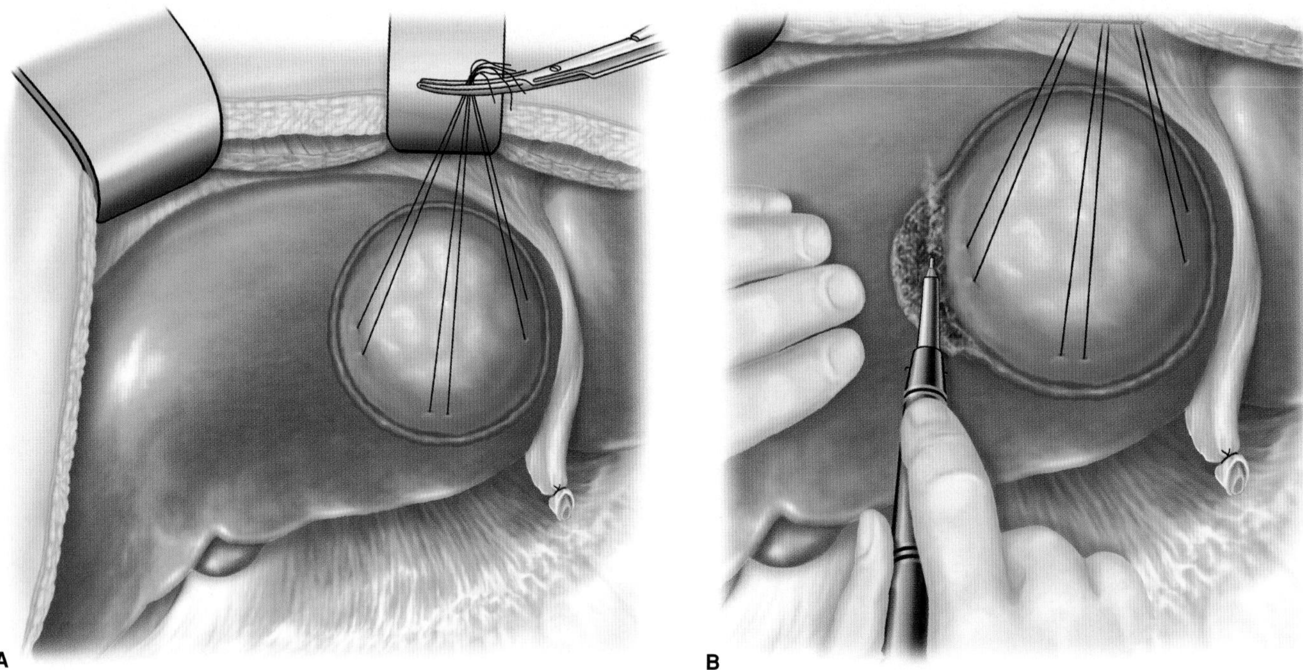


Figure 28.20 Hydatid liver cysts can be removed with a standard liver resection or "pericystectomy." Prior to "pericystectomy," stay sutures are placed in the bordering normal liver parenchyma (**A**). The line of dissection is carried out circumferentially outside of the stay sutures (**B**).

## Procedure

### Surgical Technique

Exploration of the abdominal cavity should be performed to rule out extrahepatic disease. Mobilize the liver in similar fashion to the mobilization required for hepatic resections. Povidone-iodine or hypertonic saline should be available on the surgical field in case of intraoperative rupture of the cyst. Both manual palpation and ultrasound examinations of the liver should be performed to delineate the location and number of intrahepatic cysts. Often, biliary communications between normal liver parenchyma and the cyst wall can be appreciated on ultrasound and assist with surgical planning.

Hydatid cysts that are located deep within the liver need to be treated by standard hepatic resection (see Chapters 19 to 24). If they are located superficially, however, within 2 to 3 cm of the liver surface, a pericystectomy can be performed after a hepatotomy is performed to reach the cyst wall. Cysts in the right liver often dissects free of the diaphragm but a small diaphragm resection may be required.

### Preparation for Pericystectomy

Before beginning the parenchymal transection the central venous pressure should be below 3 mm Hg. A vessel loop is placed around the porta hepatis in case a Pringle maneuver is required. The liver is packed on all borders with hypertonic soaked gauze pads in case the cyst is accidentally ruptured. Cyst contents are never drained intentionally and the cyst wall should not be manipulated. Stay sutures are placed in the normal parenchyma (not the cyst wall) to enhance retraction and exposure (Fig. 28.20A).

Liver transection is performed with a crush/clamp technique or coagulating device (Fig. 28.20B). The cyst should be removed en-bloc without rupture (Fig. 28.21).

# Polycystic Liver Disease

Patients with polycystic liver disease often have symptoms of abdominal distention and pain related to mass effect of enlargement of the cysts. Resection is indicated in selected

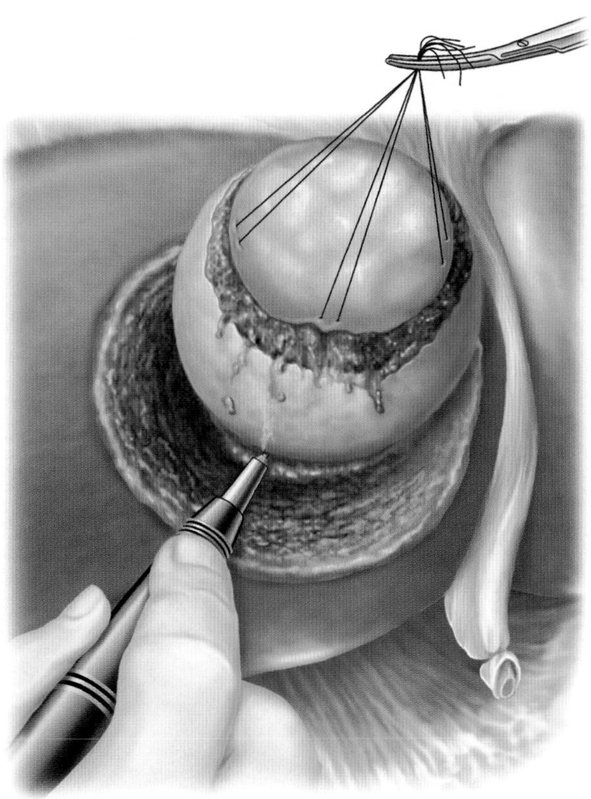

Figure 28.21 En-bloc resection of a hydatid cyst.



patients with symptoms, although it must be recognized that the efficacy of surgical decompression for polycystic disease is inferior to that for simple hepatic cysts; liver transplantation has been used in selected patients with disease that is not amenable to debulking surgery. The goals of resection is to debulk as much of the bulk of the liver as possible. Lesions with suspected bleeding or infectious complications should be evaluated prior to operation with US or MRI examination. The vascular nature of the cyst walls, and the potential of significant blood loss during resection, must be appreciated; vascular staplers are often used to maintain hemostasis.

In patients with polycystic liver disease, they frequently have renal cysts and a family history with autosomal dominant cysts. Cysts are often multiple and gradually increase in size over time. Renal failure is often what determines the prognosis in patients with this disease. Patients with polycystic liver disease type I usually have symptoms from the mass effect of the cysts and laparoscopic deroofing should be considered the first line of treatment. In patients with types II and III polycystic disease the presentation is often related to hepatomegaly. Deroofing is often not successful in reducing symptoms in patients with digestive symptoms, respiratory failure, and cachexia. Improved symptomatic relief may be achieved with a combination of hepatic resection and fenestration of cysts in the liver remnant. Although the recurrence of cysts after treatment is low, other untreated cysts can grow and become symptomatic.

## CONCLUSIONS

- Symptomatic benign liver cysts can often be treated with laparoscopic unroofing.
- Open unroofing may be required for cysts deep in the liver or near the dome of the liver.
- Biliary cystadenomas can be enucleated via open or laparoscopic approaches; however, resection is often indicated, since malignancy cannot be excluded reliably on imaging.

- Hydatid cysts should be resected avoiding spillage of contents into the peritoneum, utilizing a standard liver resection or "peri-cystectomy."
- In patients with symptomatic polycystic liver disease, debulking is warranted but symptom recurrence is common.

## Recommended References and Readings


Gamblin TC, Holloway SE, Heckman JT, et al. Laparoscopic resection of benign hepatic cysts: a new standard. *J Am Coll Surg.* 2008;207(5):731–736.

Giuliante F, D'Acapito F, Vellone M, et al. Risk for laparoscopic fenestration of liver cysts. *Surg Endosc.* 2003;17(11):1735–1738.

Katkhouda N, Hurwitz M, Gugenheim J, et al. Laparoscopic management of benign solid and cystic lesions of the liver. *Ann Surg.* 1999;229(4):460–466.

Martin IJ, McKinley AJ, Currie EJ, et al. Tailoring the management of nonparasitic liver cysts. *Ann Surg.* 1998;228(2):167–172.

Mazza OM, Fernandez DL, Pekolj J, et al. Management of nonparasitic hepatic cysts. *J Am Coll Surg.* 2009;209(6):733–739.

Morino M, De Giuli M, Festa V, et al. Laparoscopic management of symptomatic nonparasitic cysts of the liver. Indications and results. *Ann Surg.* 1994;219(2):157–164.

Regev A, Reddy KR, Berho M, et al. Large cystic lesions of the liver in adults: a 15-year experience in a tertiary center. *J Am Coll Surg.* 2001;193(1):36–45.

Spiegel RM, King DL, Green WM. Ultrasonography of primary cysts of the liver. *AJR Am J Roentgenol.* 1978;131(2):235–238.

Tocchi A, Mazzoni G, Costa G, et al. Symptomatic nonparasitic hepatic cysts: options for and results of surgical management. *Arch Surg.* 2002;137(2):154–158.

# 29 Congenital Dilations of the Biliary Tract

**Carlos U. Corvera**

##  INDICATIONS/CONTRAINDICATIONS

Choledochal cysts are abnormal dilations of the bile ducts, congenital in origin. Several classification systems have been proposed on the basis of the location, shape, or type of biliary dilation. The most widely adopted classification is Todani's modification of the original Alonso-Lej description and encompasses five types of cysts (Fig. 29.1):

- Type I—Fusiform or saccular dilation of the extrahepatic biliary tree involving both the common hepatic and common bile duct.
- Type II—A supraduodenal diverticulum of the common hepatic or common bile duct.
- Type III—Choledochoceles-intraduodenal diverticulum.
- Type IV—Intrahepatic and extrahepatic fusiform cyst involvement.
- Type V—Caroli's disease-multiple intrahepatic cysts.

However, mounting evidence suggests that choledochoceles (Type III) and Caroli's disease (Type V) are distinct clinical entities. This chapter will focus on the most common types of cysts, which represent fusiform dilations of the extrahepatic biliary tree involving both the common hepatic and common bile duct (Type I), with or without varying degrees of intrahepatic ductal involvement (Type IV). These congenital choledochal cysts are thought to be associated with yet another congenital anomaly involving the anatomy of the pancreatobiliary duct junction.

The clinical presentation of patients with choledochal cyst has changed from the classical "triad" of abdominal pain, jaundice and a right upper quadrant mass, probably as a result of modern advances in imaging technologies and widespread adoption of prenatal screening. Children are more likely to present with jaundice and/or a mass, whereas, choledochal cysts in adults may be identified incidentally or on evaluation of symptoms related to the long-term consequences/complications of the cyst, such as suppurative cholangitis, pancreatitis, cystolithiasis and/or malignancy. These well-described complications in adults have led to the evolution of surgical management from the historical simple drainage procedures to the current recommendation of complete cyst excision and biliary reconstruction.

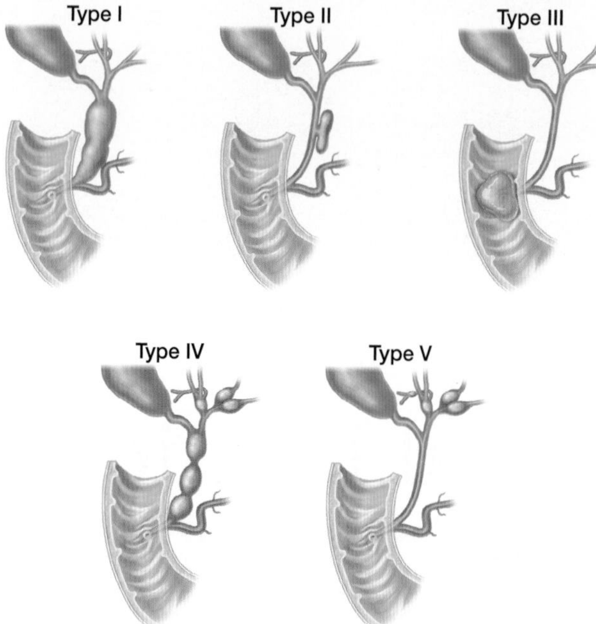


Figure 29.1 Todani's modification of Alonso-Lej classification of choledochal cysts. Type I—Solitary fusiform or saccular dilation of the common hepatic and common bile duct; Type II—Supraduodenal diverticulumof the common hepatic or common bile duct. Type III—Intraduodenaldiverticulum of the distal common bile duct –Choledochocele. Type IV—Intrahepatic and extrahepatic fusiform cysts, or multiple extrahepatic cysts. Type V—Multiple intrahepatic cysts—Caroli's disease.

The diagnosis of choledochal cysts has been simplified by contemporary high resolution, three-dimensional, abdominal imaging technologies and widespread availability of interventional radiology and endoscopy. Imaging studies should clearly define the relationship of the cyst to the other portal structures. Abdominal ultrasonography is generally the first study obtained, followed by either computed tomography (CT), nuclear medicine: hydroxyimidoacetic acid scan (HIDA), or magnetic resonance imaging (MRI) and magnetic resonance cholangiopancreatography (MRCP) (Fig. 29.2). If necessary, the diagnosis can be confirmed by more invasive studies such as percutaneous transhepatic cholangiography (PTC) or endoscopic retrograde cholangiopancreatography (ERCP) (Fig. 29.3). While these "direct" cholangiographic studies have the advantage of providing diagnostic information (i.e., cytologic brushings or biopsy), a disadvantage is that they can lead to serious periprocedural complications. PTC can be technically difficult to perform in patients with small nondilated duct require a more proximal approach, thereby increasing the risk of vascular injury. In these patients, acute pancreatitis can be precipitated more easily, probably because of the typical high insertion of the pancreatic duct into the biliary tract. Because of this, we recommend that these more invasive diagnostic studies be obtained only when the anatomy or the extent of the cyst requires further characterization.

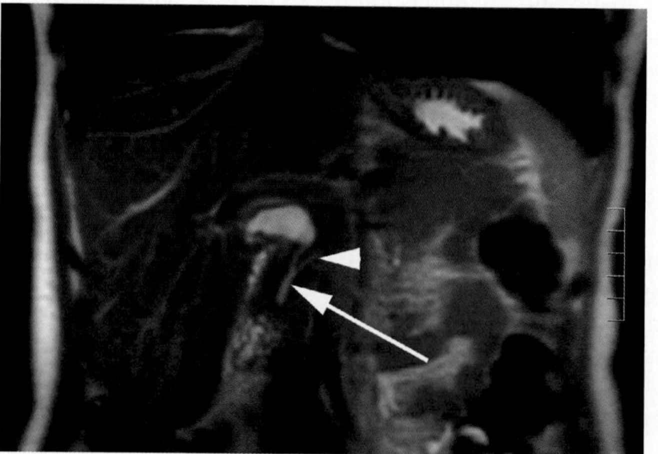

Figure 29.2 MRI (coronal T2-weighted, gadolinium enhanced) showing a choledochal cyst with long common channel (*arrow*) and main pancreatic duct (*arrowhead*) which joins the common bile duct just below the cystic dilatation.

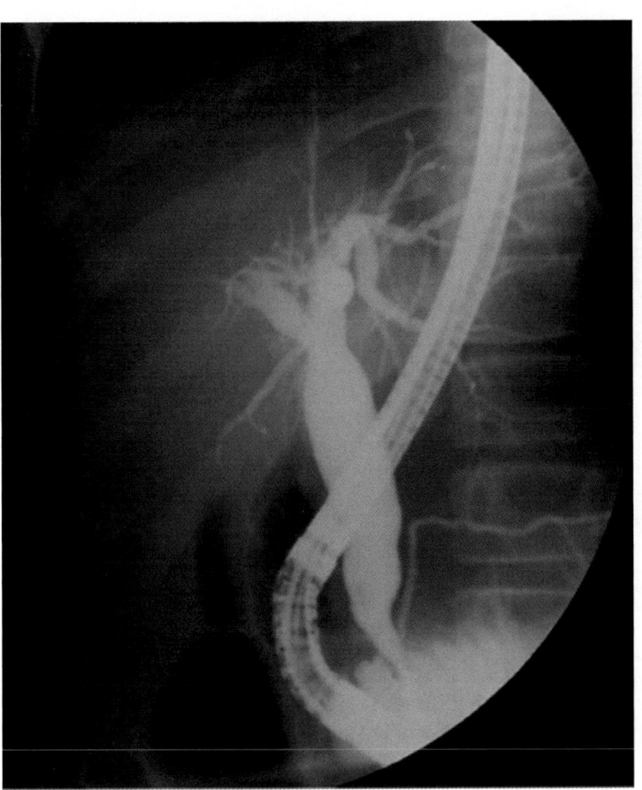

**Figure 29.3** ERCP- Showing A Todani Type IV Congenital Choledochal Cyst With Intrahepatic Fusiform Cyst Involvement.



## PREOPERATIVE PLANNING

1. Clear delineation of biliary and ampullary anatomy by direct or indirect cholangiography is critical to avoid injury to the fragile narrow tapering of the distal bile duct (pancreaticobiliary junction). If the diagnosis is made during cholecystectomy, intraoperative cholangiography should be done to delineate the entire cyst anatomy. Otherwise, complete cross-sectional preoperative imaging by CT or MRI is necessary to define the extent of intrahepatic ductal involvement (see Chapter 18). If extensive unilateral hepatic involvement (usually the left side) is found, complete cyst excision with concomitant partial hepatectomy should be planned and discussed with the patient in the preoperative setting. Finally, the possibility of encountering malignancy should always be anticipated in the adult patient. Coexisting malignancy is suspected in patients who present with weight loss, jaundice, elevated tumor markers, and/or imaging findings that show a mass or intracystic mural nodules. Appropriate planning and counseling for additional surgical procedures, (i.e., concomitant hepatectomy, pancreatectomy, and/or need for extensive lymph node dissection) should be done preoperatively (see Chapter 26).

## SURGICAL TECHNIQUE

### Choledochal Cyst Resection—Pertinent Anatomy

A clear understanding of the anatomic relationships of the liver, biliary tract, portal vessels, and pancreas is essential for safe resection of congenital choledochal cysts (see Chapter 18). In addition, knowledge of common variations in the relationship of the right hepatic artery and cystic artery to the biliary tract is critical to avoid unexpected hemorrhage or biliary injury. The following are important anatomic relationships that must be understood to safely perform this procedure (Fig. 29.4):

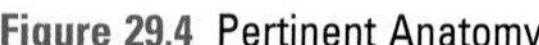
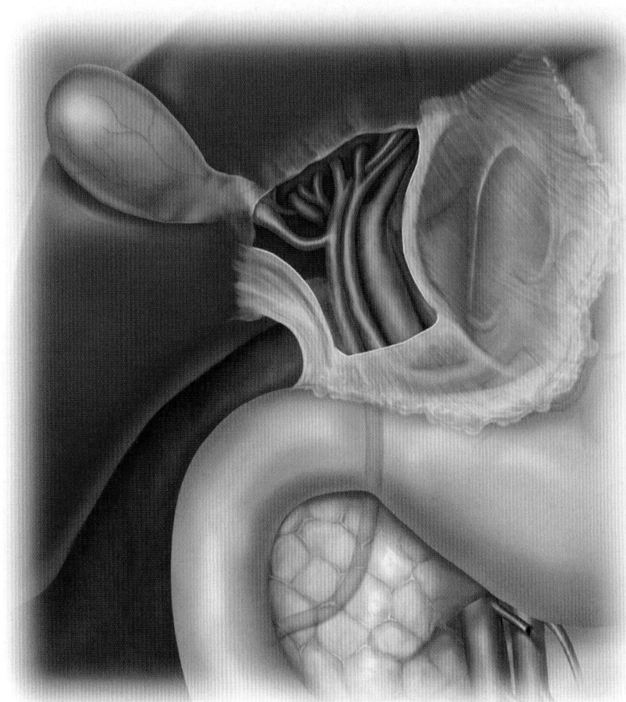

Figure 29.4 Pertinent Anatomy

- The biliary confluence is typically situated anterior to the right branch of the main portal vein.
- The right hepatic artery usually courses posterior to the common hepatic duct and gives rise to the cystic artery.
- If present, a replaced or accessory right hepatic artery originates from the superior mesenteric artery and courses toward the liver, running posterolaterally along the right side of the common bile duct and behind the cystic duct before entering into Calot's triangle.
- The posterior location of the portal vein within the hepatoduodenal ligament is important to understand since it is typically distorted or displaced posteromedially by the enlarged fusiform biliary cyst.
- Precise knowledge and identification of the portal vein is critical to avoid inadvertent injury during dissection, especially in cases associated with dense pericystic inflammation due to prior bouts of ascending cholangitis or pancreatitis.
- The distal common bile duct courses downward and posteriorly to enter directly into the pancreas, or follows an extrapancreatic course for a short segment or within a posterior groove before it enters the substance of the gland.

## Surgical Techniques for Congenital Dilations of the Biliary Tract

The surgical management of patients with congenital choledochal cysts continues to evolve. While traditional laparotomy via a midline, right transverse or subcostal incision remains popular, in the past decade, published reports of patients being treated by minimally invasive surgery (MIS) have surged worldwide. Most of these MIS experiences are laparoscopic, with a few case reports describing robot-assisted cyst excision and reconstruction. The application of MIS to treat congenital choledochal cysts is particularly attractive because the specimen is small and can be retrieved through a small port-site incision. Moreover, this disease generally affects young patients, in whom cosmetic concerns may be more important. Although the MIS approach requires further evaluation before it can be recommended as the new standard, the increasing utilization of minimally invasive surgical techniques in hepatobiliary diseases warrants description of this approach. Therefore, the traditional open and laparoscopic operative techniques for complete resection of choledochal cysts are described below.

## Traditional Laparotomy "Open" Technique

### Positioning

- Patient is positioned supine with the right arm tucked and left arm out.
- The choice of incision for exploration is based on surgeon's preference and is influenced by patient size, body habitus, or presence of incision from prior laparotomy. We prefer a right-side, modified Makuuchi incision in patients with a steep costal margin and a standard right subcostal incision in patients with a wide abdominal surface and/or costal margin.

### Complete Choledochal Cyst Excision

At exploration, the cyst should be immediately obvious bulging from the lateral edge of the hepatoduodenal ligament and distorting the first and second portion of the duodenum anteriorly.

- Cholecystectomy is started by incising the peritoneum overlying the dilated and distorted gallbladder neck. The cystic duct typically arises from the lateral midportion of the fusiform cyst wall. The cystic artery is identified, isolated, clamped, divided, and ligated. A top-down dissection is used to mobilize the gallbladder from the liver bed.
- A Kocher maneuver is done to mobilize the duodenum from the retroperitoneum.
- The peritoneum is incised on the superior border along the first portion of the duodenum and it is reflected downward and rolled inferomedially to expose the anterior cyst wall. Since inflammation is minimal, this dissection is usually straightforward and is done in a blunt and sharp fashion until the distal bile duct/cyst is circumferentially isolated.
- The lower end of the cyst is encircled with a vessel-loop or umbilical tape and used for traction. This maneuver provides excellent exposure of the adjacent portal vascular structures.
- The fusiform dilation commonly extends behind the duodenum and into the substance of the pancreas. Therefore, as the dissection progresses inferiorly along the distal common bile duct, care must be taken not to injure the underlying pancreatic duct (Fig. 29.5). A detailed understanding and interpretation of the preoperative cholangiogram is crucial in guiding this part of the dissection. In most cases, a rapid "funneling" of the cyst wall occurs with a tapering to a normal caliber bile duct and



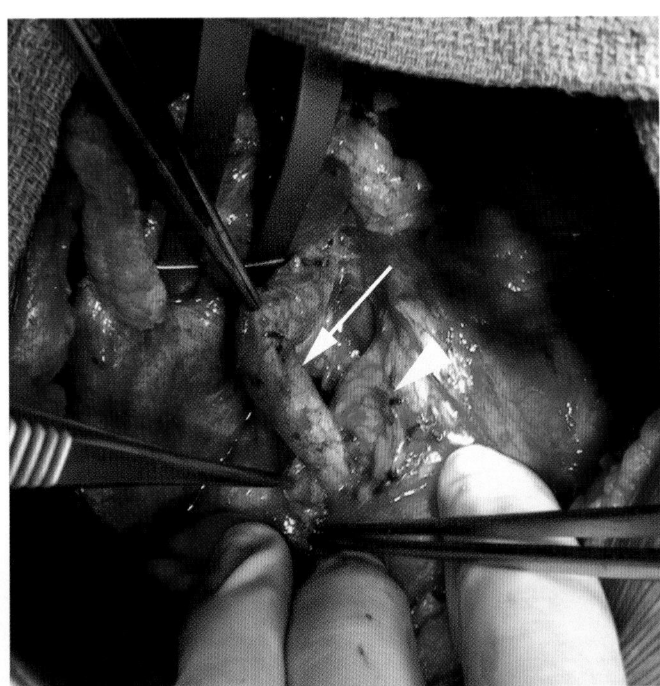

**Figure 29.5** Duodenum is rolled/retracted caudally to expose the intra-pancreatic dissection demonstrating the tapering of the distal common bile duct (*arrow*) and the pancreatic groove (*arrowhead*).

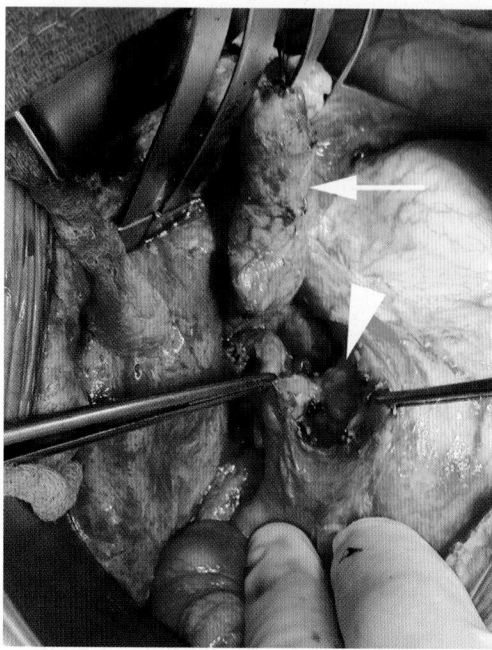

Figure 29.6 Distal Bile duct has been transected and retracted upward (*arrow*) to expose the underlying portal vein and hepatic artery. Note the intra-pancreatic dissection (groove) necessary to excise the cyst (*arrowhead*).

only a few millimeters distance from the pancreatic duct junction. In order to achieve a "complete" cyst excision, it is essential to follow the distal extent of the cyst dissection until a normal-sized common bile duct is identified (Fig. 29.5).

- Once identified, the normal-sized distal common bile duct is divided and oversewn with a 3-0 or 4-0 absorbable suture depending on the duct size. The proximal divided end of the cyst is also oversewn to avoid bile spillage.
- The choledochal cyst is then reflected upward to allow dissection away from the portal vein and the hepatic artery (Fig. 29.6). This tissue plane is generally areolar and flimsy and can be reflected by blunt finger dissection up to the hepatic bifurcation.
- ***Note:*** rarely, intense inflammation of the cyst wall is found as a result of subclinical cholangitis or pancreatitis. This makes dissection and separation of the cyst wall from the portal vascular structures extremely hazardous. In these instances, we recommended using an internal cyst dissection approach that leaves a thin protective outer wall in place over the portal vascular structures. This technique involves entering the cyst wall anteriorly and extending the opening medially toward the hepatic artery. The medial edge of the cyst wall is carefully dissected and two layers are developed consisting of inner epithelial and external fibrous layers (Fig. 29.7). After

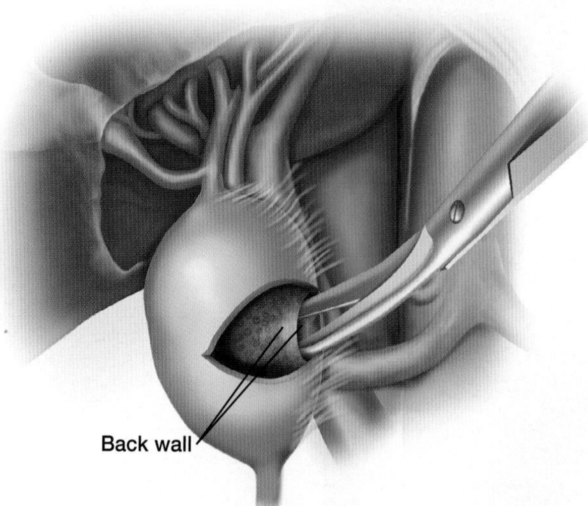


Figure 29.7 Internal Cyst Resection Approach. Recommended technique for choledochal cysts with associated intense inflammation. The cyst wall is opened, the medial edge is separated and two layers providing a safe plane of dissection.

complete cyst resection, only the thin external fibrous wall lining involving the hepatic artery and portal vein is left in place.

- If preoperative imaging and intraoperative findings demonstrate a transition to a normal caliber common hepatic duct, the specimen is divided at this point. If, however, the choledochal cyst is known to have intrahepatic extension, the hilar plate is lowered, and the hepatic bifurcation is dissected to expose both the takeoff of the right and left ducts. Under these circumstances, the hepatic confluence is included in the specimen.
- If malignancy is suspected (i.e., mural nodules, inflammation, etc. are present), a frozen section should be requested. The specimen is opened and inspected in the operating room by the pathologist. If malignancy is found, the appropriate cancer operation to achieve histologically negative margins is done along with a regional lymph node dissection.

### Biliary-enteric Reconstruction

In children, the best choice for biliary-enteric reconstruction remains controversial. While most pediatric surgeons prefer a hepaticojejunostomy using a Roux-en Y jejunal limb, others claim that reconstruction by hepaticoduodenostomy in the setting of favorable anatomy (i.e., mobile duodenum, large ductal confluence) is more physiologic and is associated with fewer long-term complications, such as small bowel obstruction. In adults, biliary reconstruction following choledochal cyst excision should be done by using a 70 cm Roux-en-Y hepaticojejunostomy (see Chapter 17). We prefer the retrocolic position for the jejunal segment brought up through the transverse mesocolon just to the right of the middle colic vessels. This location provides a comfortable lie for the Roux limb in most patients. Occasionally, the anticolic position is necessary to provide a more suitable tension-free position depending upon the degree of mesenteric fat content or length (Fig. 29.8).

- A standard hepaticojejunostomy, according to the technique of Blumgart and Kelly, is performed using absorbable 4-0 or 5-0 sutures (see Chapter 17 and Figs. 17.13–17.15; see Figs. 27.15–27.18). This technique is useful for very proximal anastomoses to small ducts. The anterior row of sutures is placed sequentially and the needles retained; the posterior row is then placed from the bowel to the bile duct (Fig. 29.8A). The bowel is then parachuted down and the posterior row is secured (Fig. 29.8B). Finally, the previously placed sutures in the anterior row of the bile duct are now placed sequentially through the anterior bowel wall and secured (Fig. 29.8C). If the duct diameter is over 1 cm, a single layer, continuous technique is used on the posterior wall, and the front wall is constructed in an interrupted manner. If the duct diameter is ≥1.5 cm, the posterior and anterior walls can be done separately using a single layer continuous suture.
- The completed biliary-enteric anastomosis should be inspected for bile leakage and repaired if necessary. An intra-abdominal drain should be left in place adjacent to the anastomosis to control a potential postoperative bile leak.

## Laparoscopic Surgical Technique

The decision to embark on an MIS approach for choledochal cysts must be made with the understanding that the fundamental principles of open surgery will not be compromised in order to extend the known benefits of the laparoscopic approach. In other words, the essential steps (i.e., exposure and maneuvers) done in the traditional open approach must be reproduced by the laparoscopic approach. Moreover, laparoscopic resection of choledochal cyst with biliary reconstruction remains technically challenging even for highly experienced laparoscopic surgeons, and therefore should not be attempted until the basic and advanced laparoscopic skill sets have been mastered.

## Equipment and Positioning

- MIS requires state-of-the-art equipment including dedicated operating rooms fitted with ceiling mounted boons, high-resolution display monitors and modern thermal energy generators.

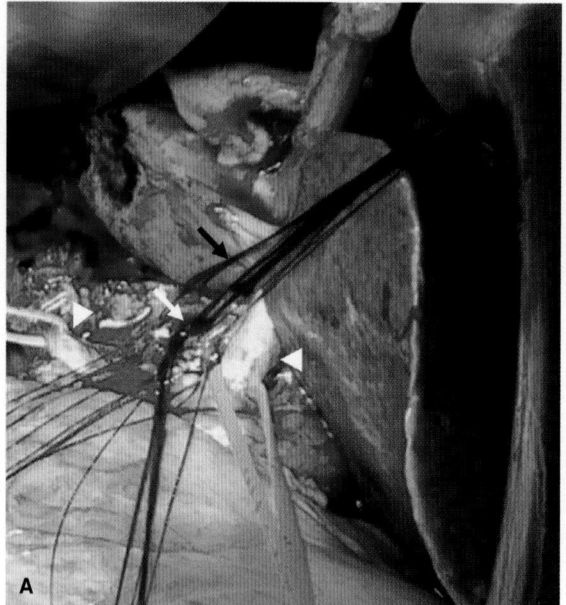

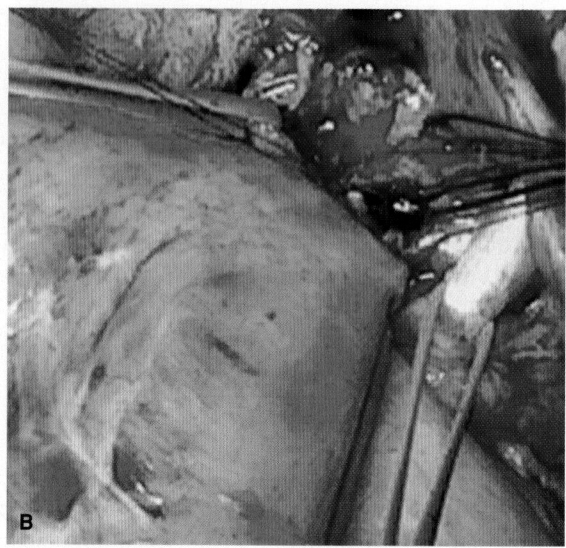

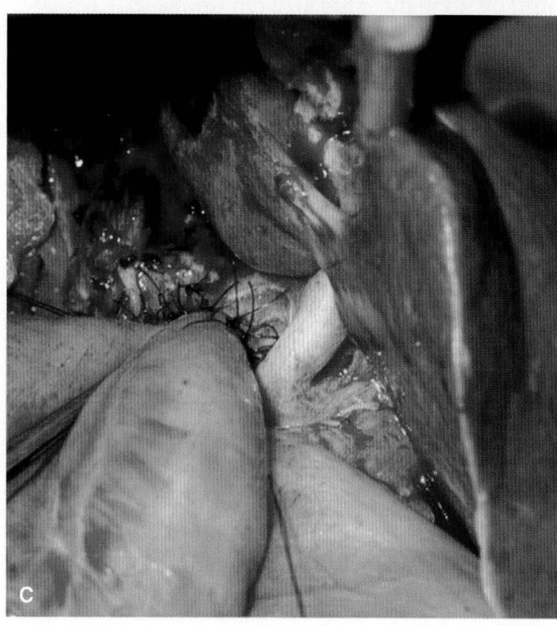

**Figure 29.8 A**: The anterior row of sutures (*black arrow*) is placed sequentially into the bile duct (*white arrow*) and the needles retained. The posterior row of sutures (*black arrowhead*) is placed from the jejunal limb (out of view) to the back wall of the bile duct. The left hepatic artery and a replaced right hepatic artery are retracted on vessel loops (*white arrowheads*). **B:** The bowel has been parachuted down the posterior row of sutures has been secured. The anterior row of sutures (*black arrow*) is now passed into the anterior wall of the bowel. The bile duct lumen is shown (*white arrow*). **C:** The completed anastomosis after the anterior row of sutures has been secured.

- Disposable laparoscopic instrumentation should be organized on a separate Mayo stand lying over or next to the patient to allow easy access (Fig. 29.9).
- As with all laparoscopic procedures, proper patient positioning is important. Generally, the choice for patient positioning depends on surgeon preference, patient body size and shape, or anticipated internal anatomy.
- For laparoscopic resections, either a partial lateral, right side-up (Fig. 29.10) or a split-legged position (Fig. 29.11) is recommended.
- The split-legged position is appropriate for the robot-assisted approach (Fig. 29.12) since the scrubbed assistant can be situated in-between the legs while the primary surgeon is working from the console and the robot is located at the head of the bed.

## Port-site Location

The most important aspect of completing this procedure laparoscopically begins with optimal port-site placement. Ideally, operating ports should be placed approximately 15 cm from the operating site and the angle between the axis of the camera/scope and the

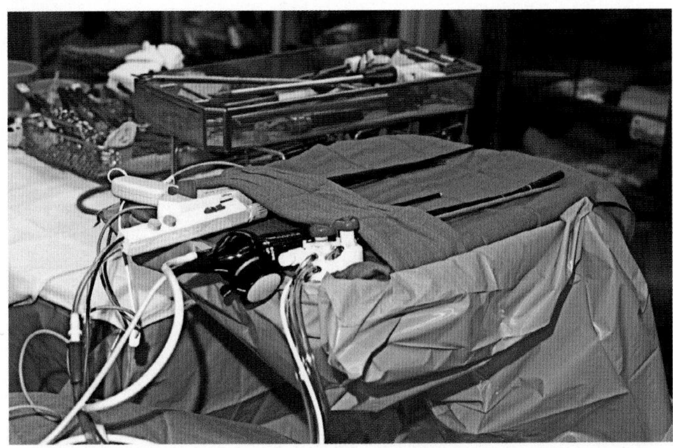

Figure 29.9 Equipment Organization. Mayo stand is used to organize and protect the multiple laparoscopic instruments, lines and cords and is positioned over the patient for easy access. The general instrument table is maintained away from the shifting patient.

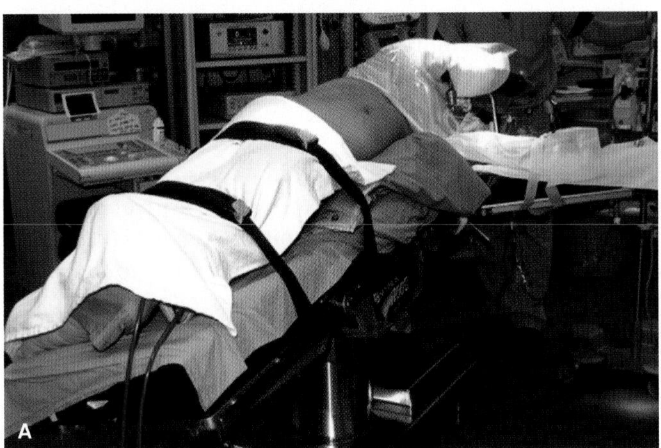

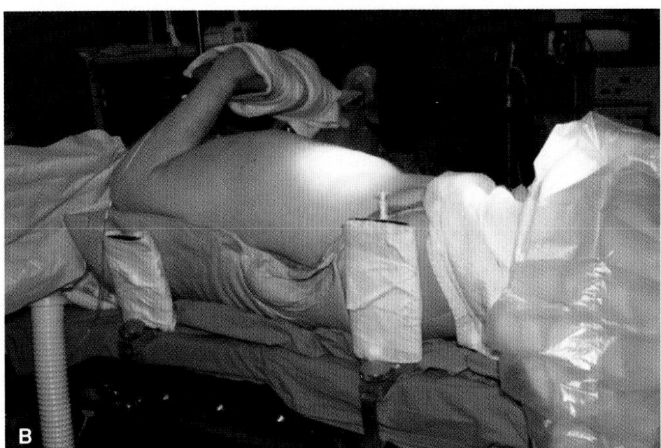

Figure 29.10 The semi-lateral, partial right-side up operating room table position: **(A)** The bed is flexed at the hip to increase exposure below the right costal margin and the patient is securely fastened. Note the near-supine position when the table is rotated fully to the right. **(B)** A viewed from the right side shows a beanbag (*arrowhead*) and two kidney rests (shoulder and hip, *arrows*) used to stabilize the patient.

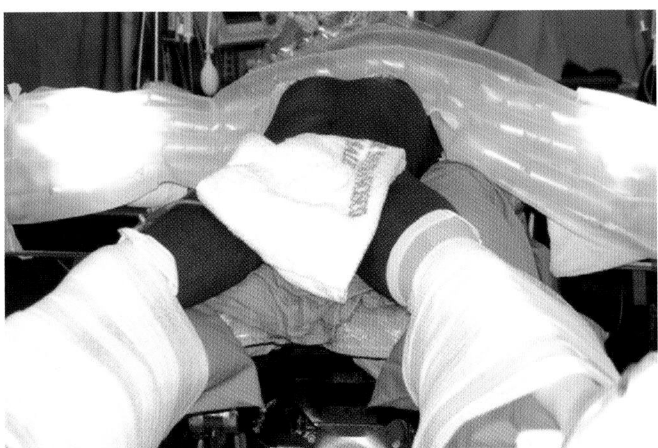

Figure 29.11 Split-leg (i.e. French or Frog-legged) operating room table position: This is a popular laparoscopic approach for upper abdominal procedures and allows the primary surgeon to stand in-between the legs and a second assistant stands on the patient's left.

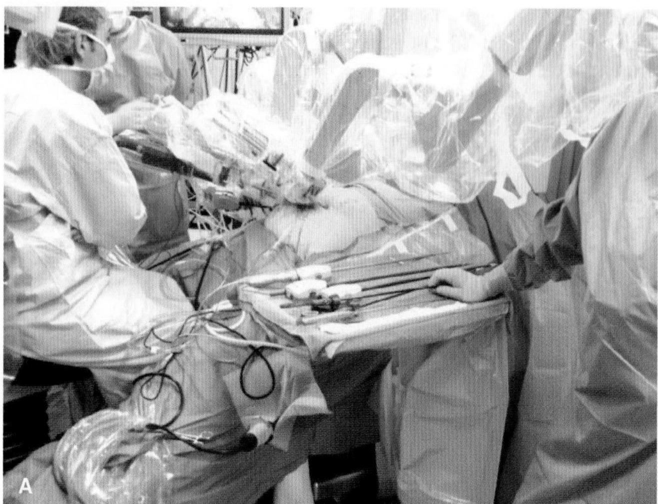


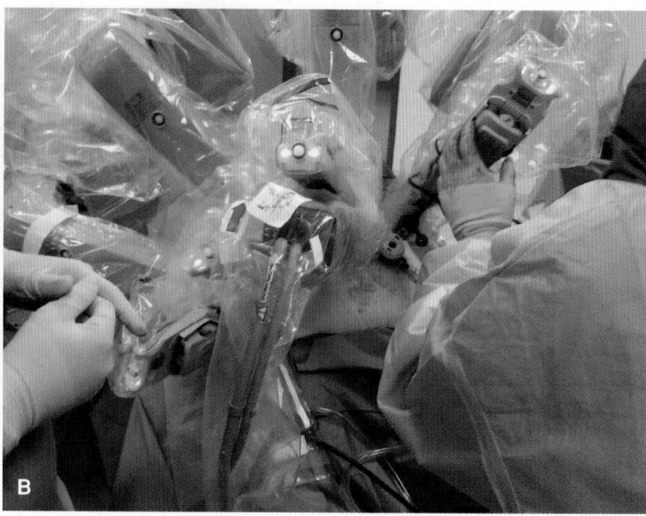


Figure 29.12 Set-up for Robot-assisted Approach: **(A)** The four-armed robot is best situated at the head of the bed just to the left of the anesthesiologist. Note that the split-legged bed position is best for a robot-assisted resection. **(B)** The scrubbed assistant is seated in-between the legs to allow rapid exchange of instrumentation. Note the Mayo stand being used to organize and secure instrumentation.

operating ports should be between 30 and 60 degrees to avoid "sword fighting". The principal goal is to allow maximal maneuverability and exposure of the critical anatomic structures. Since construction of the hepaticojejunostomy is typically the most challenging step of this procedure, the importance of the final instrument location to allow for safe dissection and ergonomic intracorporeal suturing cannot be overstated.

### Technical Details

- In children, choledochal cysts can reach large sizes that require aspiration/decompression to improve visualization for dissection, but this is rarely necessary in adults.
- The general port sites used for a laparoscopic choledochal cyst resection and biliary reconstruction are shown in Figure 29.13.
- If an extra corporeal jejunojejunostomy anastomosis is planned, we recommend starting with a gel port using a limited periumbilical incision (2 to 3 cm) (Fig. 29.13).

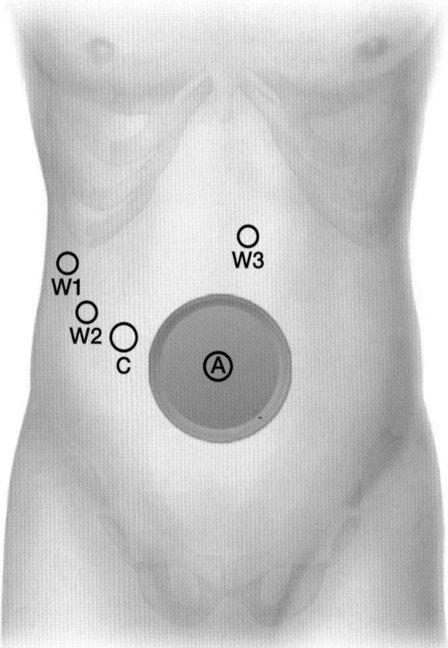


Figure 29.13 Port Site Locations for Laparocopic Approach: This diagram shows the general port site location used for a Laparoscopic choledocholcyst resection and biliary reconstruction. W1-3 = 5 mm working ports; C = 10 mm Camera port; A = Additional working port. Note, the GelPort (grey) with a limited umbilical incision is used for extra-corporeal construction of the jejuno-jejunostomy.

- The ideal scope location is to the right of the umbilicus, through the rectus muscle, thereby providing a more axial view of the hilum.
- The distance of scope from the operative site should not exceed 25 cm.
- All operating ports are placed only after a pneumoperitoneum is established and the internal anatomy has been examined.
- The technical steps for resection of the choledochal cyst by the MIS approach using either a conventional laparoscopic or by Robot-assisted method follows the same sequence as outlined above for the conventional open approach.
- Pertinent steps for the minimally invasive surgical management approach of choledochal cyst include:
  1. **Jejunojejunostomy:** To reduce the long operative times required for the MIS approach, most surgeons perform an extra corporeal jejunojejunostomy through a limited periumbilical incision when biliary reconstruction is done by hepaticojejunostomy. The proximal jejunum is marked with a stitch and grasped at approximately 20 to 30 cm distal to the ligament of Treitz and exteriorized through the umbilical port. Some surgeons prefer to do the entire procedure totally laparoscopically and perform a side-to-side jejunojejunosotomy with an endo-GIA stapling device. *Alternatively, this step can be omitted completely by choosing to instead reconstruct the biliary tract by hepaticoduodenostomy.*
  2. **MIS hepaticojejunostomy:** A 60 to 70 cm Roux jejunal limb is positioned in front of the colon and an end-to-side biliary-enteric anastomosis is constructed using a single layer interrupted or continuous technique depending on the size of the duct. The temptation to leave a small cuff of cyst wall at the hepatic duct junction to simplify the anastomosis should be resisted since there several reports that document the development of carcinoma in the retained choledochal cysts.

## POSTOPERATIVE MANAGEMENT

The immediate postoperative management of patients who underwent choledochal cyst excision and biliary reconstruction is the same routine care administered to hospitalized patients who underwent laparotomy or laparoscopic hepatobiliary procedures. Emphasis is placed on controlling postoperative incisional pain, and close observation for signs of common early complications such as bleeding, ileus, wound infection, and/or biliary leakage. The decision to remove the abdominal drainage catheter either in the hospital or in the clinic is based on surgeon preference or on the total 24-hour volume produced and fluid characteristics. We prefer to remove the drain during the postoperative check-up appointment 1 to 2 weeks after discharge and if the volume is less than 20 to 30 cc per day.

- For long-term surveillance, patients are seen in follow-up at 6 and 12 months, and annually thereafter.
- Liver function tests and a postoperative radionucleotide scan are obtained to document the patency of the anastomosis and are useful as baseline studies.

## COMPLICATIONS

Late complications after choledochal cyst excision typically result from either a stricture at the biliary-enteric anastomosis, or the formation of a primary ductal stricture. Regardless, these late strictures can be problematic, resulting in recurrent bouts of cholangitis, formation of intrahepatic stones and ultimately pyogenic abscesses requiring treatment by partial hepatectomy. Similarly, incomplete cyst excision can lead to ascending cholangitis from intrahepatic or cyst remnant stones, not to mention the persistent malignant potential.

## RESULTS

Long-term follow-up data (ranging from 17 to 25 years) from several studies has shown that primary complete cyst excision with a wide bilioenteric anastomosis is the treatment choice for choledochal cysts. However, the choice for biliary reconstruction remains a matter of ongoing debate. Early published results from Japan favored hepaticoduodenostomy because it was thought to be a more physiologic procedure than hepaticojejunostomy, however, the authors later reported that in the 97 treated choledochal cysts, the incidence of postoperative complications was higher in the hepaticoduodenostomy group. This observation influenced the authors to recommend hepaticojejunostomy as the preferred biliary reconstruction since it allows for enlargement of the hilar ducts to provide a wider stoma for anastomosis. In contrast, a report from India of 79 patients comparing hepaticoduodenostomy with hepaticojejunostomy found that hepaticoduodenostomy was associated with better outcomes after an average of 17 years of follow-up. Nevertheless, good long-term outcomes can be expected regardless of the biliary reconstruction technique chosen, as long at a complete choledochal cyst excision can be done.

## CONCLUSIONS

Choledochal cysts, which are congenital dilations of the biliary tract involving both the extra and intrahepatic ducts, carry a substantial risk for malignant transformation and should be completely excised. Over the past decade, the preferred operative management of these cysts has begun to shift toward a minimally invasive surgical approach. While the laparoscopic technique has not been universally embraced (probably because it remains technically challenging), data supporting its feasibility, safety and efficacy continues to mount. Choledochal cysts affect young females most commonly and they have the most to gain from the cosmetic benefits of this approach. While the laparoscopic approach is gradually gaining acceptance, the role of robotic-assisted resection is even more unclear, especially given its high cost and the current financial constraints of our healthcare system.

## Recommended References and Readings

Akaraviputh T, Trakarnsanga A, Suksamanapun N. Robot-assisted complete excision of choledochal cyst type I, hepaticojejunostomy and extracorporeal Roux-en-y anastomosis: a case report and review literature. *World J Surg Oncol.* 2010;8:87.

Desmet VJ. Ductal plates in hepatic ductular reactions. Hypothesis and implications. III. Implications for liver pathology. *Virchows Arch.* 2011;458(3):271–279. Epub 2011 Feb 8. Review.

Kendrick ML, Nagorney DM. Bile duct cysts: contemporary surgical management. *Curr Opin Gastroenterol.* 2009;25(3):240–244. Review.

Lenriot JP, Gigot JF, Ségol P, et al. Bile duct cysts in adults: a multi-institutional retrospective study. French Associations for Surgical Research. *Ann Surg.* 1998;228(2):159–166.

Liu SL, Li L, Hou WY, et al. Laparoscopic excision of choledochal cyst and Roux-en-Y hepaticojejunostomy in symptomatic neonates. *J Pediatr Surg.* 2009;44(3):508–511.

Mukhopadhyay B, Shukla RM, Mukhopadhyay M, et al. Choledochal cyst: A review of 79 cases and the role of hepaticodochoduodenostomy. *J Indian Assoc Pediatr Surg.* 2011;16(2):54–57.

Parada LA, Hallén M, Hägerstrand I, et al. Clonal chromosomal abnormalities in congenital bile duct dilatation (Caroli's disease). *Gut.* 1999;45(5):780–782.

Shi LB, Peng SY, Meng XK, et al. Diagnosis and treatment of congenital choledochal cyst: 20 years' experience in China. *World J Gastroenterol.* 2001;7(5):732–734.

Shimotakahara A, Yamataka A, Yanai T, et al. Roux-en-Y hepaticojejunostomy or hepaticoduodenostomy for biliary reconstruction during the surgical treatment of choledochal cyst: which is better? *Pediatr Surg Int.* 2005;21(1):5–7.

Todani T, Watanabe Y, Toki A, et al. Classification of congenital biliary cystic disease: special reference to type Ic and IVA cysts with primary ductal stricture. *J Hepatobiliary Pancreat Surg.* 2003;10(5):340–344.

Todani T, Watanabe Y, Urushihara N, et al. Biliary complications after excisional procedure for choledochal cyst. *J Pediatr Surg.* 1995;30(3):478–481.

Visser BC, Suh I, Way LW, et al. Congenital choledochal cysts in adults. *Arch Surg.* 2004;139(8):855–860; discussion 860–862.

Ziegler KM, Zyromski NJ. Choledochoceles: are they choledochal cysts? *Adv Surg.* 2011;45:211–224. Review.

# 30 Vascular Isolation and Techniques of Vascular Reconstruction

**Ian McGilvray and Alan W. Hemming**

##  INDICATIONS/CONTRAINDICATIONS

Hepatobiliary surgical and liver preservation techniques have evolved to the point that the reconstruction of critical hepatic vasculature can be performed with acceptable morbidity and mortality. As a result, the indications for surgery on tumor involving the hepatocaval confluence, inferior vena cava, and/or portal vessels are expanding—this is particularly true in centers that have a strong background in both hepatobiliary oncology and liver transplantation. The techniques described in this chapter are generally applicable to cases where the local aggression of the tumor involved—as it relates to vascular structures such as the cava and hepatic veins—does not preclude long-term survival. Examples of this concept include intrahepatic cholangiocarcinomas that are confined to the liver with no lymph node extension but invasion or encasement of major vascular structures in the liver, sarcomas that invade or impinge on major hepatic vascular structures, and selected cases of metastatic colon cancer or hepatocellular carcinoma. Whatever the diagnosis, careful patient selection is of paramount importance to ensure that the possible benefits outweigh the risks: these cases should always be approached in the context of multidisciplinary oncologic care.

The liver receives a dual vascular inflow of approximately 1500 ml/min. The portal vein provides three quarters of total hepatic blood flow while the hepatic artery provides the remaining 25%. This inflow is directed into the liver and subsequently the hepatic sinusoids. Outflow from the sinusoids is via the terminal hepatic venules, which subsequently coalesce into larger branches of the hepatic veins and then the major hepatic vein branches subsequently empty into the inferior vena cava.

During liver surgery, the hepatic parenchyma must be divided and measures to control the 1500 ml/min of blood flow through the liver must be used to minimize bleeding. The great majority of liver resections can be performed using standard techniques that control blood loss and minimize hepatocellular injury (see Chapter 18). Standard techniques include maintaining a low central venous pressure to minimize bleeding from small hepatic veins and meticulous ligation or control of small intrahepatic vessels while maintaining hepatic perfusion. However, there are instances which may require varying degrees of hepatic vascular inflow and outflow control to avoid major hemorrhage. In standard liver resection, even without vascular involvement, it may be beneficial to perform pedicle clamping (Pringle's maneuver) to reduce bleeding from the cut surface of the liver during transection. Pringle's maneuver has been shown to be tolerated best when applied intermittently, with 15 minute clamp periods interspersed with 5 minute periods of perfusion. Alternatively a period of ischemic preconditioning of the liver using a short period of clamping followed by a more prolonged clamp application of up to one hour has been shown to attenuate ischemia reperfusion injury. There are few contraindications to using hepatic inflow occlusion, or pedicle clamping during most liver surgery. In patients that have an injured liver due to biliary obstruction, chemotherapy, or steatosis, it may be wise to avoid inflow occlusion but should be used if bleeding is excessive.

Cases that involve major vascular structures that require resection and reconstruction will need additional vascular control. If possible, the surgeon can take advantage of the dual blood supply to the liver (arterial and portal) and clamp one source while maintaining the other. For example, if only the portal vein needs to be resected and reconstructed, proximal and distal control of the vein can generally be achieved while maintaining arterial flow to the liver, thus avoiding prolonged ischemia. If hepatic arterial involvement requires resection and reconstruction portal venous flow can be maintained and hepatic ischemia is minimized.

Tumors that involve or are in close proximity to the inferior vena cava or confluence of the hepatic veins may require total vascular isolation of the liver, with control of both vascular inflow and outflow. Depending on the complexity of the vascular reconstruction that is to be performed, it may be necessary to increase the acceptable period of hepatic ischemia by using cold perfusion techniques, whether in situ, or ex vivo. Historically, complete vascular isolation has not been as well tolerated by the liver or the patient as simple inflow occlusion, and major vascular reconstruction during liver surgery has been associated with increased morbidity and mortality. Patients with any significant comorbidity, including even mild renal dysfunction are likely poor candidates for hepatic resection with vascular reconstruction. This chapter will focus on techniques involved in resecting and reconstructing the IVC and hepatic veins.

## PREOPERATIVE PLANNING

As with all liver resectional surgery for malignancy, complete staging of the tumor is required. This includes both imaging of the liver and staging of any extrahepatic disease (see Chapter 18). More recently both CT (Fig. 30.1) and MRI (Fig. 30.2) have allowed volumetric assessment of the projected liver remnant. In standard liver resections a

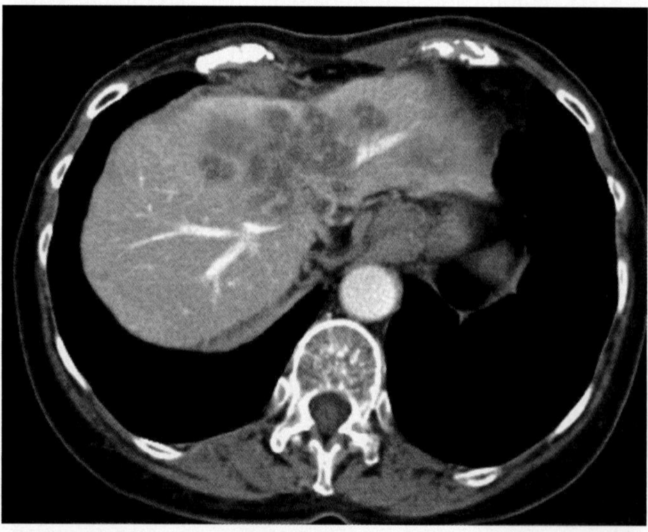

**Figure 30.1** CT demonstrating metastatic colorectal cancer involving middle and left hepatic veins that will require left trisectionectomy with resection/reconstruction of the origin of the right hepatic vein.

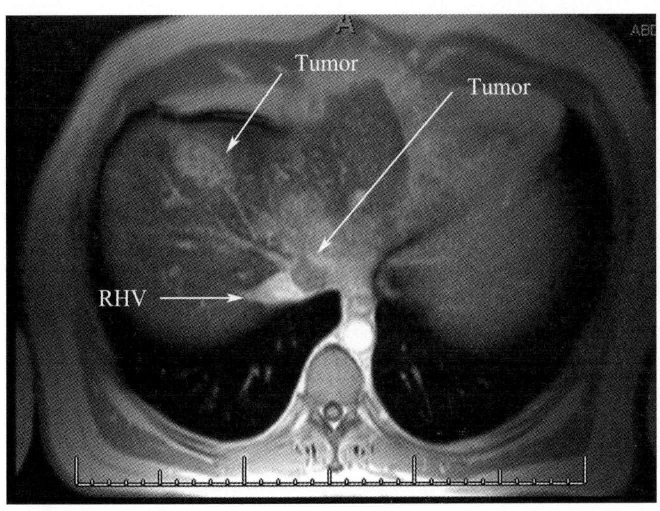


Figure 30.2 MRI demonstrating metastatic colorectal cancer invading the middle hepatic vein and extending into the inferior vena cava.



future liver remnant volume of 25% or more of total liver volume is acceptable for proceeding to resection. In cases where major vascular reconstruction is being considered we have chosen—somewhat arbitrarily—a projected liver remnant of less than 40% as an indication for preoperative portal vein embolization of the side of the liver to be resected. This recommendation is based on what is required for performing resections in the injured or cirrhotic liver. While there is no prospective data to indicate an absolute requirement, there seems little down side to providing an additional margin of safety in complex hepatic operations that require vascular reconstruction.

Preoperative assessment of the location of the liver tumor in relation to vascular structures is critical. Planning the resection with attention to major venous outflow tributaries with associated drainage areas may identify specific large venous branches that can be preserved for the sake of postoperative liver function (Fig. 30.3). The course of the operation and need for clamping, volume loading, cold perfusion, veno-venous bypass and the need and source of vascular grafts are best identified well before the procedure rather than urgently partway through the operation.

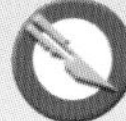

# SURGICAL TECHNIQUE

## Positioning and Incision

The patient is placed supine. Various incisions can be used, and generally involve some variation of a bilateral subcostal incision with or without a midline extension. (see Figs. 18.7,

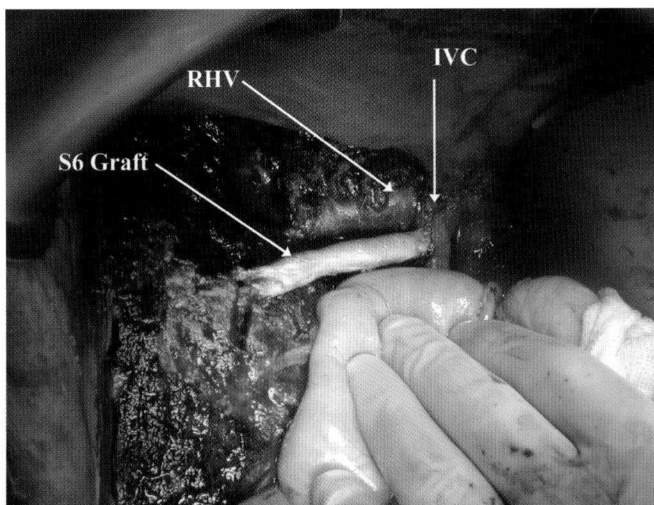


Figure 30.3 Left trisectionectomy with reconstruction of the segment 6 venous outflow using cryopreserved venous graft. IVC, inferior vena cava; RHV, right hepatic vein; S6 Graft, segment 6 vein graft.

19.3 and 21.5) Alternatively a midline incision with a right extension parallel to the costal margin, or "hockey stick incision" can be used, and either approach can be combined with a midline sternotomy for the sake of exposure of the hepatocaval confluence.

## Assessment of Resectability

The abdomen is assessed for extrahepatic disease. Portal and aortacaval nodes are assessed. The liver is mobilized by dividing right and left triangular ligaments as well as the gastrohepatic omentum. A replaced left hepatic artery running through the gastrohepatic omentum is identified and preserved if present and required for inflow to the planned liver remnant. In some cases, a large tumor of the right lobe will require an anterior approach without mobilization of the right triangular ligament until after division of the hepatic parenchyma (see Chapter 19). Intraoperative ultrasound can be used to assess tumor size, number and relation to vascular structures. An initial decision regarding resectability and the need for vascular grafts and/or techniques is made at this time, realizing that options may change as the case proceeds.

## Strategies to Achieve Vascular Control

Total vascular isolation: Tumors involving the retrohepatic IVC or the hepatic veins as they enter the IVC require various techniques to establish inflow and outflow control in order to minimize blood loss. In total vascular isolation, control of the portal vein and hepatic artery (inflow), and the suprahepatic and infrahepatic IVC (outflow) is established to minimize bleeding from the hepatic artery, portal vein, and hepatic veins. Total vascular isolation may be more damaging than hepatic inflow occlusion alone: Some evidence suggests that hepatic venous back-diffusion may minimize ischemic injury. However, most of the hepatic parenchymal division can usually be performed without total vascular isolation, and clamping of the IVC or hepatic veins can be reserved for the relatively short time period that is required to resect and reconstruct these structures. For total vascular isolation, as much mobilization of the liver off of the vena cava is performed as possible without violating tumor planes prior to hepatic parenchymal transection (see Chapter 19). In some cases, the bulky nature of the tumor inhibits the ability to rotate the liver safely and a primary anterior approach to the IVC can be taken with little or no mobilization of the liver off of the IVC.

The approach to vena caval resection depends on the extent and location of tumor involvement (Figs. 30.4–30.6). If the portion of vena cava involved with tumor is below

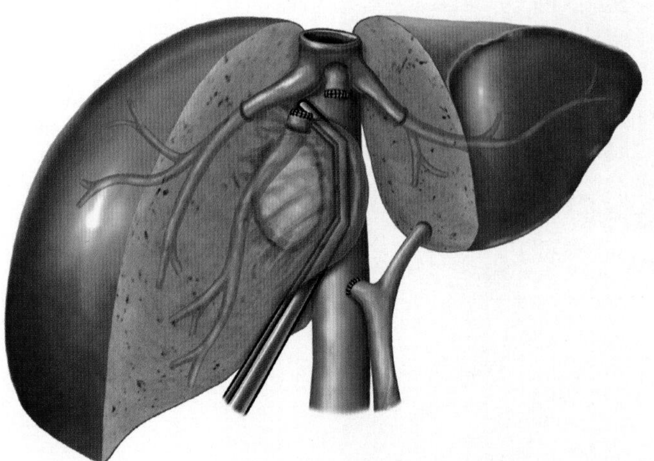

**Figure 30.4** A side biting vascular clamp can be placed tangentially on the IVC and the IVC repaired primarily if the area of involvement is small and the IVC is narrowed less than 30%.

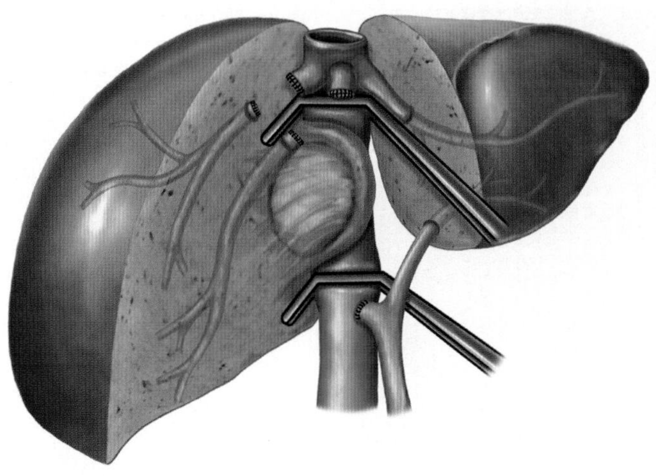

Figure 30.5 For tumors below the hepatic veins the liver can be divided with vascular clamps placed above and below the tumor on the IVC, maintaining portal inflow to the area of liver to be preserved during the caval resection/reconstruction.

the hepatic veins, then the parenchyma of the liver can be divided exposing the retrohepatic IVC. The parenchymal transection can be performed with inflow occlusion; however, if possible, the parenchymal division is done while maintaining hepatic perfusion. Central venous pressure is kept at or below 5 cm $H_2O$ during parenchymal transection to minimize blood loss. Once the IVC is exposed, portal inflow occlusion, if used, is released, the patient is volume loaded, and clamps are placed above and below the area of tumor involvement. The portion of liver and involved IVC is then removed allowing improved access for reconstruction of the IVC. The placement of clamps on the IVC inferior to the origin of the hepatic veins allows continued perfusion of the liver and minimizes the hepatic ischemic time. Cases where tumor involvement does not allow placement of clamps on the IVC inferior to the origin of the hepatic veins may require some element of cold perfusion of the liver, described below, unless the reconstruction time is expected to be short, cold perfusion techniques can be used. In general the superior anastomosis of the graft is performed first, with clamps subsequently repositioned on the graft below the hepatic veins if necessary to allow release of portal inflow occlusion and reperfusion of the liver to minimize ischemic time (Figs. 30.7–30.10).

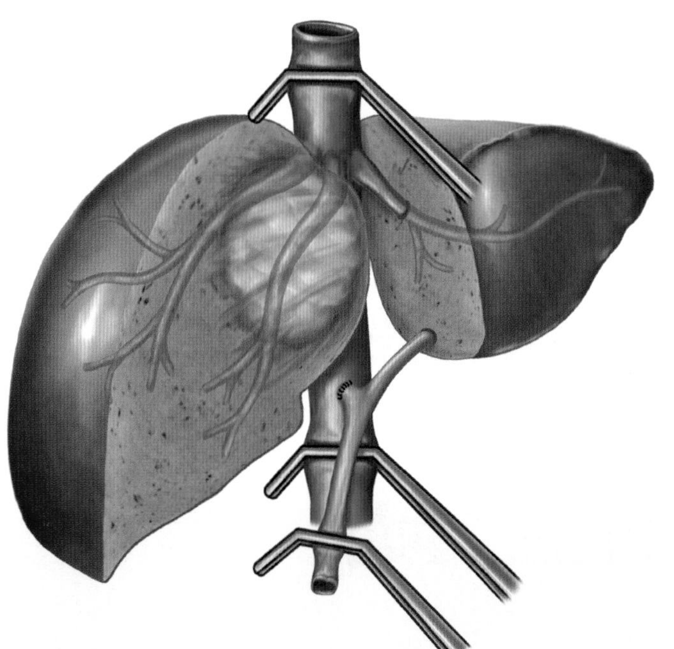

Figure 30.6 Tumors that are at the level of, or involve the hepatic veins require total vascular isolation.

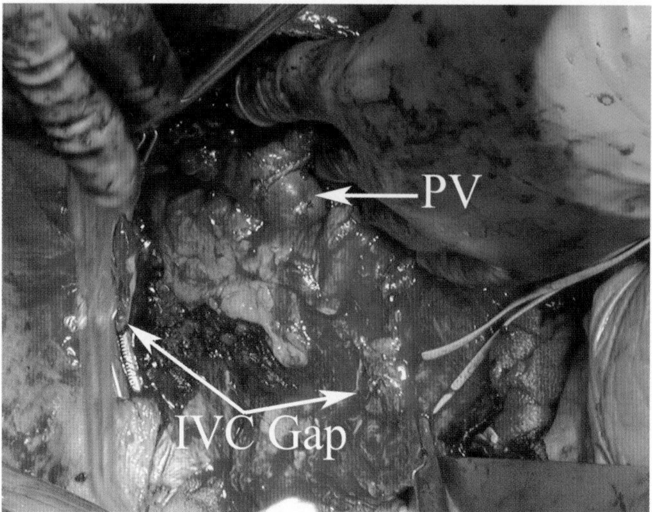


Figure 30.7 Intraoperative picture of patient with the right lobe resected en bloc with the IVC. Notice the gap between vascular clamps where the IVC has been resected. The top clamp is positioned below the left and middle hepatic veins to allow continued perfusion of the left lobe during IVC reconstruction. IVC, inferior vena cava; PV, portal vein.

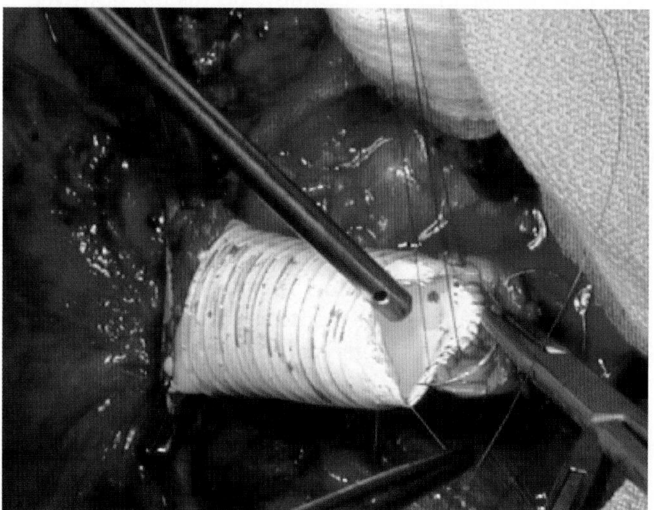

Figure 30.8 20 mm ringed Gortex graft is used to reconstruct the IVC.

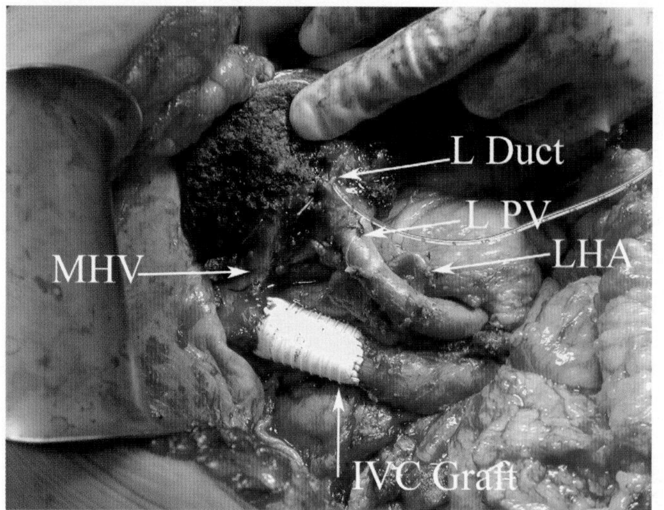


Figure 30.9 Reconstructed IVC. Notice superior edge of graft sits just below the entry of the middle hepatic vein into the IVC. IVC, inferior vena cava; L duct, left hepatic duct; LHA, left hepatic artery; LPV, left portal vein, MHV, middle hepatic vein.

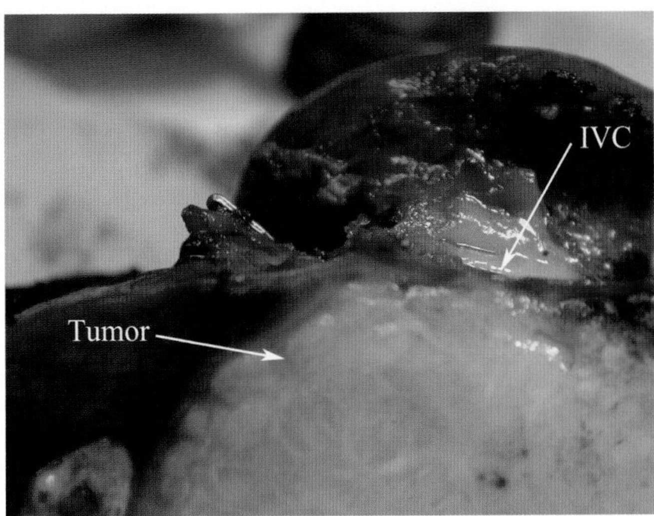


**Figure 30.10** The resected specimen from Figure 30.7. Tumor extends into the anterior surface of the IVC and is inseparable from the vein wall but does not penetrate into the lumen of the IVC.



# Cold Perfusion for Liver Resections with Vascular Reconstruction

Standard liver resection techniques are sufficient for almost every liver resection, without the use of hypothermic perfusion. However tumors that are centrally placed and involve all three main hepatic veins, with or without involvement of the retrohepatic inferior vena cava, are essentially unresectable using standard liver resection techniques. Those few patients that require complex reconstruction of hepatic venous outflow may benefit from either ex vivo or in situ hypothermic perfusion of the liver with subsequent hepatic resection and vascular reconstruction.

Fortner first described the use of hypothermic perfusion during liver resection to protect the liver from ischemic injury in 1974. In an attempt to offer resection to patients with tumors that were unresectable by conventional means and also inappropriate for liver transplantation, Pichlmayr developed hypothermic perfusion with ex vivo liver resection. During ex vivo liver resection, the liver is completely removed from the body and perfused with cold preservation solution on the back table. The liver resection is then performed on the back table in a bloodless field, allowing reconstruction of hepatic venous outflow to be performed under ideal conditions. The development of in situ hypothermic perfusion techniques followed, including the so-called in situ and ante situm procedures. In situ hypothermic perfusion uses standard liver mobilization techniques, but the liver is cold-perfused via the portal vein. In the ante situm procedure the liver is cold-perfused via the portal vein and the hilar structures are left otherwise intact. The suprahepatic IVC is divided and the liver is rotated forward, allowing improved access to the area of the liver and centered around the hepatic vein confluence. The procedure and role for each technique will be described below.

# In Situ Hypothermic Perfusion

A limited in situ cold perfusion technique can be used when a single hepatic vein or the IVC requires reconstruction. In this technique, most of the parenchymal transection can be performed without inflow occlusion, and total vascular isolation is then applied to divide and reconstruct the vascular structures only. The portal vein dissection is carried high to gain control of the right and left branches and perfusion tubing placed into the portal vein side ipsilateral to the tumor but directed into the liver remnant. The cannulated portal vein branch is then divided above the cannula while maintaining portal flow to the remnant side. Alternatively the main portal main can be used to place

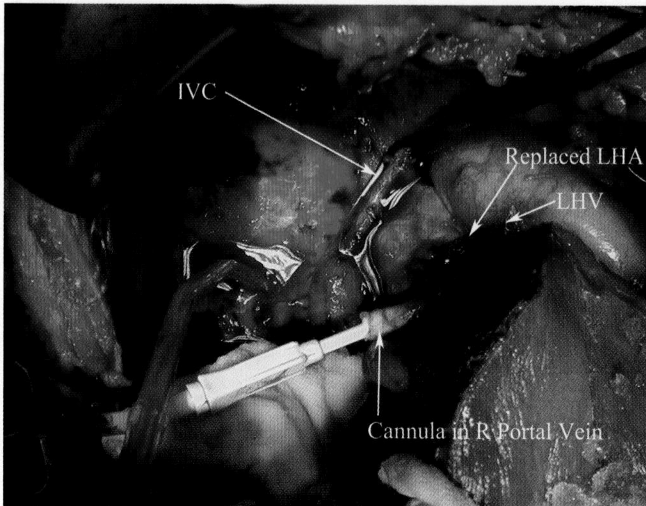


**Figure 30.11** In situ cold perfusion. The cannula has been placed in the divided right portal vein branch and the left lobe flushed with cold UW preservation solution. Note the replaced left hepatic artery (replaced LHA) clamped separately. IVC, Inferior vena cava; LHV, left hepatic vein.

the perfusion tubing but will need repair at the completion of the procedure. The patient is volume-loaded, and clamps placed sequentially on the infrahepatic cava, the portal vein, hepatic artery and then the suprahepatic IVC. If only the hepatic vein requires reconstruction, IVC flow can be maintained by clamping the trunk of the target hepatic vein tangentially and parallel to the IVC, thereby only partially narrowing the IVC. The anterior wall of the IVC or hepatic vein is incised (Fig. 30.11) and cold perfusion of the liver with organ preservation solution performed. The hepatic vein trunk is transected and the specimen is removed. The hepatic vein and/or IVC can then be reconstructed in a bloodless field, without time pressure (Fig. 30.12). Before completing the anastomosis the liver is flushed with cold 5% albumin. At completion of the vascular anastomosis, portal and hepatic arterial flow is reestablished. With the majority of the parenchymal transection being done without vascular isolation and with shorter ischemic times using these techniques, the authors do not use veno-veno bypass.

Standard in situ cold perfusion is considered for liver resections that require total vascular isolation for periods exceeding 1 hour or perhaps in injured liver for periods shorter than 1 hour. This technique is used for tumors involving the hepatic veins and/or retrohepatic IVC where longer periods of vascular isolation will be required either due to vascular involvement or due to the need for dissection of long stretches of intrahepatic vasculature that may result in excessive blood loss.

In standard in situ cold perfusion (Fig. 30.13) the liver is mobilized as for total vascular isolation, with control of supra and infrahepatic IVC and the portal structures. The portal vein (3 to 4 cm) is exposed to place a perfusion catheter and a portal venous cannula for veno-veno bypass if utilized. Although most patients tolerate total vascular

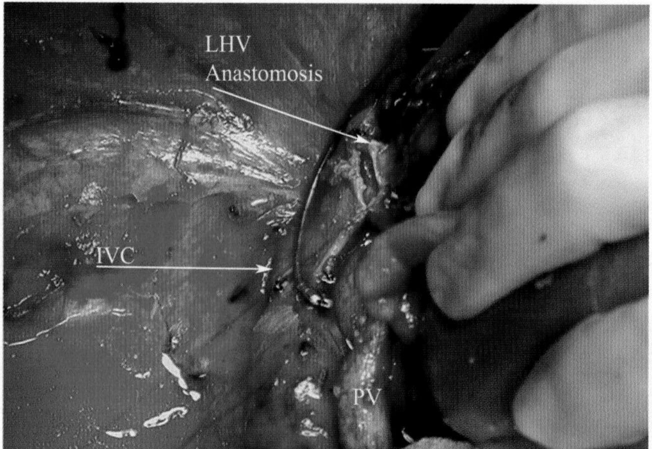


**Figure 30.12** Case from Figure 30.11 with the left hepatic vein being reimplanted into the IVC. The posterior wall of the anastomosis has been performed with the anterior wall still to be completed. IVC, inferior vena cava; LHV, left hepatic vein.

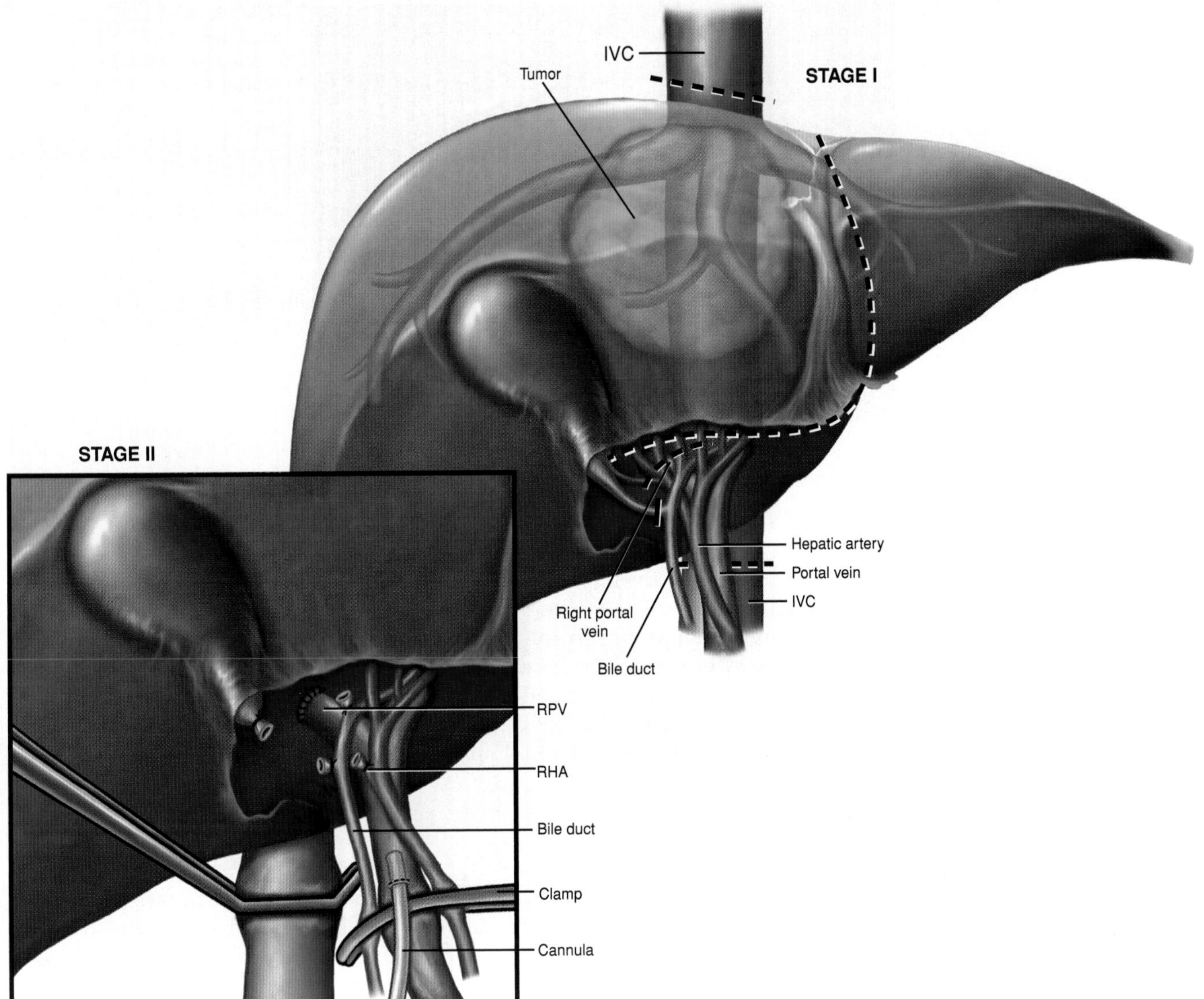


**Figure 30.13** Diagrammatic representation of standard in situ cold perfusion with the cannula placed into the main portal vein. The front wall of the portal vein will require repair prior to reperfusion of the liver. RHA, right hepatic artery; RPV, right portal vein.



isolation without it, veno-venous bypass reduces the time pressure and gut edema associated with prolonged portal clamping. The infrahepatic IVC is clamped and the patient placed on the caval portion of veno-veno bypass. A portal clamp is placed high on the portal vein with bypass instituted below. The portal cannula can be inserted down toward the superior mesenteric vein, and full veno-venous bypass is started. The liver side of the portal vein is cannulated for cold preservation and the hepatic artery clamped. The suprahepatic IVC is clamped and a transverse venotomy created in the infrahepatic IVC just above the clamp. Cold perfusion of the liver is begun with preservation solution and the effluent suctioned from the venotomy in the infrahepatic IVC. Preservation solution is either histidine-tryptophan-ketoglutarate (HTK), or University of Wisconsin solution (UW). The liver resection and hepatic vein resection/reconstruction then proceeds in a bloodless field with excellent visualization of intrahepatic structures. At completion of the liver resection, the liver is flushed of cold preservation solution through the portal vein with cold 5% albumin before restoring flow to the liver. The portal bypass cannula is removed and the portal vein is repaired or reanastomosed if divided. The infrahepatic venting IVC venotomy is closed and the suprahepatic caval clamp is removed to assess the integrity of the hepatic vein reconstruction and the presence of cut surface bleeding. Portal and hepatic arterial inflow is then reestablished. The patient is then decannulated from caval bypass.

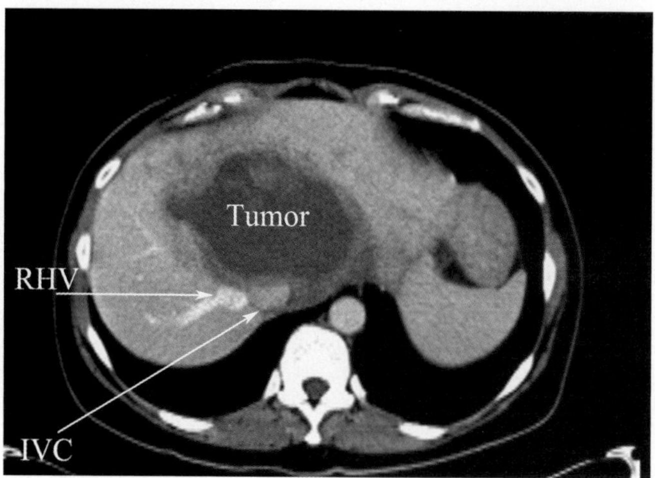


**Figure 30.14** CT of a case with a large central tumor involving IVC, middle and left hepatic veins and abutting or involving the right hepatic vein. IVC, inferior vena cava.

# Ex Vivo Liver Resection

In practice almost all liver resections can be performed without ex vivo approach. However, patients who have tumors that involve the IVC and hepatic veins that will require complex venous repair, or patients with combined hepatic vein and hilar involvement may be candidates for ex vivo resection (Fig. 30.14). During ex vivo resection, the liver is completely removed from the patient and perfused with cold preservation solution on the back table. The hepatic resection and vascular reconstructions are performed on the back table before reimplanting the remnant liver into the patient.

## SURGICAL PROCEDURE

The liver is assessed for resectability. Since the indication for ex vivo resection is generally involvement of the hepatic veins with or without cava involvement, the liver may be quite congested due to obstructed venous outflow. Thus, care must be taken not to injure the liver during mobilization: Any small breach of the liver capsule becomes an outflow route for the obstructed venous flow, and bleeding can be substantial. Large tumors may restrict the ability to rotate the liver without undue tension, and in these cases it is prudent to make an early decision regarding ex vivo resection before attempting elevation of the liver off of the IVC. A midline sternotomy can also be of use in these cases (Fig. 30.15). Intraoperative ultrasound is used to assess the level of vascular

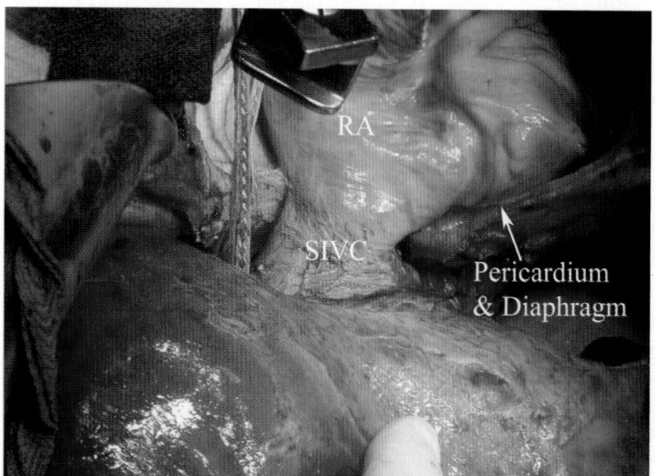


**Figure 30.15** Exposure to the hepatocaval confluence provided by median sternotomy is unsurpassed and should be considered in any difficult case requiring reconstruction near the hepatocaval junction. RA, right atrium; SIVC, suprahepatic inferior vena cava; RHV, right hepatic vein.

involvement and to confirm vascular anatomy originally identified on preoperative imaging. If a decision is made to proceed with an ex vivo approach, the following steps are performed.

A. The hilar structures are prepared. The arterial anatomy is dissected and an appropriate site is chosen for planned division. This usually is at the level of the common hepatic artery–gastroduodenal artery junction. If the tumor involves the hilar structures, the artery must be dissected far enough to determine that there is a usable, tumor-free portion of the respective hepatic artery branch to reconstruct. The portal vein is identified, and the common bile duct is encircled without skeletonization. A cholecystectomy is performed. The bile duct is reflected off the portal vein taking care to preserve its blood supply, and the neural and lymphatic tissues around the portal vein are cleared.
B. The infrahepatic IVC is dissected out down to the level of the renal veins and encircled. Planned vascular clamp placement is immediately above the renal veins, although division of the vena cava may be substantially more cephalad.
C. The liver is freed from the surrounding attachments. If the tumor is infiltrating the diaphragm, the portion of the diaphragm involved is resected en bloc with the tumor.
D. The suprahepatic IVC is prepared. The phrenic veins are divided bilaterally, allowing the diaphragm to be dissected away from the IVC and providing an increased length of intraabdominal IVC. We also open the pericardium directly anterior to the IVC and loop the intrapericardial IVC, or use a midline sternotomy for the same reason. Control of the intrapericardial IVC allows placement of the clamp on the vena cava within the pericardium as a primary option for tumors that are very large.
E. Percutaneous access of the internal jugular vein and femoral vein is achieved, the IVC is clamped, and the cava portion of bypass is started. The portal vein is clamped just below the bifurcation, and the portal cannula is inserted down toward the superior mesenteric vein and secured. The portal vein is completely transected approximately 1.5 to 2 cm below the bifurcation, and the portal flow is added to the bypass circuit. The liver continues to be perfused by arterial blood at this time.
F. The bile duct is transected sharply approximately 1 to 1.5 cm below the bifurcation. The gastroduodenal artery is ligated and divided. The common hepatic artery is clamped, and the hepatic artery is transected at the takeoff of the gastroduodenal artery. The suprahepatic IVC is clamped either below the diaphragm or within the pericardium, and the suprahepatic vena cava is transected away from tumor, leaving enough room to perform the suprahepatic cava anastomosis at the time of reimplantation. The infrahepatic IVC is divided as cephalad as possible, and the liver is removed and placed in an ice bath. Cold perfusion through the portal vein and hepatic artery is initiated on the back bench. Cold perfusion can be with either histidine-tryptophan-ketoglutarate solution or University of Wisconsin solution.
G. Bleeding is controlled, and the bypass circuit is assessed (Fig. 30.16). The abdomen is loosely packed and covered, and attention is turned to the back table.

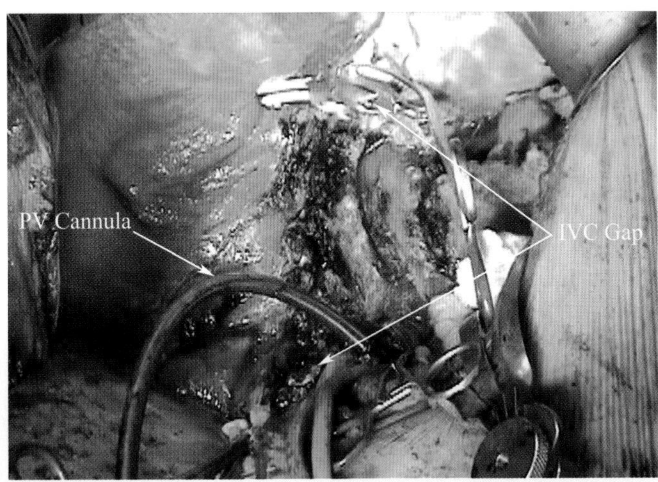


Figure 30.16 Case from Figure 30.14 with the liver and retrohepatic IVC completely removed with the patient placed on veno-veno bypass. PV cannula, the cannula for the portal flow into the bypass circuit. Notice the long gap between IVC clamps where the IVC has been removed en bloc with the liver.

An alternative method can be performed in cases that have complex hepatic vein involvement without IVC involvement with tumor that preserves the inferior vena cava and uses a temporary portacaval shunt to decompress the gut during the anhepatic phase. This option avoids bypass, but can be used only when there is no IVC involvement and when the IVC can be preserved in situ.

## Ex Situ Liver Resection

After it is removed from the patient, the liver is placed immediately in an ice bath and perfused with preservation solution through the portal vein. The hepatic artery and biliary tree are also flushed with another 200 to 300 ml of preservation solution. The liver is immersed in cold UW solution, and the resection is performed.

Hilar structures are dissected and divided. Parenchymal transection can be performed using various techniques, including ultrasonic dissection and water jet, or even sharp division with a knife. Small bile ducts and vessels are ligated or oversewn. Large hepatic veins are cut sharply and later assessed for reconstruction. At completion of the resection, it is helpful to flush the portal vein, hepatic artery, and bile duct with University of Wisconsin solution to identify leaks from the cut surface of the liver, which can be repaired before reimplantation.

## Hepatic Vein and Inferior Vena Cava Reconstruction

The hepatic veins are relatively thick-walled and straightforward to reconstruct within 2 to 3 cm of their merging with the IVC. For reconstructions of hepatic veins transected relatively close to the IVC, the liver parenchyma can be trimmed back such that direct reimplantation of the hepatic vein into the IVC or the IVC replacement can be performed. Multiple orifices of hepatic veins can be "plastied" together or implanted into venous conduits. Saphenous vein, superficial femoral vein, internal jugular vein, and cryopreserved vein grafts all have been used to reconstruct hepatic veins. Segments of uninvolved hepatic vein from the side of the liver resected can be salvaged and used for grafts, or patches. Venous grafts should be kept as short as possible, and great care must be taken to place the grafts such that they do not kink.

Ringed 20 mm Gore-Tex tube graft is used to replace the segment of IVC although, if at all possible, hepatic veins should be reimplanted into orthotopic or transposed IVC. In some circumstances, it is necessary to reimplant the hepatic veins directly into a relatively stiff artificial graft that is replacing the IVC. In this situation, it is important to make a larger opening in the Gore-Tex than one might expect and to triangulate the anastomosis to prevent anastomotic stricturing.

At completion of the back bench reconstruction, one has an autograft that is similar to that of a reduced size or split liver allograft (Fig. 30.17). Total cold ischemic time is usually 2 to 4 hours.

## Reimplantation

Reimplantation is similar to reduced size or living donor liver transplantation. The suprahepatic IVC anastomosis is performed first. When the back wall of the infrahepatic vena cava anastomosis has been completed, the portal vein is flushed with 500 ml of cold 5% albumin, which is vented through the infrahepatic cava anastomosis. The infrahepatic vena cava anastomosis is then completed. The cold rinse washes the University of Wisconsin solution out of the liver before reperfusion, which otherwise can cause dramatic cardiac dysfunction or arrest if allowed into the circulation on reperfusion.

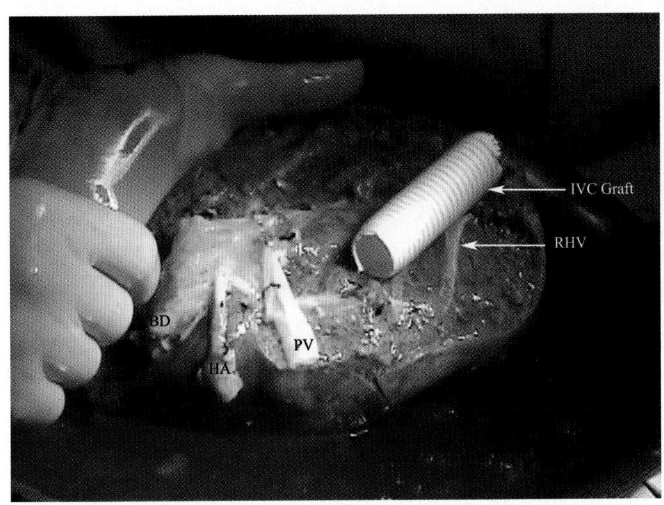


**Figure 30.17** Graft obtained after ex vivo resection and back table reconstruction of case from Figure 30.14. BD, bile duct; HA hepatic artery; IVC graft, inferior vena cava graft; PV portal vein; RHV, right hepatic vein.



After the infrahepatic cava anastomosis is performed, the portal limb of the bypass circuit is clamped and removed from the portal vein. The portal venous anastomosis is performed.

The suprahepatic cava clamp is removed, and the liver is allowed to back perfuse through the hepatic veins. Any major bleeding is controlled before reestablishing the portal flow (Fig. 30.18). The portal venous clamp is removed, and the liver is reperfused. The patient is then taken off veno-venous bypass. The arterial anastomosis is performed, and the liver is reperfused with arterial blood. Total warm ischemic time ranges from 20 to 40 minutes. After hemostasis has been achieved, the biliary anastomosis is performed whether duct to duct or with Roux-en-Y choledochojejunostomy.

# Postoperative Care

Postoperative care is similar for combined liver and caval resection whether performed warm or cold. Day 1 transaminases in the 200 to 1000 IU/L range are standard, but return to near-normal by 1 week. Hyperbilirubinemia is common and, as one might expect, seems to vary inversely with the size of the liver remnant. Hyperbilirubinemia by itself is not concerning if other markers of liver function are improving. An early sign that the autograft is functioning is the return of lactate levels to baseline in the first 12 to 24 hours after surgery. Maintenance of coagulation parameters, in particular prothrombin time or international normalized ratio, suggests recovery of liver function.

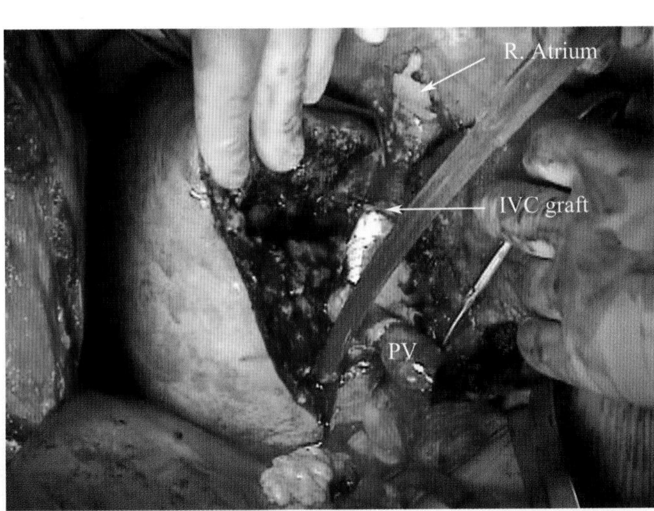


**Figure 30.18** Case from Figure 30.14 reimplanted just after portal vein reperfusion. A vascular clamp has been temporarily used to occlude venous outflow to the liver to assess the cut surface of the liver for bleeding. Notice the pericardium has been opened from below for intrapericardial access to the suprahepatic IVC. IVC graft, inferior vena cava graft; PV portal vein; R Atrium right atrium.

Hypophosphatemia can occur between postoperative days 1 and 3 as the liver regenerates and may be profound and require constant intravenous replacement. Without much evidence as to its effectiveness, we have used low-dose intravenous heparin (500 U/hr) perioperatively and attempt to maintain the hematocrit between 30% and 35%. Patients who have artificial venous caval grafts are started on low-dose aspirin before discharge. This is maintained for life, though there is no data that confirms the need for long-term anticoagulation.

## CONCLUSIONS

The role of such an extensive procedure in advanced malignancies is open for discussion. Most of the literature on ex vivo liver resections has been case reports that describe aspects of technique, and long-term follow-up is not available. Perioperative mortality even in well-selected patients is between 10% and 30%. By contrast, the perioperative mortality for patients undergoing in situ or ante situ hepatic hypothermic perfusion with vascular reconstruction is around 10% or less. Long-term survival after ex vivo liver resection is also poor—at best, the 5-year survival for ex vivo resections performed for malignancy is 15% to 30%. Oldhafer et al. reported a median survival of 21 months in patients undergoing ex vivo liver resection for colorectal metastases in the largest and longest series of ex vivo liver resections, though it might be expected that the general improvement in survival following resection for colorectal metastases seen over the last decade would apply to ex vivo liver resections as well.

Notwithstanding the considerations above, there is no doubt that the occasional patient is cured by this aggressive procedure. It is also worth noting that many patients may benefit by being considered for ex vivo liver resection or in situ cold perfusion simply because a surgeon prepared to perform ex vivo resection realizes that the resection can be performed using a less aggressive technique, whether that be total vascular isolation and vascular resection without cold perfusion or even more standard liver resection.

## Recommended References and Readings


Azoulay D, Eshkenazy R, Andreani P, et al. In situ hypothermic perfusion of the liver versus standard total vascular exclusion for complex liver resection. *Ann Surg.* 2005;241:277–285.

Clavien PA, Selzner M, Rüdiger HA, et al. A prospective randomized study in 100 consecutive patients undergoing major liver resection with versus without ischemic preconditioning. *Ann Surg.* 2003;238:843–850; discussion 851–842.

Dubay D, Gallinger S, Hawryluck L, et al. In situ hypothermic liver preservation during radical liver resection with major vascular reconstruction. *Br J Surg.* 2009;96:1429–1436.

Fortner JG, Shiu MH, Kinne DW, et al. Major hepatic resection using vascular isolation and hypothermic perfusion. *Ann Surg.* 1974;180:644–652.

Hemming AW, Reed AI. Left trisegmentectomy with reconstruction of segment 6 hepatic venous outflow using cryopreserved vein graft. *J Gastrointest Surg.* 2005;9:353–356.

Hemming AW, Reed AI, Fujita S. Ex vivo extended left hepatectomy with caval preservation, temporary portacaval shunt, and reconstruction of the right hepatic vein outflow using a reversed portal vein bifurcation graft. *J Hepatobiliary Pancreat Surg.* 2006; 13:525–529.

Hemming AW, Reed AI, Fujita S, et al. Surgical management of hilar cholangiocarcinoma. *Ann Surg.* 2005;241:693–699; discussion 699–702.

Hemming AW, Reed AI, Fujita S, et al. Role for extending hepatic resection using an aggressive approach to liver surgery. *J Am Coll Surg.* 2008;206:870–875; discussion 875–878.

Hemming AW, Reed AI, Langham MR Jr, et al. Combined resection of the liver and inferior vena cava for hepatic malignancy. *Ann Surg.* 2004;239:712–719; discussion 719–721.

Liu CL, Fan ST, Lo CM, et al. Anterior approach for major right hepatic resection for large hepatocellular carcinoma. *Ann Surg.* 2000;232:25–31.

Lodge JP, Ammori BJ, Prasad KR, et al. Ex vivo and in situ resection of inferior vena cava with hepatectomy for colorectal metastases. *Ann Surg.* 2000;231:471–479.

Oldhafer KJ, Lang H, Schlitt HJ, et al. Long-term experience after ex situ liver surgery. *Surgery.* 2000;127:520–527.

Pichlmayr R, Bretschneider HJ, Kirchner R, et al. Ex situ operation on the liver. A new possibility in liver surgery. *Langenbecks Arch Chir.* 1988;373(2):122–126.

Smyrniotis V, Kostopanagiotou G, Lolis E, et al. Effects of hepatovenous back flow on ischemic-reperfusion injuries in liver resections with the pringle maneuver. *J Am Coll Surg.* 2003;197:949–954.

# 31 Laparoscopic Partial Hepatectomy

**Michael D. Kluger and Daniel Cherqui**

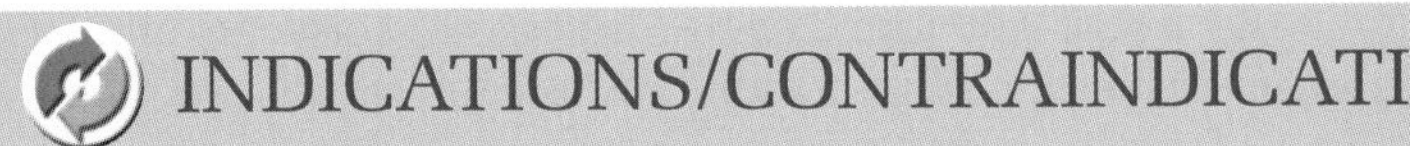

## INDICATIONS/CONTRAINDICATIONS

Although laparoscopic liver surgery was first reported nearly two decades ago, it has not received wide attention until relatively recently. Different resections require varying levels of expertise, but all require familiarity with preoperative planning and perioperative care of the liver patient, open liver surgery, hepatic anatomy, and advanced laparoscopic principles. The 2008 Louisville Statement divides these operations among pure, hand-assisted and hybrid laparoscopy. Pure laparoscopy involves complete mobilization and resection via laparoscopic ports, although an incision may be used for specimen extraction. Hand-assisted laparoscopy involves the elective placement of a hand-port for mobilization or resection, which is then used for specimen extraction. Hybrid refers to a procedure where the resection is performed through a mini-laparotomy, though laparoscopy with or without hand assistance is utilized for mobilization. We favor pure laparoscopy for all resections.

Lesion size and location are the most important determinants of when laparoscopic resection is appropriate. Although there is variation in this evolving field as to what some centers will consider for laparoscopic resection. Table 31.1 details the indications and contraindications generally supported by high volume centers. Asymptomatic lesions convincingly recognized by imaging to be benign, that do not have harmful potential and would normally not be resected by laparotomy, should not be resected because laparoscopy is feasible.

## PREOPERATIVE PLANNING

### Equipment and Instruments

All equipment must be state of the art, tested before each operation, and nursing staff should be familiar with proper set-up and functioning. In addition to an operating room

**TABLE 31.1 Indications and Contraindications to Laparoscopic Partial Hepatectomy**

| Indications | Relative Contraindications | Contraindications |
|---|---|---|
| • Solitary mass ≤5 cm, or pedunculated mass of any size that does not obscure safe working space<br>• Peripherally located lesions in segments 2 to 6<br>• Left lateral sectionectomy | • Lesions located in proximity to the major hepatic veins, the inferior vena cava or the hepatic hilum<br>• Lesions isolated to segments 7 and 8<br>• Multiple or bilateral lesions | • Patient unlikely to tolerate or recover from an open operation because of chronic medical conditions<br>• Gallbladder cancer and hilar cholangiocarcinoma<br>• Insufficient oncologic margin |

sized to accommodate the laparoscopy and liver transection instrument consoles, the following instruments and devices are necessary:

- An adjustable remote controlled electric split-leg table.
- 10 mm 30° laparoscope, high definition camera and xenon lighting. High definition monitors positioned lateral to each shoulder and above the patient's head when the patient is supine, and across from the surgeon when the patient is in the left lateral decubitus position.
- Two $CO_2$ insufflators (12 mm Hg is used for the prevention of gas embolism) with full tanks. Two insufflators are preferred, as intermittent suction is necessary to maintain a smokeless field when using diathermy instruments on liver parenchyma.
- Comfortable ergonomic laparoscopic instruments, including ratcheted fenestrated and atraumatic bowel forceps, curved and right angle dissectors, scissors, bipolar diathermy forceps, monopolar diathermy hook, needle holders and a liver retractor.
- Disposable or reusable ports (5, 10, 12, and 15 mm), laparoscopic in-line and cutting vascular staplers, ultrasonic dissector, LigaSure or Harmonic devices, clip appliers (combinations of small, large, locking, absorbable and titanium), a suction-irrigator and a large specimen bag.
- An ultrasound with B- and D-modes and a high frequency laparoscopic transducer.
- 5-0 Prolene sutures cut to 20 to 30 cm, umbilical tapes and tourniquet materials.
- Scope warmer, as smoke and splattering affect the optics.
- A set of conventional instruments and retractors for open surgery should be available.
- An adequate back-up supply of all mentioned equipment.

## Patient Preparation

A thorough history and physical examination should be performed to evaluate for medical disease or previous abdominal incisions that might complicate a laparoscopic approach. Severe cardiac, pulmonary, or renal disease should be further evaluated at the surgeon's discretion. High quality magnetic resonance or computed tomography imaging with vascular reconstruction should be reviewed in order to evaluate for intrahepatic arterial and portal anomalies and to determine if the lesion is amenable to a laparoscopic resection (see Chapter 18). Informed consent should include a thorough discussion of the risks and benefits of laparoscopic surgery relative to the risks and benefits of open surgery, with a discussion of the possibility of conversion to an open resection.

Patients are preferably admitted 1 day preoperatively and routine labs are drawn, including a basic metabolic profile, complete blood count, coagulation series, liver function tests, and tumor markers. The patient is advised to take minimal fluids for 24 hours before surgery and kept NPO past midnight with the objective of low central venous pressure during the operation.

The operation can be divided into five stages that should be planned before proceeding to the operating room: (1) patient position; (2) port placement and ultrasonography; (3) mobilization, control of inflow/outflow and marking the liver; (4) parenchymal dissection, hemostasis, and biliary stasis; and (5) specimen extraction.

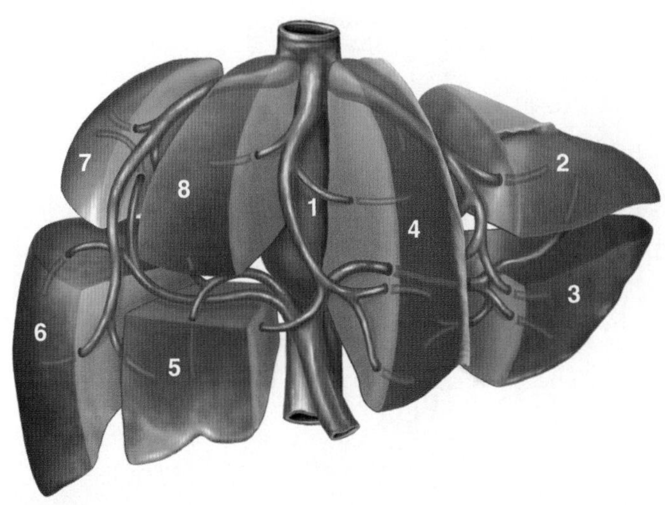


Figure 31.1 The eight Couinaud segments. Segments 2–6 are most amenable to laparoscopic resection.



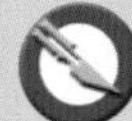

## SURGICAL TECHNIQUE I: GENERAL PRINCIPLES

### Pertinent Anatomy

The liver is divided into eight segments on the basis of the divisions of the right and left portal veins according to the nomenclature of Couinaud (Fig. 31.1). Just as in open resection, laparoscopic resection is defined by the Brisbane 2000 terminology of liver anatomy and resections. Tumors 5 cm or less in size located in the anterolateral segments (i.e., 2, 3, 4b, 5, and 6) are most amenable to laparoscopic resection (Fig. 31.1). Other lesions require more advanced expertise. Liver anatomy has been described elsewhere in this book.

### Patient Positioning

After patient and procedure confirmation, general anesthesia is induced and a central venous catheter, arterial line, large bore peripheral intravenous catheter, nasogastric tube, and Foley catheter are placed. Routine anesthesia monitoring includes heart rate, arterial blood pressure, pulse oximetry, capnometry, and esophageal temperature. Central venous pressure is measured as required and other monitoring utilized at the discretion of anesthesia (see Chapter 18). Perioperative antibiotics are given. Bilateral intermittent venous compression devices are placed and the abdomen is prepped from the neck to the groin and then covered with a steri-drape.

For all resections, the patient can be placed in the supine position with the lower limbs apart on a split-leg table. Both arms are padded and tucked at the sides. The surgeon stands between the legs, with an assistant at each side. The scrub nurse is positioned behind the surgeon along the right leg, with the instruments behind. A mayo stand positioned over the right leg holds the most commonly utilized instruments. Reverse Trendelenburg allows the bowels to drop into the lower abdomen and the table is tilted laterally as necessary to take advantage of gravity and the weight of the liver to improve exposure. An example of the room set-up and patient position is demonstrated in Figure 31.2 (see also Chapter 29 and Figs. 29.9–29.13). For masses in segments 6 or 7, the patient can be placed in the left lateral decubitus position. The arms, legs, and left shoulder are padded and placed in physiologic positions. The surgeon and one assistant stand on the patient's ventral side, with the scrub nurse opposite at the legs.

### Port Placement, Exploration, and Ultrasonography

An open technique is used to gain access to the abdomen supraumbilically and a 10 mm port is placed to serve as the camera port. The remaining four ports are placed under

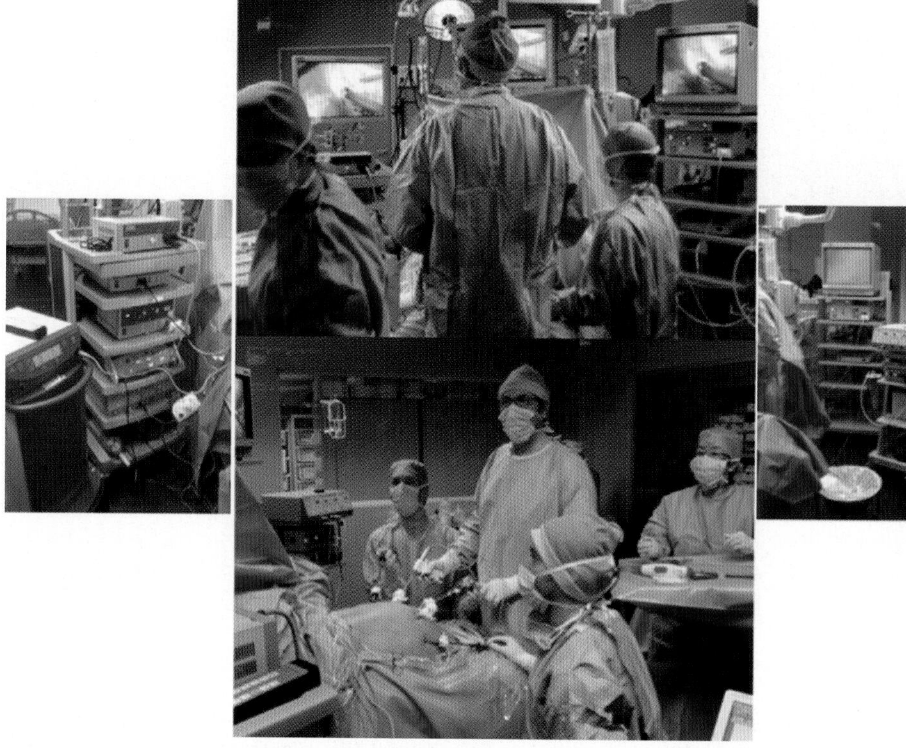

Figure 31.2 Room set-up. The patient is on a split-leg table with the surgeon between the legs and assistants seated on both sides. The scrub nurse and instruments are behind the surgeon at the patient's right leg. Monitors are placed above the patient's head and at the right and left shoulders. Instrument consoles are to the sides, with cords being draped from the chest toward the legs. For large pedunculated masses of segment 6, the patient may be placed in the left lateral decubitus position.

direct vision: Right and left para-median versa-step 5 to 12 mm working ports, and right and left lateral 5 mm ports for retraction instruments (Fig. 31.3). For left lateral decubitus positioning, four ports are used: a 10 mm in the left upper quadrant, a supra-umbilical 12 mm port, a 12 mm paraumbilical port in the mid-clavicular line, and a 10 mm trocar in the anterior-axillary line (Fig. 31.3). Port position may vary based on body habitus, but generally follow a curve from right to left similar to the profile of the liver.

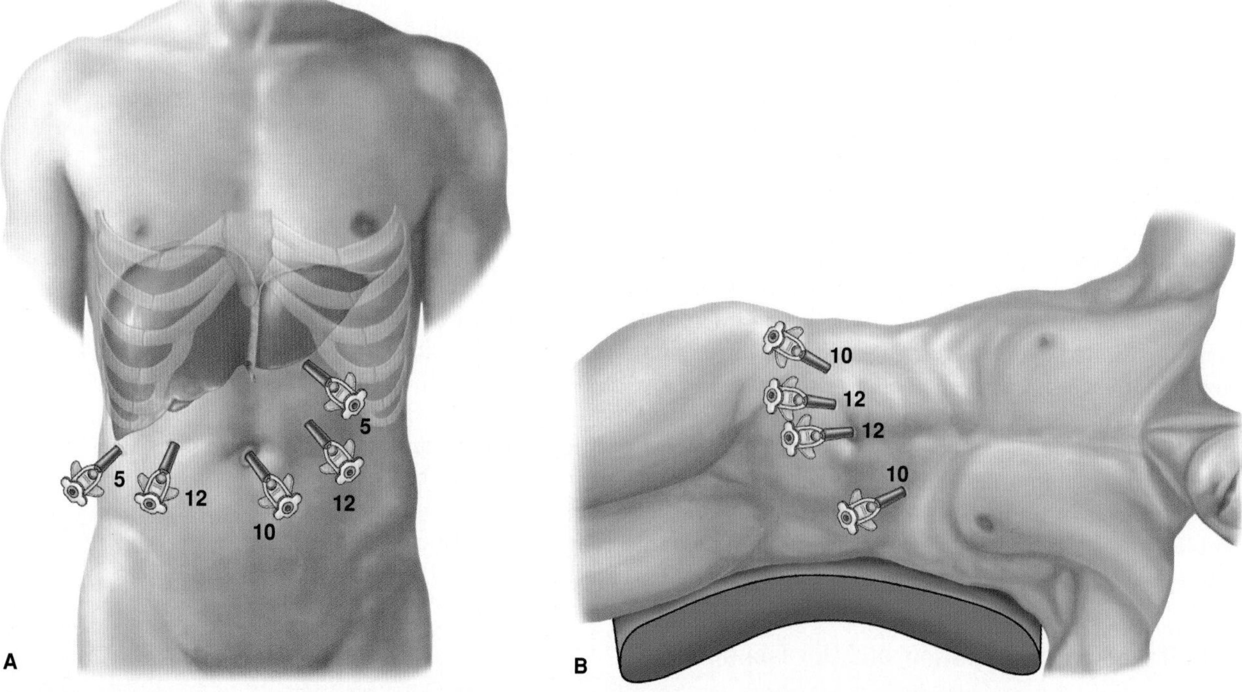


Figure 31.3 Port placement. All laparoscopic liver procedures can be performed in the supine position with ports placed as demonstrated (**Image A**). For left lateral decubitus position, four ports are used as demonstrated (**Image B**). Numbers refer to port sizes.

After a thorough inspection of the peritoneal cavity for ascites, carcinomatosis, and signs of portal hypertension, attention is turned to the liver for signs of superficial lesions, steatosis, cholestasis, cirrhosis, or other gross pathology. Laparoscopic ultrasound is systematically performed to confirm the location of the lesion, vascular anatomy, verify margins, and identify sub-centimeter lesions.

## Mobilization, Control of Inflow/Outflow, and Marking the Liver

Liver mobilization requires freeing the liver's ligamentous attachments from the diaphragm. Use of diathermy prevents bothersome bleeding, though the diaphragmatic and hepatic veins must be carefully avoided. The degree of liver mobilization is determined by the type of resection to be performed (see Chapters 19, 20 and 23):

- For right or left hemihepatectomy and left lateral sectionectomy, the round ligament is divided and the falciform ligament is taken down from the abdominal wall along its length to the confluence of the hepatic veins and vena cava. It is important that these ligaments are transected close to the abdominal wall as to prevent dangling remnants from obstructing the view or soiling the scope.
- For left hemihepatectomy and left lateral sectionectomy, the left triangular and coronary ligaments are divided close to the liver from laterally to medially, as is the attachment of the lesser omentum. If a replaced or accessory left hepatic artery is present, it should be transected between clips. The middle and left hepatic venous confluence with the vena cava is exposed medial to lateral with cold sharp dissection (Fig. 31.4).
- For right hepatectomy, the right triangular and coronary ligaments are divided before or after the parenchymal transection, depending on whether a conventional or anterior approach is chosen, respectively.
- For right or left hemihepatectomy, or any right-sided resection larger than a metastasectomy, the gallbladder and distal cystic ducts can be used as handles to improve exposure of the transection plane after ligation of the cystic duct and artery. For left liver lesions the gallbladder is left in situ so that it can be used to retract the right liver to the right. For right liver lesions the gallbladder is dissected from the gallbladder plate with the exception of the fundus, so that it can be used to retract the liver to the left. If the patient is status-post cholecystectomy, the liver is retracted using atraumatic graspers.

If pedicle occlusion is anticipated, the pars flaccida is opened and an instrument passed behind the portal triad in order to encircle it with an umbilical tape. The ends

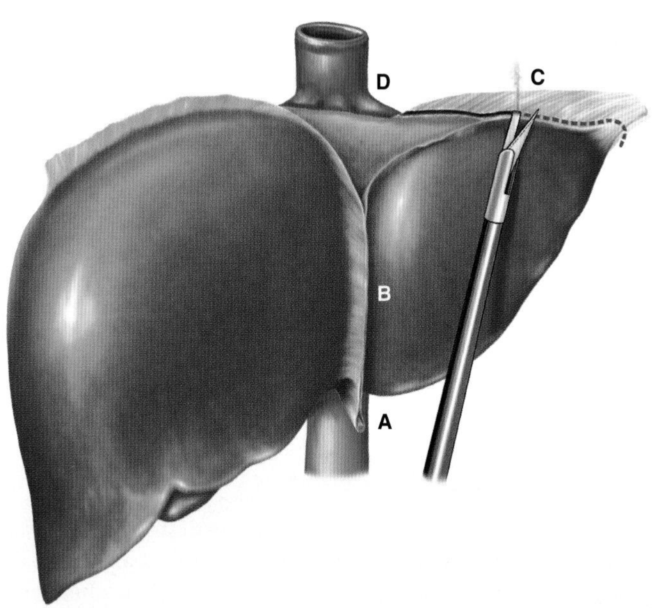


**Figure 31.4** An example of mobilization of the left lateral segment. The round (**A**) and falciform ligaments (**B**) are taken close to the abdominal wall so that there are no hanging remnants. The left triangular (**C**) and coronary ligaments are taken down with diathermy close to the liver's surface in order to avoid injuries to the diaphragm and contents of the lesser sac. Finally, the middle and left hepatic veins are exposed with cold sharp dissection (**D**).

Part II: Liver

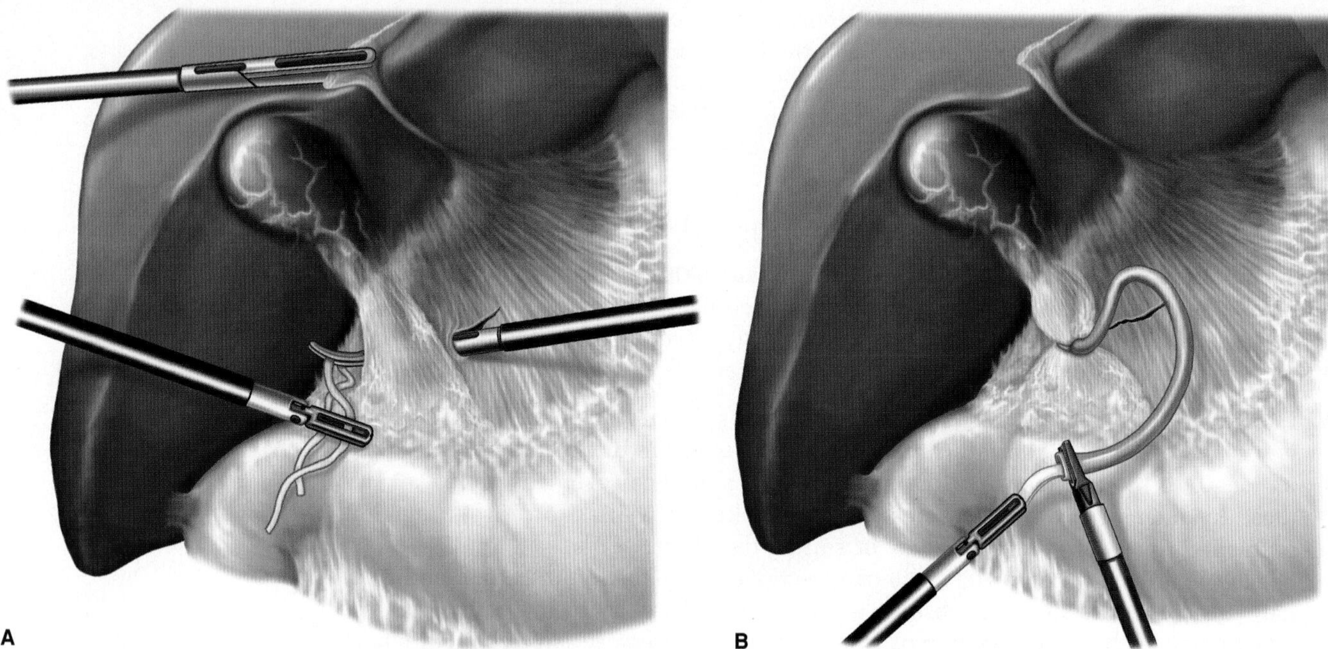


Figure 31.5 Hepatic inflow can be controlled by creating an intracorporal tourniquet by first passing an umbilical tape around the pedicle (**Image A**). This is then passed through a 16 Fr rubber tube extracorporeally, returned to the abdomen through a port and clipped taught if occlusion is necessary (**Image B**).

of the tape are then extracorporeally passed through a 16 French rubber tube of approximately 4 to 5 cm and returned to the abdomen. If pedicle clamping is required, a laparoscopic instrument grasps the ends of the tape taught while a laparoscopic locking-clip applier pushes the tubing toward the pedicle and applies a clip, thereby maintaining the Pringle (Fig. 31.5). We favor 15 minutes of clamping interrupted by 5 minutes of pedicle flow.

On the basis of the laparoscopic ultrasonography or demarcation lines when hepatic artery and portal vein flow are interrupted, the transection plane is outlined on the liver capsule with monopolar diathermy.

## Parenchymal Transection

From a simplistic view, the operator dissects through three layers of liver parenchyma perfused and drained by varying sized vascular and biliary structures. The first layer, the capsule, is easily penetrated and made hemostatic using monopolar diathermy. The second layer is comprised of the superficial 2 to 3 cm of parenchyma that can be transected with Harmonic ultrasonic shears (Ethicon Endosurgery; Cincinnati, OH, USA) or the LigaSure vessel-sealing device (Valleylab; Boulder, CO, USA). For the deep parenchyma, dissection is best accomplished with an ultrasonic dissector (Integra; NJ, USA; Olympus; Tokyo, Japan). Vascular and biliary structures encountered during the dissection of the superficial and deep parenchyma are ligated and transected with different devices based on their diameter. Vascular and biliary structures less than 3 mm are ligated and transected using the Harmonic, LigaSure, or bipolar diathermy. Larger arteries (i.e., hepatic artery) and bile ducts are ligated using plastic locking clips (Hem-o-lok, Teleflex Medical; NC, USA). Laparoscopic staplers with 2.5 mm depth loads are used for Glissonian pedicles, portal branches and hepatic veins (Fig. 31.6).

## Conversion to Laparotomy

Conversion rates in the literature range from 0% to 55%, with the most cited reasons for conversion being hemorrhage, adhesions and anatomic difficulties. Hand-assisted laparoscopy can be utilized as needed for failure of case progression or to aid in obtaining

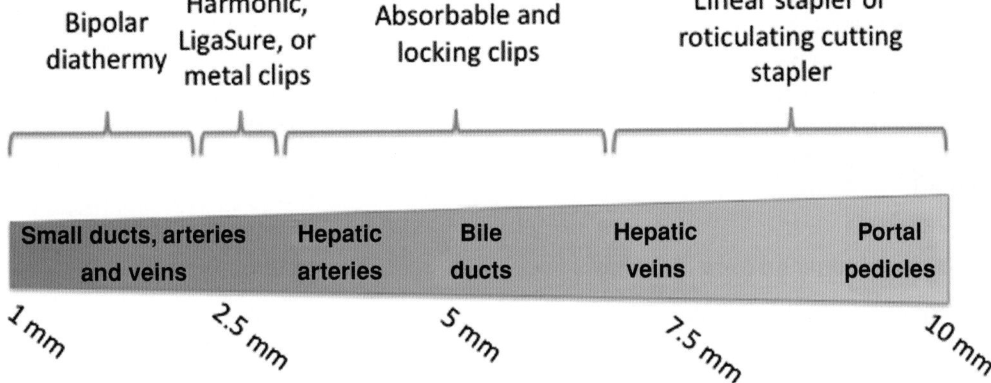


Figure 31.6 Schematic of average vessel and duct diameters encountered during laparoscopic partial hepatectomy and the respective instruments used to ligate, transect, and obtain hemo- and biliary stasis.

hemostasis. A gas-tight port is placed in the right lower quadrant and the incision is later used for specimen extraction. Conversion should not be considered failure and should be performed without hesitation when a patient's wellbeing is at risk.

## Extraction, Drainage, and Closure

Large lesions can be removed through preexisting scars, hand-port incisions, or in the virgin abdomen, through a 5 to 8 cm Pfannenstiel incision. Regardless of the chosen incision, the abdominal wall is incised to the fascia and a 15 mm trocar is inserted at the center of the incision. A large capacity endoscopic bag is introduced and the specimen retained. The specimen is then retracted against the fascia, and the fascia and peritoneum are opened only as much as necessary for retrieval (Fig. 31.7). The fascial layers are anatomically reapproximated with absorbable sutures and the pneumoperitoneum reintroduced. Smaller lesions can be removed through extension of trocar incisions after placement in an endoscopic bag. The operative site is lavaged and examined for hemo- and biliary stasis.

A cholangiogram catheter can be inserted through the cystic duct for formal radiographic cholangiography or methylene blue injection if necessary. Drains are usually omitted except after right hepatectomy where a 10 Fr closed circuit suction drain is placed in the subphrenic space. The skin and port-site incisions are closed with absorbable subcuticular sutures.



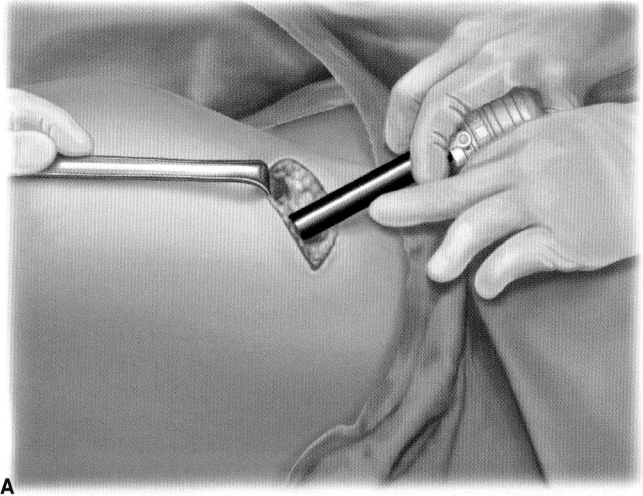


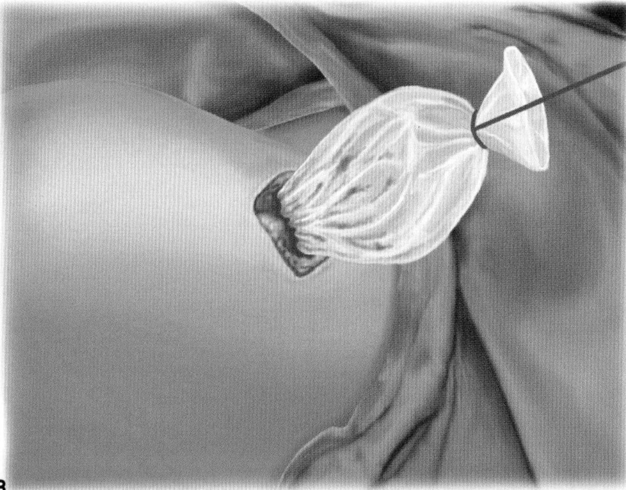


Figure 31.7 Specimen extraction. A 15 mm port is inserted through the fascia at the center of the chosen extraction incision, in this case a Pfannenstiel incision (**Image A**). After the specimen is retained within a protective endoscopic bag, it is pulled flush with the abdominal wall and the fascia is opened only wide enough for the specimen to be retrieved (**Image B**).

## SURGICAL TECHNIQUE II: SPECIFIC PROCEDURES

This section describes specific principles necessary to perform the most common procedures and is structured such that the technical skills described build upon those detailed in the preceding less complex resections and in the section, Surgical Technique I.

### Metastasectomy or Tumorectomy

Although the least complex of the laparoscopic resections, attention to hemostasis, biliary stasis, and oncologic principles remain essential.

- Superficial lesions in segments 2 to 6 are most amendable to this procedure and liver mobilization is rarely necessitated.
- For malignant lesions, 10 to 20 mm margins are measured using ultrasonography and marked using diathermy. For benign lesions, a wide margin is not required.
- Parenchymal transection is performed with the Harmonic scalpel or LigaSure and follows the marked margins. Hemostasis is achieved by bipolar diathermy and clips (Fig. 31.8).
- Avoid digging a hole in one area, because depth may be underappreciated and vascular or biliary structures inadvertently violated. A 4-0 Prolene can be used to lift the lesion away from the surrounding parenchyma to promote circumferential, consistent-depth dissection.
- If significant veins, ducts or sectoral pedicles are encountered, a segmentectomy should be considered to prevent necrosis or biliary fistula.

For all of the resections to be described in the subsequent sections, it is useful for the surgeon to operate with the following instrument combinations: For superficial parenchyma, electrosurgical (Harmonic or LigaSure) instrument in one hand and suction irrigator in the other; and for deeper parenchyma, ultrasonic dissector in one hand and bipolar forceps in the other. A right angle clamp is important for effective dissection of medium and large vessels and ducts. The assistants may need to change their grasp and traction on both sides of the dissection plane to keep it continually open to the surgeon.

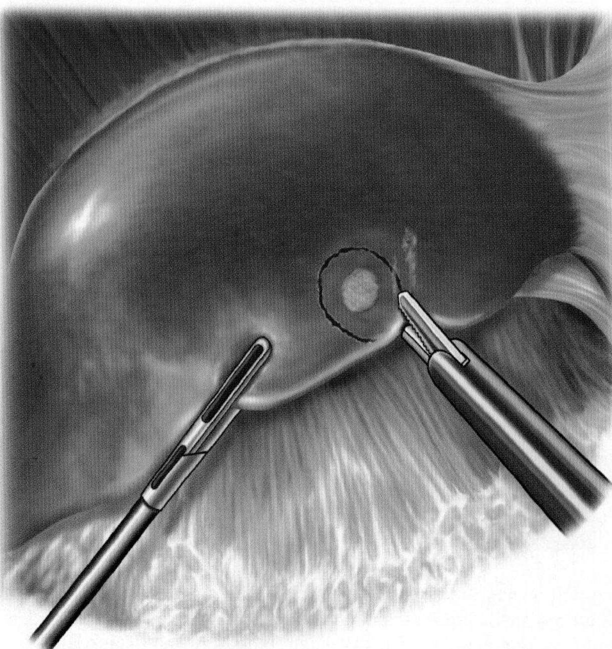

**Figure 31.8** A superficial malignant lesion is outlined with monopolar diathermy with a 1 to 2 cm margin. Harmonic shears or the LigaSure are used to transect the liver parenchyma.

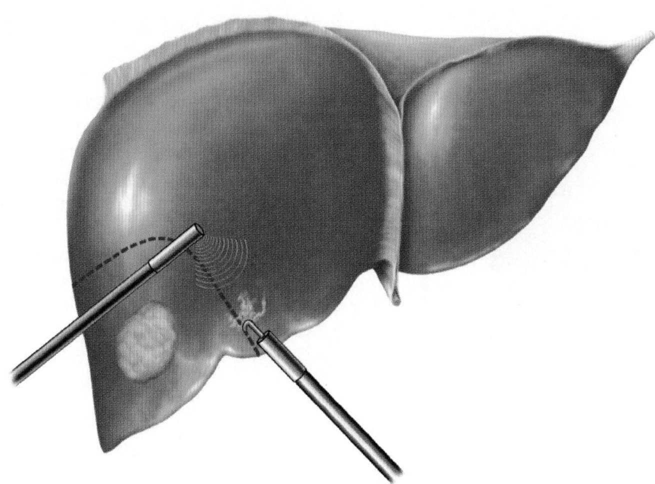

**Figure 31.9** Example of preparing for segmentectomy of segment 6. The laparoscopic ultrasound confirms the position of the lesion and identifies the feeding triad. Monopolar diathermy traces the transection plane on the surface of the liver to incorporate the mass and feeding pedicle, while not violating the pedicles of segments 5 and 7.



## Segmentectomy (see Chapter 24)

These resections require a thorough knowledge of hepatic anatomy and laparoscopic ultrasonography in order to isolate the feeding pedicle. Dissecting beyond anatomical borders or too proximal on the hepatic pedicle may interfere with the arterial/portal inflow and biliary outflow of bordering segments.

- Laparoscopic segmentectomy is most suitable for segments 3 to 6, and liver mobilization is necessary for these resections. Isolated 1, 7, and 8 segmentectomies are beyond the scope of this chapter.
- Rather than reliance on surface anatomy, ultrasonography is used to determine Couinaud segmental anatomy and then marked on the liver's surface (Fig. 31.9).
- Bilateral traction maintained by the assistants with atraumatic graspers allows the parenchymal transection plane to be visualized by the operating surgeon.
- As discussed in the *Equipment and Instruments*, a combination of ultrasonic and electrosurgical instruments is used to dissect the parenchyma. Sectorial pedicles are ligated with locking clips and other vessels or ducts are ligated with metal clips as they are encountered. Additional hemostasis is obtained by using bipolar diathermy.

## Left Lateral Sectionectomy (see Chapter 20)

Laparoscopic left lateral sectionectomy is the emerging standard for lesions in segments 2 and 3.

- The left lateral section is mobilized and a parenchymal bridge over the inferior surface of the round ligament is divided with diathermy if present.
- The transection plane is visualized by retracting the round ligament superiorly and to the patient's right, and the left lateral segment superiorly and to the left with atraumatic forceps.
- The transection is performed to the left of the patient's falciform ligament (to avoid injury to the segment 4 pedicle) progressing cranially from anterior to posterior (Fig. 31.10).
- Transection is continued until the portal pedicles to segments 2 and 3 are visualized posteriorly. These are divided with 2 to 3 firings of a laparoscopic stapler (Fig. 31.11).
- Parenchymal transection continues cranially until the left hepatic vein is visualized, at which point it is divided with a roticulating cutting linear stapler proximal to its confluence with the middle hepatic vein.

## Hemihepatectomy

These are more complex procedures because they involve deep parenchymal transection and deal with major vascular structures both in the hilum and at the level of the

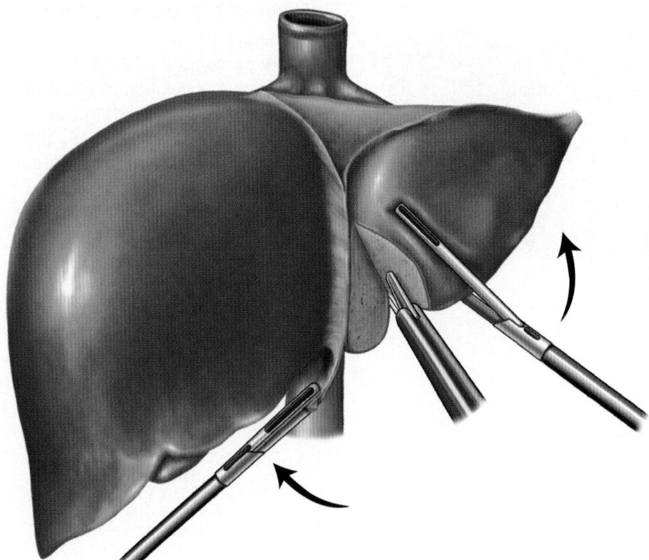

**Figure 31.10** For left lateral sectionectomy, by grasping opposite liver edges with atraumatic forceps and retracting to their respective sides, the assistants open the transection plane for the surgeon. The superficial 1 to 3 cm of parenchyma can be transected with a Harmonic scalpel or LigaSure. Transection must be carried out to the left of the patient's falciform ligament.

main hepatic veins. The laparoscopic approach to these procedures is not fully standardized, and requires preliminary mastering of the minor laparoscopic resections. These major resections require preparation of inflow occlusion, differing degrees of liver mobilization and dissection of the respective vascular pedicles and hepatic veins as previously discussed. The right and left bile ducts are not approached during ligation of the portal vein and hepatic artery, but are dealt with intraparenchymally when the transection line has reached the hilum.

## Right Hemihepatectomy (see Chapter 19)

This procedure can be performed from an anterior or posterior approach. Although the hilar dissection is the same for both approaches, the latter entails extensive pretransection mobilization and extrahepatic control of the right hepatic vein; the use of a hand-port may be useful in this setting. The pure laparoscopic anterior approach is our preference:

- After minimal mobilization as discussed, the distal cystic duct is retracted to the patient's left and the gallbladder to the right, exposing the short course of the extrahepatic right pedicle.

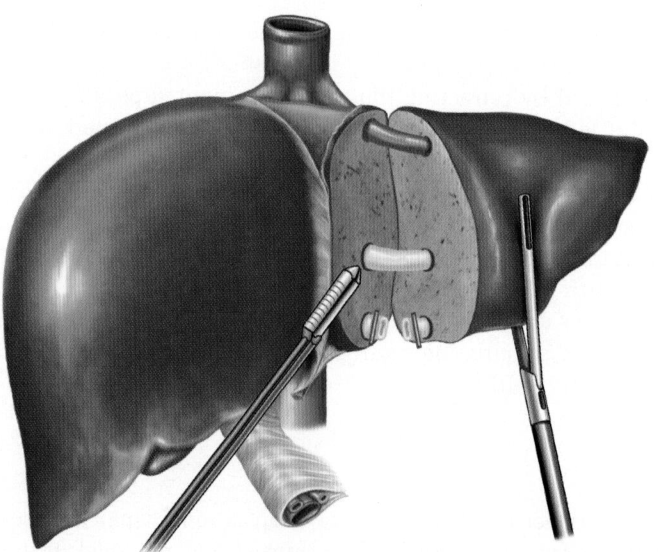

**Figure 31.11** As transection progresses from caudad-to-cephalad, the pedicles for segments 2 and 3 are encountered and stapled, and finally the left hepatic vein is stapled proximal to the confluence with the middle hepatic vein.

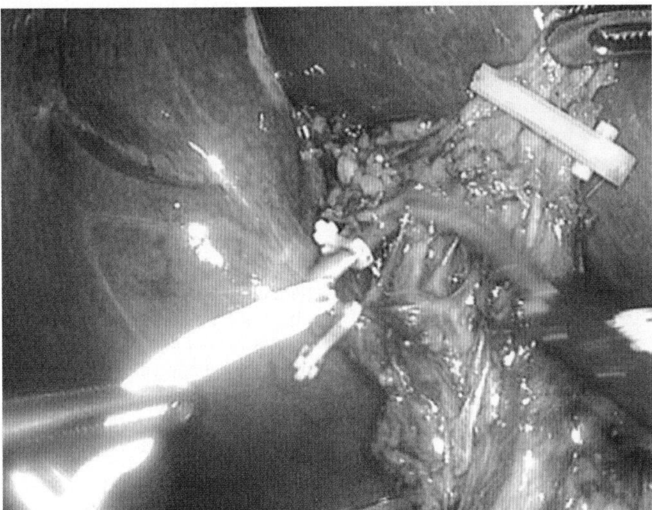

**Figure 31.12** Transection of the right hepatic artery. The distal cystic duct (large clip) is retracted to the left thereby rotating the hepatoduodenal ligament and exposing the pulsating right hepatic artery. The right hepatic artery is then mobilized free of connective tissue for a distance of 1 to 2 cm with the aid of a right angle clamp and an umbilical tape for retraction. After test clamping, the artery is ligated between two locking clips and transected.



- The right hepatic artery is circumferentially dissected for a distance of 1 to 2 cm and encircled with a tape to retract it away and protect the other hilar structures. After visualization of the contralateral arterial branch, it is divided between plastic locking clips (Fig. 31.12).
- The right portal vein is visualized posterior to the artery and dissected and taped in a similar manner. The bifurcation and left portal branch must be clearly visualized. When transecting the right portal vein with a linear stapler, the tape should be pulled to the patient's left so as to displace the bifurcation to the left and lengthen the right branch (Fig. 31.13). This prevents narrowing of the left portal branch. It will be necessary to ligate a vein branch to the caudate process (the right extent of segment 1) from the right portal vein with an electrosurgical device to safely dissect the right portal branch.
- Parenchymal transection is started at the inferior edge of the liver in the anterior-to-posterior and caudad-to-cephalad directions along the demarcation line. At the hilar plate the right bile duct is circumferentially dissected until the anterior and posterior branches are visualized, at which point the duct can be divided with locking clips or the stapler. Division of the hilar plate allows the dissection plane to be opened wide for easier parenchymal transection.

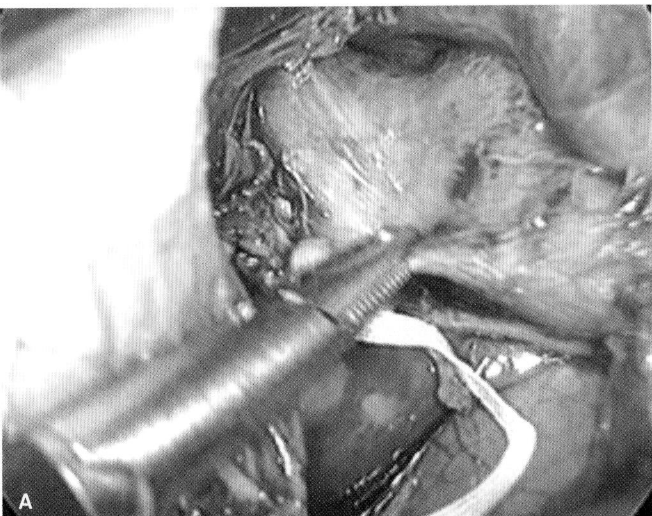


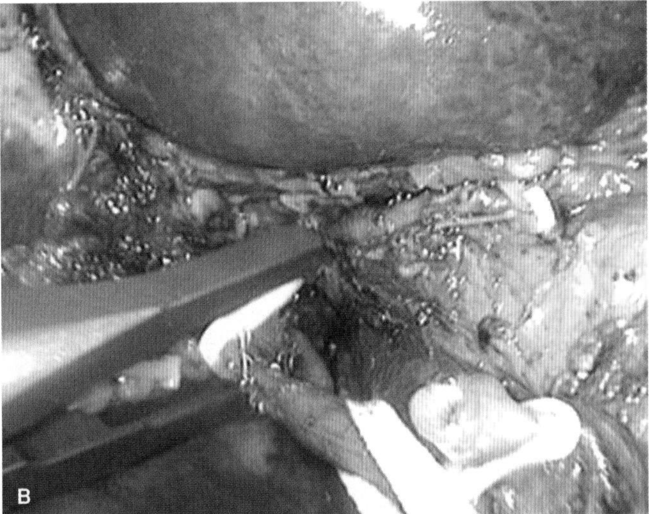


**Figure 31.13** The portal vein is mobilized until the bifurcation of the right and left veins is visualized and an umbilical tape is placed around the bifurcation **(Image A)**. The umbilical tape is used to retract the bifurcation to the patient's left. This prevents narrowing of the left portal vein when the right vein is stapled. As can be seen, the vein is stapled proximally and clipped distally.

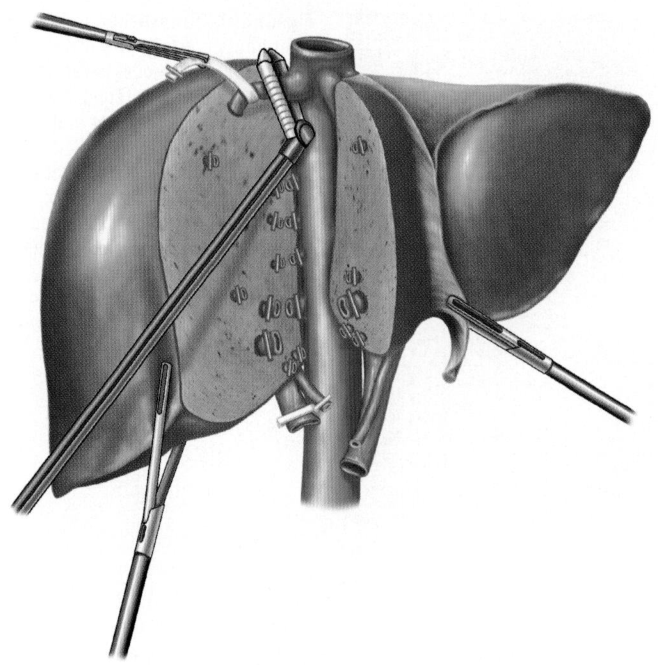

Figure 31.14 Right hemihepatectomy. Parenchymal transection continues from anterior-to-posterior and caudad-to-cephalad with the ultrasonic dissector. Vessels and ducts are sealed with bipolar diathermy or clipped depending on their size both within the parenchyma and between the parenchyma and cava. As can be seen, the branches of the middle hepatic vein draining segments 5 and 8 are clipped. A roticulating stapler is best used to transect the right hepatic vein, with an umbilical tape retracting the distal vein and cava to the right in order to prevent caval damage.

- It will be necessary to next divide the connective tissue junction between the right lobe and segment 1 with electrosurgery to fully expose the retro-hepatic cava. As parenchymal transection progresses, Glisson's capsule is divided along the anterior surface of the cava while systematically clipping and dividing the small bridging veins.
- As progress is made cranially, the proximal hepatic veins draining segments 5 and 8 toward the middle hepatic vein are exposed, clipped and divided (Fig. 31.14).
- The right hepatic vein is identified at its insertion into the cava, taped, retracted to the patient's right and transected with a roticulating linear stapler (Fig. 31.14).
- The specimen is now retracted to the right and to the left as the attachments of the right hemiliver are freed from the diaphragm with electrosurgical instruments (Fig. 31.15), and the cava and hepatocaval ligament with clips and staplers, respectively.

## Left Hemihepatectomy (see Chapter 20)

- The left lateral segment is mobilized and suprahepatic cava cleared of fibrous tissue as previously discussed (Fig. 31.4). The insertion of the hepatic veins into the vena cava must be identified.

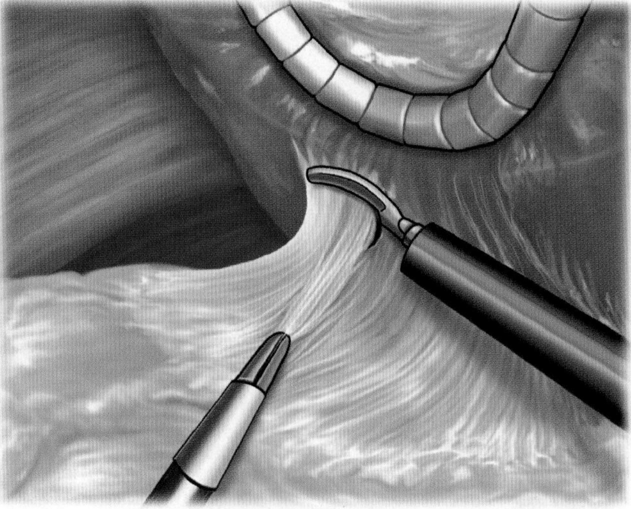

Figure 31.15 After the right hemiliver is devascularized, it is retracted to the left and to the right in order to free it from all of the ligamentous attachments to the diaphragm.

- Optionally, the common trunk of the left and middle hepatic vein can be controlled extrahepatically. For this, the left lateral segment is retracted superiorly and to the right to expose the caudate lobe. The peritoneum above the caudate is next opened to expose the cava. The insertion of the left hepatic vein into the cava is then visualized. The avascular plane between the cava and the liver is dissected with a blunt right angle dissector toward the space between the common trunk and right hepatic vein. An umbilical tape is grasped in this space, withdrawn and the common trunk encircled.
- The extra-hepatic left Glissonian pedicle is exposed and carefully dissected using endoscopic scissors and bipolar diathermy. The left hepatic artery and left portal vein are individually isolated using right-angled forceps, elevated with umbilical tapes and ligated with locking clips and a linear stapler, respectively.
- The extra-hepatic vessel ligation delimits the plane that intersects the gallbladder and inferior vena cava fossa. Parenchymal transection proceeds anterior-to-posterior and caudad-to-cephalad.
- Once dissection enters the hilar plate, the left bile duct is divided with a linear stapler or between clips. Parenchymal transection continues cranially until the insertion of the left hepatic vein into the common trunk. The previously placed umbilical tape is retracted to the patient's right, facilitating division of the left hepatic vein with a roticulating stapler without encroaching upon the middle hepatic vein.

## POSTOPERATIVE MANAGEMENT

Depending on the resection and underlying medical conditions, patients are maintained in the post anesthesia care unit or intensive care unit for at least the first postoperative night. Postoperative studies include a complete blood count, basic metabolic profile, liver function tests, and coagulation panel. As long as there are no unexpected gross abnormalities, labs are thereafter performed daily. Patients are extubated when typical criteria are met. Intravenous hydration is provided until liquids are tolerated orally. No postoperative prophylactic antibiotics are given. Patients are maintained on subcutaneous heparin for 4 weeks, and encouraged to ambulate as early as postoperative day 1. Analgesia initially consists of patient-controlled analgesia, followed by an oral agent. Diet is advanced as tolerated and patients are discharged when tolerating a regular diet, ambulating comfortably and have sufficient analgesia with oral agents. Follow-up is scheduled for 2 weeks.

## COMPLICATIONS

The mortality and morbidity rates in studies of laparoscopic partial hepatectomy are at least equivalent if not better than those of large series of open liver resections. In their review of 127 published papers on laparoscopic hepatic resection, Nguyen and colleagues found a cumulative mortality rate of 0.3%. This compares favorably to the 0% to 5.4% reported in an open resection literature from high volume centers. All deaths were postoperative and most often caused by liver and multiorgan system failure. Of 2,804 patients, a total of 295 morbid complications were reported (10.5%). Liver-specific complications included bile leaks (1.5%), transient liver failure/ascites (1%) and abscess (2%). The remaining 6% were those common to all operations, including hemorrhage, wound infection, hernia, bowel injury, arrhythmia and urinary or respiratory tract infections.

In our 11-year series of 166 consecutive patients, there were no deaths and low morbidity, with early postoperative complications occurring in 14%. There were eight complications specific to liver resection, including 6 Clavien grade 1 complications (jaundice or ascites), 1 grade 3a (bile leak requiring percutaneous drainage), and 1 grade 3b (hemoperitoneum requiring laparotomy 12 hours after surgery). There were three abdominal wall complications including 2 grade 1 wound complications and 1 grade

3b (early incisional hernia). There were 3 grade 1 pulmonary complications and 1 grade 4 (respiratory failure with 7-day mechanical ventilation). There were eight miscellaneous grade 1 complications. Two patients (1.2%) developed late incisional hernias.

Barriers to the wide acceptance of laparoscopic surgery such as threat of gas embolism, violation of oncologic principles, port-site metastases, peritoneal dissemination, and significant bleeding have not been evidenced in the literature.

## RESULTS

Laparoscopic partial hepatectomy provides the benefits that laparoscopy has offered to patients undergoing many other abdominal operations. Case-control studies have demonstrated shorter lengths of hospitalization, less operative blood loss, less transfusion requirements, less analgesic requirements, quicker return to oral consumption, less morbidity and less postoperative adhesions. Studies have demonstrated decreased costs when accounting for shorter hospitalizations. There are also the benefits of better cosmesis, maintenance of the sensory, and motor integrity of the abdominal wall and earlier access to adjuvant therapy.

Perhaps more important than demonstrating perioperative benefits is confirmation that oncologic principles are obeyed. With regard to margins, recurrence and survival, comparable results between open and laparoscopic resections have been well demonstrated in the literature.

## CONCLUSIONS

Despite close to 10 years of development, this remains an emerging field that should be approached by surgeons experienced in both liver and laparoscopic surgery. Laparoscopic partial hepatectomy is a safe procedure for selected patients, with considerable perioperative benefits compared to laparotomy, and oncologic principles are maintained. Although the indications for laparoscopic surgery can be somewhat rigid in relation to lesion size and location, greater experience and newer technology are continually expanding the possibilities of this procedure.

## Recommended References and Readings


Bryant R, Laurent A, Tayar C, et al. Laparoscopic liver resection-understanding its role in current practice: the Henri Mondor Hospital experience. *Ann Surg.* 2009;250(1):103–111.

Buell JF, Cherqui D, Geller DA, et al. The international position on laparoscopic liver surgery: The Louisville Statement, 2008. *Ann Surg.* 2009;250(5):825–830.

Buell JF, Thomas MT, Rudich S, et al. Experience with more than 500 minimally invasive hepatic procedures. *Ann Surg.* 2008; 248(3):475–486.

Chang S, Laurent A, Tayar C, et al. Laparoscopy as a routine approach for left lateral sectionectomy. *Br J Surg.* 2007;94(1):58–63.

Cherqui D, Husson E, Hammoud R, et al. Laparoscopic liver resections: a feasibility study in 30 patients. *Ann Surg.* 2000;232(6): 753–762.

Cherqui D, Soubrane O, Husson E, et al. Laparoscopic living donor hepatectomy for liver transplantation in children. *Lancet.* 2002; 359(9304):392–396.

Gigot JF, Glineur D, Santiago Azagra J, et al. Laparoscopic liver resection for malignant liver tumors: preliminary results of a multicenter European study. *Ann Surg.* 2002;236(1):90–97.

Kluger MD, Cherqui D. Minimally invasive techniques in hepatic resection. In: Jarnagin WR, ed. *Blumgart's Surgery of the Liver, Biliary Tract, and Pancreas.* 5th ed. Philadelphia, PA: Elsevier.

Koffron AJ, Auffenberg G, Kung R, et al. Evaluation of 300 minimally invasive liver resections at a single institution: less is more. *Ann Surg.* 2007;246(3):385–392.

Lesurtel M, Cherqui D, Laurent A, et al. Laparoscopic versus open left lateral hepatic lobectomy: a case-control study. *J Am Coll Surg.* 2003;196(2):236–242.

Nguyen KT, Gamblin TC, Geller DA. World review of laparoscopic liver resection-2,804 patients. *Ann Surg.* 2009;250(5):831–841.

Vigano L, Laurent A, Tayar C, et al. The learning curve in laparoscopic liver resection: improved feasibility and reproducibility. *Ann Surg.* 2009;250(5):772–782.

Vigano L, Tayar C, Laurent A, et al. Laparoscopic liver resection: a systematic review. *J Hepatobiliary Pancreat Surg.* 2009;16(4): 410–421.

# Index

Note: Page numbers followed by f and t indicates figure and table respectively.